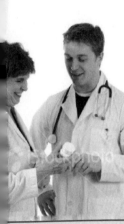

PHARMACY MANAGEMENT

ESSENTIALS FOR

ALL PRACTICE SETTINGS

Notice

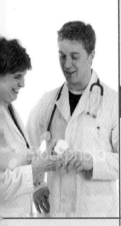

PHARMACY MANAGEMENT

ESSENTIALS FOR

ALL PRACTICE SETTINGS

SECOND EDITION

Shane P. Desselle, PhD, RPh, FAPhA
Professor and Associate Dean for
   Tulsa Programs
Chair, Department of Clinical and
   Administrative Sciences-Tulsa
University of Oklahoma
College of Pharmacy
Tulsa, Oklahoma

David P. Zgarrick, PhD, RPh
John R. Ellis Distinguished Chair
   of Pharmacy Practice
Professor of Pharmacy Administration
Drake University
College of Pharmacy and Health Sciences
Des Moines, Iowa

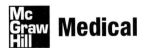 **Medical**

New York Chicago San Francisco Lisbon London Madrid Mexico City
Milan New Delhi San Juan Seoul Singapore Sydney Toronto

Pharmacy Management: Essentials for All Practice Settings, Second Edition

Copyright © 2009 by The McGraw-Hill Companies, Inc. All rights reserved. Printed in the United States of America. Except as permitted under the United States Copyright Act of 1976, no part of this publication may be reproduced or distributed in any form or by any means, or stored in a data base or retrieval system, without the prior written permission of the publisher.

3 4 5 6 7 8 9 0 DOC/DOC 12 11 10 9

ISBN 978-0-07-149436-6
MHID 0-07-149436-7

This book was set in Adobe Garamond by Aptara®, Inc.
The editors were Michael Weitz and Kim J. Davis.
The production supervisor was Sherri Souffrance.
Project management was provided by Sandhya Joshi, Aptara®, Inc.
The designer was Cathleen Elliott, the cover designer was Aimee Davis.
RR Donnelley was printer and binder.

This book is printed on acid-free paper.

Library of Congress Cataloging-in-Publication Data
Pharmacy management: essentials for all practice settings/[edited by] Shane P. Desselle,
    David P. Zgarrick. — 2nd ed.
        p. ; cm.
    Rev. ed. of: Pharmacy management / Shane P. Desselle, David P. Zgarrick. c2005.
    Includes bibliographical references and index.
    ISBN 978-0-07-149436-6 (pbk. : alk. paper) 1. Pharmacy management.   I. Desselle, Shane P.
        II. Zgarrick, David P.   III. Desselle, Shane P. Pharmacy management.
    [DNLM: 1. Pharmacies—organization & administration. QV 737 P5357 2009]
    RS100.D47 2009
    615′.1068—dc22
                                                                        2008005181

DEDICATION

To Deborah and Brittney (S.P.D.)
and
To Michelle, Miles, Grace, and Elle (D.P.Z.)

CONTENTS

CONTRIBUTORS

Michelle Belsey
Vice President for College Relations and Professional Recruitment, Rite-Aid Corporation, Camp Hill, Pennsylvania

John Bentley, PhD
Associate Professor, Department of Pharmacy Administration, School of Pharmacy, University of Mississippi, University, Mississippi

Joseph Bonnarens, PhD
Dean of Student Affairs, Associate Professor, Pharmacy Administration, School of Pharmacy, Pacific University, Hillsboro, Oregon

Michelle A. Chui, PharmD, PhD
Associate Professor of Pharmacy Administration, Midwestern University of Wisconsin, College of Pharmacy, Glendale, Arizona

Bartholomew E. Clark, RPh, PhD
Associate Professor Pharmacy Sciences Department, School of Pharmacy and Health Professions, Creighton University, Omaha, Nebraska

Edward Cohen, PharmD
Director, Clinical Services, Clinical Education and Immunization Services, Walgreens Health Services, Deerfield, Illinois

Michael R. Cohen, RPh, MS, ScD, FASHP
President, Institute for Safe Medication Practices, Horsham, Pennsylvania

Shane P. Desselle, PhD, RPh, FAPhA
Professor and Associate Dean for Tulsa Programs, Chair: Department of Clinical and Administrative Sciences-Tulsa, University of Oklahoma, College of Pharmacy, Tulsa, Oklahoma

William Doucette, PhD
Associate Professor, College of Pharmacy, University of Iowa, Iowa City, Iowa

Kevin Farmer, PhD
Associate Professor, University of Oklahoma College of Pharmacy, Oklahoma City, Oklahoma

Karen B. Farris, PBS Pharm, PhD
Associate Professor, Division of Clinical and Administrative Pharmacy, College of Pharmacy, University of Iowa, Iowa City, Iowa

Bill G. Felkey, MS, RPh
Professor, Department of Pharmacy Care Systems, Auburn University, Auburn, Alabama

Caroline A. Gaither, BS Pharm, MS, PhD, FAPHA
Associate Professor and Director of Graduate Studies, Department of Clinical, Social and Administrative Sciences, College of Pharmacy, University of Michigan, Ann Arbor, Michigan

David A. Gettman, RPh, MBA, PhD
Associate Professor, Pharmaceutical, Administrative, and Social Sciences, University of Appalachia College of Pharmacy, Oakwood, Virginia

Vincent J. Giannetti, PhD
Professor, Social and Administrative Sciences in Pharmacy, Mylan School of Pharmacy, Duquesne University, Pittsburgh, Pennsylvania

William A. Gouveia, MS, FASHP, DHL
Director of Pharmacy, Tufts-New England Medical Center; Associate Professor of Medicine, Tufts University School of Medicine, Boston, Massachusetts

Matthew Grissinger, RPh, FASCP
Medication Safety Analyst, Institute for Safe Medication Practices, Huntington Valley, Pennsylvania

Dana P. Hammer, RPh, MS, PhD
University of Washington School of Pharmacy, Seattle, Washington

Donald Harrison, BS, MS, PhD
Associate Professor, Department of Clinical and Administrative Sciences, College of Pharmacy, University of Oklahoma, Oklahoma City, Oklahoma

David A. Holdford, RPh, MS, PhD
Associate Professor, Department of Pharmacy, School of Pharmacy, Virginia Commonwealth University, Richmond, Virginia

David A. Latif, MBA, PhD
Professor and Chair, Department of Pharmaceutical and Administrative Sciences, University of Charleston School of Pharmacy, Charleston, West Virginia

Frank Massaro, PharmD
Pharmacy Practice Manager, Tufts-New England Medical Center, Boston, Massachusetts

Randal McDonough, MS, PharmD, CGP, BCPS
Co-owner and Director of Clinical Services, Towncrest and Medical Plaza Pharmacies, Iowa City, Iowa

Rashid Mosavin, RPh, PhD, MBA
Associate Professor, Department of Pharmacotherapy and Outcome Science, School of Pharmacy, Loma Linda University, Loma Linda, California

Glen T. Schumock, PharmD, MBA, FCCP
Associate Professor, Department of Pharmacy Practice; Director, Center for Pharmacoeconomic Research, University of Illinois at Chicago, Chicago, Illinois

Virginia (Ginger) G. Scott, PhD, MS, RPh
Professor and Director of Continuing Education, Department of Pharmaceutical Systems and Policy, West University School of Pharmacy, Morgantown, West Virginia

Kathleen Snella, PharmD, BCPS
Assistant Dean, Vice-Chair and Associate Professor, Division of Pharmacy Practice, University of Missouri-Kansas City School of Pharmacy, Columbia, Missouri

Margaret R. Thrower, PharmD
Assistant Professor, Auburn University Harrison School of Pharmacy, Auburn, Alabama

Bradley P. Tice, PharmD, RPh, CDM, PMP
Chief Clinical Officer, PharmMD Solutions, LLC, Brentwood, Tennessee

David J. Tipton, PhD
Associate Professor, Mylan School of Pharmacy, Duquesne University, Pittsburgh, Pennsylvania

Julie M. Urmie, PhD
Assistant Professor, Program in Pharmaceutical Socioeconomics, College of Pharmacy, University of Iowa, Iowa City, Iowa

Terry L. Warholak, PhD, RPh
Clinical Assistant Professor, Pharmacy Practice and Science, University of Arizona College of Pharmacy, Tuscon, Arizona

Donna West, RPh, PhD
Associate Professor, Division of Pharmaceutical Evaluation and Policy, University of Arkansas for Medical Sciences College of Pharmacy, Little Rock, Arkansas

Noel E. Wilkin, RPh, PhD
Interim Vice Provost, Pharmacy Administration; Research Associate and Professor, Research Institute of Pharmaceutical Sciences; Director, Center for Pharmaceutical Marketing and Management, University of Mississippi School of Pharmacy, Oxford, Mississippi

Godwin Wong, PhD
Visiting Associate Professor, Lester Center for Entrepreneurship and Innovation, University of California Berkeley Haas School of Business, Berkeley, California

David P. Zgarrick, PhD, RPh
John R. Ellis Distinguished Chair of Pharmacy Practice, Professor of Pharmacy Administration, Drake University College of Pharmacy and Health Sciences, Des Moines, Iowa

PREFACE

WHAT'S NEW IN THIS EDITION!!

In planning for the second edition, we started by listening to our fellow educators, pharmacists, and students. Through surveys, e-mails, and conversations we learned about what users liked about the first edition, and what they would like to see added or changed in the future. Using what we learned, we worked with the chapter authors not only to improve the ease of use for faculty and students, but also to reflect the changes in pharmacy practice and management that have occurred in the last 4 years.

- **Every chapter has been updated** to reflect the fluid nature of their respective management topic.
- **New content has been added to reflect major events in our profession**, such as the implementation of the Medicare Modernization Act and subsequent addition of an outpatient prescription drug benefit (Medicare Part D).
- **New trends in the management literature and research studies** are reflected in each of the chapters.
- Four chapters have been added to the second edition. Since effective managers must also have leadership skills,

  We have added a chapter on the **role of leadership in management**.

  Medicare Part D represents probably both the biggest challenge an opportunity to pharmacy practice in the last 20 years. We have added a chapter dedicated to the management implications of this program, as well as updated other chapters to describe the impact of this program on other areas of practice.

  Pharmacy practice and health care delivery inherently involves risk. We have added a chapter devoted to describing and managing the risks commonly seen in operating a pharmacy practice. The ability to take advantage of the opportunities in today's pharmacy practice requires not only management skills but also a mindset that can think strategically about the risks and benefits of new programs. We have added a chapter on **entrepreneurship** to describe how having an entrepreneurial spirit can improve a pharmacy practice and to describe how entrepreneurship skills can be acquired.

WHY DID WE CREATE THIS TEXTBOOK?

This is a very exciting time for pharmacists, pharmacy students, educators, and others associated with the profession of pharmacy. A number of factors have come together to provide new opportunities for pharmacists, especially in patient care and expanded professional roles. But with the new opportunities also comes challenges, including the challenge of how to manage the personal and professional resources necessary to succeed in today's ever-changing environment.

Educators must not only keep up with changes in pharmacy practice, but also anticipate and prepare our students for opportunities and contingencies that will arise throughout their professional careers. In our efforts to best prepare students, pharmacy management educators have increasingly had to gather teaching materials from a variety of textbooks, journals and other educational resources. This is due to the fact that many resources only focus on a specific management function (marketing, personnel, accounting and finance) or a specific practice setting (independent pharmacies, hospital pharmacies). We believed that there would be value in a comprehensive pharmacy management textbook that covered many content areas and gathered a variety of resources into one text. We also wanted to develop a resource that could be applied in a wide variety of practice settings. Our colleagues throughout the profession also agreed that a comprehensive management textbook was needed. Our desire to meet these needs sparked our interest to develop this text.

WHAT HAS CHANGED FROM THE FIRST EDITION?

In planning for the second edition, we started by listening to our fellow educators, pharmacists, and students. Through surveys, e-mails, and conversations we learned about what users liked about the first edition, and what they would like to see added or changed in the future. Using what we learned, we worked with the chapter authors not only to improve the ease of use for faculty and students, but also to reflect the changes in pharmacy practice and management that have occurred in the last 4 years.

Every chapter has been updated to reflect the fluid nature of their respective management topic. In many cases, new content has been added to reflect major events in our profession, such as the implementation of the Medicare Modernization Act and subsequent addition of an outpatient prescription drug benefit (Medicare Part D). New trends in the management literature and research studies are reflected in each of the chapters.

Four chapters have been added to the second edition. Since effective managers must also have leadership skills, we have added a chapter on the role of leadership in management. Medicare Part D represents probably both the biggest challenge an opportunity to pharmacy practice in the last 20 years. We have added a chapter dedicated to the management implications of this program, as well as updated other chapters to describe the impact of this program on other areas of practice. Pharmacy practice and health care delivery inherently involves risk. We have added a chapter devoted to describing and managing the risks commonly seen in operating a pharmacy practice. The ability to take advantage of the opportunities in today's pharmacy practice requires not only management skills but also a mindset that can think strategically about the risks and benefits of new programs. We have added a chapter on entrepreneurship to describe how having an entrepreneurial spirit can improve a pharmacy practice and to describe how entrepreneurship skills can be acquired.

WHAT WILL THE READER FIND IN THIS TEXTBOOK?

This textbook is organized to reflect all of the major management functions performed by pharmacists in any practice setting. The book is divided into sections representing each function, and is further divided into chapters that detail the various components of each function.

Our experience as educators has taught us that students are the most effective learners when they are "ready" to learn. Many students selected pharmacy as a major in part from the desire to help people, but also due to their fascination and intrigue with how such small amounts of various medicinal substances have such profound effects on the body. Many of these students also believe that they only need to learn about management after they graduate, and then only if they take on a managerial or administrative position at their pharmacy. The first section of this book makes the case that management skills are important for all people and pharmacists, regardless of their position or practice setting. After establishing the need for management in both our personal and professional lives, the next four sections describe the management functions and resources that are common to all pharmacy practice settings (operations, people, money, traditional pharmacy goods and services). Chapters within each section focus on important aspects of each function or resource.

As pharmacy practice evolves from a product to a patient orientation, there are unique challenges that arise in managing the value-added services that pharmacists are developing to meet patient needs (e.g., cholesterol screening, diabetes education, drug therapy monitoring, etc.). A section of this book is dedicated to the planning, implementation, reimbursement and evaluation of these new patient care services offered by pharmacists.

Several chapters are dedicated to describing the risks inherent in pharmacy practice, and the impact that laws, regulations, and medication errors have on pharmacy management. The final section outlines the role of entrepreneurship, and how management functions are applied in specific pharmacy practice settings (independent, chain, and hospitals).

HOW EACH CHAPTER IS ORGANIZED?

Each chapter is divided into several sections to facilitate the reader's understanding and application of the material. Chapters begin with a list of learning objectives that outline the major topics to be addressed. A brief scenario is used to describe how a pharmacy student or pharmacist may need or apply the information described this chapter in their daily lives or practice. Questions at the start of each chapter provide direction and assist the reader in understanding what they can expect to learn.

The text of each chapter provides comprehensive coverage of the content and theory underlying the major concepts. References to the management and pharmacy literature are commonly used to provide readers with links to additional background information. Explanations and applications are also used to help readers better understand the need to master and apply each concept. Questions at the end of each chapter encourage readers to think about what they have just learned and apply these concepts in new ways.

WHAT WE HOPE YOU WILL GAIN FROM THIS BOOK

If you are a pharmacy student, we hope that using this book will help you gain an appreciation for the roles of management in pharmacy practice, regardless of your future position or practice setting. This book will also provide you with a variety of management theories and tools that you can apply in your daily life as well.

We realize that many pharmacists have not had much management coursework in their formal education or professional training. We hope that this book serves as a valuable guide to pharmacists who may require some assistance dealing with matters they did not anticipate when embarking on their careers. For those pharmacists with formal management education and experience, we hope that this book serves as a valuable reference or as a source of new ideas that can be applied in daily practice.

For educators, this book has been designed as a comprehensive pharmacy management textbook. As a whole, it is meant to be used in survey courses that cover many areas of pharmacy management. The section format also allows the book to be used in courses that focus on specific pharmacy management functions or topics. The sections and content of each chapter are meant not only to provide valuable information that is easy for students to understand, but also to stimulate further discussion and motivate students to learn more on their own.

WE WOULD LIKE TO HEAR FROM YOU!

Textbooks today have great deal in common with computer software programs. The creators of each have put a great deal of time and effort into getting their final outputs ready for consumers, but it rarely can be considered a "finished product". Textbooks, like computer software, are "works in progress" that can always be improved. The best way to improve these products is to seek input from their users. As you use this book, we would like to learn what you like about it, what could be improved, and what topics or features you would like to see to be included in the future. Please feel free to share your thoughts at any time by reaching us through *pharmacy@mcgraw-hill.com.* We plan to improve this book over future editions by listening to your feedback and continuing to reflect changes in the management sciences and pharmacy practice.

ACKNOWLEDGMENTS

We would like to thank the pharmacy administration colleagues who have played an important role in our development throughout our undergraduate and graduate studies, as well as at our institutions. Over the years, we have also come to know many other colleagues in our discipline who have shared their knowledge and provided advice. We have learned a great deal about our discipline and about teaching from our colleagues, and feel fortunate that they have been willing to share their knowledge and experience with us.

Thanks must also go to all the faculty, staff and administrators at the University of Oklahoma and Drake University who have provided an environment that makes this type of endeavor possible. We would also like to thank all of the students we have taught who have inspired us to continue to strive to become better educators.

We would like to thank everyone at McGraw-Hill, and in particular the editor of the first edition, Michael Brown, and of the current edition, Michael Weitz, for working with us to make our idea for a comprehensive pharmacy management textbook a reality.

Finally, we would like to acknowledge of efforts of each of our chapter authors. We chose our authors not only because of their expertise, but also because of their dedication to teaching and the professional development of pharmacy students and pharmacists. There is no way in which we could have completed this textbook without their efforts.

SECTION I

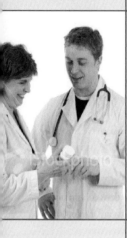

WHY STUDY MANAGEMENT

IN PHARMACY SCHOOL?

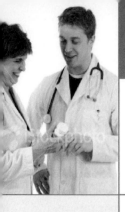

PHARMACEUTICAL CARE AS A MANAGEMENT MOVEMENT

Shane P. Desselle

About the Author: Dr. Desselle is Professor, Associate Dean for Tulsa Programs, and Chair, Department of Pharmacy: Clinical and Administrative Sciences—Tulsa at the University of Oklahoma College of Pharmacy. Dr. Desselle received a B.S. degree in pharmacy and a Ph.D. in pharmacy administration from the University of Louisiana at Monroe. He has practice experience in both community and hospital pharmacy settings. Dr. Desselle teaches courses in American health care systems, health care economics, social and behavioral aspects of pharmacy practice, and research methods. His research interests include performance appraisal systems in pharmacy, quality of work life among pharmacy technicians, direct-to-consumer prescription drug advertising, Web-based pharmacy services, and pharmacy benefit design. Dr. Desselle won the Duquesne University School of Pharmacy's President's Award for Teaching in 2003 and President's Award for Scholarship in 2004 and was recognized for his contributions to pharmacy by being named a Fellow of the American Pharmacists Association in 2006.

■ LEARNING OBJECTIVES

After completing this chapter, students should be able to

1. Identify changes in the roles of pharmacists since the early 1900s.
2. Describe how pharmacy practitioners and educators viewed the need for management skills as the roles of pharmacists evolved.
3. Identify principal domains of pharmacy care. Describe the practices of pharmaceutical care and medication therapy management as a series of management functions.
4. Identify myths surrounding the practice of pharmacy and health care as a business.
5. Evaluate the need for a management perspective to better serve patients and improve outcomes to drug therapy.
6. List the managerial sciences, and describe their use as tools to assist pharmacists in practice.

SCENARIO

Mary Quint has just completed the first 2 years of a doctor of pharmacy curriculum, and despite many long hours of hard work and a few anxious moments preparing for examinations, she has been pleased with her educational experience thus far. She also perceives that as she continues progressing through the curriculum, the upcoming courses will be more integrated and directly applicable to pharmacy practice. She is especially excited about taking courses in pharmacology and therapeutics so that she can "really learn about how to be a pharmacist." She glances down at her schedule and sees that she is enrolled in a required course in pharmacy management, and her enthusiasm becomes somewhat tempered. She immediately consults with fellow students on what they have heard about the course, and they tell her that the course is about "finance, accounting, and marketing." Despite some positive comments provided by students having already completed the course, she is concerned. "What do I have to take this course for? I did not come to pharmacy school for this. I'm very good at science. If I liked this kind of stuff, I would have majored in business. How is this going to help me to become a better pharmacist?" she asks herself.

After some thought, she comes to realize that, at worst, taking this course will not be the end of the world, and even better, it simply might be a moderate intrusion in her Monday-Wednesday-Friday routine. She begins to focus on other issues, such as her part-time job at Middletown South Pharmacy. Lately, she has dreaded going to work there. The staff consistently seems rushed and impatient. There always seems to be conflict among the employees, and as soon as one fire has been put out, another larger one begins to burn. She regrets her decision to quit her job at Middletown North Pharmacy 3 months ago, even though it took 20 minutes longer to get there. Things always seemed to run smoothly at Middletown North.

CHAPTER QUESTIONS

1. How have pharmacists' roles in delivering pharmaceutical products and services evolved over the past few decades? What roles and functions do pharmacists perform today?
2. What is the significance of management within the context of the pharmaceutical care and medication therapy management movements? Why has its significance typically been overlooked by pharmacists and pharmacy students?
3. What are some of the myths surrounding the confluence of business practices and the provision of patient care by pharmacists?
4. What evidence exists that a business perspective is critical to providing effective pharmacy services to patients?
5. What are the managerial sciences, and how can pharmacy practitioners use them effectively?

INTRODUCTION

The preceding scenario, though perhaps overly simplistic, properly captures the feelings of many students who select pharmacy as a major. They generally are interested in science, have a desire to help people in need, and prefer a career offering long-term financial security. Given that the pharmacy curriculum consists of courses that apply knowledge from physics, chemistry, anatomy, physiology, and therapeutics, most pharmacy students achieved success in science and math courses throughout their prepharmacy studies. Second, students selecting pharmacy as a major typically are attracted to health care fields and may have contemplated nursing, medicine, or other health professions. Research has demonstrated that people in health care are caring and empathic and seek personal reward and self-actualization through the helping of others (Bell, McElnay, and Hughes, 2000; Carmel and Glick, 2001; Fjortoft and Zgarrick, 2003; Kunyk and Olsen, 2001). Finally, many pharmacy students have also considered the relatively high salaries of their chosen profession prior to making their 6-year educational commitment. While few fields guarantee graduates a job, and certainly not one with entry-level salaries approaching a six-digit figure, pharmacy students take comfort in knowing that employment in their profession will provide them with a generous and steady stream of income. It comes as no surprise that pharmacists and pharmacy students have been shown to be risk-averse individuals who do not deal with uncertainties particularly well (Curtiss, 1980; Gaither, 1998a; Latif, 2000). This further explains their gravitation toward science-oriented courses that offer straightforward solutions to problems.

Unbeknown to many pharmacy students is that the actual practice of pharmacy does not present a succession of problems that can be resolved along such clear demarcations. While the sequential processes involved in community pharmacy practice have remained the same—patients present with prescriptions, pharmacy personnel fill them, and the necessary counseling is offered or provided by the pharmacist—a careful introspection reveals that the profession has undergone a rapid, head-turning transformation over just the past few decades. Pharmacists now are increasingly involved with providing services in addition to medications and are taking greater responsibility for patients' outcomes arising from drug therapy. Pharmacists have become more integrated into health care delivery teams that coordinate patient care through the implementation of guidelines and treatment algorithms. Pharmacists operate as part of a health care delivery system largely driven by reimbursements from third-party payers who insist on obtaining high-quality patient care at the lowest possible cost.

For pharmacy students to better understand the way that pharmacy is practiced today, time should be devoted to understanding the major forces that have shaped the profession. This chapter begins with a brief history of the evolution of pharmacy practice in the twentieth century. This history, coupled with a snapshot of contemporary pharmacy practice, will make it clear that the pharmaceutical care and medication therapy management movements are as much about management as they are about clinical pharmacy practice. The chapter proceeds by pointing out some myths about the exclusivity of the pharmacy business and patient outcomes and by providing evidence that what is best for the operation of a pharmacy business often is what is best for the patients that it serves. The chapter concludes with a brief discussion of the managerial sciences—tools that every practitioner will find useful at one point or another regardless of the practice setting. This chapter and all succeeding chapters use an *evidence-based approach* to discuss pharmacy management, relying on recent literature and research findings to describe and explain what is happening in practice today. Students are encouraged to explore readings of interest among the references cited throughout the text.

■ A BRIEF HISTORICAL OVERVIEW OF PHARMACY PRACTICE

Pharmacy Practice Prior to the 1940s

There have been several noteworthy efforts to describe the evolution of pharmacy practice. Some have described the process within the context of "waves," or shifts, in educational and industrial forces (Hepler, 1987), another through identifying stages of professional identity (Hepler and Strand, 1990), and still another through describing momentous occurrences in the health care delivery system whose effects rippled throughout the pharmacy profession (Broeseker and Janke, 1998). While these approaches appear quite disparate, their descriptions of the principal drivers of change closely mirror one another. The approach taken here is simply to describe these changes in the early, middle, and late twentieth century.

Pharmacy in the Early Twentieth Century

Pharmacy in the United States began in the twentieth century much like it existed in the latter 1800s. Pharmacy was, at best, a "marginal" profession. Most practitioners entered the occupation through apprenticeship rather than formal education. The pharmacist's principal job function was described as the "daily handling and preparing of remedies in common use" (Sonnedecker, 1963, p. 204). Pharmacists, or "apothecaries," often were engaged in the wholesale manufacture and distribution of medicinal products. Pharmacists' roles during this time were considerably different from what they are today. In the early twentieth century, pharmacists' primary roles were to procure raw ingredients and extemporaneously compound them into drug products for consumer use. While pharmacists had not yet achieved recognition as health care professionals, they often had considerable autonomy in their practice. There was no clear distinction between "prescription" and "nonprescription" drugs. Although physicians were engaged in the process of writing prescriptions, pharmacists were not precluded from dispensing preparations without a physician's order. Consumers commonly relied on their pharmacists' advice on minor ailments and often entrusted the nickname of "doc" to their neighborhood pharmacist (Hepler, 1987).

Pharmacists had little choice but to have sharp business acumen to survive. Because few of the products they dispensed were prefabricated by manufacturers, pharmacists had to be adept at managing inventories of bulk chemicals and supplies used in compounding the preparations they dispensed. They also had to have a keen sense of how to manage time and people to accomplish a series of complex tasks throughout the workday.

A series of studies commissioned by the U.S. government in the early 1900s produced what became known as the Flexner Reports in 1915. These reports were critical of health care professionals and their education, including pharmacists. The reports questioned the validity and necessity of pharmacists as health care professionals. Shortly thereafter, the American Association of Colleges of Pharmacy (AACP) commissioned a study directed by W. W. Charters that ultimately served as the basis for requiring a 4-year baccalaureate degree program for all colleges of pharmacy (Hepler, 1987). These and other forces led to dramatic changes in pharmacy in the coming years.

Pharmacy in the Middle of the Twentieth Century

The 1940s through the 1960s often have been referred to as the "era of expansion" in health care (Relman, 1988). The Flexner Reports paved the way for a more scientifically sound, empirically based allopathic branch of medicine to become the basis by which health care was practiced and organized. The federal government invested significant funds to expand the quantity and quality of health care services. The Hospital Survey and Construction (Hill-Burton) Act of 1946 provided considerable funding for the renovation and expansion of existing hospitals and the construction of new ones, primarily in underserved inner-city and rural areas (Torrens, 1993).

Ironically, pharmacists began to see their roles diminish during this era of expansion. Among the factors responsible for this decline were advances in technology and the pharmaceutical sciences and societal demands that drug products become uniform in their composition. These brought changes about the mass production of prefabricated drug products in tablet, capsule, syrup, and elixir dosage forms, thus significantly reducing the need for pharmacists to compound prescription orders. The passage of the Durham-Humphrey Amendment to the Food, Drug, and Cosmetic Act in 1951 created a prescription, or "legend," category of drugs. Pharmacists did not have the ability to dispense these drugs without an order from a licensed prescriber. Finally, pharmacy's own Code of Ethics, promulgated by the American Pharmaceutical Association (APhA), stated that pharmacists were not to discuss the therapeutic effects or composition of a prescription with a patient (Buerki and Vottero, 1994, p. 93). This combination of forces relegated the role of the pharmacist largely to a dispenser of preprepared drug products.

The response of schools and colleges of pharmacy to these diminishing roles was the creation of curricula that were more technical, scientific, and content-driven. A fifth year of education was added to the 4-year baccalaureate degree by colleges and schools of pharmacy during the late 1940s and early 1950s following the AACP Committee on Curriculum report entitled, "The Pharmaceutical Curriculum" (Hepler, 1987). It was during this time that pharmacology, pharmaceutics, and physical chemistry matured as disciplines and became the fabric of pharmacy education. Pharmacy students were required to memorize an abundance of information about the physical and chemical nature of drug products and dosage forms. Courses in the business aspects of pharmacy took a secondary role, whereas education in patient care (e.g., communications and therapeutics) was for all intents and purposes nonexistent.

With the Code of Ethics suggesting that pharmacists not discuss drug therapies with their patients, the profession lost sight of the need for pharmacists to communicate effectively with patients and other health care professionals. As the number of hospital and chain pharmacies expanded, resulting in pharmacists being more likely to be employees rather than business owners, the importance of practice management skills was not stressed in schools of pharmacy. Ironically, studies such as the Dichter Report commissioned by the APhA revealed that consumers regarded pharmacists more as merchants than as health care professionals (Maine and Penna, 1996).

Pharmacy in the Latter Part of the Twentieth Century

The era of expansion slowed in the 1970s when society began experiencing "sticker shock" from the monies being spent on health care. Congress passed the Health Maintenance Act of 1973, which helped to pave the way for health maintenance organizations (HMOs) to become an integral player in the delivery of health care services. Governments, rather than the private sector, took the lead in attempting to curb costs when they implemented a prospective payment system of reimbursement for Medicare hospitalizations based on categories of diagnosis-related groups (Pink, 1991).

The Millis Commission's report in 1975, *Pharmacists for the Future: The Report of the Study Commission on Pharmacy* (Millis, 1975), suggested that pharmacists were inadequately prepared in systems analysis and management skills and had particular deficiencies in communicating with patients, physicians, and other health care professionals. A subsequent report suggested including more of the behavioral and social sciences in pharmacy curricula and encouraged more faculty participation and research in real problems of practice (Millis, 1976).

Prior to these reports, the American Society of Hospital Pharmacists had published *Mirror to Hospital Pharmacy,* stating that pharmacy had lost its purpose, falling short of producing health care professionals capable of engendering change and noting that frustra-

tion and dissatisfaction among practitioners was beginning to affect students (Hepler, 1987, p. 371). The clinical pharmacy movement evolved in the 1970s to capture the essence of the drug use control concept forwarded by Brodie (1967) and promoted the pharmacist's role as therapeutic advisor. The clinical pharmacy movement brought about changes in pharmacy education and practice. After being introduced in 1948, the 6-year Doctor of Pharmacy (Pharm.D.) degree became the only entry-level degree offered by a small number of colleges of pharmacy during as early as the late 1960s and early 1970s. The additional year was devoted mostly to therapeutics or "disease-oriented courses" and experiential education. Eventually, the Doctor of Pharmacy degree become the entry-level degree into the profession, and colleges of pharmacy eventually began to phase out baccalaureate programs (American Association of Colleges of Pharmacy, 1996).

The trends begun by leaders and academicians in the field toward a more clinical practice approach may appear to be an ill-conceived response to recent changes in the delivery of health care. These changes emphasize a heightened concern over spiraling costs and have resulted in the deinstitutionalization of patients and the standardization of care using such tools as protocols, treatment algorithms, and critical pathways. It also may appear to fly in the face of changes in the organization of the pharmacy workforce and current market for pharmaceuticals. With the proportion of independently owned community pharmacies at an all-time low in the year 2000, chain, supermarket, and mass-merchandiser pharmacies had garnered nearly 64 percent of the outpatient prescription drug market (National Association of Chain Drug Stores, 2003). Studies have long suggested that pharmacists willing and clinically knowledgeable enough to provide pharmaceutical care face significant barriers when practicing in a chain environment (Miller and Ortmeier, 1995). Additionally, two relatively new venues for outpatient pharmacy services that virtually exclude face-to-face consultation with patients have evolved. In the year 2005, mail-order pharmacy operations had secured 19.1 percent of the market share (in sales revenue) for outpatient prescription drugs (National

Association of Chain Drug Stores, 2006). The new millennium also saw the implementation of Internet pharmacy sites, many of which are owned and operated by traditional "brick and mortar" chain pharmacy corporations.

■ PHARMACEUTICAL CARE AS A MANAGEMENT MOVEMENT?

With these changes in mind, adopting pharmaceutical care as a practice philosophy would appear "a day late and a dollar short" for both the profession and the patients it serves. Indeed, this may be the case if the concept of pharmaceutical care were entirely clinical in nature. The originators of the concept fervently stressed that pharmaceutical care is not simply a list of clinically oriented activities to perform for each and every patient but is, in fact, a new mission and way of thinking that takes advantage of pharmacists' accessibility and the frequency to which they are engaged by patients—a way of thinking that engenders the pharmacist to take responsibility for managing a patient's pharmacotherapy to resolve current and prevent future problems related to their medications.

It has been argued that the focus on preventing and resolving medication-related problems is simply an extension of *risk management* (Wiederholt and Wiederholt, 1997; see also Chapter 28). Risks are an inherent part of any business activity, including the provision of pharmacy services. Common risks to business practice include fire, natural disasters, theft, economic downturns, and employee turnover, as well as the fact that there is no guarantee that consumers will accept or adopt any good or service that is offered to them. The practice of pharmacy involves additional risks, specifically the risk that patients will suffer untoward events as a result of their drug therapy.

These events are significant because they may result in significant harm and even death to a patient and can also pose serious detriments to pharmacists, such as feelings of guilt and stress, the potential for litigation from patients and their families, the threat

of punitive action by state boards of pharmacy, and the loss of social esteem enjoyed by the profession as a whole. Risk management suggests that risk cannot be avoided entirely but rather that it should be assessed, measured, and reduced to the extent feasible (Tootelian and Gaedeke, 1993, p. 163).

The idea that pharmaceutical care should be viewed strictly as a clinical movement has been called into question (Wilkin, 1999). Evidence that pharmaceutical care exists in part as a management movement was provided in a recent study that sought to identify standards of practice for providing pharmaceutical care (Desselle and Rappaport, 1996). A nationwide panel of experts identified 52 standards of pharmacy practice, only to have a statewide sample of pharmacists judge many of them as infeasible to implement in everyday practice (Desselle, 1997). Of the practice standards that were judged to be feasible, further research yielded a system of "factors" or "domains" in which these standards could be classified (Desselle and Rappaport, 1995). These practice domains can be found in Table 1-1. Figuring very prominently into this classification was the "risk management" domain, which included activities related to documentation, drug review, triage, and dosage calculations. However, the contributions of the managerial sciences do not stop there. The remaining four domains connote significant involvement by pharmacists into managerial processes. Two of the domains ("services marketing" and "business management") are named specifically after managerial functions.

■ FROM PHARMACEUTICAL CARE TO MEDICATION THERAPY MANAGEMENT

While the pharmaceutical care movement made an indelible mark on the profession, its terminology is being replaced with more contemporary language that reflects pharmacists' growing roles in the provision of public health services. In recognizing the morbidity and mortality resulting from medication errors as a public health problem, the profession has begun to

Table 1-1. Pharmaceutical Care Practice Domains

I. *Risk management*
   Devise system of data collection
   Perform prospective drug utilization review
   Document therapeutic interventions and activities
   Obtain over-the-counter medication history
   Calculate dosages for drugs with a narrow therapeutic index
   Report adverse drug events to FDA
   Triage patients' needs for proper referral
   Remain abreast of newly uncovered adverse effects and drug–drug interactions

II. *Patient advocacy*
   Serve as patient advocate with respect to social, economic, and psychological barriers to drug therapy
   Attempt to change patients' medication orders when barriers to compliance exist
   Counsel patients on new and refill medications as necessary
   Promote patient wellness
   Maintain caring, friendly relationship with patients
   Telephone patients to obtain medication orders called in and not picked up

III. *Disease management*
   Provide information to patients on how to manage their disease state/condition
   Monitor patients' progress resulting from pharmacotherapy
   Carry inventory of products necessary for patients to execute a therapeutic plan (e.g., inhalers, nebulizers, glucose monitors, etc.)
   Supply patients with information on support and educational groups (e.g., American Diabetes Association, Multiple Sclerosis Society)

IV. *Pharmaceutical care services marketing*
   Meet prominent prescribers in the local area of practice
   Be an active member of professional associations that support the concept of pharmaceutical care
   Make available an area for private consultation services for patients as necessary
   Identify software that facilitates pharmacists' patient care–related activities

V. *Business management*
   Use technicians and other staff to free up the pharmacist's time

embrace the concept of medication therapy management (MTM). MTM represents a comprehensive and proactive approach to help patients maximize the benefits from drug therapy and includes services aimed to facilitate or improve patient compliance to drug therapy, educate entire populations of persons, conduct wellness programs, and become more intimately involved in disease management and monitoring. The MTM movement has been especially strengthened by language in the Medicare Prescription Drug, Improvement and Modernization Act (MMA) of 2003 (Public Law Number 108-173), which mandates payment for MTM services and proffers pharmacists as viable health professionals who may offer such services. As such, MTM is now considered a key component in the provision of pharmacy care services.

MYTHS CONCERNING THE CONFLUENCE OF BUSINESS PRACTICE AND PHARMACY

Despite evidence that would suggest otherwise, the need for a management perspective in pharmacy is often overlooked and even shunned by some pharmacy students and practitioners. Common misconceptions about the need for a management perspective have been documented (Tootelian and Gaedeke, 1993, p. 23):

- *The practice of pharmacy is ethically inconsistent with good business.* The origin of this myth probably evolved from the unethical business practices of some organizations. Scandals involving abuses by corporate executives at large international firms in the early 2000s have done little to mitigate these perceptions. The incident involving a pharmacist in Kansas City, Missouri, diluting chemotherapeutic drugs to spare inventory costs demonstrated that health care professions are not without unscrupulous members (Stafford, 2002). Furthermore, some people believe that companies involved in the sale of health care goods and services should be philanthropic in nature and are upset that companies profit from consumers' medical needs. Despite occasional examples of misconduct, most companies and persons involved in business operations conduct themselves in an appropriate manner.

- *Business is not a profession guided by ethical standards.* Pharmacists and pharmacy students generally are cognizant of the vast number of rules and regulations that govern pharmacy but are less aware of the standards governing practice in advertising, accounting, and interstate commerce. Many of the rules and regulations governing pharmacy practice were borrowed from legislation existing in sectors other than health care.

- *In business, quality of care is secondary to generating profits.* This misconception likely results from the efforts by payers of health care and by managers to control costs. In light of the fact that in 2005 health care accounted for approximately 16 percent of the nation's gross national product and cost over $5000 per person (Kaiser Family Foundation, 2005), health care consumers have little choice but to become more discerning shoppers of health care services. Because resources are limited, the number of services and products provided to consumers cannot be boundless. Conscientiousness in the allocation of resources helps to ensure that more of the right people receive the right goods and services at the right time and place. Many people do not stop to think that if a company in the health care business is not able to pay its own workforce and cover its other costs of doing business, it will have little choice but to close its doors, leaving a void in the array of services previously afforded to consumers. Even nonprofit entities have to pay the bills because if they cannot break even, they too have to shut down operations. Students may be surprised to learn that most nonprofit companies in health care compete quite fiercely against companies that are structured on a for-profit basis.

- *The good pharmacist is one who is a "clinical purist."* This is perhaps a manifestation of the other misconceptions, in addition to a false pretense that the complexities of modern drug therapy do not allow time for concern with other matters. On the contrary, a lack of knowledge on how to manage resources and a lack of understanding on how to work within the current system of health care delivery will only impede the pharmacist's goal to provide MTM services. Pharmacists who "don't want to be bothered with management" face the same logistical constraints, such as formularies, generic substitution, prior authorizations, limited networks, employee conflict and lack of productivity, breakdowns in computer hardware and software, budgetary limitations, and changes in policy that all other pharmacists face. The problem with the "don't want to be bothered with management" pharmacists is that they will be less likely to operate efficiently within the system, becoming frustrated and ultimately less clinically effective than the pharmacists who accept these challenges as part of their practice.

The United States has been facing an acute shortage of pharmacists in the wake of an ever-increasing number of prescription drugs dispensed (Gershon, Cultice, and Knapp, 2000). At the same time, the profession has come under more intense pressure to reduce the incidence of medication errors in both institutional and ambulatory settings (Thompson, 2001; Institute of Medicine, 2006). This is placing a burden on pharmacists to be especially productive, efficient, and error-free. Productivity is a function of a pharmacist's ability to manage workflow, technology, the quality and efficiency of support personnel, phone calls, and other problems that arise in day-to-day practice.

Moreover, pharmacy administrators reward pharmacists who can manage a pharmacy practice. New graduates often obtain entry-level administrative positions (e.g., pharmacy department manager, area manager, or clinical coordinator) after just 2 to 3 years in practice. It is not uncommon to see pharmacy graduates move up into even higher-level administrative positions (e.g., district or regional manager of a chain or associate director or director of a hospital pharmacy department) within 5 to 10 years of graduation. Pharmacists who can manage a practice successfully (i.e., increase volume, reduce errors, engender customer satisfaction, improve profitability, and reduce employee turnover) are in the best position for promotions.

A final point to consider is that even if a pharmacist does not ascend to an administrative position, he or she inherently "manages" a practice the instant he or she takes a position as a pharmacist. Staff pharmacists in every practice setting manage technicians and clerks every hour of every day. They also manage the flow of work through their sites and the use of medications by patients. Closely tied to this issue is the issue of personal job satisfaction. The pressures on the modern pharmacist are unmistakable. Satisfaction with one's job and career is important because they are closely related to one's satisfaction with life (Sumer and Knight, 2001). Pharmacists' ability to manage their work environment can have a significant impact on their ability to cope with the daily stressors of practice, increasing job satisfaction, and diminishing the likelihood of career burnout or impairment through the abuse of alcohol and drugs.

■ GOOD MANAGEMENT PRACTICE AND MEDICATION THERAPY MANAGEMENT—A WINNING COMBINATION

Evidence of the success of a management perspective in pharmacy practice abounds. A series of studies examined the use of strategic planning by pharmacists in both community and hospital settings (Harrison and Bootman, 1994; Harrison and Ortmeier, 1995, 1996). These studies showed that among community pharmacy owners, those who fully incorporated strategic planning saw higher sales volume and profitability than did those who did not or who did so just partially. Pharmacies owned by "strategic planners" also were significantly more likely to offer clinical or value-added services than pharmacies run by owners who were not. Likewise, better administrative, distributive, and clinical performance among hospital pharmacies also was associated with their respective directors' involvement in the strategic planning process.

Another study pointed out that support from supervisors and colleagues had a positive impact on the commitment that pharmacists display toward their respective organizations, thus enhancing the likelihood that these pharmacists would not quit their jobs (Gaither, 1998b). Other studies suggest that pharmacists' perceived ability to adhere to standards of pharmacy practice hinged considerably on the effectiveness of supervisors to provide them with feedback and facilitate their satisfaction on the job (Desselle and Tipton, 2001). The same study also demonstrated that pharmacists designating themselves as "managers" were less satisfied with their own jobs, likely as a result of their lack of training in such areas.

Surveys of pharmacists commonly indicate that looking at their practices today, they wish they had more training in management during their professional education. One study suggested that a business/work orientation was the skill most critical in implementing a successful practice (Speedie, Palumbo, and Leavitt, 1980). It was suggested in another survey that lack of time and poor communication were primary obstacles to delivering pharmacy care services (Ciancanglini, Waterhouse, and D'Elia, 1994). Still another study concluded that it would benefit practicing pharmacists to seek continuing education in management, health care systems and policy, and pharmacotherapeutics (Desselle and Alafris, 1999). It has been argued that to achieve excellence in the implementation of MTM services, pharmacists must obtain and properly allocate resources, design efficient distribution systems, select and train adequate support staff, develop systems for disseminating knowledge on new drugs and technology, and document and evaluate the cost-effectiveness of the services provided—all of which are tasks that require management skills (Smith, 1988).

Table 1-2 summarizes many of the principal factors that affect the delivery of pharmacy care services and is used to further illustrate the existing synergy between pharmacy care and good business practice. First, the demographic composition of the patient population has changed dramatically. The mean age of Americans continues to increase, as does their life expectancy. This results in a greater proportion of patients presenting with multiple disease states and complex therapeutic regimens. Although many of our nation's seniors lead normal, productive lives, their visual acuity, hearing, mobility, and ability to use and/or obtain viable transportation may be comprised. Pharmacists must take on additional responsibilities in managing these patients' care and coordinating their services. Also, the population of patients that pharmacists serve is becoming more ethnically diverse. Good pharmacy managers will benefit from a heightened sensitivity toward the needs of all patients and efforts to carry products that appeal to specific populations.

The shift in the demographic composition of patients also brings to bear the varying beliefs people have about treating their disease states and taking medications and their trust in the health care delivery system. All the clinical and scientific knowledge in the world

Table 1-2.	Factors Affecting the Delivery of Pharmacy Products and Services

Patient demographics
   Aging population
   Females as decision makers
   Ethnic composition of patients
Attitudes and belief systems
   Beliefs about disease, sick role, and
      medication-taking
   Trust in the health care delivery system
   Direct-to-consumer advertising of prescription
      drugs
Third-party payers and coverage issues
   Complexity/differences among payers' policies
   Formularies
   Limited networks
   Limited access for some patients
   Lack of knowledge by patients
Competitive markets
   Diminished margins
   Diversity in the types of providers offering
      products and services
Technology
   Software
   Automated dispensing technology

is rendered useless if pharmacists lack basic knowledge about the patients whom they serve. Even the most carefully devised and therapeutically correct pharmaceutical care plan will not work if the patient does not put faith in the pharmacist's recommendations. Good pharmacists are able to relate to patients of all persuasions and convince them to put faith in the consultation they provide. An additional consideration is the increased marketing of health care products directly to consumers. This has resulted inevitably in an increase in the frequency of medication-specific queries from patients. Good pharmacists do not bias their answers but are able to triage their patients' requests with appropriate information and recommendations.

A management perspective is indispensable when it comes to issues dealing with third-party payers (e.g., private insurers, government-sponsored programs; see Chapter 16). Unlike other countries, whose health care systems are founded on single-payer reimbursement structures, practitioners in the United States face a mix of payers, including individual patients, private insurers, employers, and government health plans. Each payer differs in its formularies (list of approved drugs), rules for reimbursement, and the network of pharmacists qualified to accept its coverage. The management-minded pharmacist is able to identify payers that afford the pharmacy the opportunity to provide quality patient care while maintaining an appropriate level of profit. Pharmacists must provide appropriate information about coverage to patients, who often do not know about the intricacies of their plans and the health care system (Fronstin, 2000). Additionally, pharmacists must coordinate therapeutic plans for cash-paying patients whose financial situation may preclude them from receiving certain therapies and services.

An additional challenge facing pharmacies and pharmacists is that of shrinking profit margins. A pharmacy's profit margin is the excess of revenues after covering expenses that it secures as a percentage of its total revenues. As the percentage of prescriptions paid for by sources other than patients has increased, profit margins have decreased. In addition to selecting the right mix of plans in which to participate, the management-minded pharmacist looks for other opportunities to bring in additional revenues and decrease expenses, such as implementing cognitive services, selling ancillary products, effectively purchasing and maintaining proper levels of inventory, effective marketing, and having the appropriate amount and type of personnel needed to do the job. This is especially important in light of the fact that consumers have more choices than ever in seeking health care solutions, ranging from nontraditional sources (e.g., complementary and alternative medicine) to more traditional sources (e.g., grocery stores, convenience stores, gift shops, and the Internet).

The management-minded pharmacist also maintains software and automated dispensing technologies that free up time formerly spent in the dispensing process. This gives pharmacists more time to provide patient care and perform other practice and management functions.

The arrival on the scene of MTM and the complexities of Medicare legislation further underscore the need for practice management skills among pharmacists. In addition to knowledge required to help patients navigate the health care system, pharmacists must be able to maximize efficiency in human, capital, and technological resources to serve patients, provide services, and take advantage of the unique opportunities to gain reimbursement for MTM services.

■ THE MANAGERIAL SCIENCES

Although mentioned throughout this chapter, a more formal examination of the managerial sciences should put into perspective their use as tools to implement pharmacy services effectively. The managerial sciences are summarized in Table 1-3. The reason they are referred to as *sciences* is because their proper application stems from the scientific process of inquiry, much the same as with other pharmaceutical sciences. The science of *accounting* (see Chapter 15) involves "keeping the books," or adequately keeping track of the business's transactions, such as sales revenues, wages paid to employees, prescription product purchases from suppliers, rent, and utility bills. This must be done to ensure that the company is meeting its debts and achieving its financial goals. Accounting is also used to determine the amount of taxes owed, to make reports to external agencies and/or auditors, and to identify areas where the company's assets could be managed more efficiently. While accounting is used to evaluate a company's financial position, *finance* is more concerned with the sources and uses of funds (e.g., Where will the money come from to pay for new and existing services? Which services are most likely to enhance profitability for a pharmacy?).

The other managerial science commonly associated with managing money is *economics*. However, the use of economics transcends financial considerations. Economics is a tool to evaluate the inputs and outcomes of any number of processes. It can be used to determine

Table 1-3.   The Managerial Sciences

Accounting
   Keep the books
   Record financial transactions
   Prepare financial statements
   Manage cash flows
   Analysis of profitability
   Determine business strengths and weaknesses
   Compute taxes owed to federal, state, and local
      governments
Finance
   Determine financial needs
   Identify sources of capital
   Develop operating budgets
   Invest profits
   Manage assets
Economics
   Determine optimal mix of labor and capital
   Determine optimal output
   Determine optimal hours of business operation
   Determine levels of investment into risk
      management
Human resources management
   Conduct job analyses
   Hire personnel
   Orient and train personnel
   Motivate personnel for performance
   Appraise personnel performance
   Allocate organizational rewards
   Terminate employment
Marketing
   Identify competitive advantages
   Implement competitive advantages
   Identify target markets
   Evaluate promotional strategies
   Implement promotional strategies
   Evaluate promotional strategies
   Select proper mix of merchandise
   Properly arrange and merchandise products
   Price goods and services
Operations management
   Design workflow
   Control purchasing and inventory
   Perform quality assurance initiatives

the right mix of personnel and automated dispensing technologies, the optimal number of prescriptions dispensed given current staffing levels, whether or not a pharmacy should remain open for additional hours of business, and how much to invest in theft deterrence. It is also used to determine the most appropriate drugs to place on a formulary or to include in a critical pathway.

Human resources management (see Chapter 9) is used to optimize the productivity of any pharmacy's most critical asset—its people. It involves determining the jobs that need to be done, recruiting people for those jobs, hiring the right persons for those jobs, training them appropriately, appraising their performance, motivating them, and seeing that they are justly rewarded for their efforts. It also involves issues such as determining the right mix of fringe benefits and retirement programs, setting vacation and absentee policies, assistance with career planning, ensuring employees' on-the-job safety, and complying with laws and rules established by regulatory bodies.

It may be easy to assume that *marketing* is simply another word for *advertising* (see Chapters 20 and 21). However, while promotional activities are a significant component of marketing, its activities include identifying the company's strengths over its competitors, properly identifying consumer bases to which marketing strategies will be directed, carrying the right mix of goods and services, arranging these products for optimal "visual selling," and establishing the right prices for goods and services. Price setting is critical not only for products but also especially for services. It is here that pharmacists often make mistakes when trying to establish cognitive or value-added services. Services priced too low are unprofitable, perhaps even a money-losing proposition, whereas services priced too high will fail to attract customers.

Operations management (see Chapter 5) involves establishing policy delineating the activities of each employee on a day-to-day basis, what tools they will use to accomplish their tasks, and where those tasks will be performed (i.e., workflow design). It also entails maintaining the proper inventory of prescription and nonprescription products so that, on the one hand, the pharmacy is not consistently running out of drug products that patients need and, on the other hand, there are not excess amounts of products reaching their expiration date prior to sale or otherwise taking up valuable space that could be used for other purposes.

"SMOOTH OPERATIONS"— REVISITING THE SCENARIO

The preceding discussion of the managerial sciences, especially the issue of workflow design in operations management, brings us back to the scenario involving Mary Quint. Pharmacy students questioning the significance of management and the importance of having a management perspective need not look much further than this case. Mary is faced with a dilemma probably all too common to pharmacy students and practitioners. Students who have worked in numerous environments probably can recall that in some of these places things just seemed to be "going well." Both the customers and the employers were happy, and it was not completely unpleasant to have to show up at work. At other places, there always appears to be a crisis. Immediately on waking up in the morning, one's first thoughts are of dread at having to go to work that day. While this may be somewhat of an oversimplification, the latter places are not being managed well, whereas the former ones probably are. The tremendous variability that exists from one workplace to another is indicative of how critical management is for both the employees working there and the patients they serve. Now ask yourself, Where do you think that you would rather work, and where do you think that patients are receiving the best care, Middletown North Pharmacy or Middletown South Pharmacy?

CONCLUSION

Contrary to popular belief, good business and good patient care are not mutually exclusive. In fact, they are almost entirely mutually dependent. Superior patient care and the implementation of clinical services are made possible by pharmacists who are skilled in management. Pharmacists must be attuned to the internal and external forces that shape the practice of pharmacy. The managerial sciences of accounting, finance, economics, human resources management, marketing, and operations management are indispensable tools for today's practitioner.

QUESTIONS FOR FURTHER DISCUSSION

1. Would you be willing to extend your commute or make other similar sacrifices to work at a place where you enjoyed your job? Why or why not?
2. How do you feel about the role that management plays in the practice of pharmacy?
3. Can you identify someone in a managerial position who is very good at what he or she does? What is it that makes him or her effective?
4. Do you believe that you are going to be an effective pharmacist? What makes you think so?
5. Do you think that you are going to ascend eventually to a managerial position? Why or why not?

REFERENCES

American Association of Colleges of Pharmacy. 1996. Paper from the Commission to Implement Change in Pharmaceutical Education: Maintaining our commitment to change. *Am J Pharm Educ* 60:378.

Bell HM, McElnay JC, Hughes CM. 2000. Societal perspectives on the role of the community pharmacist and community-based pharmaceutical services. *J Soc Admin Pharm* 17:119.

Belluck P. 2001. Prosecutors say greed drove pharmacist to dilute drugs. *New York Times,* August 18.

Brodie DC. 1967. Drug-use control: Keystone to pharmaceutical service. *Drug Intell* 1:63.

Buerki RA, Vottero LD. 1994. *Ethical Responsibility in Pharmacy Practice.* Madison, WI: American Institute of the History of Pharmacy.

Broeseker A, Janke KK. 1998. The evolution and revolution of pharmaceutical care. In McCarthy RL (ed), *Introduction to Health Care Delivery: A Primer for Pharmacists,* p 393. Gaithersburg, MD: Aspen.

Carmel S, Glick SM. 2001. Compassionate-empathic physicians: Personality traits and social-organizational factors that enhance or inhibit this behavior pattern. *Soc Sci Med* 43:1253.

Ciancaglini PP, Waterhouse GA, E'Elia RP. 1994. Pharmaceutical care skills evaluation. Paper presented at the American Association of Colleges of Pharmacy Annual Meeting, Albuquerque, NM, July 8.

Curtiss FR. 1980. Job stress, job satisfaction, anxiety, depression, and life happiness among female versus male pharmacists. *Contemp Pharm Pract* 3:264.

Desselle SP. 1997. Pharmacists' perceptions of pharmaceutical care practice standards. *J Am Pharm Assoc* NS37:29.

Desselle SP, Alafris A. 1999. Changes in pharmacy education sharpen counseling skills. *US Pharmacist* 24:78.

Desselle SP, Rappaport HM. 1996. Establishing standards of care in the community setting. *J Pharm Care* 1:1.

Desselle SP, Rappaport HM. 1995. Feasibility and relevance of identified pharmaceutical care practice standards for community pharmacists. Paper presented at the American Association of Pharmaceutical Scientists Annual Meeting, Miami, FL, November 7.

Desselle SP, Tipton DJ. 2001. Factors contributing to the satisfaction and performance ability of community pharmacists: A path model analysis. *J Soc Admin Pharm* 18:15.

Fjortoft N, Zgarrick D. 2003. An assessment of pharmacists' caring ability. *J Am Pharm Assoc* 43:483.

Fronstin P. 2000. Confidence and confusion: The health care system in the United States. *Stat Bull* 81:18.

Gaither CA. 1998a. Investigation of pharmacists' role stress and the work/nonwork interface. *J Soc Admin Pharm* 15:92.

Gaither CA. 1998b. Predictive validity of work/career-related attitudes and intentions on pharmacists' turnover behavior. *J Pharm Market Manag* 12:3.

Gershon SK, Cultice JM, Knapp KK. 2000. How many pharmacists are in our future? The Bureau of Health Professions Projects Supply to 2020. *J Am Pharm Assoc* 40:757.

Harrison DL, Ortmeier BG. 1995. Levels of independent community pharmacy strategic planning. *J Pharm Market Manag* 11:1.

Harrison DL, Ortmeier BG. 1996. Predictors of community pharmacy strategic planning. *J Pharm Market Manag* 11:1.

Harrison DL, Bootman JL. 1994. Strategic planning by institutional pharmacy administrators. *J Pharm Market Manag* 8:73.

Hepler CD. 1987. The third wave in pharmaceutical education: The clinical movement. *Am J Pharm Educ* 51:369.

Hepler CD, Strand LM. 1990. Opportunities and responsibilities in pharmaceutical care. *Am J Hosp Pharm* 47:533.

Institute of Medicine. 2006. *Preventing Medication Errors: Quality Chasm Series.* Washington, DC: National Academy of Sciences.

Kaiser Family Foundation. 2005. United States spends more per capita than other nations study finds. Available at www.kaisernetwork.org_dailyreports; accessed on April 25, 2007.

Kunyk D, Olson JK. 2001. Clarification of conceptualizations of empathy. *J Adv Nurs* 35:317.

Latif DA. 2000. Relationship between pharmacy students' locus of control, Machiavellianism, and moral reasoning. *Am J Pharm Educ* 64:33.

Maine LL, Penna RP. 1996. Pharmaceutical care: An overview. In Knowlton C, Penna R (eds), *Pharmaceutical Care,* p 133. New York: Chapman & Hall.

Miller MJ, Ortmeier BG. 1995. Factors influencing the delivery of pharmacy services. *Am Pharm* NS35:39.

Millis JS. 1975. *Pharmacists for the Future: The Report of the Study Commission on Pharmacy.* Ann Arbor, MI: Health Administration Press.

Millis JS. 1976. Looking ahead: The Report of the Study Commission on Pharmacy. *Am J Hosp Pharm* 33:134.

National Association of Chain Drug Stores. 2006. 2006 Foundation Industry Profile. Alexandria, VA: National Association of Chain Drug Stores.

Pink LA. 1991. Hospitals. In Fincham JE, Wertheimer AI (eds), *Pharmacists and the U.S. Healthcare System,* p 158. Binghamton, NY: Pharmaceutical Products Press.

Relman AS. 1988. Assessment and accountability: The third revolution in medical care. *N Engl J Med* 319:1220.

Smith WE. 1988. Excellence in the management of clinical pharmacy services. *Am J Hosp Pharm* 45:319.

Sonnedecker G. 1963. *Kremers and Urdang's History of Pharmacy.* Philadelphia, PA: Lippincott.

Speedie SM, Palumbo FB, Leavitt DE. 1974. Pharmacists' perceptions of the antecedents of success in pharmacy. *Contemp Pharm Pract* 3:189.

Stafford M. 2002. Ex-pharmacist gets 30 years for diluting cancer drugs. Associated Press, December 5.

Sumer HC, Knight PA. 2001. How do people with different attachment styles balance work and family? A personality perspective on work-family linkage. *J Appl Psychol* 86:653.

Thompson CA. 2001. Health care system needs overhaul, IOM report says. *Am J Health Syst Pharm* 58:556.

Tootelian DH, Gaedeke RM. 1993. *Essentials of Pharmacy Management.* St. Louis: Mosby.

Torrens PR. 1993. Historical evolution and overview of health service in the United States. In Williams JS, Torrens PR (eds), *Introduction to Health Services,* 4th ed, p 3. Albany, NY: Delmar.

Wiederholt JB, Wiederholt PA. 1997. The patient: Our teacher and friend. *Am J Pharm Educ* 61:415.

Wilkin NE. 1999. Pharmaceutical care: A clinical movement? *Mississippi Pharm* 26:13.

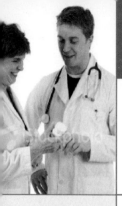

2

MANAGEMENT FUNCTIONS

David P. Zgarrick

About the Author: Dr. Zgarrick is John R. Ellis Distinguished Chair of the Department of Pharmacy Practice and Professor of Pharmacy Administration at Drake University's College of Pharmacy & Health Sciences. Dr. Zgarrick received a B.S. degree in pharmacy from the University of Wisconsin and an M.S. and Ph.D. in pharmaceutical administration from The Ohio State University. He has practice experience in both independent and chain community pharmacy settings. Dr. Zgarrick teaches courses in pharmacy operations management, business planning for professional services, and drug literature evaluation. His research interests are in pharmacist compensation and workforce issues, professional service development, and the use of evidence-based medicine by pharmacists.

◼ LEARNING OBJECTIVES

After completing this chapter, students should be able to

1. Define the terms *management* and *manager.* Describe how concepts in management figure into our everyday lives.
2. Compare and contrast *management* and *leadership.*
3. Compare and contrast classical views of management with modern views.
4. Describe the management process within the contexts of what managers do, resources they manage, and levels at which managers perform their roles.
5. Integrate modern views of management with the management process.
6. Apply the management process to all personal and professional activities.

◼ SCENARIO

Krista Connelly is a second-year pharmacy student. Like most second-year students, she describes her life as "incredibly stressed out." A typical day consists of getting up at 6 a.m., getting dressed and running out the door by 7 a.m., and driving to school to get to her first class by 8 a.m. (making sure to avoid the accident on the expressway that she heard about on her way out the door). While at school, she finds time to squeeze in cups of coffee and snack bars between the lectures, labs, and workshops that usually last until at least 4 p.m. She also makes a point to go to the library to prepare upcoming assignments, as well as to meet with her professors to review how she did on her exams.

After class today, Krista has an Academy of Students of Pharmacy (ASP) meeting. Krista is the vice president of her chapter. As vice president, she is in charge of working with all the committee chairs. In the past few weeks she has had to help the new professional service chairperson develop a brown bag seminar, talk her fund-raising chairperson out of quitting, and write a report on each committee's activities for the chapter Web site. While she really enjoys her leadership role in ASP, she finds some of the people she works with to be frustrating and wonders how she can motivate them to do a better job.

After her meeting, Krista drives to a fast-food restaurant to grab a quick dinner on her way to her part-time pharmacy technician job. If she's not working, she'll head to a friend's house to study for an upcoming exam. She usually gets back to her apartment by 10 p.m. and mentally prepares for what she needs to do in the next few days. She might catch a little bit of TV before heading to bed by midnight.

On weekends, Krista catches up on what one might call "activities of daily living." She'll do her laundry, pay her bills, surf the Internet, call her parents and friends back home, and get together with her friends on Saturday night. When Krista and her friends (most of whom are also pharmacy students) go out, they'll often talk about their plans after they graduate from pharmacy school. They talk about how exciting it will be to counsel patients, work with other health care professionals, and finally start making those high salaries they have heard so much about. None of them says that they want to be pharmacy managers. "The pharmacy manager at my store is always on my case about coming in late or having to arrange my hours around

my exam schedule," said Krista. "I don't see how being a manager can help me do the things I want to as a pharmacist."

▓ CHAPTER QUESTIONS

1. Why is it that all pharmacists should be considered managers regardless of their titles or positions?
2. Why should pharmacy students study management?
3. What is the difference between management and leadership?
4. How does management affect every aspect of our daily lives?
5. Will the same approach to management be effective for all types of situations encountered by pharmacists?

▓ WHAT IS MANAGEMENT?

For many people, a distinct set of images comes to mind when they hear the word *management*. First and foremost, they think of a person (or possibly a group of people) who is "the boss" to whom they report at work. While some people view their relationships with management as positive, many of us have had experiences where this has not been the case. This is why when you ask people what they think of management, they often provide negative views and experiences. Ask pharmacy students what they think about entering careers in pharmacy management, and you'll likely get answers similar to those provided by Krista Connelly and her friends in the scenario.

Perhaps it may be better to start by looking a bit more closely at the term *management*. The stem of the word is *manage*, which according to *Webster's Dictionary* is a verb meaning "to control the movement or behavior of, to lead or direct, or to succeed in accomplishing" (Allee, 1990). Think about how this definition applies to your daily life. Have you ever controlled the movement or behavior of someone or something (even if it was just yourself)? Have you ever succeeded in accomplishing a task (even if it was just getting to an examination on time)?

According to Tootelian and Gaedeke (1993), *management* is "a process which brings together resources and unites them in such a way that, collectively, they achieve goals or objectives in the most efficient manner possible." Contrary to what many people believe, management is a *process,* which is simply a method of doing something. Processes are used to perform simple everyday tasks (e.g., swinging a golf club or driving to school) as well as more complex activities (e.g., hiring a pharmacy technician or dosing an aminoglycoside drug). People perform processes because they want to achieve a goal or objective. Goals and objectives can be personal (e.g., a low golf score or getting to school on time) or professional (e.g., a smoothly operating pharmacy or high-quality patient care). Because processes require resources, and resources are scarce (they are not present in unlimited supply), it is important that resources be used in such a way as to achieve goals and objectives in the most efficient manner possible. While one could achieve one's goal of getting to school on time by driving 90 miles an hour, one also could argue that this would not be the most efficient use of the driver's resources, especially if there is a sharp turn ahead or a police officer waiting around the corner.

Managers are simply people who perform management activities. While people whom we think of as "the boss" and those with administrative appointments within an organization certainly are managers, the fact is that anyone who has a task to accomplish or a goal to achieve is a manager as well. Pharmacy students and pharmacists who say that they do not want to be managers may not desire the authority and responsibilities of having an administrative position, but there is no getting around their need to use resources efficiently to perform the tasks related to their jobs. Thus all pharmacists, regardless of their job responsibilities or position, should view themselves as managers.

Another term that is used commonly when thinking about management is *leadership*. While some people use the terms interchangeably to describe characteristics that are expected of people who are "in charge" of organizations, leadership is a distinctly different skill from *management*. Leadership involves the ability to inspire or direct others. While it certainly is desirable that all managers also have leadership skills, they do not necessarily go hand in hand.

■ CLASSICAL AND MODERN VIEWS OF MANAGEMENT

While management and managers have been with us since humans have had tasks to perform and goals to accomplish (e.g., gathering food or finding shelter), the study of management as a scientific and academic curriculum is relatively new. Before the industrial revolution of the eighteenth and nineteenth centuries, most people lived and worked alone or in small groups. While people at that time still had goals and objectives that needed to be accomplished efficiently, there was little formal study of the best ways to do so. The advent of the industrial revolution brought together groups of hundreds and thousands of people who shared a common objective. In order to get large groups of people to work together effectively, industrialists and academics established hierarchies and systems that allowed large industrial organizations to accomplish their goals (especially those related to growth and profitability).

Around the turn of the twentieth century, an American industrialist and a French engineer began to publish observations in what would become known as the *classical,* or *administrative, school* of management thought. F. W. Taylor, an executive with Bethlehem Steel, published *The Principles of Scientific Management* in 1911. He was among the first to espouse applying scientific principles to management of the workplace. Henri Fayol, a French mining engineer and corporate executive, published *Administration Industrielle et Generale* in 1916. Both Taylor and Fayol argued that all organizations, regardless of size or objective, had to perform a standard set of functions to operate efficiently. Fayol's five management functions (i.e., forecasting and planning, organizing, commanding, coordinating, and controlling) became widely accepted throughout the industrialized world. Both Fayol's five management functions and 14 principles for organizational design (Table 2-1) are still used by managers today. For example, while in the scenario Krista Connelly has the responsibility for working with her ASP chapter's

---

Table 2-1. **Classical Management Theory (Fayol)**

Fayol's 5 management functions:
1. Forecast and plan
2. Organize
3. Command
4. Coordinate
5. Control

Fayol's 14 principles for organizational design and effective administration:

- *Specialization/division of labor.* People should perform tasks specific to their skills. No one person should be expected to perform all the skills needed to run an organization.
- *Authority with corresponding responsibility.* People with responsibility also have sufficient authority within an organization to ensure that a task is performed.
- *Discipline.* People should follow rules, with consequences for not following rules.
- *Unity of command.* The organization has an administrator who is recognized as having the ultimate authority (e.g., CEO or president).
- *Unity of direction.* The organization has a sense of direction or vision that is recognized by all members (e.g., mission statement).
- *Subordination of individual interest to general interest.* The goals of the organization supercede the goals of any individuals within the organization.
- *Remuneration of staff.* Employees should be paid appropriately given the market for their skills and their level of responsibility.
- *Centralization.* Performing similar tasks at a single location is more effective than performing these tasks at multiple locations.
- *Scalar chain/line of authority.* Each employee has one, and only one, direct supervisor.
- *Order.* Tasks should be performed in a systematic fashion.
- *Equity.* Supervisors should treat employees with a sense of fairness.
- *Stability of tenure.* Benefits should go to employees who have stayed with an organization longer.
- *Initiative.* Organizations and employees are more effective when they are proactive, not reactive.
- *Esprit de corps.* Teamwork, harmony.

---

committee chairs, she cannot be effective in her ability to carry out her responsibilities unless her position provides her with authority that is recognized by the committee chairs. Chapter 8 provides more information on Fayol's principles of organizational design.

Much of Taylor's and Fayol's work was developed based on the workplace conditions of the eighteenth, nineteenth, and early twentieth centuries. The great industries of those times focused primarily on the mass production of tangible goods. Very few people were educated beyond grammar school. The few people with

higher levels of education (almost always men) generally were given administrative positions. They were expected to supervise large numbers of less educated production-line employees. In this hierarchy, the role of administrators generally was to command and control their employees, and the role of workers was to carry out the tasks at hand without question.

On the other hand, the workforce and workplace of the late twentieth and early twenty-first centuries have evolved into something quite different. According to the U.S Bureau of Labor Statistics (2007), more than five times the number of people are involved in the provision of services than in the production of tangible goods. Today's workforce is much better educated and more highly skilled than workers had been in the past. In many cases, today's administrators have less formal education and fewer technical skills than the people they are supervising.

These trends have led many to question the relevance of classical management theories in today's rapidly changing world. Walk down the "Business" aisle of practically any bookstore and you'll find literally hundreds of books written by management "gurus" such as Covey, Drucker, Peters, and many others espousing modern management techniques and offering "hands on" advice about how to deal with day-to-day workplace issues. Researchers apply scientific methods to the study of management and publish their results in scholarly journals, similar to what we see in pharmacy and medicine. These books and research studies make important contributions to management science, given the continued need to use scarce resources to achieve goals and objectives in an ever-changing business climate. However, as will be discussed below, classical management theory still has a place in today's pharmacies, as well as in our personal lives.

■ THE MANAGEMENT PROCESS

Figure 2-1 describes one way in which Fayol's management functions can be adapted to describe what managers do in today's world. There are three dimensions of management: (1) activities that managers perform, (2) resources that managers need, and (3) levels at which managers make decisions. Every action taken by a manager involves at least one aspect of each of the three dimensions.

Management Activities

Fayol's five management functions have been adapted to describe four activities that all managers perform. While managers who hold administrative positions in their organizations may have formal ways of performing these activities (and are evaluated on their ability

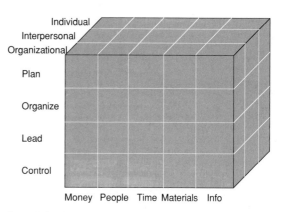

Figure 2-1. The management process.

to get them done), all managers (which means all of us!) perform each of these activities every day, whether we are thinking of them or not.

The first of these four activities is planning. *Planning* is predetermining a course of action based on one's goals and objectives. Managers must consider many factors when planning, including their internal and external environments. The chief pharmacist at a community pharmacy or the director of a hospital pharmacy will develop plans to predetermine which drug products he wishes to carry or what professional services he might offer. Some pharmacists will even go so far as to develop formal strategic and business plans for their pharmacies (see Chapters 5, 6, and 24 through 27). On the other hand, planning can also be very informal. Anyone who goes to work or school in the morning develops a plan for how they will get there (i.e., What time do I need to arrive? What form of transportation should I take? What route should I follow?).

The next management activity is organizing. *Organizing* is the arrangement and relationship of activities and resources necessary for the effective accomplishment of a goal or objective. Once a pharmacist has decided which drug products or services she should offer, she needs to ask herself *what* resources she needs to provide them, *how* she will go about obtaining these resources, and then determine *when* she will need to obtain them. Once the person going to work or school has a plan, he needs to think about what else he may need to do to accomplish his goal (e.g., check the weather and traffic reports, get gas in his car, drop his kids off with a child care provider, etc.).

The next step is the leading or directing step. This step combines Fayol's command and coordinate steps to provide a better description of what managers actually do in today's world. *Leading* or *directing* involves bringing about purposeful action toward some desired outcome. It can take the form of actually doing something yourself (the person going to work or school just needs to get up and go) or working with others to lead them to where you want your organization to be. A pharmacist eventually may offer the goods and services described in her plans, but almost certainly she will need to work with a number of other people within her organization to accomplish this task. In the scenario, Krista Connelly, in her role has vice president of her ASP chapter, is responsible for seeing that the chapter's committees work effectively to accomplish their objectives. Working with others often requires leadership skills, which will be discussed in Chapter 14.

The fourth step is the control or evaluation step. *Control* or *evaluation* involves reviewing the progress that has been made toward the objectives that were set out in the plan. This step involves not only determining *what* actually happened but also *why* it happened. Performing quality-control checks to help ensure that patients are receiving the desired medication in the appropriate manner is a very important function of a pharmacy practice. Pharmacists can also ask themselves if the goods and services they offered met their goals. These goals can be from the perspective of their patients (e.g., Did the goods and services result in high-quality patient care or improved clinical outcomes?), as well as from other perspectives (e.g., Did the service improve the pharmacist's job satisfaction? Did it improve the profitability of the pharmacy or organization?). The person going to work or school not only should ask himself if he arrived on time but should also know why he did or did not (e.g., the traffic accident on the expressway, hitting the snooze button that third time before getting up, etc.). Chapters 9 and 28 review some of the methods that pharmacists use to help ensure the quality of their operations and reduce the occurrence of medication errors.

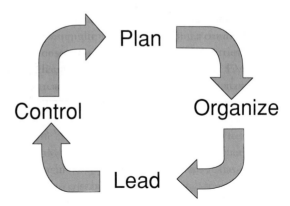

Figure 2-2. Management activities cycle.

Management activities should be performed in order, starting with the planning step. They are also meant to be cyclic, meaning that what a manager learns in the control and evaluation step should be incorporated into the planning step the next time she needs to accomplish that objective (Fig. 2-2). For example, if a pharmacy student receives a score on an examination that did not meet his goal, he should use what he learned in the evaluation step (e.g., what questions he got wrong, time spent studying, etc.) to help him plan for the next examination.

Resources That Are Managed

Regardless of their level or position within an organization, managers must use resources to achieve their goals and objectives. Keep in mind that resources are scarce, meaning that they are not available in unlimited supply. Both organizations and individuals must use resources efficiently to achieve their goals and objectives.

The first resource that many managers think of is money. Customers generally provide money to pharmacies and pharmacists in exchange for goods and services. Employers generally pay their employees money in exchange for the services they provide to the organization. Managing money is important to any organization or individual, and several chapters of this book are dedicated to explaining how pharmacies and pharmacists manage money and use economic information to make decisions (see Chapters 15 through 19). Money in and of itself can be an important yardstick for measuring the success of an organization or an individual. However, most managers value money for its ability to allow them to obtain additional resources that are necessary to achieve other goals and objectives.

Another resource that is very important to managers is people. In pharmacy practice, there is very little that any one person can accomplish on his or her own, regardless of the practice setting. Pharmacists must work with other employees in their pharmacies, other health care professionals, and especially the patients and customers they serve. Given the importance of this topic, an entire section of this book (Chapters 8 through 14) is dedicated to the management of people.

How many times have you heard someone say, "I'd have got that done if I'd have had more time"? Of all the resources managers have at their disposal, time can be the most limiting. After all, there are only 24 hours in a day! Time management is essential for today's busy pharmacist, as well as for most other people. In the scenario, Krista Connelly is a great example of a pharmacy student who could benefit from time and stress management. Chapters 13 and 14 are dedicated to time management, stress management, and organizational skills that can help you to get the most out of this precious resource.

When many people think of pharmacy, they still think of a pharmacist standing behind a counter compounding drug products and dispensing prescriptions. While pharmacy practice continues to evolve from a product to a patient orientation, managing material resources is still a very important function in a pharmacy. Community pharmacies filled 3.4 billion prescriptions in 2005, an increase of almost 70 percent over the past decade (NACDS, 2006). The costs of these drug products, as well as the costs of the equipment and supplies necessary to dispense them safely and efficiently to patients, continues to rise in all practice settings. Just as people need to assess their needs and supplies of material goods (e.g., food, clothing, household supplies, etc.) before going on a shopping trip, pharmacies need to make the same assessments before purchasing drug products, equipment, and supplies. Chapters 7, 22, and 23 are all designed to help readers learn more about managing material resources.

While the eighteenth and nineteenth centuries were known as the time of the industrial revolution, the twenty-first century certainly will be known as the information age. The advent of the computer and the Internet in the late twentieth century has resulted in an explosion of information that is literally at most people's fingertips. This already has had a tremendous impact on pharmacy practice, providing pharmacists with information about drugs and patients that they did not have only a few years ago. While it is not certain what implications this will have for pharmacy practice in the future, it is certain that information management is becoming an important job for pharmacists. Chapter 8 provides an overview of technologies that pharmacists use to manage information, as well as insights into what role information management may have in the future of pharmacy practice.

Levels of Management

When managers perform management activities, they can do so at a number of levels with a variety of different purposes in mind. While some people think of management activities as only occurring at a corporate or organizational level, management activities occur much more frequently at lower levels.

There is not a person reading this book who has not performed self-management activities. Just the fact that you are a pharmacy student or pharmacist attests to the fact that you have performed a number of activities on your own just to get to this point. Self-management is the most frequently occurring level of management, if for no other reason than that practically every decision we make every day (both professional and personal) requires self-management. For example, pharmacists must prioritize and manage their time efficiently so that they can accomplish the wide variety of tasks, from ensuring that every prescription is dispensed accurately to making sure that they have time to counsel their patients.

Next to self-management, the most frequent level on which managers find themselves performing is the interpersonal level. Interpersonal management occurs between the manager and one other person. In a pharmacy, this might involve a pharmacist counseling a patient about a medication or training a technician on how to adjudicate a claim with a third-party payer. Our personal lives are full of interpersonal relationships, including those with our parents, siblings, spouse, children, friends, and significant others.

The level of management that occurs less frequently is organizational management. This involves actions that affect groups of people. We frequently think of this occurring at work, especially when a pharmacist needs to develop a policy or make a decision that may affect many people at the pharmacy. High-level administrators in large organizations (e.g., pharmacy chains, hospitals, etc.) often make decisions that affect everyone within the organization. Keep in mind that people who hold administrative positions are not the only ones who perform organizational management. Anyone who has ever had to make an "executive decision" among a group of classmates who are studying for an examination or deciding where to go for lunch can relate to the kinds of organizational-level decisions that business leaders make every day.

■ INTEGRATING MODERN AND CLASSICAL VIEWS OF MANAGEMENT

Much of what was first described by Taylor and Fayol at the beginning of the twentieth century is still applied today by managers at all levels of administration in all types of organizations. However, much has changed in both pharmacy practice and the workplace over that time, and management science has exploded to keep up with those changes.

One hundred years ago, the relationship between an administrator and a worker was very hierarchical. The authority of the administrator generally went unquestioned, and workers simply did what they were told. In today's workplace, there is much more of a partnership between administrators and workers. While administrators are still responsible for achieving organizational goals and objectives, workers generally expect to have input as to how goals and objectives will be accomplished and also expect to share in the rewards when those goals are accomplished.

Health care organizations such as hospitals and pharmacies present a number of managerial challenges to administrators. Unlike the workers of Taylor's and Fayol's day, most health care workers are highly educated and skilled professionals. Trends toward specialization among health care professionals often create situations where staff-level health care workers have more knowledge and expertise of their particular area than their administrators. As you can imagine, administrators of health care professionals who attempt to use their authority to command and control these employees may find this not to be an effective way to achieve organizational goals and objectives.

Modern views of management suggest that managers must adapt their management activities to their workers. These functions generally occur in addition to the classical management functions. According to Nelson and Economy (2003), today's manager also needs to

- *Energize.* Today's managers need to have a vision of what they want to create and the energy to make it happen. When you think of good managers with whom you have worked in the past, they are probably not the kind of people who just want to keep doing the same thing every day for the rest of their lives. They generally have ideas about what they would like to see their organizations become in the future and the energy to attract others who want to join in. They are always trying to make the best of what often can be stressful situations, especially when the level of resources available may be less than they desire. In pharmacy today, good managers are often pharmacists who want to see the profession move forward by developing new professional services and opportunities to provide pharmaceutical care. Their energy and enthusiasm generally attract motivated pharmacists and other personnel who share their vision and want to work with them. These managers also seem to find the resources they need to carry out their vision or make the most of what they already have. Not only does the power of energy and enthusiasm work for pharmacists, but it also benefits pharmacy students as well. Do you think that Krista

Connelly would be as an effective leader if she did not have a high level of energy and enthusiasm for ASP's goals and objectives?

- *Empower.* If you are a highly educated and skilled health professional, the last thing you probably want is to have an administrator questioning your decisions and telling you how you should do your job. In today's environment, managers should empower their employees to do what needs to be done. In many ways, today's manager is very much like the coach of a team. Coaches develop a game plan; select players; provide them with training, resources, and advice; and then step back and let the players execute the game plan. Good coaches empower their players to carry out their game plan. Managers who empower their employees provide them with training, resources, and advice and then let the employees get the job done. Krista Connelly can empower her ASP committee chairpersons by providing them with goals, resources, and advice and then letting them get to work.

  This is not to say that managers do not need to supervise their employees. Managers are still responsible for seeing that their organizations' goals are met, which may mean having to intervene with workers. Just as coaches need to provide resources and advice to their players during a game, and occasionally replace a player who is not executing the game plan, managers need to provide resources, advice, and occasionally discipline to see that their organizations' goals are met.

- *Support.* After a manager has empowered her employees to do their jobs, she should not just leave them on their own, especially when things start to go wrong. Today, good managers need to be coaches, collaborators, and sometimes even cheerleaders for their employees. Providing support for employees does not mean that managers should be willing to do their employees' work or always agree with the decisions their employees make on the job. It does mean that managers need to provide their employees with the training, resources, and authority needed to do their jobs. Managers also need to be good coaches, letting their employees know when they have done

a good job, as well as helping them to learn when things are not going so well. Even pharmacy students like Krista Connelly know that a few kind words to her committee chairpersons will help her ASP chapter in the long run.

  In providing support, managers must also be mindful to balance the needs and resources of their organizations with what their employees need. As much as a manager may wish to give a valued employee a big raise, the manager must also consider how much money is available for a raise and other potential uses of his financial resources.

- *Communicate.* In today's information-laden environment, communication between managers and employees is more important than ever. While managers can energize, empower, and support their employees, if they cannot communicate their messages, they will not be effective, and their organizations will suffer. The cornerstone of communications in any environment is trust. If employees feel that they can bring up any question or concern to a manager, they probably will be much more receptive to what the manager has to say.

  One major challenge for managers and employees today is the vast number of ways in which they can communicate with each other. Communication that used to take place between managers and employees in person now can take place over the telephone, via voice mail, or even by means of text messaging and e-mail. While these additional methods can make it easier for managers and employees to communicate with each other, care must be taken in using these methods. As you can imagine, not every method of communication is appropriate for every type of message (e.g., disciplining or firing an employee in a text message on a cell phone is *not* a good idea).

■ WHY SHOULD I STUDY MANAGEMENT?

After reading the first two chapters of this book, you still may be asking yourself, "Why should I study management?" You may think that being a good manager just involves using your common sense and applying the Golden Rule (act toward others as you would have others act toward you). After all, you probably have done a good job managing yourself up to this point without taking a management course or reading a management textbook. Can managing a pharmacy practice be that much different?

While there is certainly a role for applying self-management skills, most pharmacy managers agree that managing a pharmacy practice successfully requires a unique set of skills. Some of these skills can be quite technical [e.g., financial management (see Chapters 15 through 19) and marketing (see Chapters 20 through 23)], requiring a knowledge base that goes beyond what many pharmacists bring to their practices. These skills should be studied just as one would study medicinal chemistry, pharmacology, or therapeutics.

Something else to keep in mind is that in today's workplace, what might be common sense to you may not make sense at all to the other people you encounter. Pharmacists today work with employees, other health professionals, and especially patients who come from a wide variety of racial, ethnic, cultural, and educational backgrounds. People from diverse backgrounds bring with them an incredible amount of insight and experience. Pharmacists who do not take this into account when working with diverse groups of people may find themselves frustrated and not able to achieve their goals and objectives effectively.

In this book we make an effort to present material that is relevant to both pharmacy students and pharmacists. Pharmacy students who use this book will find that many of the scenarios that start each chapter are directed toward experiences to which they can relate. There may be some of you right now who think that your life has a lot in common with Krista Connelly's. We anticipate that this is the case. The information provided in each chapter not only will help students to better deal with management issues they are currently experiencing but will also help to prepare them for what to expect in the future as pharmacists.

Pharmacists who use this book often have a good idea of why they need to have management skills. After all, they are living pharmacy practice management on a daily basis! The information provided in this book should help to provide pharmacists with the skills they will need to better meet the challenges they face every day. In addition, the last four chapters of this book (Chapters 31 through 34) describe how pharmacists in a variety of practice settings apply management skills on a daily basis.

■ QUESTIONS FOR FURTHER DISCUSSION

Listed below are three scenarios that represent how pharmacists use the management process on a daily basis. For each scenario, please describe (1) the level of management being performed, (2) the type of management activity being performed, and (3) the resources that the pharmacist needs to perform this activity.

Scenario 1: Sabin Patel, R.Ph., is trying to decide what form of education (nontraditional Pharm.D., certificate program, continuing education) would best allow her to maintain her practice skills.

Scenario 2: Doug Danforth, Pharm.D., is training a technician regarding information that needs to be collected during an initial patient interview.

Scenario 3: Casey Kulpinski, Pharm.D., is reviewing her pharmacy's financial statements to determine if her diabetes care center met her chain's financial goals.

REFERENCES

Allee JG (ed). 1990. *Webster's Dictionary.* Baltimore: Ottenheimer Publishers.

National Association of Chain Drug Stores (NACDS). 2006. *The Chain Pharmacy Industry Profile: 2006.* Alexandria, VA: National Association of Chain Drug Stores.

Nelson B, Economy P. 2003. *Managing for Dummies,* 2d ed. New York: Wiley.

Tootelian DH, Gaedeke RM. 1993. *Essentials of Pharmacy Management.* St Louis: Mosby.

U.S. Bureau of Labor Statistics. 2007. www.bls.gov/news.release/empsit.nr0.htm; accessed on April 11, 2007.

SECTION II

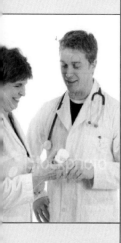

MANAGING OPERATIONS

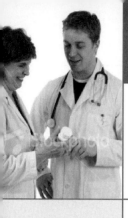

3

STRATEGIC PLANNING IN PHARMACY OPERATIONS

Glen T. Schumock and Godwin Wong

A **bout the Authors:** Dr. Schumock is a graduate of Washington State University (B.Pharm.), the University of Washington (Pharm.D.), and the University of Illinois at Chicago (MBA). He also completed a residency and a research fellowship. Currently, Dr. Schumock is Director of the Center for Pharmacoecomic Research and Associate Professor in the Department of Pharmacy Practice at the University of Illinois at Chicago. Dr. Schumock teaches in courses on pharmacy management, pharmacoeconomics, and business planning for pharmacy services. Dr. Schumock has published over 100 articles, book chapters, and books. He is on the editorial boards of the journals *Pharmacotherapy* and *PharmacoEconomics*. Dr. Schumock is a board-certified pharmacotherapy specialist and is a Fellow in the American College of Clinical Pharmacy.

Dr. Wong has been on the faculty of the Haas School of Business at the University of California, Berkeley, for 20 years. His areas of interests are corporate strategic planning, entrepreneurship, information technology management, and venture capital. He has conducted leadership and strategic planning workshops for various health care groups, hospital administrators, and pharmaceutical companies and has lectured to executives in 20 countries. He has served on the boards of directors of several California banks, Silicon Valley companies, and international corporations. He received a B.S. from the University of Wisconsin, an M.S. from UCLA, and a Ph.D. from Harvard University.

■ LEARNING OBJECTIVES

After completing this chapter, students should be able to

1. Provide an overview of planning activities conducted by pharmacy and health care organizations.
2. Describe the general process common to all types of planning.
3. Describe the purpose of strategic planning, and illustrate the specific steps to develop a strategic plan.

4. Differentiate a vision statement from a mission statement.
5. Highlight examples of strategic planning in pharmacy organizations.
6. Identify barriers and limitations to planning.

SCENARIO

Ted Thompson graduated from pharmacy school magna cum laude 2 years ago with a doctor of pharmacy degree and successfully passed the licensing examination, making him a registered pharmacist. After graduation, Ted completed a pharmacy practice residency at a prestigious teaching hospital with a reputation for having an excellent pharmacy department and advanced clinical pharmacy services. Following his residency, Ted took a job as a clinical pharmacist in a community hospital in his hometown. In hiring Ted, the hospital pharmacy department fulfilled an interim objective toward their goal of developing contemporary pharmacy services.

The hospital is located in a town of approximately 100,000 people, and a large portion of the population is elderly. Partly because of both the favorable payer mix (mostly Medicare) and the fiscal savvy of the chief financial officer (CFO),[1] the hospital has done very well from clinical and economic perspectives. The pharmacy department has a good drug distribution system and a director of pharmacy (DOP) who, while not trained clinically, understands the value of these services.

The hospital is growing rapidly and, as such, has become increasingly reliant of pharmacy services. Because of the many opportunities that confront the pharmacy department, the DOP has decided that the department should develop a plan to guide its priorities

---

[1] In a business or organization, the CFO is the individual who is responsible for the financial decisions and investments made by the company. In a hospital or health system, the CFO is likely to have several departments and functions reporting to him or her, including general accounting, accounts receivable and accounts payable, payroll, budgeting, and finance.

over the next 5 years. To accomplish this, the DOP has determined that over the next several months, the department will undergo a strategic planning effort. This effort will begin with a selected group of individuals from within the department, each representing key functions and constituencies. Ted was asked to be part of this group because of his clinical role and expertise and because expansion of the clinical pharmacy services provided by the department is recognized as a goal that likely will be part of this strategic plan.

Having no real management training or experience, Ted recognized the need to learn more about the purpose of strategic planning and the process that will be required to develop the departmental strategic plan.

CHAPTER QUESTIONS

1. What are the different activities that pharmacies and health care organizations engage in when they plan for the future?
2. What is the purpose of strategic planning, and how is it different from other types of planning?
3. What are the steps typically taken by a pharmacy organization when developing a strategic plan?
4. What is a vision statement, and for whom is it written?
5. What is a mission statement, and for whom is it written?
6. What are the barriers or limitations associated with planning that should be kept in mind while undertaking this process?

INTRODUCTION

The scenario illustrates an important activity within pharmacies and health care organizations that is rarely considered by new pharmacy graduates. In this scenario, Ted is asked to participate in the development of a strategic plan. Strategic planning is one of the most common types of planning that is conducted by health care organizations. However, strategic planning is not unique to pharmacies or health care organizations; in fact, it represents a core management activity that is employed by all businesses.

This chapter begins with a general discussion of management planning by pharmacy organizations. Pharmacies and health care organizations, like many businesses, are involved in, or should be involved in, many different types of planning for different purposes within the organization. This chapter provides an understanding of where the responsibility of planning lies within organizations and the general structure or process involved in planning efforts. These general concepts are applicable to all types of planning in all different types of organizations, including pharmacies.

Next, this chapter discusses one specific type of planning—strategic planning. The intent of this discussion is to provide a general understanding of the role of strategic planning and to identify its key steps or components. While the material in this chapter is applicable to almost any type of organization, examples pertinent to the profession of pharmacy or pharmacy practice within health care organizations are provided. For readers interested in a more complete understanding of planning, there are many options for obtaining information beyond what is presented here. There are literally hundreds of textbooks addressing both general and specific topics within this field. Several good texts are included in the reference list at the end of this chapter (Koteen, 1997; Martin, 2002; Porter, 1980, 1985; Stoner, Freeman, Gilbert, 1995; Thompson and Strickland, 1983).

▪ PLANNING IN GENERAL

In the broadest sense, *planning* represents the purposeful efforts taken by an organization (for our purposes, a pharmacy organization) to maximize its future success. Planning, as it is referred to here, is sometimes called *management planning* because it is typically part of the duties of managers. Planning has been described as one of the four key functions of managers (along with organizing, leading, and controlling). In fact, of the four functions, planning is crucial because it supports the other three (Stoner, Freeman, and Gilbert, 1995). However, planning may involve more than just managers at high levels; in fact, in smaller companies or in companies with fewer levels of management, front-line employees often are involved in planning.

Many different types of planning activities occur within pharmacy organizations. The most common types include business planning, financial planning, operational planning, resource planning, organizational planning, and strategic planning. The purpose of each type of planning is different. It is not the intent of this chapter to cover all these types of planning. Instead, a brief description of the purpose and characteristics of each is outlined in Table 3-1. Some of these types of planning activities have subtypes within them. For example, one type of resource planning deals specifically with human resources (Smith, 1989). Another type of resource planning that has gained increasing importance is information technology planning. This type of planning focuses specifically on the present and future information needs of an organization and the technologies and systems to meet those needs (Wong and Keller, 1997; Breen and Crawford, 2005).

Because of the importance of effective planning, many organizations invest significant time and resources in these efforts. Ultimately, the chief executive officer (CEO) or president of a company is responsible for making certain that the organization is successful—ensuring that success largely depends on planning that occurs within the organization.[2] However, in large companies, given the scope of planning activities that must take place, much of the work involved in planning is delegated to a special department dedicated entirely to planning. Often, outside

---

[2] The CEO is the top administrator of an organization, reporting only to the board of directors. The CEO is responsible for the overall success of the organization and is the key decision maker.

Table 3-1. Types of Planning

Type	Purpose	Characteristics
Strategic planning	To ensure that the organization is doing the right things. Addresses what business the organization is in, or ought to be in, provides a framework for more detailed planning and day-to-day decisions.	Long term (5–20 years); scope includes all aspects of the organization; viewpoint is external—how the organization interacts with or controls its environment.
Operational planning	To ensure that the organization is prepared perform the immediate tasks and objectives to meet the goals and strategy of the organization. To ensure that the organization is doing things right.	Short term (1–5 years); scope is specific to the immediate actions that need to be taken to move the organization forward; viewpoint is internal—day-to-day accomplishment of tasks.
Business planning	To determine the feasibility of a specific business or program. Business planning is used to make a decision about investing in and moving forward with a program.	Short term (1–5 years); can be used to make decisions to start a new business, expand a business, or terminate a business.
Resource planning	To ensure the resources necessary to achieve the goals and strategy of the organization. Resource planning can be comprehensive (all resources needed to achieve goals and strategic plan of the organization) or can focus on a specific type of resource.	Midterm (1–10 years); scope is specific to the resource or resources defined in the plan—specific resources may include human resources, information/technology resources, financial resources, capital and facilities, and others; viewpoint is internal—the resource needs of the organization.
Organizational planning	To ensure that an organization is organized appropriately to meet the challenges of the future. Key elements include reporting relationships, definition of responsibilities, and definition of authorities.	Midterm (1–10 years); scope specific to the structural aspects of the organization including divisions, reporting relationships, coordination, control; viewpoint is internal—how the company organizes itself.
Contingency planning	To provide a fallback option or direction should the original strategy of the organization fail or should something unexpected occur. Contingency planning can occur for a specific anticipated situation, the most common of which are business-related crises (such as a labor strike), natural disasters, and changes in management personnel.	Short to long term (1–20 years); scope is specific to the particular situation that may occur; viewpoint is both external (if the situation is created in the environment) and internal.

consultants are employed to assist organizations in their planning efforts.

The actual process of planning may vary by the type of planning being conducted and by the size of the organization or system. Here, the term *system* refers to the entity for which planning is being conducted. That entity may be the entire pharmacy organization or a program or function within it. Programs can be considered subunits or specific services within an organization. An example of a program within a pharmacy organization would be a clinical pharmacy service program. A *function* is an activity that cuts across different subunits of an organization. An example of a function within a pharmacy organization would be the function of information management.

Regardless of the system for which planning is being conducted, planning varies in terms of sophistication. In some cases, planning can be relatively simple and straightforward. In other cases, it may involve extensive analyses of data with complicated forecasting, decision-making models, and algorithms. Nevertheless, all planning processes share a few basic characteristics, as shown in Table 3-2.

The eight steps shown in Table 3-2 define the general process that is followed in most planning efforts. These general steps in some cases may be expanded or condensed depending on the situation or presented in a slightly different fashion. Nevertheless, the key components of understanding the purpose, assessing the situation, establishing goals, and devising a method to accomplish those goals should be common to all planning activities.

As shown in the table, the planning process should begin with consideration of the purpose of the organization or system and of the planning effort itself. This is followed by an analysis of the present situation or status of the system. Next, specific future goals are determined, and then a strategy for bridging the gap between the present and future is developed. Interim objectives that measure progress toward the goals are then identified, and responsibilities and timelines for each objective are assigned. The plan then needs to be communicated, implemented, and monitored.

▇ STRATEGIC PLANNING

The purpose of strategic planning is to ensure that the organization is doing the right things now and in the future. Strategic planning addresses what business the organization is in or ought to be in and helps to determine long-term goals for the organization. For example, what is the business of a particular community pharmacy? Does the pharmacy want to be in the "prescription business" or the "health care business"? Does a health system want to be in the "hospital business" or a "business that provides a continuum of care"? Obviously, how a pharmacy organization answers these questions may influence how it views itself and how it conducts its business, thus providing a framework for more detailed planning and day-to-day decisions.

Strategic planning has been defined as the process of selecting an organization's goals, determining the policies and programs (strategies) necessary to achieve specific objectives en route to those goals, and establishing methods necessary to ensure that the policies and strategic programs are implemented (Steiner, Miner, and Gray, 1982). More broadly, strategic planning can be considered an effort that enables the optimal deployment of all organizational resources within current and future environmental constraints. The result

Table 3-2.   Steps in the Planning Process
1. Define or orient the planning process to a singular purpose or a desired result (vision/mission).
2. Assess the current situation.
3. Establish goals.
4. Identify strategies to reach those goals.
5. Establish objectives that support progress toward those goals.
6. Define responsibilities and timelines for each objective.
7. Write and communicate the plan.
8. Monitor progress toward meeting goals and objectives.

of this optimization is to increase the likelihood that the organization will survive, and preferably thrive, in the future.

In evaluating the performance of a company, it is often informative to look at its strategy historically over time. While many factors can influence organizational performance, companies that engage in long-range strategic planning are often more successful than those that do not. Again, this is true for pharmacy organizations as well as other types of businesses. Strategic planning can be either reactive or proactive. Reactive strategic planning is not the ideal, but it is often necessary, especially in industries that are changing rapidly (such as health care). Preferably, proactive strategic planning enables an organization to control its environment instead of vice versa.

Beyond proactive planning, organizations that are able to think and plan in a provocative or "out of the box" manner may position themselves not only to control the business environment but also to actually create or recreate the business environment. This type of strategic thinking has been considered the pinnacle of planning efforts by organizations—ideal for companies to position themselves to be most competitive. Using strategy to create an environment that puts the company at an advantage compared with its competitors is integral to this effort (Porter, 1980, 1985). An example outside the health care industry is Apple, Inc., and its iPod product. The October 2001 introduction of the iPod was the direct result of Apple's strategy to create a whole new category of portable entertainment—a strategy that obviously has been extremely successful. A similar example is that of the Web site Facebook, which, together with similar sites, has developed a new market for interaction via the Internet that did not exist previously.

The time horizon of strategic planning helps to distinguish it from other types of planning. Strategic planning has also been called *long-term planning*. The actual timeline used by organizations may vary or in some cases may not be known. Because the future is unknown, it is often difficult to predict with any accuracy the amount of time it will take for an organization to reach its long-term goals. Nevertheless, a key component of strategic planning is to identify time periods within which goals are to be reached.

The time horizon for strategic planning may be as long as 10 to 20 years or as short as 2 years. In a survey conducted by the Net Future Institute, managers were asked what time period they considered to be long term (Martin, 2002). The most common response was 2 years (40.2 percent), followed by 5 years (32.7 percent) and 1 year (17.9 percent). Admittedly, many of the companies involved in this survey were in high-tech industries, where rapid change may impair longer-term planning. However, health care is also an industry of rapid change, and thus planning must be done similarly to that in other fast-growing industries.

The problem with strategic planning, even in 5-year time periods, is that it is not likely to result in any truly sustainable competitive advantages or a significant organizational metamorphosis. Further, because strategic goals are based on the company's vision for the future, goals that incorporate new paradoxes or visionary changes may be difficult for employees to believe if the time period for accomplishing those goals is too short. Nevertheless, these are the types of goals that should be created in strategic planning, so it is the time period that must be congruent with these goals, not vice versa. The worst mistake would be to "dumb down" the goals to make them consistent with a shorter time period.

Vision and Mission

An important part of the process of strategic planning is to create momentum and to motivate personnel within the pharmacy organization. Strategic planning has a lot to do with defining what a company is all about and creating a "story" about the organization. The communication of the organization's story occurs across a number of different statements that may be products of strategic planning. Most essential of these statements are the vision statement and the mission statement.

The *vision* is what the pharmacy organization wants to be at some future time point. The vision may be complex and multidimensional, but the vision statement should be short. The *vision statement* should make people think and should motivate people to strive for something greater. A company vision statement should inspire employees to create a different future for the organization. The vision of the organization is used in the strategic planning process as both the beginning point and the end point. That is, once the vision is set, then strategic planning is about how to reach that end point. The vision is also used to define the mission of the organization. For example, the vision statement of Baptist Health Care in Pensacola, Florida, is "To be the best health system in America" (see www.elakeviewcenter.org/BHC/Mission.aspx). This vision drives both the mission of the organization and its values, and presumably, these together guide the daily business decisions made by Baptist Health Care.

The *mission* is the purpose of the company. The *mission statement* defines what the company does or is. It is a statement of the present going ahead into the near future. It is a document written to create a sense of purpose for customers and employees. The mission statement should be short—usually no more than two sentences. It focuses on the common purpose of the organization and may draw from the values or beliefs held by the organization. The mission statement should help to differentiate the company from others that provide the same products or services. Some organizations include in the mission statement not only what the company does but also how it does it— essentially the differentiating point.

The following elements have been suggested in developing a mission statement for a community pharmacy: the intended (or target) customers, the core values of the pharmacy (such as compassion, respect, and confidentiality), the key services and products provided by the pharmacy, the benefits incurred by customers (such as improved health and improved safety), and the desired public image of the pharmacy (Hagel, 2002).

All pharmacy organizations should have a mission statement. Kerr Drugs, a chain of pharmacies in the Carolinas, provides a good example of a mission statement that focuses on the key services of the organization. The mission of Kerr Drugs is "To be the most comprehensive provider of community pharmacy and related health care services, offering our customers quality merchandise, value for their money and the most exceptional customer service in the industry." (see www.kerrdrug.com/about_kerr.html). The mission statement of the Wyeth (www.wyeth.com) Pharmaceutical Company emphasizes the benefits incurred to its customers. It reads, "We bring to the world pharmaceutical and health care products that improve lives and deliver outstanding value to our customers and shareholders." Similarly, the mission of Novartis (www.novartis.com/about-novartis/our-mission/index.shtml) Pharmaceuticals is to "discover, develop and successfully market innovative products to prevent and cure diseases, to ease suffering and to enhance the quality of life."

As noted earlier, the mission statement creates a sense of purpose for both the employees and customers of the organization. Employees of Kerr Drug know that their customers will expect reliable and comprehensive services and therefore that they should strive to provide that each day. This chapter later discusses how pharmacies such as Kerr Drug that have well-defined missions and that engage in strategic planning are more likely to be successful.

In addition to the mission statement, some businesses use a *company slogan* to convey a message to customers about the organization. The company slogan generally is more marketing-driven than is the mission statement, but in some cases the company slogan serves a similar role. Like the mission statement, the company slogan sends a message to both customers and employees, and it must be congruent with the actions of the organization or else it will not be credible. A great example of a company slogan is that of the Nike Company. The slogan "Just Do It!" has energy and a sense of action. It is easy to see how the slogan and the company's mission, "To bring inspiration and innovation to every athlete in the world," combine to create a powerful image of what this company is all about. A good example of a slogan for a pharmacy organization is that of the Walgreens Company, which reads, "Walgreens. The Pharmacy America Trusts." Again, this slogan is brief yet conveys a meaningful message.

The vision, mission, and other statements that form the company story are critical elements in strategic planning. If these elements already exist in the organization, then the process of strategic planning starts with these as its foundation or modifies them as necessary. If these elements do not already exist, then the process of strategic planning must include their conception.

Process of Strategic Planning

The process of strategic planning does not vary significantly from the process used in other types of planning. This chapter highlights only the aspects of the steps shown in Table 3-2 that are distinctive to strategic planning compared with other types of planning efforts.

Preplanning Phase

Preplanning can be defined as the steps necessary to organize the strategic planning effort—or "planning for the planning." Strategic planning is a significant undertaking that consumes much time and energy. A pharmacy organization choosing to engage in a strategic planning effort should not take this lightly. Strategic planning is a financial investment—in the personnel time required and in the payment of consultants, if used. These costs should be weighed against the value to be gained by the effort. If strategic planning is performed correctly, its value will greatly exceed any costs. On the other hand, if strategic planning is done in a superficial or hurried manner, its costs will exceed its benefits. Preplanning should include a careful assessment of this balance.

Preplanning should also define the objectives of the planning efforts and the procedures that will be used to accomplish those objectives. Preplanning should define who should be involved, where the planning process will occur, and how much time will be allotted to the effort. Preplanning should also consider any political purposes and ramifications of the undertaking. In laying out the scope of the planning effort, preplanning should orient the activity to the vision of the organization, if one exists.

Planning Phase

In the *planning phase* of strategic planning, ideas are actively generated for the pharmacy organization. This may be referred to as *strategizing*. As in any planning process, it is usually best to start with the destination in mind, as in planning a trip by viewing a map. Once the destination is clear, one must find the starting place on the map. The next step is to determine the different routes or options to get from here to there. Among the different routes, one should select that which best meets the needs within the constraints of limited resources. If speed is important, then one selects the quickest route. If scenery is important, then one selects the most scenic route. Besides the route, the mode of transportation needs to be determined. Options might include taking a train, driving a car, or flying in an airplane (or a combination of any of these). Once the route and method of transportation are known, one selects key milestones, or places to stop, along the way. Knowing these intermediate points helps to keep the journey on track. The process of strategic planning is very similar, except strategic planning is, or should be, a group effort involving all levels of the organization.

In strategic planning, the "destination" is the vision of the organization in the future. However, it is also necessary to identify where, what, and how the organization is in the present. This is called *situation analysis,* and it should consider both the past performance and the current situation. This is the starting point on the journey. Based on the vision (destination), along with the present situation (starting point), planners next should identify the goals for the organization. These goals could be considered synonymous with the things considered important in the map example, such as speed and scenic beauty. Once the goals are identified, the course is plotted to get from the present to the future. For this, it is crucial to identify and select preferred strategies that will accomplish the goals. Strategies are synonymous with the routes and the modes and costs of transportation in the travel example. Last, one should determine objectives that will help to reach the goals. Objectives are like the intermediate points, or places to pass through on the map. These objectives provide a shorter-term milestone and, in implementation, help to measure progress toward the goal. The relationship between vision, goals, strategy, and objectives is shown graphically in Fig. 3-1.

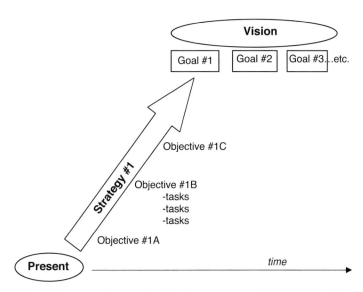

Figure 3-1. Relationship between vision, goals, objectives, strategy, and mission. To reach a certain vision, or future state, the organization must set and reach one or more goals. Each goal is associated with a specific strategy or method of reaching that goal. The strategy can be defined by the objectives that are necessary intermediate accomplishments toward the goal. A set of tasks, or actions, may be associated with each objective. Collectively, these tasks are also called *tactics* that the organization employs to meet an objective. *(Adapted from Coke, 2001, with permission from the publisher.)*

Considering the preceding overview, the steps in the planning process can be examined more closely. After crafting a vision statement, planners must analyze and define the current situation. As is the case with any system, history helps to define the present. Therefore, part of the situation analysis is to evaluate the past performance of the organization. This evaluation should include all measures of performance, including customer satisfaction and financial indicators.

The situation analysis also should define the present. A common method for conducting the situation analysis is to evaluate the internal strengths and weakness of the organization and the external opportunities and threats to the organization. This is known as a *SWOT (Strength, Weaknesses, Opportunities, Threats) analysis.* Categories of internal strengths and weaknesses to consider may include profitability, quality of pharmacy service, customer service, competence and ability of pharmacy staff, and the efficiency of the pharmacy operations. Categories of external opportunities and threats to consider may include the extent of competition from other pharmacy organizations, the availability of technology, regulations that may help or hinder the business, availability of reimbursement for services provided (i.e., clinical or cognitive pharmacy services), costs incurred by the pharmacy organization, political issues having an impact on health delivery, and changes in the market and types of customers served by the organization.

By comparing the results of the situation analysis with the desired future state (vision), the extent and nature of the gap between the two begins to become clear. The next steps in the planning phase attempt to bridge that gap. First, strategic planning serves to define goals for the organization that are consistent with the vision. These goals should also capitalize on the organization's strengths and opportunities while minimizing the threats and mitigating the weaknesses.

The last part of the planning process deals with organizing to *operationalize* the strategy. Because the goals and vision are a desired future state that may be unachievable in the short term, intermediate objectives are needed to help advance toward that target. In the planning process, the objectives pertinent to each goal are identified and usually are accomplishable in the short term (1 year), whereas goals are in the longer term (3 to 5 years). Because objectives are short term, a budget, schedule, and responsibility can be assigned to each.

There is no common or standard way to organize the written strategic plan. However, most contain the following key elements: (1) the organization's vision, (2) strategies, (3) goals for each strategy, (4) objectives required to meet those goals, and (5) tasks or action plans to compete the objectives. Examples of strategic plans for pharmacy organizations can be found in the references listed at the end of this chapter, and Table 3-3 is an excerpt from one of those references (Hutchinson, Witte, and Vogel, 1989). The original strategic plan published by these authors included eight major strategies with multiple goals for each. Note that the tasks listed also should include a planned date for completion of the task and a party responsible for each task.

Postplanning Phase

Once the major pieces of the planning phase have been developed, the *postplanning phase* begins. This phase includes three vitally important steps: (1) communicating the plan, (2) implementing the plan, and (3) monitoring progress once the plan is implemented.

While strategic planning is a process, the strategic plan is a document that communicates the plan. The strategic plan should be written such that it communicates all aspects of the plan effectively.

The actual implementation of the strategic plan requires managers and executives of the pharmacy organization to understand the long-range goals while at the same time determining and taking the steps necessary to accomplish the shorter-range objectives. The process of mapping out the actions necessary to accomplish short-term objectives is called *operational planning,* which focuses on determining the day-to-day activities that are necessary to achieve the long-term goals of the organization. One can differentiate strategic planning from operational planning by viewing the primary focus of each. Strategic planning focuses on doing the right thing (effectiveness), whereas operational planning focuses on doing things right (effi-

Table 3-3. Example Strategic Plan
Strategy: The department will achieve an organized approach to cost containment and cost reduction.
Goal: Develop an ongoing workload-monitoring system based on a system of pharmacy service units.
Objectives:
• To develop a workload-monitoring system that identifies distributive and clinical workload by satellite area
• To use the workload statistics to predict staffing needs
• To evaluate overuse and underuse of staff based on the need for the activities performed
Tasks/action plans:
• Determine what distributive and clinical indicators will be used
• Develop a method for collecting the workload statistics
• Collect hours worked by staff category and satellite area
• Develop a monthly productivity report by area
• Analyze staffing patterns in comparison with workload statistics

Source: Adapted from Hutchinson, Witte, and Vogel, 1989, with permission from publisher.

ciency). In other words, strategic planning defines what to do, and operational planning defines how to do it.

The operational plan is an outline of the tactical activities or tasks that must occur to support and implement the strategic plan—sometimes called *tactics.* The relationship between tasks or tactics (operational planning) and the key elements of strategic planning is shown in Fig. 3-1. Managers in an organization focus their day-to-day work on tactics. Their perspective, therefore, tends to relate to the short term. Yet it is important that, on a periodic basis, an attempt be made to step back from day-to-day activities and reorient oneself to the bigger picture (the vision, goals, and strategy of the organization). For example, a pharmacy manager may receive a request from a physician or a nurse to have the department begin to provide a new service in a hospital. Before agreeing to do so, it is important that the manager consider how this new service fits into the vision and goals of the pharmacy department.

Another key element of the postplanning phase is *monitoring*. A plan for monitoring should be created. This monitoring should evaluate the extent of implementation in comparison with the planned schedule. Monitoring should also evaluate the effectiveness of the organization in meeting its objectives and ultimately its goals, especially in the deployment of limited resources, both human and financial. In other words, have both the plan and its implementation been effective? Intrinsic to this monitoring process is the possibility that changes to the plan may be necessitated by changes in the environment or by changes in the organization. As such, the strategic plan should be considered a fluid document.

STRATEGIC PLANNING EXAMPLES IN PHARMACY ORGANIZATIONS

There are plenty of published examples and descriptions of strategic planning in pharmacy organizations, although a majority come from the hospital practice setting (Anderson, 1986; Birdwell and Pathak, 1989; Guerrero, Nickman, Bair, 1990; Harrison, 2005, 2006; Harrison and Bootman, 1994; Harrison and Ormeier, 1996; Hutchinson, Witte, Vogel, 1989; Kelly, 1986; Linggi and Pelham, 1986; Newberg and Banville, 1989; Portner et al., 1996; Shane and Gouveia, 2000). For chain drug stores, independent pharmacies, or other for-profit pharmacy organizations, it would be counterproductive to publish, and thus make available to competitors, the company strategy and objectives. Rather, these plans frequently are guarded fiercely so that they do not fall into the hands of competitors. Nevertheless, there are some general publications designed to assist community pharmacies in strategic planning (Hagel, 2002).

A survey of 1,500 randomly selected community pharmacies published in 1996 found that only a small proportion (30.8 percent) of respondents re-

Table 3-4. Steps Used in the Strategic Planning Process by Community Pharmacies

Step	Percentage*
Develop mission statement	76.9
Identify strengths and weaknesses	94.2
Identify threats and opportunities	90.2
Formulate and select strategies	83.8
Review pharmacy structure and systems	60.1
Implement strategies	86.1
Evaluate implemented strategies	76.3

*N = 173 community pharmacies that reported use of strategic planning; values represent the percentage that incorporate each specific step of the strategic planning process.
Source: Adapted from Harrison and Ortmeier, 1996, with permission from the publisher.

ported having conducted strategic planning in their pharmacies (Harrison and Ormeier, 1996). For those that did conduct strategic planning, an average of 5.9 (of 7) different steps in the strategic planning process were used, and 45.7 percent incorporated all seven steps (Table 3-4). The authors also reported that community pharmacies that conducted strategic planning had significantly higher self-rated performance on clinical services, dispensing services, and financial performance—suggesting that strategic planning can improve organization success. In 2005, an update of the survey showed little change. As in the previous survey, increased use of strategic planning was associated with improved organizational performance (Harrison, 2005, 2006).

A similar study conducted in the hospital pharmacy environment found that 63 percent of respondents (hospital pharmacy directors) conducted strategic planning in their pharmacies and followed 4.7 (of 6) steps in the strategic planning process. This supported the belief that strategic planning within hospital pharmacies is more commonplace than previously thought (Harrison and Bootman, 1994). In the hospital environment, many published descriptions of strategic planning activities have focused specifically on planning for clinical pharmacy services (Anderson, 1986; Kelly, 1986; Linggi and Pelham, 1986).

Strategic planning, when used by hospital pharmacy departments, appears to have positive results. A study was conducted of pharmacy directors at hospitals in the United States to determine if more sophisticated planning resulted in improved departmental outcomes (Birdwell and Pathak, 1989). Pharmacy departments were categorized into levels of strategic planning sophistication based on different steps in that were employed the planning process. In departments with high levels of planning, outcomes such as satisfaction by hospital administrators, professional image among hospital administrators, number of clinical pharmacy programs, and the quality of clinical pharmacy programs were rated higher by pharmacy directors than in departments with lower levels of sophistication in planning. In other industries, strategic planning also has been shown to improve company performance and has yielded positive results (Hodges and Kent, 2006–2007).

Consistent with these findings was another study that described the impact of strategic planning conducted in the Department of Veterans Affairs Medical Center pharmacies. Strategic planning resulted in more Veterans Affairs Medical Centers with increased pharmacist involvement in patient care, increased involvement in specific types of clinical services, more efficient drug distribution systems, and increased involvement in pharmacy education (Portner et al., 1996).

Strategic planning in pharmacy is particularly important when there are changes that occur in the practice environment. The Medicare Modernization Act (MMA) of 2003 is a good example of such a change. This legislation, which went into effect in 2006, created the Medicare prescription drug benefit (also known as Medicare Part D) and established the requirement that medication therapy management (MTM) be provided to high-risk Medicare beneficiaries (see Chapter 17). Successful pharmacy organizations used strategic planning to predict the impact of the MMA and to develop practice plans for provision of MTM (Lewin Group, 2005). Another example of change in the pharmacy practice environment is the increased emphasis on

medication errors promoted by the Joint Commission, the body responsible for accrediting hospitals and other health care organizations. By monitoring the literature, successful hospital pharmacy departments were able to predict this movement and then developed and implemented plans to establish the technologic and human resources necessary to improve patient safety (Shane and Gouveia, 2000).

■ BARRIERS AND LIMITATIONS TO PLANNING

Effective planning requires a serious commitment of time and resources. For a variety of reasons, organizations may not be successful in their planning efforts. Lack of success may stem from failure to recognize and minimize common barriers to planning efforts or failure to understand inherent limitations in planning.

Barriers

Organizations must overcome several barriers to ensure a successful strategic planning process, as shown in Table 3-5. The most serious barrier is lack of endorsement by the top executive(s). Buy-in and participation by top corporate executives and the board of directors are

Table 3-5. Barriers to Effective Planning

1. Failure to commit sufficient time to the planning effort
2. Interpersonal issues such as struggles over power or politics and individual or group resistance to change
3. Lack of planning skills
4. Failure to plan far enough into the future
5. Constantly changing environment
6. Failure to implement owing to lack of time or lack of resources
7. Failure to monitor progress
8. Lack of support of top executive and/or board of directors

critical to strategic planning. Without these, the whole planning effort could be a waste of time and resources.

A frequent barrier to effective planning is failure to commit sufficient time to the planning process. Good planning requires significant management and staff time. Ideally, some of the more creative aspects of planning should be accomplished during uninterrupted time. Pharmacy organizations commonly hold retreats, where those involved in the planning process meet in a location outside the usual work environment. The time and expense associated with such events require a huge commitment on the part of both the organization and the personnel involved.

Sometimes interpersonal issues, such as organizational culture or struggles for power and politics, become barriers to effective planning. Individuals who are involved in planning or implementation may be resistant to change (for a variety of reasons) and thus consciously or subconsciously sabotage the planning effort. Likewise, if the organization or personnel lack the skills necessary to conduct planning, the results may be less than optimal and even harmful to the organization. In the same context, failure to plan far enough into the future can be problematic, especially for certain types of planning. Strategic planning in particular is intended to guide the organization over the long term.

The environment also can pose a barrier to effective planning. In an environment such as health care, where things are changing constantly or are ambiguous, effective planning is more difficult and uncertain. For example, consider all the changes that may affect pharmacy organizations that make planning for the future difficult. These include changes in technology and automation, new drugs and therapies, changes in payment rates of prescriptions and availability of reimbursement for clinical pharmacy services, changes in regulations, and fluctuations in the labor market for pharmacists.

Organizations operating in rapidly changing environments may put off or avoid planning altogether. Unfortunately, failure to plan, even when it is difficult, may be even more detrimental in the long term.

Another barrier to the planning effort is failure to communicate the plan effectively to the employees of the pharmacy organization. Written plans must be drafted in such a way that the messages are communicated clearly to the appropriate audience. Plan documents sometimes have the tendency to use jargon or terminology, so-called plan-speak, that is not consistent with that which would be most beneficial to clear and accurate interpretation by the audience. Besides the written document, verbal presentations and other forms of communication are often important.

The most common barrier to effective planning is failure to implement, so-called analysis but no action. Three causes of failure to implement plans include the unavailability of resources, lack of time, and failure to monitor or measure progress. Implementation of strategy often involves the mobilization of resources. If organizations do not have the necessary resources or are unwilling to commit those resources, then implementation will be jeopardized. In today's ever-increasing speed of business, managers often cannot find the time to use adequately the results of planning already conducted to guide their daily activities. The term *management by crisis* is used often to describe the modus operandi of busy managers, meaning that their work is directed more by the problems they face at the immediate moment than by any careful consideration of the actual goals of the organization. In the long term, this may result in failure of the company to meet its goals (Martin, 2002). Finally, the failure to monitor, for whatever reason, the progress made toward goals developed in the planning process can be a significant barrier to success of the planning effort.

Limitations

Besides the barriers to planning just listed, certain limitations to planning must also be acknowledged. Managers often are caught up in the notion that planning is a magic bullet for the ills of an organization. They must acknowledge the fact that planning is no cure-all.

First, planning is, to some degree, guesswork (but educated and experienced guesswork, hopefully). While decisions are based on evidence available about the past and the likelihood of events in the future, risk is still involved. Nothing is certain. Even with good data and good strategy, negative things may happen that were unpredictable and thus unavoidable.

Second, plans and predictions are only as good as the data and information that go into them. Poor data will result in poor strategy. What pharmacy organizations get out of the planning activity will be correlated directly with the degree of effort, creativity, time, and resources they put into it. Organizations that adopt boilerplate or "cookie cutter" approaches to planning most likely will fail.

Two additional limitations of planning deal with how an organization implements the plan. Planning is not a substitute for action. Organizations that are all about planning but neglect to take the actions dictated will not be successful. To the opposite extreme, the plan should not be considered as static or unyielding. Planning should be a continuous process, and plans should change as the environment dictates. To follow a plan blindly without consideration of changes in the environment that may make the plan obsolete is foolhardy.

CONCLUSION

The scenario of Ted Thompson that began this chapter illustrates how knowledge of planning-related concepts may be applicable to the work activities of a recent pharmacy graduate. Knowledge of concepts in the chapter should better position Ted to participate in the strategic planning initiative being organized by the DOP. Ted should now clearly appreciate the importance of this type of planning to the future of the hospital and to the pharmacy department. Ted should also be able to anticipate the process that might be followed. Ted also should anticipate certain questions that will need to be addressed in the planning process. For example, given the pharmacy described in the scenario, what might be a suitable vision for the department? What goals and objectives might the department establish during its strategic planning exercise?

The concepts discussed in this chapter become only more important as one advances through a career and assumes higher levels of leadership and responsibility in a pharmacy or health care organization. It is also important for students and new practition-

ers to understand the process involved in establishing and maintaining the viability of the organization for which they work. A good understanding of management concepts, and planning in particular, will allow the pharmacy practitioner to better appreciate the context from which management operates. This will then better enable pharmacy practitioners to have input into and be able to influence the direction and decisions of a pharmacy organization.

QUESTIONS FOR FURTHER DISCUSSION

1. Select a specific pharmacy practice setting (i.e., hospital practice, community practice, or managed care). What barriers do you believe would limit the ability of pharmacists and pharmacy managers to conduct effective planning in that setting?
2. Write a vision statement for a hypothetical pharmacy organization. Explain how you selected the language and message of the statement.
3. Conduct an Internet search of vision and mission statements of health care organizations. Identify and compare the statements from at least three different organizations. What are the strengths and weakness of these statements?
4. Describe changes that have occurred in the practice of pharmacy over the past 20 years. How would strategic planning have enabled a pharmacy organization to better position itself for those changes?

REFERENCES

Anderson RW. 1986. Strategic planning for clinical services: The University of Texas M.D. Anderson Hospital and Tumor Institute. *Am J Hosp Pharm* 43:2169.

Birdwell SW, Pathak DS. 1989. Use of the strategic-planning process by hospital pharmacy directors. *Am J Hosp Pharm* 46:1361.

Breen L, Crawford H. 2005. Improving the pharmaceutical supply chain: Assessing the reality of e-quality through e-commerce application in hospital pharmacy. *Int J Qual Reliab Manag* 22:572.

Coke A. 2001. *Seven Steps to a Successful Business Plan.* New York: American Management Association.

Guerrero RM, Nickman NA, Bair JN. 1990. Using pharmacists' perceptions in planning changes in pharmacy practice. *Am J Hosp Pharm* 47:2026.

Hagel HP. 2002. Planning for patient care. In Hagel HP, Rovers JP (eds), *Managing the Patient-Centered Pharmacy.* Washington, DC: American Pharmaceutical Association.

Harrison DL. 2006. Effect of attitudes and perceptions of independent community pharmacy owners/managers on the comprehensiveness of strategic planning. *J Am Pharm Assoc* 46:459–64.

Harrison DL. 2005. Strategic planning by independent community pharmacies. *J Am Pharm Assoc* 45:726–33.

Harrison DL, Bootman JL. 1994. Strategic planning by institutional pharmacy administrators. *J Pharm Market Manag* 8:73.

Harrison DL, Ortmeier BG. 1996. Strategic planning in the community pharmacy. *J Am Pharm Assoc* NS36:583.

Hodges H, Kent T. 2006–2007. Impact of planning and control sophistication in small business. *J Small Bus Strat* 17:75.

Hutchinson RA, Witte KW, Vogel DP. 1989. Development and implementation of a strategic-planning process at a university hospital. *Am J Hosp Pharm* 46:952.

Kelly WN. 1986. Strategic planning for clinical services: Hamot Medical Center. *Am J Hosp Pharm* 43:2159.

Koteen J. 1997. *Strategic Management in Public and Nonprofit Organizations,* 2d ed. Westport CT: Praeger.

Lewin Group. 2005. Medication therapy management services: A critical review. *J Am Pharm Assoc* 45:580–7.

Linggi A, Pelham LD. 1986. Strategic planning for clinical services: St Joseph Hospital and Health Care Center. *Am J Hosp Pharm* 43:2164.

Martin C. 2002. *Managing for the Short Term: The New Rules for Running a Business in a Day-to-Day World.* New York: Doubleday.

Newberg DF, Banville RL. 1989. Strategic planning for pharmacy services in a community hospital. *Am J Hosp Pharm* 46:1819.

Porter ME. 1980. *Competitive Strategy: Techniques for Analyzing Industries and Competitors.* New York: Free Press.

Porter ME. 1985. *Competitive Advantage: Creating and Sustaining Superior Performance.* New York: Free Press.

Portner TS, Srnka QM, Gourley DR, et al. 1996. Comparison of Department of Veterans Affairs pharmacy services in 1992 and 1994 with strategic-planning goals. *Am J Health-Syst Pharm* 53:1032.

Shane R, Gouveia WA. 2000. Developing a strategic plan for quality in pharmacy practice. *Am J Health-Syst Pharm* 57:470–4.

Smith JE. 1989. Integrating human resources and program-planning strategies. *Am J Hosp Pharm* 46:1153.

Steiner GA, Miner JB, Gray ER. 1982. *Management Policy and Strategy.* New York: Macmillian.

Stoner JAF, Freeman RE, Gilbert DR. 1995. *Management,* 6th ed. Englewood Cliffs, NJ: Prentice-Hall.

Thompson AA, Strickland AJ. 1983. *Strategy Formulation and Implementation: Tasks of the General Manager.* Plano, TX: Business Publications.

Wong G, Keller U. 1997. Information technology (IT) outsourcing: An alternative to re-engineer your IT. In Berndt R (ed), *Business Reengineering.* Heidelberg: Springer-Verlag.

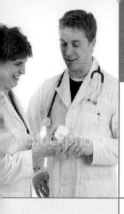

4

BUSINESS PLANNING FOR PHARMACY PROGRAMS

Glen T. Schumock and Godwin Wong

About the Authors: Dr. Schumock is a graduate of Washington State University (B.Pharm.), the University of Washington (Pharm.D.), and the University of Illinois at Chicago (MBA). He also completed a residency and a research fellowship. Currently, Dr. Schumock is Director of the Center for Pharmacoeconomic Research and Associate Professor in the Department of Pharmacy Practice at the University of Illinois at Chicago. Dr. Schumock teaches courses on pharmacy management, pharmacoeconomics, and business planning for pharmacy services. Dr. Schumock has published over 100 articles, book chapters, and books. He is on the editorial boards of the journals *Pharmacotherapy* and *PharmacoEconomics*. Dr. Schumock is a board-certified pharmacotherapy specialist and is a Fellow in the American College of Clinical Pharmacy.

Dr. Wong has been on the faculty of the Haas School of Business at the University of California, Berkeley, for 20 years. His areas of interests are corporate strategic planning, entrepreneurship, information technology management, and venture capital. He has conducted leadership and strategic planning workshops for various health care groups, hospital administrators, and pharmaceutical companies and has lectured to executives in 20 countries. He has served on the boards of directors of several California banks, Silicon Valley companies, and international corporations. He received a B.S. from the University of Wisconsin, an M.S. from UCLA, and a Ph.D. from Harvard University.

▪ LEARNING OBJECTIVES

After completing this chapter, students should be able to

1. Describe the purpose of business plan planning.
2. Discuss the important components of a business plan.
3. Review important aspects of communicating and implementing a business plan.
4. Highlight examples of business plan planning within pharmacy organizations.

■ SCENARIO

The scenario begun in Chapter 3 continues here. In brief, Ted Thompson is a clinical pharmacist at a medium-sized community hospital. Ted has just finished participating in the process of developing a strategic plan for the pharmacy department. Included in the 5-year plan is a goal for the department to develop successful clinical pharmacy service programs and, where possible, to generate revenue from those programs.

After his first year at the hospital, Ted has formulated several ideas for new clinical pharmacy services that the department could offer that might generate revenue. During his annual performance evaluation, he discusses these ideas with his boss, the director of pharmacy (DOP). The DOP is happy that Ted has come forward with his ideas and encourages him to investigate these options further. One idea that is of particular interest is to develop a service or business to provide "consultant pharmacy services" to area nursing homes.

As a clinical pharmacist serving the general medicine area of the hospital, Ted has developed a high level of interest and expertise in the care of the elderly. His duties often involve contacts with area nursing homes, especially when patients are discharged to these facilities and when there are issues with continuity of drug therapy. Because of this, and because of his concern for patients, Ted has developed a good reputation with the physicians and nursing staff not only in the hospital but also within area nursing homes. Ted tells the DOP that during his contacts with these homes, he has heard that most are unhappy with the quality of the medication reviews currently provided by an outside consultant pharmacist. They have asked repeatedly if he or the hospital would consider providing these services.

The DOP indicates that he thinks that the consultant pharmacy service idea is a good one. He suggests that Ted develop a "business plan." Ted has heard of the term *business plan* before but really does not know what it entails. However, he is willing and prepared to learn and to do whatever is necessary to accomplish the proposed idea.

■ CHAPTER QUESTIONS

1. What is the primary objective of business planning in the pharmacy environment?
2. What are the important components of a business plan of a proposed clinical pharmacy service?
3. What are the principal factors to include in an analysis of the potential financial performance of a proposed new program?
4. For whom is a business plan written?

■ INTRODUCTION

Chapter 3 discussed general concepts of planning by pharmacy organizations and reviewed a specific type of planning—strategic planning. This chapter discusses another key type of planning that is used by pharmacy organizations. The distinguishing characteristic of *business planning* is that it focuses on a specific program or business within the organization. Here the term *business* is used synonymously with *program*. For example, in a pharmacy organization, the business or program may be a new clinical service. In a large corporation, such as a chain pharmacy, the business or program may be a drive-through prescription service or a disease management program in selected stores. Business planning also can be used for startup companies, where the proposed program or business comprises the totality of the organization.

The purpose of business planning is to provide data and proposed actions necessary to answer a business question, usually in the form, "Should we invest in the proposed business?" As this question illustrates, business planning is used most commonly when an organization wishes to project the future risks and benefits of a proposed new business venture. For example, in the scenario faced by Ted, the business question relates to the proposed new program that will provide consultant pharmacy services to nursing homes. However, business planning also may be used to make decisions about expanding or terminating an existing program.[1]

---

[1] Here it may be useful to distinguish the terms *business Plan, business planning,* and *business plan planning.* Business plan

As with strategic planning, the process of business planning produces a written plan. A key point to clarify here is that the business plan needs to be written with the "audience" in mind. If the decision maker is the chief executive officer (CEO) and/or chief financial officer (CFO), then the plan should be written so that it is applicable to and appropriate for that audience. Business plans that do not consider the audience are less likely to be acted on favorably. A common mistake by authors of business plans (including pharmacists) is to write in a manner that is too technical or detailed, thus failing to hold the attention of executives, who might be the decision makers.

This chapter will discuss practical issues in the development of a pharmacy-related business plan. Because business planning is an activity that is commonly employed by organizations of all sizes, there are ample resources on this topic. Some excellent general guides to business planning are listed in the reference section of this chapter (Bangs, 1998; Cohen, 2001; Coke, 2001; O'Hara, 1995; Pinson and Jinnet, 1999). There are also several references specific to business planning in pharmacy organizations (Hagel, 2002; Phillips and Larson, 2002; Schneller, Powell, and Solomon, 1998; Schumock, Stubbings, and McBride, 2004; Tipton, 2001). A more detailed, workbook-style resource for business planning for clinical pharmacy services is also available and may be especially useful to those who are in the position of developing an actual business plan (Schumock and Stubbings, 2007).

◼ THE BUSINESS CONCEPT

The practice of pharmacy is a unique combination of the provision of patient care and the running of a business, and there are many opportunities for pharmacists to create new and innovative services that both fulfill

---

planning culminates in the development of a business plan and is the primary topic of this chapter. Business planning encompasses not only the development of the business plan but also the ongoing monitoring and review of the success of a program.

patient needs and generate profits. Pharmacists should not lose the "entrepreneurial" spirit that is necessary to promote and nurture pharmacy business and that has driven many of the advances in the profession. Business planning is a means by which pharmacists can do this.

The place to start with any new business idea is to conduct a preliminary evaluation. This is called *exploring the business concept.* The purpose of this preliminary exploration is to determine if the idea merits the development of a complete business plan. As with other planning processes, business planning is a not a trivial undertaking. For this reason, it is advisable to be sure that the concept is one that is reasonable prior to investing time and energy into developing the business plan.

The preliminary evaluation usually begins with a literature search. Literature searches yield the best results when conducted using electronic databases such as that of the National Library of Medicine, which can be searched using PubMed. Other databases and search engines are also available in most medical libraries. Search terms should be consistent with the area of interest. For example, to identify articles that describe consultant pharmacy services in nursing homes, Ted (from the scenario) might use the following search terms: *clinical pharmacy, consultant pharmacy, pharmacy services, nursing homes,* and *long-term care.* Literature searches can be made more specific by limiting the search to certain date ranges, types of articles (i.e., reviews or descriptive reports), or specific journals of publication (i.e., pharmacy journals), if appropriate.

Another way to identify primary literature of interest is to obtain systematic literature reviews that have been published. These reviews usually provide extensive citations and may categorize articles based on types of pharmacy services or other classifications that are of interest. A number of very comprehensive reviews have been published and are included in the reference list of this chapter (Hatoum and Akhras, 1993; Hatoum et al., 1986; Plumridge and Wojnar-Horton, 1998; Schumock et al., 1996, 2003; Willett et al., 1989).

A further source of information is the Internet. Using the search terms listed earlier, it is possible to identify additional resources pertinent to the subject of interest. For example, by typing *consultant pharmacy services* into a search engine such as Google, Ted will identify the Web site of the American Society of Consultant Pharmacists (ASCP), which will lead to a host of resources available on this topic. However, as most experienced Web users will recognize, Internet searches can produce an inordinate amount of "noise" in the form of unrelated sites or references and, from that standpoint, may be inefficient. Some Web sites will have links to other related sites that are very helpful.

One Web site that may be particularly useful for gaining access to information on many different types of clinical pharmacy services is maintained by the Center for Pharmacoeconomic Research at the University of Illinois at Chicago College of Pharmacy. The site is called *VClinRx,* short for "The Value of Clinical Pharmacy Services," and it is a searchable database of literature on clinical pharmacy services. It can be accessed at http://www.uic.edu/pharmacy/centers/pharmacoeconomic_research/.

Primary and secondary literature identified in these searches can provide a variety of information to assist in exploring the business concept. First, some publications will serve primarily to describe the experiences of others in providing the program or service. Other publications may provide an actual evaluation of the program or service. For example, an article may evaluate the impact of the service on the health outcomes of patients or may provide evidence of the financial impact of the program. Obviously, this type of information will be extremely valuable to anyone proposing to implement similar services. In fact, part of the process of exploring the business concept may include the generalization of results found in the literature. For example, it is possible to combine the results of published studies and estimate the clinical and economic outcomes that may be expected if the service were to be implemented in a different setting (Schumock, 2000; Schumock and Butler, 2003; Schumock, Michaud, and Guenette, 1999). Resources are also available for developing and establishing certain types of pharmacy services (American College of Clinical Pharmacy, 1994; Cooper, Saxton, and Cameron, 2004).

Besides gaining experience from literature, exploration of the business concept should consider the size and receptivity of potential customers of the service. A preliminary analysis of the demand that may exist for the service should be conducted. This should include a clear description of the need for the service and the number of potential customers that may exist in the market. Information about the market can come from a variety of sources. Demographic data related to trends in the population in the community usually are available from county or city Web sites or from the U.S. Census Bureau. Local, state, and federal public health agencies will be able to provide information on disease patterns and statistics. Information can even be gathered from existing or potential customers by conducting interviews or surveys. Consulting companies also may be available to assist in assessing the market for the proposed program.

Once information on the market is obtained, it then can be used to consider the revenue that may be generated by the program. It should be noted that some programs will not generate revenue; rather, they may reduce costs—which can be equally important. Further, while most programs are required to provide a financial benefit, in some cases other, nonquantifiable benefits may be considered of equal or greater importance (i.e., clinical benefits).

Given that the proposed program appears to have a potential market and that it may create a financial benefit (or some other form of benefit) for the organization, the remaining issue is the ability of the program to address a specific goal(s) in the organization's strategic plan. For example, if a hospital's strategic plan includes a goal of expanding vertically into related health care markets, such as long-term care, then the pharmacy's proposal to initiate a consultant pharmacy service would be consistent with and supportive of that goal.

Having conducted the preliminary exploration of the business concept, it is probably prudent to seek the advice of others before moving forward with the complete business planning process. Here, Ted may consider discussing the idea with key stakeholders in the organization, including the individual or individuals who will make the ultimate decision to more forward with the concept. For example, Ted should broach the idea of the consultant pharmacy service proposed in the scenario with senior executives in the hospital, such as the CEO and CFO. Ted may also wish to get input from key stakeholders in the local nursing homes, such as the physician medical directors, nursing directors, and administrators of those facilities. If the reception to the concept is positive, the development of a complete business plan can begin.

STEPS IN THE DEVELOPMENT OF A BUSINESS PLAN

The process of business planning is similar to other types of planning and, as such, is consistent with the general steps discussed in Chapter 3. This section describes the usual steps taken in the business planning process.

Define the Business or Program

As with other types of planning, the initial step of business planning is to define the business or service proposed. After exploring the business concept (see above), Ted likely already will have developed a clear idea of the business proposal. To formalize a definition of the business, he should develop a specific statement of the purpose of the program. This statement is also called a *mission statement* and was discussed in Chapter 3. The mission will crystallize the aims of the program and help to steer the direction taken in other steps of the planning process.

Conduct Market Research and Analysis

The next steps in business planning (evaluating the market, evaluating competitors, and assessing clinical and quality requirements) are part of the situation analysis described in the general planning process (see Chapter 3). The term *market* refers to the customers of the program. An analysis of the potential customers of the business is clearly an important exercise, and this can be done in a number of ways. First, the market can be described geographically. For example, the organization may collect data that would give projections of the number of customers in different local regions. In

the scenario, Ted would want to identify the different nursing homes in the region surrounding his hospital. For each nursing home, he will also want to identify the number of patients, the types of patients, and the different characteristics of each facility. These homes and the patients within them will comprise the potential market for the service.

In addition to the information on area nursing homes, Ted should also be interested in demographics of the population in the region. Ted will want to know the number and percentage of elderly people in the region and the trends with respect to the age of the population. If he finds that the people in area are growing older or that older people are moving into the area, then this would bode well for the proposed business.

It is important to note that the term *customers* is not always synonymous with *patients* when speaking of health care programs. In particular, the customers of pharmacy programs may be something or someone other than patients. In many cases, the customers of pharmacy programs are physicians or other health care professionals. In the scenario, the customers are actually the individual nursing homes because the proposed service would be paid for by the homes. In analyzing the market, Ted should identify the segment of the market to which the program or business is most apt to appeal. This is commonly known as the *target market*. The target market may be based on a special market niche that the program fulfills and/or a special customer need.

Conduct Competitor Analysis

A key component of analyzing the external environment is to identify and gauge potential competitors. The goal of the competitor analysis is to understand the characteristics of other providers so that the business can be positioned favorably compared with competitors. Data about competitors sometimes are difficult to obtain. Surveys of customers, price comparisons, and publicly available information (i.e., Web sites) should be investigated.

A comparison should be made of the characteristics and market share of each competitor with those of the proposed program. Characteristics such as years in business, number of customers, percentage of the market (i.e., market share), and product or service niche should be compared. The strengths and weaknesses of each competitor should also be reviewed and compared with those of the proposed business. Categories of strengths and weakness to consider include service quality, staff competence and credentials, customer service, customer access, price, technology or innovation, and delivery mechanisms.

In health care, our definition of *competitors* sometimes has to be broadened beyond that which is most obvious. For example, in the hospital environment, a new pharmacy program actually may compete with other professions within the hospital. Many of the advanced clinical services that pharmacists provide replace functions of other health care professionals, especially physicians. This is true even in the outpatient environment. For example, a pharmacy-run immunization clinic may compete with physician offices that also administer vaccines.

In the case of the proposed consultant pharmacy service (scenario), Ted should consider as competitors any other organizations that provide the same service (consultant pharmacy service). In the nursing home environment, local retail pharmacies or large regional or national long-term care pharmacies that provide medications to nursing homes may also provide consultant pharmacy services. In some cases, individual pharmacists provide these services to one or two homes on an independent consultant basis.

Assess Clinical and Quality Requirements

The health care market more than most others is highly regulated. Clearly, anyone proposing a new business in a regulated environment must be aware of these regulations and have a plan to comply with them. Thus part of the business planning process is to analyze applicable regulations and requirements. This analysis should extend beyond just the mandatory legal rules or requirements. It should include voluntary standards, such as those endorsed by professional organizations and societies; it also should include standards of accrediting bodies and any other guidelines or expectations with respect to the service proposed. Obviously, pharmacy is not immune to regulations. On the legal side, there are federal, state, and city/county ordinances, laws,

statutes, and regulations that must be followed when applicable.

In the proposed consultant pharmacy service (scenario), there are many different sources of regulatory guidelines. First, regulations of the Centers for Medicare and Medicaid Services (CMS) require that long-term care facilities employ consultant pharmacy services in order to be eligible for Medicare reimbursement. Clearly, this and similar state regulations should be reviewed. Because the practice of pharmacy is regulated primarily at the state level, the state pharmacy practice act must be complied with. Some states provide regulations that specifically deal with consultant pharmacy services in nursing homes, whereas others address the nondispensing services of pharmacists more generally. Last, the ASCP provides guidelines and other resource materials (i.e., practice standards or guidelines) to it members (Cooper, Saxton, Cameron, 2004).

Assessing clinical and quality requirements of the proposed program also means planning for how to comply with these standards. Compliance should be considered both on an initial basis and over the long term. Clinical and quality requirements may necessitate the hiring of certain (qualified) staff, the development of work processes to monitor quality, and the implementation of technology or procedures to ensure compliance.

Define Processes and Operations

The business planning process shifts from the initial situation analysis to more of a projection and goal-setting approach in the next four steps. Defining the details associated with the planned operations of the business is the first of these steps. This step includes planning of the optimal organizational structure (with a link to the larger organization), the staffing levels, personnel requirements, and the reporting relationships of the program. Personnel job titles, job descriptions, and the number of full-time equivalents[2] (FTEs) needed in each position should be determined.

---

[2] A *full-time equivalent* (FTE) is a value used to measure the actual or budgeted work hours in an organization. One FTE is equal to 2080 hours per year (or 40 hours per week,

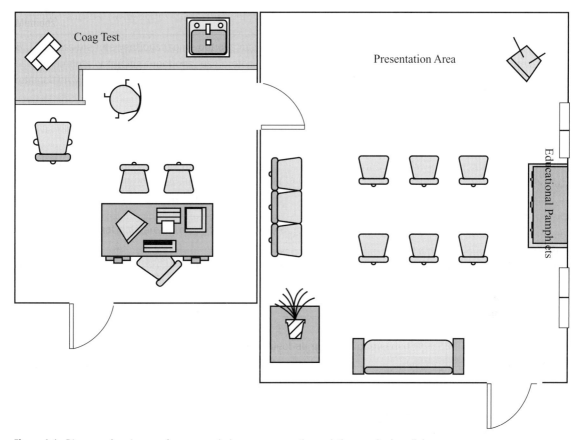

Figure 4-1. Diagram of work area of a proposed pharmacy-run anticoagulation monitoring clinic.

Planning should also elicit the physical structure, equipment, and resources required to operate the program. This includes planning for the types of equipment, physical layout, furniture, and information systems. Last, the work processes should be planned. This can be done using flowcharts and other tools to design the customer interface and delivery of the proposed service. Diagrams can be used to show workflow within a space, if appropriate; an example of a workspace for a pharmacy-run anticoagulation monitoring clinic is shown in Fig. 4-1. The planned operations should be

sufficient to determine the workload capacities of the program. From this, strategies should be devised to deal with extremes in demand (either insufficient or excess workload).

Planning of the processes and operations helps to clarify the practical, day-to-day activities that will occur in the program. This type of planning provides critical information needed in later steps of the business planning process (i.e., for development of financial projections).

In the consultant pharmacy proposal, planning of processes and operations will include estimation of the number and types of pharmacists (or other staff) that will be needed to provide the proposed services. Ted will also need to determine the job requirements (i.e., must have completed a geriatrics certificate program)

---

52 weeks per year). Part-time employees are counted as less than a full FTE. For example, an employee who works 20 hours per week is equal to 0.5 FTE.

and have a rough idea of the job descriptions for each position. With respect to the organizational structure, he will need to determine to whom the consultant pharmacist(s) should report and where within the hospital pharmacy department organizational structure this business will reside. The work processes of the consultant pharmacists will need to be defined, along with any work aids that may be required in this process (i.e., electronic drug information or documentation systems). Important policies or procedures that govern the activities and decision making of the program and staff also should be determined. Methods for communication between the consultant pharmacist(s) and the nursing home personnel (i.e., physicians, nurses, and administrators) should be defined. This planning process should also include identification of a system for workload monitoring and for billing the nursing homes for the services provided. Many other details of the operation also will need to be developed in this planning process.

Develop a Marketing Strategy

The second of the goal-setting steps is to define a marketing strategy. The marketing strategy should be based on information gathered in the previous steps of the business planning process, especially the market and competitor analyses. The marketing strategy should identify the target market for the program and develop a plan for gaining the business of that market. This plan should include the means of communicating to customers and the message that should be communicated to them. The strategy for a new business should be separated into the initial marketing plan and the ongoing marketing plan. The initial marketing plan defines the promotional activities and market goals for the period directly before and immediately after implementation of the new program. The ongoing marketing plan defines the promotional and market goals over the longer term. Resources are available to assist in the development of pharmacy-related marketing plans (Doucette and McDonough, 2002; Holdford, 2003).

The marketing strategy for the consultant pharmacy service (scenario) largely will depend on the current status of such services in area nursing homes. It is likely that the market comprises all the nursing homes in a limited geographic region surrounding the hospital. However, it may be Ted's wish to target the service only to the largest homes (i.e., those over 500 beds) or to those with the highest acuity (or some other target characteristic). Usually, nursing home administrators make the decision to contract with a consultant pharmacy service (with input from medical and nursing staff); therefore, the communication plan should focus on those individuals. The best method of communicating information about the program likely will be face-to-face visits by Ted with those administrators responsible for homes in the target market. The marketing plan may call for obtaining contracts with only a couple homes in the first 6 months of the program but then to increase gradually by one home every 6 months. The ongoing marketing strategy would be in accordance with this.

Develop Financial Projections

Perhaps the most critical step in the business planning process is the development of financial projections for the program. Most programs that do not have a positive benefit-to-cost ratio usually will not be approved. That is, the program must be profitable. While it is preferable that programs generate revenue, it is possible that pharmacy services are justifiable based on reducing expenditures. For example, a clinical pharmacy antibiotic dosing service in a hospital may reduce expenditures on antibiotics and reduce patient length of stay but generate no revenue. If the financial benefit of the dosing service (i.e., reduced expenditures) exceeds the costs associated with providing the program (i.e., pharmacist salary), then the program can be considered financially viable. Obviously, there may be additional benefits from the dosing service, such as improved patient outcomes, that also would favor its approval.

The business planning process must include an analysis of both the costs that will be incurred to provide the service and the financial benefits that may occur as a result of the program. More detailed descriptions of the methods to project these figures are available elsewhere (Schumock, 2000). The calculations involved in this planning process may be aided by the use of financial spreadsheets. A set of financial spreadsheets designed for creating financial projections is available to those in the position of having to develop a business plan (Schumock and Stubbings, 2007). The revenue and expense statement, which lists revenue by category, expenditures by category, and net profit each year for a 3- to 5-year period, is the most useful of these. An example of a revenue and expense projection for consultant pharmacy services (scenario) is shown in Table 4-1.

In developing the financial projections, revenue (if it exists) should be based on the anticipated volume of business, changes to that volume expected over time, and the income per unit of service. Information on billing for pharmacy services may be helpful in estimating potential revenue of the proposed service (American College of Clinical Pharmacy, 1999; Larson, Uden and Hadsall 2000; Vogenberg, 2006). Discounts to income (contractual agreements) should be factored into these calculations, as should future increases in the amount charged for the service. Expenditures must also be projected. If the program requires significant capital investment, those expenditures should be depreciated over the life of the item and accounted for appropriately. Other investments required to initiate the program also should be shown in the financial estimates. Ongoing costs, such as salaries and benefits, minor equipment, supplies, rent, and other overhead, should be categorized and accounted for. Costs that are considered variable should be increased proportionate to the changes in volume expected. All costs should be increased annually based on inflation, the consumer price index (CPI), or other evidence of expected increases in the costs of goods or services.

Identify an Action Plan

The next step in the business planning process is to define major milestones and an action plan of implementation and operation of the program. This action plan should detail the start and finish dates and list responsible individual(s) for each task necessary to accomplish the objectives of the business plan. The action plan should include periodic monitoring and assessment of the performance (i.e., clinical, financial, or other) of

the program. A Gantt chart is one method to depict the action plan visually. An example of a Gantt chart for a long-term consultant pharmacy services is shown in Fig. 4-2.

Assess Critical Risks and Opportunities

Another key step in the business planning process is to determine the critical risks and opportunities of the proposed program. This is essentially the same as the SWOT analysis presented in Chapter 3, except that the business being evaluated is proposed rather than already existing. While it may seem more reasonable to conduct the SWOT analysis earlier in the business planning process, as was done in strategic planning, because the program is in the proposal stage, some of the key considerations for this analysis must come from the previous steps, such as the financial analysis, and thus it is done later in the process.

An example of a SWOT analysis for a proposed long-term care consultant pharmacy services program is shown in Tables 4-2 and 4-3. Strengths and weakness are internal characteristics, whereas opportunities and threats are characteristics of the external business environment. A number of factors can be considered when conducting this analysis. The factors considered will vary based on the nature of the business and the business environment.

Establish an Exit Plan

The last step of the planning process is to develop an exit plan. The *exit plan* is a formal protocol for determining when and why a decision would be made to terminate the program. The exit plan also defines the steps that would be taken if such a decision were to be made.

A decision to exit a program usually is based on failure of the business to meet predetermined goals (financial or otherwise). Typically, any new business is given a certain amount of time to meet its goals (18 to 24 months). Many organizations fail to have a mechanism in place to make a termination decision and instead let the business flounder and perhaps continue to lose money. It is much more preferable to have a definitive benchmark to which the program can be compared and a decision made promptly and decisively.

Table 4-1. Example Revenue and Expense Projections for Consultant Pharmacy Services Program, Most Likely Scenario, Years 1–5

	Year 1	Year 2	Year 3	Year 4	Year 5	Total
Operating revenue						
Patient revenue	504,000	1,008,000	1,176,000	1,260,000	1,764,000	5,712,000
Deductions from revenue	0	0	0	0	0	0
Net patient revenue	504,000	1,008,000	1,176,000	1,260,000	1,764,000	5,712,000
Operating expenses						
Salaries	312,000	426,400	561,600	595,296	1,017,120	2,912,416
Employee benefits	81,100	110,900	146,000	154,800	264,500	757,300
Medical director	0	0	0	0	0	0
Medical supplies	6,000	6,890	7,420	7,950	8,500	36,760
Office supplies	0	0	0	0	0	0
Education and travel	0	0	0	0	0	0
Maintenance/repair	300	318	337	357	757	2,069
Consulting	0	0	0	0	0	0
Contracted services	0	0	0	0	0	0
Marketing	5,000	2,500	2,650	2,809	5,300	18,259
Dues and subscriptions	3,585	3,780	3,975	3,975	4,170	19,485
Rent	12,500	12,700	13,500	14,300	15,150	68,150
Postage	3,500	4,200	4,800	5,300	6,900	24,700
Equipment expense	13,000	1,272	1,348	0	1,515	17,135
Utilities/telephone	8,300	8,798	9,326	9,886	10,479	46,789
Insurance	900	1,166	1,248	1,323	1,826	6,463
Other expenses	16,500	3,090	3,285	12,423	8,894	44,192
Bad debt expense	0	0	0	0	0	0
Building depreciation	0	0	0	0	0	0
Equipment depreciation	0	0	0	0	0	0
Total operating expenses	462,685	582,014	755,489	808,419	1,345,111	3,953,718
Net income (loss)	41,315	425,986	420,511	451,581	418,889	1,758,282
Net assets at beginning	350,000	391,315	817,301	1,237,812	1,689,393	4,485,821
Net assets at end	391,315	817,301	1,237,812	1,689,393		

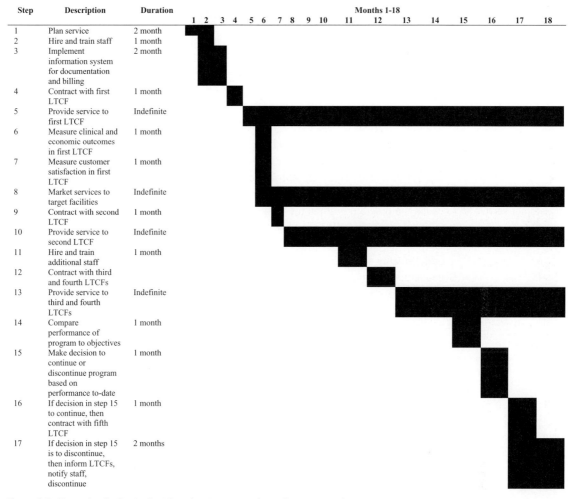

Step	Description	Duration	Months 1-18

Figure 4-2. Example of a Gantt chart for a log-term consultant pharmacy services program.

If a decision is made to terminate a program, then there should be clear actions for how the business will be dissolved. First, there should be a plan for when and how customers will be notified. Further, in some cases it may be important to provide customers with information about others who can provide the service and then schedule a seamless transition. Second, there should be a plan for how employees will be notified. The plan may include efforts to place employees in other areas of the organization or what, if any, compensation package may be available. Third, there should be a plan for how the facilities, equipment, and other capital (*capital* will be discussed in Chapter 18) will be sold or transferred. An exit plan for a program could involve transferring the control of the program from one organization or one administrative unit to another.

■ COMMUNICATION OF THE BUSINESS PLAN

Typically, there are two key components to communicating the work accomplished in planning. The first is to create a written document—the actual business

Table 4-2. Internal Strengths and Weaknesses of Consultant Pharmacy Services Program

Factor	Strength	Weakness
Profitability	As a new program associated with a hospital, overhead expenses are minimal and thus profitability is high. The program is also able to share staff with the hospital, thus reducing salary expenses.	
Quality	As a new program, the organization has limited experience specific to the long-term care environment. This may jeopardize quality initially.	
Customer service	Because the program is small (at least initially), it will be able to provide more attention to customers and thus better-quality service.	
Staff	Because the pharmacist(s) included in the program have hospital experience, their level of clinical knowledge is beyond that of most competitors.	
Operations	Because the program is associated with a hospital, it can rely on the hospital pharmacy department for backup during off hours.	Because the program is small and new in this business, efficiency may be limited.

plan. The second is to present the business plan orally, usually as part of a formal decision-making process.

Writing the Business Plan

As stated previously, writing the business plan is an extremely important part of business planning. The business plan should be informative and balanced in its presentation of the proposal. The document should be written with a specific audience in mind (the financial decision maker). It should be both easy to read and easy to understand and therefore must possess proper organization, grammar, punctuation, and sentence structure.

The contents of a business plan typically follow a sequence of items that are unique to this type of planning. An example of the table of contents of a simple business plan is shown in Table 4-4. It should be noted that the contents of the business plan will vary based on the industry, the business proposed, and the needs of the organization. More detailed plans may be required in certain industries.*

The business plan should begin with an *executive summary.* This summary should be short (one or two pages) but should hit the main points of the proposal. The executive summary needs to capture the attention of the reader. In a poorly written business plan, the reader may form a negative opinion of the program

---

* As another example, the proposed contents of a business plan for a for-profit venture include executive summary, introduction/synopsis, venture idea, overall industry, market research/competition, production/sourcing plan, service/delivery plan, marketing/sales plan, management plan, human resources plan, ownership/organization plan, financial plan, financing plan, growth/exit plan, implementation plan, contingency plan, and assessment/evaluation plan.

Table 4-3. External Opportunities and Threats of Consultant Pharmacy Services Program

Factor	Opportunities	Threats
Competition	Because the competitors also provides pharmaceutical products, they could be considered biased in the clinical recommendations they make. Alternatively, the proposed program does not provide pharmaceutical products and is therefore more objective.	Competitors are well established, large, and financially sound. Competitors also provide pharmaceutical products, which may be desirable. New competitors may enter the local market in the future.
Technology	Competitors have advanced information systems and experience with these systems.	
Regulation	Consultant pharmacy services are mandated by state law. Thus nursing homes must contract with a provider of these services.	
Reimbursement	With worsening of the economy, both the federal and state governments may cut back on Medicare and Medicaid reimbursement to nursing homes. Thus these facilities may go out of business or have insufficient funds to reimburse us for the services of the program.	
Costs	Pharmacist salaries are rising rapidly due to a labor market shortage. These salaries will drive up costs, making it more difficult for the program to generate profit.	
Market/customers	The population continues to age, and as such, there may be more nursing homes in the future.	

and read no further than the executive summary. This illustrates the importance of a writing style that is engaging and error-free. Because of its position in the document, the executive summary is clearly the most critical section of the plan. In addition to the executive summary, the plan should also begin with a *table of contents*. This will both help the writer organize the plan and assist the reader in navigating the document.

The second section of the business plan is the *background and description*. Here, in a logical sequence, the plan should define the rationale for the program or service (i.e., the patient care need) and provide an explanation of why the organization is prepared to fill this need. The *service opportunity* provides the reader with a picture of the purpose of the proposed program and should lead directly to a description of the formal

Table 4-4.   Typical Table of Contents of the Business Plan

1. Executive summary
2. Background and description
3. Market analysis and strategy
4. Operational structure and processes
5. Financial projections
6. Milestones, schedule, and action plan
7. Critical risks and opportunities
8. Exit strategy
9. Conclusion
10. Supportive documents (include financial pro forma statements, letters of support)

mission of the business. Last, this section should provide other details that will help to illustrate the service, including data that may have been obtained from literature or other sources.

The next section of the business plan is the *market analysis and strategy.* In some cases, the market analysis is presented as a separate section from the marketing strategy. In either case, the market analysis is part of the situation analysis conducted during planning, whereas the marketing strategy is part of the goal-setting and strategy-development elements of planning. In the business plan document these are sometimes presented together because they address the same general topic.

The fourth major section of the business plan is the *operational structure and processes.* In brief, this section describes how the program will be run. This section of the document should provide details on how the service will be provided and by whom—in other words, the work processes that will occur. It should include information on how customers will interface with the program. The organizational structure, number and types of employees, and equipment and other resources used in operation of the program should be described. This section should also include definitions of the regulatory, clinical, and quality requirements that may be applicable to the business and a description of how these requirements will be met.

The fifth major section of the plan is the *financial projections* or *financial pro forma.* This section identifies the estimated expenditures and revenue over the first 3 to 5 years of the program. Investments required to begin and operate the program should be described as either startup costs or ongoing costs (or operating costs) and should be organized by cost categories (e.g., salaries, equipment, capital, etc.). The financial data are best presented in a revenue and expense statement (sometimes referred to as the *profit and loss statement*), as shown in Table 4-1.

The sixth section of the business plan defines the *milestones, schedule, and action plan* for the program. A timeline should be defined that includes the major accomplishments and goals of the program for implementation and through the first 3 to 5 years and may include long-range growth and expansions objectives. The action plan may also include responsibility assignments and is often presented as a Gantt chart.

The next section of the business plan defines the *critical risks and opportunities* of the business. Here, the plan should outline the major strengths and weakness of the proposed business and describe the opportunities and risk associated with the program if implemented (as formulated in the SWOT analysis). This information, both positive and negative, must be presented in an unbiased manner so that an informed decision can be made about moving forward with the program.

The business plan should include a brief discussion of what will happen if the business should fail. This *exit strategy* or *contingency strategy* should define specifically when and how a decision would be made to exit the business. The section then should outline a plan for exiting the business. This plan might include issues such as what to do with existing patients or customers (i.e., refer to other providers), what will happen with existing staff (i.e., reassign to other divisions of the organization or terminate), and how equipment and resources may be disposed of.

The last section of the business plan is the *conclusion.* The conclusion should be short. It should quickly summarize the document. Most important, the conclusion should provide a recommendation with respect to the proposed business decision. Following the conclusion are any *attachments* or *additional materials.* Supportive documentation, tables, figures, financial statements, and/or letters of support should be attached to the business plan to collaborate the written text or to present the material in a more detailed fashion.

Presenting the Plan

The oral presentation of the business plan may be as important as the written document. In most organizations, those seeking to implement new programs must present the business plan before a group, usually consisting of senior leaders in the company.

A good oral presentation can go a long way toward garnering positive support for the business plan. The personal nature of the oral presentation may add dynamics to the decision-making process that do not exist with the written document. These issues, which include politics, group dynamics, and personal interactions, can be either positive or negative. In either case, these dynamics should be anticipated and either reinforced or preempted depending on the situation.

CONCLUSION

After reading this chapter, our friend Ted Thompson should be prepared to address the charge given him in the scenario. Ted, being an intelligent person, will recognize quickly that developing a business plan for the proposed consultant pharmacy services program will be a significant undertaking. Ted would be well advised to seek assistance from others as he begins this planning process. For example, Ted may want to establish a team that would include representatives from the hospital finance department, other pharmacists who might be involved in the program, and perhaps even a physician or nurse with experience in long-term care. The assembled team then could begin the business plan planning process as outlined in this chapter. When this process is complete, Ted and his boss (the DOP) will need to follow the appropriate administrative channels within the organization to gain approval from key hospital decision makers.

Obviously, business planning is an important tool for gaining further acceptance and penetration of con-temporary pharmacy services. New pharmacy graduates must understand and be able to write business plans that will justify new or continued investments in these services. It is very likely that most new graduates will be expected to develop or help to develop a business plan for a pharmacy program at some point in their careers. Clearly, the ability to do so will benefit the pharmacist, the employer, and patients. If accepted, the new program may be an opportunity to provide new or unique services—thus heightening job satisfaction. Likewise, the new program may generate revenue or save costs elsewhere in the system—thus benefiting the employer. Patients, physicians, nurses, and others who are the recipients of the program will also benefit.

QUESTIONS FOR FURTHER DISCUSSION

1. Conduct a literature search to identify articles that may be pertinent to the business proposal described in the scenario. How many articles did you find, and how useful are they to understanding the business concept?

2. Conduct a hypothetical market and competitor analysis, and develop a marketing strategy for the consultant pharmacy services program. What are the market segments that may be important to this business? What are the strengths and weaknesses of the proposed service compared with those of its potential competitors?

3. What are important costs that would be incurred if the consultant pharmacy services program were implemented? Classify these costs as fixed or variable.

4. Explain why you think an understanding of business planning is important for pharmacists. What changes are occurring in the health care environment that make business planning even more important?

REFERENCES

American College of Clinical Pharmacy. 1994. Establishing and evaluating clinical pharmacy services in primary care. *Pharmacotherapy* 14:743–58.

American College of Clinical Pharmacy. 1999. *How to Bill for Clinical Pharmacy Services.* Kansas City, MO: American College of Clinical Pharmacy.

Bangs DH. 1998. *The Market Planning Guide: Creating a Plan to Successfully Market Your Business Product or Service,* 5th ed. Chicago: Upstart Publications.

Cohen DJ. 2001. *The Project Manager's MBA: How to Translate Project Decisions into Business Success,* 1st ed. San Francisco: Jossey-Bass.

Coke A. 2001. *Seven Steps to a Successful Business Plan.* New York: American Management Association.

Cooper JK, Saxton C, Cameron KA, eds. 2004. *Developing a Senior Care Pharmacy Practice: Your Guide and Tools for Success.* Alexandria, VA: American Society of Consultant Pharmacists.

Doucette WR, McDonough RP. 2002. Beyond the 4Ps: Using relationship marketing to build value and demand for pharmacy services. *J Am Pharm Assoc* 42:183.

Hagel HP. 2002. Planning for patient care. In Hagel HP, Rovers JP (eds), *Managing the Patient-Centered Pharmacy.* Washington, DC: American Pharmaceutical Association.

Hatoum HT, Catizone C, Hutchinson RA, Purohit A. 1986. An eleven-year review of the pharmacy literature: Documentation of the value and acceptance of clinical pharmacy. *Drug Intell Clin Pharm* 20:33.

Hatoum HT, Akhras K. 1993. A 32-year literature review on the value and acceptance of ambulatory care provided by clinical pharmacists. *Ann Pharmacother* 27:1108.

Holdford DA. 2003. *Marketing for Pharmacists.* Washington, DC: American Pharmaceutical Association.

Larson TA, Uden DL, Hadsall RS. 2000. Practice models used by pharmacists in rural Minnesota to obtain Medicare reimbursement. *J Am Pharm Assoc* 40:554.

O'Hara PD. 1995. *The Total Business Plan: How to Write, Rewrite, and Revise,* 2d ed. New York: Wiley.

Phillips CR, Larson LN. 2002. Creating a business plan for patient care. In Hagel HP, Rovers JP (eds), *Managing the Patient-Centered Pharmacy.* Washington, DC: American Pharmaceutical Association.

Pinson L, Jinnet J. 1999. *Anatomy of a Business Plan,* 4th ed. Chicago: Dearborn.

Plumridge RJ, Wojnar-Horton RE. 1998. A review of the pharmacoeconomics of pharmaceutical care. *Pharmacoeconomics* 19:1349.

Schneller LW, Powell MF, Solomon DK. 1998. Using the business plan to propose revenue-generating pharmacy services. *Hosp Pharm* 23:806.

Schumock G. 2000. Methods to assess the economic outcomes of clinical pharmacy services. *Pharmacotherapy* 20:243S.

Schumock G, Stubbing J. 2007. *How to Develop a Business Plan for Pharmacy Services.* Lenexa KS: American College of Clinical Pharmacy.

Schumock G, Butler M. 2003. Evaluating and justifying clinical pharmacy services. In Grauer D, Lee J, Odom T, et al. (eds), *Pharmacoeconomics and Outcomes: Applications for Patient Care,* 2d ed. Kansas City, MO: American College of Clinical Pharmacy.

Schumock G, Michaud J, Guenette A. 1999. Re-engineering: An opportunity to advance clinical practice in a community hospital. *Am J Health-Syst Pharm* 56:1945.

Schumock G, Stubbings J, McBride SJ. 2004. Business planning and marketing. In *Developing a Senior Care Pharmacy Practice: Your Guide and Tools for Success.* Alexandria, VA: American Society of Consultant Pharmacists.

Schumock G, Meek P, Ploetz P, Vermeulen LC. 1996. Economic evaluations of clinical pharmacy services: 1998–1995. *Pharmacotherapy* 16:1188.

Schumock G, Butler M, Meek P, et al. 2003. Evidence of the economic benefit of clinical pharmacy services: 1996–2000. *Pharmacotherapy* 23:113.

Tipton DJ. 2001. A tool for corporate decision making about cognitive pharmaceutical services. *J Am Pharm Assoc* 41:91.

Vogenberg FR. 2006. *Understanding Pharmacy Reimbursement.* Bethesda, MD: American Society of Health System Pharmacists.

Willett MS, Bertch KE, Rich DS, Ereshefsky L. 1989. Prospectus on the economic value of clinical pharmacy services. *Pharmacotherapy* 9:45.

5

GENERAL OPERATIONS MANAGEMENT

Noel E. Wilkin

About the Author: Dr. Wilkin is Interim Associate Provost, Associate Professor of Pharmacy Administration, and Research Associate Professor in the Research Institute of Pharmaceutical Sciences at The University of Mississippi. He received a B.S. in pharmacy in 1989 and a Ph.D. in 1996, both from the University of Maryland, Baltimore. Dr. Wilkin has generated substantial grant and contract support, has published in numerous peer-reviewed and professional journals, and teaches at both the graduate and undergraduate levels. His areas of research include practical reasoning and its role in decision making, pharmacy entrepreneurship and management, issues facing professional education, and mechanisms to enhance optimal drug therapy.

▪ LEARNING OBJECTIVES

After completing this chapter, students should be able to

1. Describe the concepts of operations and operations management.
2. Identify typical inputs and outputs involved in pharmacy operations.
3. Describe the operations used by a pharmacy to transform inputs into outputs.
4. Identify decisions that need to be made in typical pharmacy operations.
5. Describe the relationship between efficient operations and profitability.

▪ SCENARIO

Marie Lassiter just left her doctor and does not feel well. She stops at Cataldo's Pharmacy to have the prescription that the doctor wrote for her filled. Joe Cataldo is a pharmacist who owns Cataldo's Pharmacy. The pharmacy fills prescriptions for patients, helps diabetic patients manage their disease, offers a full line of durable medical equipment, and fills prescriptions for a local nursing home. Joe or one of his two staff pharmacists order their goods from a wholesaler. The wholesaler delivers these goods—over-the-counter (OTC) products, prescription drugs, and the other products sold in the pharmacy—on a daily basis. When the medications are delivered, the prescription medications are placed on the shelf by one of the pharmacy technicians. One of the three store clerks places the OTC items on the displays in the front of the pharmacy. When Marie enters the pharmacy to have a prescription filled, she approaches the counter and is greeted by a clerk. The clerk gathers information from her and gives the information and written prescription to the technician. The technician enters the information into the computer, which connects to another computer to verify Marie's insurance coverage and the amount of money that she should pay. The pharmacy's computer then prints a label that will be placed on the prescription vial, which is placed in a staging area to be filled. In this instance, Marie's prescription is a compounded prescription, a prescription that must be prepared by mixing several ingredients together. One of the pharmacists prepares the prescription and places it into a special vial. The pharmacist then checks it for accuracy and assurance that what was prepared matches what was ordered on the written prescription. The pharmacist then gives Marie the prescription and provides information about how to use the medication properly while the clerk rings her up and processes her credit card.

CHAPTER QUESTIONS

1. What is the importance of operations management in pharmacy practices today?
2. What resources are used in the process of creating goods and services?
3. What categories are helpful in devising strategies to manage the resources used in operations?
4. How do the differences between goods and services influence the decisions made in operations management?
5. How does scheduling affect the profitability of a pharmacy?

INTRODUCTION

Businesses exist to offer goods and services to consumers.* Businesses must use resources (*inputs*) to create the goods and services (*outputs*) that are offered. This creation process is referred to as *transformation* (Heizer and Render, 1999; Johnson, 1998). The resources are transformed into things that are needed, wanted, and demanded by consumers. Consumers then pay for these outputs because the desire to satisfy their want or need is equal to or greater than the amount of value they place on the money used to buy it. This process of creating goods and services is referred to as *operations*. It encompasses the activities or operations performed by the organization to transform resources into valued, profit-generating goods and services. To manage these activities is to perform *operations management*.

THE LINK BETWEEN OPERATIONS AND PROFITABILITY

Given that businesses perform many operations to produce goods and services, the efficiency of those operations will affect the profitability associated with the goods and services offered by the business. It costs money to develop/create goods, and it costs money to provide services. In the scenario, the pharmacy is compounding a product from multiple active ingredients. It is evident that there are a multitude of inputs, all of which have associated costs. The pharmacy must pay for the

- Ingredients, both active and inactive
- Container that will hold the final compound

---

* These goods and services, also called *offerings,* can be divided into five categories, including pure tangible good, tangible good with accompanying services, hybrid, major service with accompanying goods and services, and pure service (Kotler and Keller, 2006). There is some debate about the usefulness of distinguishing goods from services, particularly for the purposes of marketing the offerings of a business (Vargo and Lusch, 2004). For the purposes of this chapter, the terms *goods* and *services* are used in their classic sense.

- Computer that creates the label and bills the insurance company
- Software run by the computer
- Fee charged to verify and bill the prescription over the phone line
- Bag that the prescription is placed in so that the patient can carry it home
- Cost of electricity that lights, heats, and cools the work area
- Rent on the facility in which the prescriptions are prepared
- Salary and benefits for the pharmacist who compounds the prescription
- Salary and benefits for the technician who enters the prescription order into the computer
- Salary and benefits for the clerk who rings up the prescription

This is not a complete list, but it demonstrates that there are a number of costs associated with creating a product that is then sold to a patient. The pharmacy covers these costs by collecting money for the goods and services it produces. Simply put, after deducting all the costs or expenses associated with operating and creating the goods and services that are sold, the money left over is *profit*. If the owners, managers, and employees are not prudent in the purchasing and managing the inputs used to create the goods and services sold by the pharmacy, the pharmacy will not be as profitable. However, being profitable is not just about finding the inputs with the lowest cost, and it is not a matter of simply raising the prices to cover the costs.

Maximizing the efficiency of creating goods and services sold by a pharmacy requires careful planning, analysis, and management. If the pharmacist uses inferior ingredients or vials, the patient may never return to the pharmacy for another prescription. If the pharmacist is paid too little, she may not take pride in her work, she may not be as efficient as she could be, or she may end up taking more sick days—all these cause the pharmacy to pay the salary of the pharmacist without benefiting from her productivity. If an inferior computer system is purchased at a lower cost and it crashes regularly, preventing the pharmacist from being able

to fill prescriptions, this decreases the profitability of the pharmacy. This connection to profitability makes operations management a critical, multifaceted area of interest to any business.

▓ TYPICAL PHARMACY OUTPUTS (GOODS AND SERVICES)

The scenario refers to the creation of a product for Marie Lassiter. The concept of managing operations for a business that creates goods is relatively easy to comprehend. The inputs are tangible; one can see them and touch them, and often their quality can be evaluated. This is not to say that management of operations to create goods is simple, as will soon become apparent. Instead, the concept of managing the operations used to assemble a product is more comprehensible. As the scenario illustrates, even in the creation of goods, there are many intangible, nonproduct inputs. In this example, the speed and proficiency with which the pharmacist, clerk, and technician can perform their duties will influence how many prescriptions can be compounded by the pharmacy in a day. Their interactions with the patients who are having prescriptions filled will influence whether the patients return to have prescriptions filled in the future. Their ability to interact with patients will be influenced by how much assistance they have in filling the prescriptions. The scenario refers to the creation of a product, one that did not exist prior to the transformation performed by the pharmacist with the assistance of the technician and the clerk.

A common example of a service in a community pharmacy is the filling of a prescription that is not compounded. In this case, a pharmacist, with the assistance of technicians and clerks, is adding value to the product that was made by a pharmaceutical company. The pharmacist is packaging the exact amount needed by the patient, adding information that will help the patient to take it appropriately, and billing the patient's insurance company for the cost of the prescription. Pharmacists may add additional value to this product, and these value-added services illustrate the similarities to product creation.

Resources also must be expended to provide services, and pharmacists still should be concerned about their quality.

The transformation of resources to create services is not always as easily understood. This is so in part because the transformation of resources may not be tangible. For example, think about the transformation that takes place to provide information to a patient. The pharmacist must recall the information or look it up in a reference, understand its relevance to the situation and the patient, and communicate this information to the patient in a way that the patient will understand.

Managing the operations of a pharmacy to create the highest-quality goods and services for the lowest cost requires some knowledge of typical pharmacy inputs and outputs. While the outputs created by a business are the final step in operations, it is useful to learn about the typical pharmacy outputs at this point to fully appreciate the resources used to create those outputs. In other words, with knowledge of these outputs, the operations that take place within a pharmacy will be more easily understood, and the strategies used to manage those operations will have more meaning.

Community and institutional pharmacy practices generally offer a variety of medication-related goods and services. A representative list can be found in Table 5-1. The list of goods and services given in this table is by no means comprehensive. Some pharmacies have ice cream parlors, some have nail salons, and some sell gifts and collectibles. So how does one choose what goods and services a business should offer?

The outputs of the business justify the existence of the business. While this leads some consumers to identify the business by its goods and services, this is not to say that it defines the business. The company BASF, for example, is a chemical company that identified itself as a company that adds value. The company ran an advertising campaign in the late 1990s that made the claim, "We don't make many of the things you buy. We make many of the things you buy better." This advertising campaign did not make consumers believe that the company made chemicals, but rather it com-

Table 5-1. Typical Pharmacy Outputs

Community pharmacy practice

Filling of prescription medications based on physicians' orders

Compounding of prescription medications

Over-the-counter medications

Nutritional supplements

Offering and fitting durable medical equipment

Information about prescriptions medications

Information about OTC medications

Information about nutritional supplementation

Health and beauty aids

Greeting cards

Disease-state management

Prospective drug utilization review

Counseling on prescription drug use

Adjudication of claims with third-party payers

Provision of medications to nursing home residents

Special convenience packaging (e.g., bubble packs)

Screening for drug interactions

Institutional pharmacy practice

Filling of prescription medications based on physicians' orders

Compounding of prescription medications

Preparation of intravenous medications and solutions

Delivery of medications to floors

Oversight and inventory of controlled substances

Collection of orders from hospital floors

Drug event monitoring

Formulary management

Therapeutic interchange

Prescription medication counseling

Medication use evaluation

Filling of prescription medication carts

Drug information to physicians and other health care providers

Total parenteral and enteral nutrition

Stocking of emergency crash carts

Pharmacokinetic dosing

Clinical drug trials

municated to consumers that BASF was a company that added value to the everyday goods that consumers used. Despite the fact that companies can influence the perceptions of their businesses and their goods and services through marketing, many consumers categorize businesses by what they provide. Pharmacies fill prescriptions, fast-food restaurants serve inexpensive food quickly, pharmaceutical companies make drugs, and car dealers sell cars. This consumer-driven categorization of businesses can lure one to believe that goods and services offered by a business are predetermined based on the category of business. Instead, the goods and services are driven by decisions made by the people who own or operate the business. Certainly, the owners or decision makers of businesses consider consumer opinions about their businesses, and yet the outputs that a business will offer are under the control of the owners or decision makers. The mission of the business is the basis for these decisions. The mission defines the business's reason for existence. It delineates what the business does and communicates the unique advantages it has in creating the goods and services that it offers.

Opportunities to decide which products and services to offer are available to both community and institutional pharmacies. The environments are slightly different, and the decisions are important in both settings. For example, hospital pharmacies frequently are within larger infrastructures of the hospitals they serve. Many, however, still function to add value to various inputs. They serve patients and internal customers—the physicians, nurses, and other health care professionals who practice in the institution.

As a result, owners or operators of businesses can add, enhance, eliminate, or change the goods and services offered. To make these decisions, a process of strategic planning should be used. This process of planning can assist in identifying the internal and external factors—the strengths, weaknesses, opportunities, and threats—faced by a business. Once these factors are understood adequately, a pharmacy can more easily choose goods and services that have the best chance of being profitable for the business in a given geographic area (see Chapters 3 and 4).

■ TYPICAL PHARMACY INPUTS (RESOURCES)

Operations are the activities performed to transform resources (inputs) into valued, profitable goods and services. In the scenario, what are the resources that went into the filling of Marie's prescription? The obvious resources are the several active ingredients produced by pharmaceutical manufacturers that were mixed together to formulate the prescription. However, these constitute only one of the many resources that were used to fill the prescription.

Others are listed in Table 5-2, and this is not a comprehensive list. As you can see, many resources are used to fill a prescription, and not all of them are as

Table 5-2.	Resources Used to Fill Marie Lassiter's Prescription

- Prescription medications
- Pharmacist who ordered the prescription medications
- Delivery service provided by the wholesaler
- Technician who placed them on the shelf in the pharmacy in a place where the pharmacist would find them
- Shelf that they sat on until the pharmacist used them
- Vial in which the pharmacist placed the finished proeduct
- Computers used to process the prescription
- Adjudication service offered by the insurance company
- Label printed by the computer
- Software used by the computer
- Phone line used to connect the computers for the purpose of adjudication
- Clerk who rung the prescription up
- Register used by the clerk to ring it up
- Counter that the register sits on
- Facility that houses the pharmacy
- Electricity and other utilities that are available in the pharmacy

obvious as others. However, they each play a critical role in being able to transform the medication received from the wholesaler into a medication that Marie can take appropriately. Many of these resources are transparent to or are taken for granted by the ultimate consumers of the product or service, and this does not diminish their importance to activities involved in filling the prescription. A pharmacist only has to have the electricity go out once to learn how critical this resource is to the service of filling prescriptions. The lights will go out, the computer will not be able to process or adjudicate the prescription, and the cash register will not function. Some of these activities can be performed even when the electricity is out. The pharmacist can use battery-operated emergency lights or a flashlight to see. He can use reference materials to look up interactions. He can use a manual typewriter to create a label. He cannot, however, determine the amount of the patient's copay, which is calculated during the adjudication process. If the pharmacy uses a register that determines the prices of goods by scanning the Universal Product Code (UPC) of the product (POS system), then he may not even know how much to charge the patient for the goods in the store. This resource influences the efficiency of and ability to perform the activities in filling the prescription.

It is evident that electricity contributes to the efficiency of filling prescriptions. By powering the computer, it makes checking interactions, storing patient information, and printing labels much more efficient. However, it also is critical to filling prescriptions because without it some of the activities necessary to create the output of the process are not possible (e.g., real-time adjudication). Other resources in this process may not be critical to the process but increase the efficiency of the process. For example, the shelving units chosen to hold the stock prescription bottles come in different forms. Choices can range from not having shelving at all and simply stacking goods on the floor in big piles to using shelving that maximizes storage space and access to the bottles. Without any shelving, which would save the pharmacy the expense of shelves, the process would be terribly inefficient. Can

you imagine digging around in piles of bottles looking for the correct stock bottle of medication? While the pharmacy would save money by not buying shelves, it would cost the pharmacy money because extra pharmacists and technicians would have to be hired just to dig through the piles and pull out the correct medication. On the other end of the spectrum, the expense of having shelves that maximize storage space and access, as compared with simple, standard shelves, may not be warranted if the floor space of the pharmacy is conducive to having simple shelving that does not detract from efficiency. This example, although simple, illustrates how even a resource as basic as shelving can influence efficiency and, ultimately, profitability.

Each of these resources can be grouped or categorized according to many different strategies. They can be grouped into categories based on whether they are a product or service, for example. Using this categorization scheme, goods are tangible and would include (and are not limited to) shelving, computers, prescription vials, labels, software, and drugs. Services can include the tasks performed by the people involved, the wholesaler's service, the phone service, and the adjudication service. This broad categorization scheme, while illustrative, may not be helpful to the manager or owner in deciding how to choose the resources used in creating the goods and services of the business and determining how to maximize the efficiency of the process. Instead, operations management uses more specific categories to describe, analyze, and manage the operations of a business. One strategy is to consider the issues faced in operations as strategies or tactics (Mantel and Evans, 1992). Also, different businesses will categorize resources differently for purposes of managing them. While a uniform categorization scheme would be helpful, it is not necessary in understanding how various strategies can be employed to manage these resources to maximize their efficiency in the operations of the business. Instead, it is helpful to think of operations management in terms of the critical decisions that need to be made by operations managers (Heizer and Render, 1999). The 10 decisions under the purview of operations management are the following (Heizer and Render, 1999):

- Designing goods and services
- Process strategies
- Managing quality
- Location strategies
- Layout strategies
- Human resources
- Scheduling
- Supply-chain management
- Inventory management
- Maintenance

If you reconsider the scenario, it is possible to see the influence that these decisions will have on the breadth of activities involved in the operations of a pharmacy. The design of goods and services that are needed and wanted by consumers (and that offer a competitive advantage over other pharmacies) must be created. Once the goods and services are designed, the processes that will be used to create and offer them must be implemented and managed. The quality of the goods created and services offered must be maintained. The location and layout of the pharmacy need to be conducive and appropriate given the goods and services offered. Pharmacies rely heavily on personnel; human resources management and scheduling of those resources are important parts of operations management of a pharmacy. Supply-chain management is management of the supply of inputs used to create the outputs. Having an efficient supply of prescription products is critical to the service of filling prescriptions. And once the products are delivered, the inventory must be managed to minimize the costs associated with having an inventory necessary to fill prescriptions and offer OTC products. Finally, maintenance of the resources that go into operations must be considered and managed. If the resources are not functioning properly, this can create inefficiencies that decrease profitability. Each of these factors and the strategies that can be employed to maximize their efficiency are relevant to both community and institutional pharmacies. These decisions and

the strategies used to make good decisions in each of these areas are covered in more detail in other chapters. Before going into depth, however, it is helpful to understand how these areas of operations management are related to the resources used in pharmacy operations and how these operations decisions can influence profitability.

DESIGNING GOODS AND SERVICES

Designing goods and services that are in line with the needs and wants of consumers requires analysis and planning. As indicated previously, goods are tangible—they can be held and touched. Services are not tangible—they are experienced by the consumer. Except in the instance of compounded prescriptions, the design of the good is largely up to the manufacturer; however, with the advent of medication therapy management (MTM), there are increased opportunities to design innovative and creative services to accomplish these objectives. Services can be designed to have three different approaches—customer service, product service, and service products. These approaches are similar and have differences that influence how they are implemented, managed, and marketed. Customer service is aimed at improving the customer's experience with the pharmacy and is geared toward improving overall sales. As a result, these are perceived as overhead costs (Mathieu, 2001). Product services are linked to a specific product, add value to the product, and are offered in an effort to enhance sales of that product. This type of service is consumed after the product is purchased (Mathieu, 2001). The final category is a service product. This is a service that is independent of the company's tangible offerings and can be consumed separately.

Planning will play a critical role in the development of new goods and services. Analyses of the internal and external environments will play a role in determining the capabilities of the pharmacy and the needs in the market. Offering goods and services that are consistent with consumer needs and wants will increase the chances of profitability. The offering of services will affect multiple aspects of the pharmacy's operations, including marketing, production, delivery, and internal communications (Brax, 2005). Each of these has the potential to influence the day-to-day processes used to offer the goods and services to customers.

PROCESS STRATEGIES

The operations process involves many steps. The scenario at the beginning of this chapter can be broken down into over a dozen steps. The order in which those steps are performed will influence the efficiency of operations and, ultimately, the quality of the goods and services produced. As a result, it will influence the profitability of the pharmacy. For example, if a pharmacist tries to fill a prescription with a medication that has not been placed on the shelf yet, she may find herself digging through totes full of medications that were delivered from the wholesaler. In this instance, the process of filling prescriptions is affected by the inventory, when the order was placed, when the order was delivered, and when the order was put on the shelves. Similarly, prescriptions that are brought in by patients who will wait to have them filled need to be filled before prescriptions that are not going to be picked up until the next day. Patients will be influenced directly by the efficiency of this process. In processes used to create goods, the customer is not likely to be involved. In services, however, the customer may be integrally involved, as is the case with the customer service provided to patients who are waiting to have their prescriptions filled. Often patients will express their dissatisfaction at having to wait a long time to have their prescriptions filled, and this may affect whether they come again to have their prescriptions filled. Whether the patient is involved or not, decisions about the process used to create goods and services need to be designed to maximize efficiency.

The processes used by the pharmacy to create goods and provide services have specific capacities. For example, technicians can enter only so many prescriptions into a computer in an hour, and pharmacists can fill only so many prescriptions in an hour. Capacity is determined by the resource that imposes the greatest limitation on the process (Bruner, Eakes, and Freeman, 1998). This limiting resource is referred to as the *bottleneck*. To increase capacity, the bottleneck must be identified and eliminated. For example, if Marie entered the pharmacy at a time when another pharmacist was on duty, the other pharmacist might come over to fill prescriptions while the first pharmacist compounds Marie's prescription. This would prevent a bottleneck in filling other prescriptions that are dropped off while Marie's prescription is being prepared. Bottlenecks and other obstacles to efficient creation of a good or provision of a service will influence profitability by decreasing the quantity of a good created or limiting the number of services provided. For example, when Dr. Michael Kim realized that many patients were waiting for refills in the limited space in his pharmacy, he implemented a refill system. In this system, a report is generated of the upcoming refills. Patients are contacted to determine if the medication is needed. Prescriptions for medications that are needed by patients are filled and scheduled for delivery. This process change decreased the traffic in his store and allows the pharmacists to focus on the new prescriptions presented by patients who visit the pharmacy (Wilkin, 2006). Stanley Devine and Robert Beardain of Winona, Mississippi, take this process change a step further. They line up each patient's medication refills so that the patient can get all his or her medications once a month, and they contact *every* patient before the prescriptions are due to be filled. This affords them the opportunity to discuss with their patients any problems or issues that the patients may be experiencing with their medications. It also decreases the need to maintain a large inventory because the medications can be ordered just in time to refill the prescriptions for patients, affords them more control over the pace at which they fill prescriptions, increases their contact with patients, and significantly decreases the patient traffic in the pharmacy (Wilkin, 2006).

A flowchart of the process that is used by the business to create its offerings can be helpful in analyzing and designing the process. A flowchart is a diagram of the steps involved in creating the good or offering the

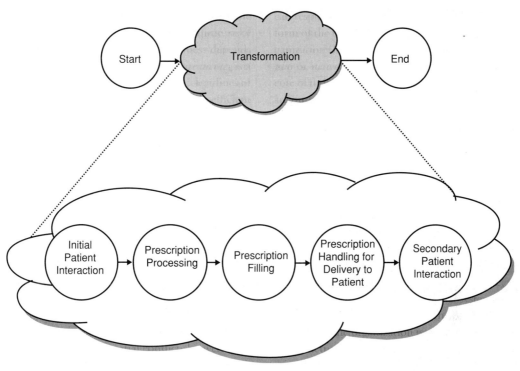

Figure 5-1. Operations performed in a community pharmacy to fill prescriptions.

service. This visual representation can be helpful in analyzing the resources used in the transformation process and can be used to improve the processes performed within the pharmacy. To diagram the process, geometric shapes are used to represent each of the steps in the process (Robson, 1991). The operations performed to fill prescriptions are depicted in Fig. 5-1. The level of detail within a flowchart can vary. This depiction outlines a series of operations that are performed within the transformation process of filling prescriptions. Multiple tasks are performed within each of these operations, and these tasks will use a number of different individuals and resources. The more detailed the diagram is, the easier it will be to evaluate the time and resources necessary at each step of the process.

The flowchart is a helpful tool in identifying and evaluating the capacities of each element of the process and areas of the process that can be improved (e.g., areas that are causing bottlenecks for improved efficiency). A clear understanding of the process used to create all the product and service offerings of the business is not only important in identifying areas where efficiency can be improved, but it can also be used to manage quality.

MANAGING QUALITY

Being able to offer goods and services that are of high quality to customers is important to any business. Ensuring quality, more specifically, *measuring* quality, will differ depending on whether a product or service is being created. The decisions made about the quality of a product produced by pharmacy operations can be based on objective standards. For example, a compounded prescription should have a certain amount of the active ingredient in the product. The quality of a product can be evaluated by measuring the quantity of the active ingredient and using other objective standards. The quality of a service, on the other hand, is determined by more subjective standards. Marie Lassiter, in the scenario, may be assessing the quality of the information she was provided. This is likely to be based on her subjective assessment of the information and the manner in which it was communicated. Services, despite their intangible nature, still need to be evaluated to determine if the intended outcomes are being achieved.

There are two types of costs associated with quality—the cost of maintaining quality and the cost associated with poor quality (Mudie and Cottam, 1999). In maintaining good quality, there are prevention costs and appraisal costs. *Prevention costs* result from the use of resources (time and personnel) to prevent errors from occurring. For example, these can include the cost of training employees and the cost of technologies (e.g., robotics, computers, and software) used to decrease the likelihood of errors. In addition to prevention costs, there are appraisal costs. *Appraisal costs* result from the use of resources to inspect, test, and audit to identify a drop in the quality of a service or product. In addition to these costs of maintaining good quality, there are costs associated with poor service quality. These costs result from internal and external failures. *Internal failures* are errors or defects that are identified and rectified before consumers receive the product or service. For example, if a pharmacist places brand-name medication in a bottle that is labeled to contain the generic medication, realizes the mistake, and corrects it, this would be considered an internal failure. It cost the pharmacy money because it consumed the pharmacist's time to correct the problem. The managers of the pharmacy would be wise to determine what factors led to the internal failure, take steps to eliminate or modify those factors, and prevent it from occurring again. *External failures* are errors or defects in goods or services that are actually delivered to consumers. Frequently, external failures are the ones identified by consumers. For example, if a consumer realizes that she has received a different medication than the one indicated on the label, this is an external failure. More often than not, this will take much more time and money to correct than an internal failure. It may

involve delivery of a new medication to the patient, loss of the product that was dispensed incorrectly because it will have to be discarded, and a potential lawsuit if harm was done to the patient (see Chapter 11 for more information on service failures). Production of quality goods and services does not occur in a vacuum. Instead, it is closely tied to the processes employed to create those goods and services.

▪ LOCATION

The location of the pharmacy can affect several aspects of operations. The location of the pharmacy can affect the following:

- How easily and efficiently the inputs for operations can be acquired
- How easily the outputs of operations can be transferred to the consumers of those outputs
- Which outputs are chosen to be offered by a given business (designing of goods and services)

In a pharmacy, there are certain skilled positions that need to be taken into consideration when locating the business. Operating a pharmacy in a location that is conducive to attracting qualified pharmacists to work there is important. The pharmacy must also be able to receive deliveries of the various products sold by the pharmacy. Proximity to consumers and the preferences of consumers will play a role in how easily the pharmacy's goods and services are transferred to the consumers of those services. For example, a chain pharmacy in a busy metroplex whose customers rely on public transportation to get to the pharmacy to have their prescriptions filled will be greatly inconvenienced if the pharmacy does not have in stock all the medications necessary to fill their prescriptions. This, therefore, affects the operations of the pharmacy. It may cause the pharmacy to have a larger inventory than otherwise needed or a delivery service to minimize the inefficiency or customer dissatisfaction that may result from not being able to fill the prescriptions while patients wait. Or the pharmacy could be located in an area with a large population of people who want to pick up their medications at a drive-through window (e.g., mothers with sick infants).

The market factors that are influenced by location will influence the operations of the pharmacy. The goods and services themselves also may make one location more profitable than another. The design of goods and services is part of operations, and if a business is located near people who want and need its products and services, it may enhance the business's chance of attracting them to the store. For example, a pharmacy located in an ethnic neighborhood that has a population of people who rely on natural products to maintain health might decide to offer such products to those consumers. The proximity of these people to the store and their desire to have such products may increase the chance of those items being profitable for the pharmacy. The location of the pharmacy certainly can affect operations, and so can the location of various goods and services within the pharmacy.

PHARMACY LAYOUT

A pharmacy needs to be designed to maximize the efficiency of the processes conducted to create the goods and services. For example, when filling a prescription, the path that the prescription takes from the patient to the pharmacist who will fill it needs to be efficient. A layout that decreases efficiency is likely to contribute to decreased profitability. Steps that require the prescription to "backtrack in the process" need to be eliminated or minimized by designing an efficient layout. The layout can also affect the efficiency with which services are provided. Having a counseling area that is readily accessible to the pharmacist and patients will increase the efficiency of providing information to patients. And it even may increase the likelihood that patients will ask for information when they need it.

In addition to the efficient operations of the pharmacy, the layout of the pharmacy will affect the patients' movement through the store. This has implications for product placement and pharmacy design (see Chapter 23).

HUMAN RESOURCES

Human resources are one of the most important resources in a pharmacy. The goods and services offered by pharmacies are transformed using personnel. These individuals perform the operations of the business and rely heavily on technologies to increase the efficiency of their tasks (e.g., computers, robotics, counting machines, and software programs). Their efficiency and ability to interact with patients will influence the efficiency of pharmacy operations. Many factors need to be evaluated when determining the human resources needed to accomplish the operations of the pharmacy. To conduct these evaluations, many tools (e.g., job design and job analyses) are available to make good decisions about the human resources needs of specific operations. The human resources and the ability to acquire them will also be affected by environmental factors. The supply and demand for pharmacists, for example, may prevent a pharmacy from finding enough pharmacists to perform the operations of the pharmacy efficiently. This may cause owners and managers to seek other mechanisms to increase the efficiency of the staff that they have (e.g., robotics or increased use of readily available personnel). These environmental factors also may cause businesses to offer higher salaries, more attractive working hours, and better benefits. However, these items need to be evaluated in light of how they will affect the profitability of the pharmacy.

The types of people attracted to work at the business also will affect operations. Motivated, productive, and competent individuals are likely to contribute to greater profitability than unmotivated, unproductive, and incompetent individuals. Hiring just the right people for the operations within the pharmacy is important. Training those people on their responsibilities is just as important. If the phone rings and no one thinks that it is their job to answer it, the pharmacy may lose a sale. Likewise, if the phone rings and the staff begin to argue over whose turn it is to answer it, this contributes to a lack of efficiency and possibly to customer dissatisfaction. In a pharmacy, human resources play a big role in the transformation of inputs to outputs. This makes human resources management an important aspect of operations management.

SCHEDULING

Given this heavy reliance on human resources, scheduling of personnel is a critical aspect of operations. Regulations state that a licensed pharmacist must be present when the pharmacy is open to fill prescriptions. This makes scheduling of pharmacists coincide with the hours that the prescription department is open. Other considerations need to be given to the pharmacists' preferences for work schedules. Given the importance of this resource and the costs associated with replacing a pharmacist, the schedule should be created in light of individuals' work preferences to whatever extent it is possible. The scheduling of support staff, for example, technicians and clerks, should be driven by the demand for goods and services. Ideally, the pharmacists will have the most help when the demand for having prescriptions filled is at its greatest. This takes careful planning and evaluation of sales and volume trends. Graphic and charting methods can be used to determine the demand for having prescriptions filled and for receiving disease-state management services. To chart the demand, however, the pharmacy must collect the data. Most computer systems will allow decision makers to track the number of prescriptions filled on a given day, and some will allow them to track the number by sales volume. By looking at the number of prescriptions filled at given times during the day, a manager can plan to have enough help to meet the demand efficiently.

Many pharmacies use what is called a *chase strategy* (Heizer and Render, 1999). In essence, they chase the demand by having personnel available to handle the demand when they predict the demand will be the greatest. For example, if a pharmacy predicts that the Monday after a holiday weekend will be busier than usual, then more pharmacists and support help are scheduled to work. If the prediction is wrong and the demand is not as high as was predicted, then the pharmacy overspends and cuts into profitability. Sometimes the influence of this error on profitability can be offset by having the "extra" staff perform tasks that could help increase efficiency at other times—for example, pull outdated drugs off the shelves and return them for credit. If the demand is in excess of what was predicted, this is no less problematic. In this case, the staff is overworked, patients wait a long time to have their prescriptions filled with the potential of harming customer relations, and the likelihood of mistakes may increase. This inefficiency can also lead to job dissatisfaction for the personnel involved. If the prediction is right, then the demand is met efficiently.

Another scheduling strategy is called *level scheduling* (Heizer and Render, 1999). This strategy is used to provide a level amount of production so that a constant workforce can be employed to handle the demand day after day and week after week. This method is employed more easily in the creation of goods where the business can create surplus in times of low demand. For example, an institutional pharmacy can compound a constant number of intravenous solutions that are used commonly in the hospital. The demand for the solutions will change over the course of the day or the week, but as long as the supply produced does not grow too small (so that the pharmacy runs out) or too large (so that the prepared solutions start to expire before they are used), this strategy can be employed effectively. This is not as easily employed in a service such as filling prescriptions. Through marketing and technology, however, a pharmacy may be able to encourage its customers to call in prescription refills during off-peak hours and even to come in at a particular time in an attempt to level off the demand across the course of the day. By lining up the prescription refill dates and contacting patients before refills are due, the pharmacy will be able to schedule the refilling of prescriptions, schedule the delivery of inventory, and schedule the other resources necessary to handle the demand. All these strategies rely on having a good estimate of demand.

Demand can be estimated using *forecasting*. "Forecasting is a necessary prerequisite for many of the methods and procedures used in operations management" (Lewis, 1981, p. 241). Forecasting demand for goods and services requires the use of information, mathematical functions, and statistical analyses.

Equally important as personnel scheduling is the scheduling of the resources used to create goods and provide services. In community and institutional pharmacy settings, the scheduling of product delivery is important. Ideally, the goods will be sitting on the shelves where they can be accessed efficiently when the orders for prescriptions come in. Scheduling of the delivery of these orders so that they come in at times when the demand is not at its peak will ensure that staff members are available to put the inventory in its proper place. Some businesses go so far as to schedule delivery and restocking of shelves at night when the store is either closed or not busy. To schedule deliveries in a manner that helps pharmacies to be efficient requires relationships with suppliers.

▥ SUPPLY-CHAIN MANAGEMENT

The *supply chain* is the chain of businesses that supply pharmacies with necessary inputs. It is important to build relationships and have agreements with other companies that will maximize the efficiency of receiving the goods needed to fill prescriptions. Wholesalers are the primary vendors for pharmacies (Lobb et al., 2002). They distribute the majority of prescription drugs in the United States. Some chain pharmacies receive goods from distributors that they own and also have relationships with wholesalers. This is done so that they can get goods that may not be available from their own distributors or so that they can get goods quickly if the wholesaler delivers more frequently than their own distributors. These relationships need to be established with reputable companies that can provide reliable service particularly in times of need, such as during natural disasters. These relationships can take different forms and entail different levels of service. By signing a contract with a pharmacy, a wholesaler agrees to provide the pharmacy with products and services that may help the pharmacy to operate efficiently. These services can include electronic order submission, next-day delivery service, private-label programs, co-operative advertising programs, special-handling services, pharmacy computer systems, pricing, and store

planning. Management of the supply chain is of great importance in the creation of goods or the provision of services that involve goods. The key elements of the decision in choosing suppliers for the pharmacy are the timely delivery of needed and properly stored medications by a licensed and reputable wholesaler at the best price. In making this decision, there are a number of wholesalers from which to choose.

According to the Healthcare Distribution Management Association (HDMA—formerly the National Wholesale Druggists' Association), there are thousands of wholesalers. Fewer than a half dozen are responsible for a majority of sales. These full-line or full-service wholesalers obtain medications directly from the manufacturers and distribute the medications to pharmacies (both independent and chains), institutions, and other wholesalers. Some chain pharmacies have regional or local distribution centers that receive medications from the wholesaler in large quantities and repackage the medications into package sizes that are more feasible at the store level.

Large, full-service wholesalers are only one type of wholesaler available to supply pharmacies and other health care institutions with medications. There are also regional wholesalers, smaller wholesalers, and secondary wholesalers (Eastern Research Group, 2001). The main distinguishing features of the different types of wholesalers include services provided, their authorization status according to the Prescription Drug Marketing Act (21 CFR Parts 203 and 205), and their sales volume. Under strict interpretation of 21 CFR Parts 203 and 205, only the large, full-service wholesalers are authorized. This designation is reserved for distributors who have formal, written distribution contracts with the manufacturers and conduct more than two transactions with the manufacturers in any 24-month period of time. The other types of wholesalers may conduct business with the manufacturers and do not have formal, written distribution contracts. If not authorized, they must provide documentation of the products' pedigree as stipulated in 21 CFR Part 203.

Different types of wholesalers may be used to meet different needs within the pharmacy. For example, one wholesaler may offer a better delivery schedule, a more efficient service, or better pricing. Additionally, the smaller and secondary wholesalers may not be able to meet all the needs of a pharmacy with regard to product line and in times of emergency. Once the inputs are obtained from suppliers, managing the inventory of those goods is important in a pharmacy.

INVENTORY MANAGEMENT

Inventory is the largest expense that a community pharmacy has (as measured as a percentage of sales) (West, 2002). This makes the management of inventory particularly important to a pharmacy. Too much inventory is seen as money sitting on the shelf, and too little causes inefficiency in the system. Imagine a scenario in which you are paid on a weekly basis. You go the grocery store to buy food. Would you buy all the milk that you would need to get through the entire month? Probably not, because it might go sour before you use it, and why would you spend money to buy all that milk when you are probably going to get paid again before you need to buy milk again. You could use the money for something other than for milk that is going to sit on your shelf for a whole month. Now imagine similar situations with medications costing more than a gallon of milk. The management of inventory will receive more extensive treatment in Chapter 22, but it is important to see the connection between the operations used to provide goods and services and the efficient management of inventory. Having money sitting on the shelf in the form of inventory may prevent a pharmacy from being able to pay for other resources within the business. This inability to pay may cause the pharmacy to incur additional charges that then decrease the profitability of the business.

MAINTENANCE

Maintenance of the resources used to create goods and provide services must be provided, or the risk of resource failure in operations increases. It is easy to understand how the maintenance of a machine used to create goods could be linked directly to the efficiency of operations. If the machine breaks down and requires costly repairs, profitability suffers. The link to services is not quite as clear, but it is just as important. When you walk into a restaurant, do you want to eat at a dirty, wobbly table? The answer is most likely no. Patients do not want to buy goods that are covered with dust. They do not want to walk up to a counter to learn how to test their blood glucose level on a test device that has not been cleaned properly or that is not functioning properly. Maintenance of the areas in which services are provided will affect the satisfaction of patients and ultimately affect the patronage of the business for its offerings.

CONCLUSION

When Marie Lassiter walked into the pharmacy to have her prescription filled, it is not likely that she considered the multitude of resources that had been assembled to provide her with that service. She is not likely to appreciate the complexity of operations that go into providing her with that service, and Marie does not necessarily have to know, ever. Pharmacists, particularly those in positions to make operations decisions, not only need to be aware of these issues, but they also stand to be more profitable by knowing how to analyze these issues and manage them effectively.

QUESTIONS FOR FURTHER DISCUSSION

1. Are the following business outputs goods or services?
   a. Filling a prescription
   b. Compounding a prescription
   c. Selling OTC medications
   d. Helping a patient to understand how to manage his illness
   e. Helping a patient to understand how to take her medication
2. How does one choose whether to offer a product or service when it has the potential to be profitable

but might be harmful to the health of the patients (e.g., selling alcohol or tobacco)?

3. Think about filling a prescription as being a service. How does a pharmacist add value? How has the product been changed by the pharmacy?

4. Categorize the services provided by a community pharmacy into the following three categories—customer service, product service, and service product.

5. List the personnel who play a role in the profitability of a community pharmacy.

6. List the personnel who play a role in the profitability of an institutional pharmacy.

■ SMALL GROUP DISCUSSION TOPICS

1. Consider the following scenario in an institutional setting. Develop a process diagram for the following scenario. What are the key resources used in each step of the process? What operations management opportunities to do you see?

> Marie is not feeling well, and on examination by her physician, she is admitted to the local hospital. The physician stops by and orders some prescriptions for Marie. He writes an order for the prescriptions on a duplicate form. One is placed in a bin and picked up by a pharmacy technician; the other is placed in Marie's chart. Once the order arrives at the pharmacy, a pharmacist enters the order into the computer, and the medication is pulled from inventory to be sent to the floor on the next round of floor deliveries. The next day, this order for Marie's medications, along with all the other medication orders for the patients in the hospital, is printed so that a cart can be filled with that day's medications. A technician fills the bins in the cart, and a pharmacist checks the filled bins. After the bins are checked, the cart is delivered to the floor. That afternoon the clinical pharmacist visits

Marie in her room to go over the medications that she is receiving.

2. The scenario in the chapter is illustrative of the inputs and outputs consumed and managed when filling a compounded prescription. What are the resources and outcomes that might be associated with providing a disease-state management service to diabetic patients? Can each of these be managed? Prioritize them based on which inputs add the most value to the output of this service. How did you decide which had the most value?

3. Pick a disease-state management service. Develop a process diagram for this service. What stages of this process do you expect to create bottlenecks? What resources would be necessary in each step of the process?

REFERENCES

Brax S. 2005. A manufacturer becoming service provider: Challenges and a paradox. *Manag Service Qual* 15:142–55.

Bruner RF, Eaker MR, Freeman, RE, et al. 1998. Operations management: Implementing and enabling strategy. In *The Portable MBA,* p. 125. New York: Wiley.

Eastern Research Group, Inc. 2001. Profile of the Prescription Drug Wholesaling Industry: Examination of Entities Defining Supply and Demand in Drug Distribution. Final Report. Task Order No. 13; Contract No. 223-98-8002. Rockville, MD: Food and Drug Administration, www.fda.gov/oc/pdma/report2001/attachmentg/toc.html.

Heizer J, Render B. 1999. *Operations Management,* 5th ed. Upper Saddle River, NJ: Prentice-Hall.

Johnson R. 1998. *Managing Operations.* Boston: Butterworth Heinemann.

Kotler P, Keller KL. 2006. *Marketing Management,* 12th ed. Upper Saddle River, NJ: Pearson Prentice-Hall.

Lewis CD. 1981. Forecasting. In Lewis CD (ed), *Operations Management in Practice.* New York: Wiley.

Lobb W, Shah M, Bonnarens J, Wilkin NE. 2002. Contributions to buyers. *J Pharm Market Manag* 14:87.

Mantel SJ, Evans JR. 1992. *Operations Management for Pharmacists: Strategy and Tactics.* Cincinnati, OH: Institute for Community Pharmacy Management.

Mathieu, V. 2001. Service strategies within the manufacturing sector: Benefits, costs and partnership. *Int J Serv Indus Manag* 12:451–75.

Mudie P, Cottam A. 1999. Service quality. In *The Management and Marketing of Services,* 2d ed. Boston: Butterworth Heinemann.

Robson GD. 1991. *Continuous Process Improvement.* New York: Free Press.

Vargo SL, Lusch RF. 2004. The four service marketing myths: Remnants of a goods-based, manufacturing model. *J Serv Res* 6:324.

West D, ed. 2002. *NCPA Pharmacia Digest.* Alexandria, VA: National Community Pharmacists Association.

Wilkin NE. 2006. *Profiles of Innovation in Community Pharmacy: Final Report.* Alexandria, VA: National Community Pharmacists Association.

SUGGESTED READINGS

Bassett G. 1992. *Operations Management for Service Industries: Competing in the Service Era.* Westport, CT: Quorum Books.

Greasley A. 1999. *Operations Management in Business.* Cheltenham, Glos, Great Britain: Stanley Thornes.

Vondle DP. 1989. *Service Management Systems.* New York: McGraw-Hill.

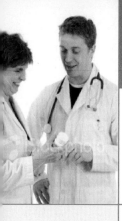

6

MANAGING TECHNOLOGY AND PHARMACY INFORMATION SYSTEMS

Margaret R. Thrower and Bill G. Felkey

About the Authors: Dr. Thrower is Regional Clinical Coordinator for McKesson Medication Management. She received a B.S. in biology from Southeast Missouri State University and a B.S. and postbaccalaureate Pharm.D. at St. Louis College of Pharmacy in 2001. She completed a postdoctoral specialty residency in drug informatics with DrugDigest.org, Express Scripts, Inc., and the St. Louis College of Pharmacy.

Mr. Felkey is Professor of Pharmacy Care Systems at the Harrison School of Pharmacy at Auburn University. Professor Felkey received a B.A. in psychology and communication through media (dual major) from the University of Maine in 1975 and an M.S. in instructional systems technology from Indiana University in 1977. He is an internationally recognized resource for the information and computer industry, health systems, pharmacy organizations, and the pharmaceutical industry, having authored over 1,100 presentations and publications. He is the Founding Editor of *Computer Medicine for the Hospital Pharmacist*. He earned the Professor the Year Award and the Outreach Award for Excellence at Auburn University in addition to numerous national and international accolades.

▪ LEARNING OBJECTIVES

After completing this chapter, students should be able to

1. Understand the importance of technology and automation in managing the information that pharmacists use in practice.
2. Identify technology needs and a process that can be used for selecting appropriate vendors for technology products.
3. Identify key components of pharmacy support technology.
4. Identify the roles of technology at the point of care.
5. Describe the functions and purposes of the Internet that facilitate management of a pharmacy care practice.
6. Understand the need for and evaluation of information on the Internet.
7. Evaluate the need for technology and automation in the practice of pharmacy.
8. Understand the importance of integration in systems used in the practice of pharmacy.

▩ SCENARIO

Jennifer Russo completed the doctor of pharmacy curriculum and then went on to complete a pharmacy practice residency and a specialty residency in infectious disease. She has just accepted a position as a clinical specialist with a large teaching hospital. She took this particular job because she wanted to have a direct impact on appropriate medication use to improve patient outcomes through educating physicians and other prescribers. Her primary responsibility is to implement an antimicrobial stewardship program in collaboration with the chief of infectious disease. She writes orders to obtain cultures and sensitivities to antibiotics, makes recommendations on appropriate drug and dose, educates physicians on appropriate drug use, and writes orders for dosage adjustments for patients in the institution. She also oversees the charging of patients and maintains an inventory of the drugs used. To accomplish these tasks effectively, she must bounce back and forth between five different computer systems. One system houses data on laboratory levels, another is used for hospital billing, and a third has a drug inventory database. She has a pharmacokinetic software program that assists her in calculating doses and estimating frequency intervals for obtaining the next drug level and also contains a drug information database. She then must enter data from these four systems into a pharmacy-based system that the central pharmacy uses for patient management. Relevant data then are extracted from this application and housed on a health information exchange (HIE) repository that enables other providers who see this patient to have pharmacy information available for decision making. She spends hours per day accessing and collecting data from the various databases and even more time entering orders and combining data from the different sources into the central pharmacy's database. After a couple of weeks, Jennifer becomes frustrated and feels that she did not go to pharmacy school to spend most of her time collecting and processing data. She is exasperated and blurts out to the pharmacy director, "There has got to be an easier way!"

▩ CHAPTER QUESTIONS

1. How has the use of technology changed the practice of pharmacy?
2. How have pharmacists' roles in delivering pharmaceutical goods and services evolved over the past few decades?
3. What role does technology play in the management of information?
4. How can the pressure of increased prescription volume be balanced with the increased focus on patient care and access to patient information necessary to providing pharmaceutical care?
5. How has the Internet and e-commerce affected the practice of pharmacy?
6. What is the importance of systems integration among the technologies used in pharmacy practice?
7. What are the main barriers to the use of technology by pharmacy employees?

▩ TECHNOLOGY IS ESSENTIAL TO MANAGING DATA AND OPERATIONS

Historically, adoption and investment in information systems in health care have lagged significantly behind those in other industries. However, the gap is narrowing. This is evidenced by the fact that in 1999, 46 percent of hospitals still used handwritten medication administration records (MARs), but this had decreased to 24 percent in 2005 (Pedersen, 2006). However, there is still considerable opportunity because implementation of electronic MARs has replaced handwritten and printed MARs in approximately 20 percent of hospitals. (Sandborn, 2007). Effective management of even moderately sized pharmacy operations quickly can exceed the capacity of the unaided human mind. Therefore, technology must be used appropriately in a systems approach that is designed to support the operation of a pharmacy. Pharmacists need to become knowledgeable users of the technology available. They need to understand both the capabilities and limitations of technology. This chapter will focus on technology concepts, skills, and attitudes that pharmacists must acquire to become effective information managers. Information is the common denominator in all health care systems, disciplines, and specialties today.

Managing the increasingly vast amount of information available to health care practitioners can be challenging. Primary literature continues to grow very quickly, with over 20,000 biomedical journals published annually (Lowe and Barnett, 1994). To keep up with this massive amount of information, an individual would need to read 6,000 articles each day (Arndt, 1992). In addition to the large amount of published medical information, pharmacists must manage large numbers of patient profiles containing information about disease states and medications. On a given day, community pharmacists typically access hundreds of the thousand to tens of thousands of patient profiles managed by their pharmacies. Similarly, it is not uncommon for a hospital patient to have his or her record amended with dozens of medication-related orders in just a day or two. An appropriate information management system needs to be employed through the adoption and diffusion of technology.

For the purposes of this chapter, *technology* is defined as "anything that replaces routine or repetitive tasks that were previously performed by people or which extends (or enhances) the capability of people to do their work" (Rough, 2001, p. 85). The term *automation* refers to "any technology, device or machine that is linked to or controlled by a computer and used to actually do work that was previously done by humans" (Rough, 2001, p. 85). It is important to appreciate this difference right from the start and to keep in mind that all automation is technology, but the reverse is not necessarily true. In addition to distinguishing between technology and automation, some cursory knowledge of data processing is a necessary prerequisite to understanding the impact of technology on pharmacy practice.

LEVELS OF DATA PROCESSING

Computers use many levels of data processing in the day-to-day operations of a pharmacy. The simplest level

of data processing is called *transaction processing.* Accepting payment for a prescription would constitute a single transaction. Processing a prescription from receipt to dispensing involves several transactions. The next level of data processing is *management information systems.* Data processing at this level groups transactions into meaningful sets. This allows administrators the ability to identify trends that predict the success of the organization. Additionally, the management information systems level can aid in determining appropriate needs for such things as staffing hours, inventory management, and third-party reimbursement. *Decision support,* the next level of data processing, occurs when the computer functions to provide support while transactions are occurring. An example of decision support would be drug utilization review (DUR) modules that alert pharmacists to potential drug-related problems while they are filling a prescription or medication order. Currently, the highest level of data processing uses *artificial intelligence* and/or *expert systems.* Expert systems can be used to help guide caregivers through complex therapy decisions or even to help providers determine when patients diagnosed with a terminal condition lack a high enough quality of life to justify continuing extraordinary life-support systems. An expert system is a program that can use a set of given rules to make decisions. Expert systems consist of a knowledge base and an inference engine. The objective of an expert system such as an electrocardiogram (ECG) diagnostic program or a drug formulary product selection program is to collect the rules and knowledge human experts employ in the knowledge base so that diagnosing or selecting would occur in a highly consistent and reliable manner.

HARDWARE

The term *hardware* encompasses computer equipment used to perform input, processing, and output activities. An increased understanding of how computers perform data processing functions can be achieved by a basic understanding of both the visible and invisible hardware that is necessary for a computer to operate individually or within a network of computers. Visible hardware includes things that one can see when walking into a work area, such as mainframe computers, servers, workstations, and dispensing devices. Many hardware systems are located "behind the scenes," including networks that connect two or more workstations, routers that pass information along on a network, gateways, and switches. Additional peripheral hardware that is used specifically in a pharmacy operation can include document and barcode scanners, robotics, and high-quality laser printers.

■ SOFTWARE

Dispensing and Drug Utilization Review

Software is available in two major categories: operation systems and application software. Every hardware system must employ an operation system software to control the operation of the devices contained in the system. The software that makes up all the applications that users employ to actually do their work makes up the second category of software. Software used to manage the drug dispensing and distribution process is an example of an application software and has been in existence since the 1970s. In addition to storing prescription information, maintaining patient profiles, and monitoring inventory levels, distribution-related software also includes DUR functions that aid pharmacists by providing messages alerting them of potential drug-related problems while filling prescriptions. First DataBank, a provider of electronic drug information, supplies knowledge bases for integration into health care applications. The modules listed in Table 6-1 incorporate clinical decision support and are a subset of available content for licensing to pharmacy information systems vendors to use within their software applications, such as DUR and pharmaceutical dispensing.

Pharmaceutical Care Software

Clinical information systems that stand alone or do not integrate into other systems are common in clinical pharmacy practice. They may involve pharmacists manually entering patient-specific data for use in managing patients' pharmacotherapy (Felkey, 1997). *Point-*

of-care software may be defined as "software used at the place where a pharmacist provides pharmaceutical care to a patient or when assisting a colleague (pharmacist, physician, or nurse) in providing care to patients." Clinical pharmacy software should be integrated with all other aspects of a pharmacy, including management and distribution programs, to ensure that care can be coordinated fully (Felkey and Fox, 2003a). Pharmacy management systems, such as Etreby, QS/1, and PDX, which are primarily pharmacy distribution systems, have added the necessary screens and resources to do pharmaceutical care management. Other companies, such as CarePoint, started their products as pharmaceutical care programs and then later added the pharmacy management system attributes to support distribution.

■ POINT-OF-CARE DEVICES

The use of point-of-care technologies allows health care professionals to be more effective and efficient in everyday practice. Point-of-care devices include, but are not limited to, notebook computers, desktops, and personal digital assistants (PDAs). To be useful to the practitioner, the computer should contain patient-oriented drug information, including appropriate mixtures of tertiary, secondary, and primary literature references on pharmacy and medical topics. These devices can use Internet access to retrieve patient-specific data from remote databases. This helps to integrate available data that are generated as a by-product of rendering patient care into data warehouses and clinical data repositories. These data warehouses then are able to populate decision-support applications at the point of care and reduce pharmacists' uncertainty during decision making. Data warehouses collect information such as patient demographics, diagnostic information, adverse drug reactions and drug allergies, laboratory results, and drug profiles to make them available for use by clinical decision makers.

Wireless networks afford health care professionals greater flexibility to render patient care because they allow care to be moved to patients instead of having to bring patients to the care. PDAs are used to interface with wireless networks, which makes delivery of

Table 6-1. Sample of Modules Available for Licensing to Pharmacy Information System Developers from First Data Bank

- *Dosage Range Check Module* Identification of safe dosage levels and frequency of administration based on patient-specific parameters.
- *Drug Allergy Module* Identification of potential allergic reactions and cross-sensitivities between drugs and specific patient-known allergens.
- *Drug Images Module* High-resolution digital images of prescription and OTC products for visual verification of correct dispensing and administration.
- *Drug Imprints Module* Physical descriptions of over 30,000 prescription and OTC products for correct dispensing and administration.
- *Drug Indications Module* Identification of all drug products available to treat a specific condition.
- *Drug Precautions Modules* Minimization of potential contraindications between drug use, medical conditions, age (pediatric and geriatric), pregnancy, and lactation. Includes Pediatric Precautions Module, Geriatric Precautions Module, Pregnancy Precautions Module, and Lactation Precautions Module.
- *Drug–Alternative Therapy Interactions* Alerts of drug interactions with herbals, dietary supplements, and other alternative-therapy agents.
- *Drug–Disease Contraindications Module* Assessment of drug use in patients who have specific diseases or health-related conditions or who have had certain procedures or diagnostic tests.
- *Drug–Drug Interaction Module* Alerts to help prevent harmful drug–drug interactions; reports only drug interactions that are clinically significant. Full-text monographs for professionals included.
- *Duplicate Therapy Module* Accurate, timely alerts to potential duplications of drug therapy, drug ingredients, and prescription refills.
- *Intravenous Compatibility Module* Data for automatic screening of physiochemical compatibility and incompatibility of IV preparations.
- *MedTeach Monographs* Database of detailed patient education information that allows health care professionals to offer patients easy-to-use written instructions on drug therapy.
- *Prescriber Order-Entry Module* Common dosage order database of standardized inpatient and outpatient medication orders, ready for integration into providers' order-entry or prescription-writing systems; helps prevent prescribing errors.
- *Side-Effects Module* Decision-support tool to quickly identify and monitor side effects.

information at the time it is most needed much more feasible (Felkey and Fox, 2003b).

Programs that are updated frequently, even daily, are available, and they can be put onto a PDA to give pharmacists access to the most up-to-date information. Clinical evaluation of the new PDA drug information programs has begun but is complicated by the constant updating of databases and the lack of a certification board. However, evaluations are useful for the publishers of these programs because they provide valuable feedback and have the potential to improve the quality of drug information.

ePocrates RxPro is a software program that is available for PDAs that contains comprehensive drug information, including alternative medicines and infectious diseases (Fig. 6-1). It is updated on a daily basis. One helpful advantage of this software is that it includes region-specific formulary information to aid clinicians in selecting a product that is covered by the patient's insurance. LexiComp Platinum (Fig. 6-2) is another

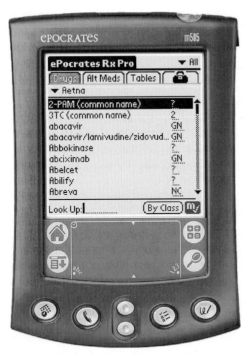

Figure 6-1. Screen shot of ePocrates RxPro software for PDAs.

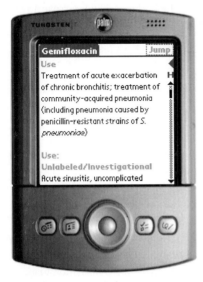

Figure 6-2. Screen shot of LexiComp Platinum software for PDAs.

comprehensive program available for PDA download and in one evaluation was named the "most clinically dependable" and was cited as offering the "greatest breadth of information" of the programs evaluated (Enders, Enders, and Holstad, 2002). Monographs that are of higher quality than most pharmacy management systems provide can be printed at the point of care and are available through the Micromedex electronic package of products.

Over 26,000 health and medication sites exist on the World Wide Web. DrugDigest.org is an evidence-based Web site for consumers that contains a comprehensive drug database and aims to empower consumers by providing nonbiased drug and health information. Unique to this site are drug–drug comparisons, side-effect comparisons, and a drug-interaction checker that is written in consumer language. In addition, the site has streaming video to instruct patients on the proper administration of insulin and eye and ear drops and the proper use of inhalers.

There is technology emerging that could facilitate provider reimbursement for dispensing what has been described as "prescription-strength information" (Kemper, 2002, p. 116) or information resources that can be "prescribed" for patients. These resources can be used to motivate patients to pursue and manage their own care. It is possible to equip patients with self-care management information to help them determine when professional care is needed and how to self-treat simple injuries and maladies. Patients traditionally have depended on learned health professionals to sort out what is important for them to know and in what sequence they should perform changes in their health behaviors. Thus, dispensing information of this sort some day may become reimbursable.

■ SELECTION PROCESS

It is important that pharmacy and the pharmacy director be involved in the selection and implementation process, even though in reality sometimes information system (IS) decisions are made at the health system level (Sanborn, 2007). The responsibility of fully realizing the benefits remains an important key to success and should not be overlooked after selection of the appropriate system (Clark, 1999). The addition of new technology for a pharmacy organization is a considerable investment in time and money and may be relatively long term. The selection of new technology may not be reversible and thus is a critical decision not to be taken lightly. The process used for selecting new technology should not be initiated until an organization determines what the technology needs to accomplish. The organization should answer the following specific questions prior to selection/addition of new automation/technology (Lewis, Albrant, and Hagel, 2002):

- *What do we need it to do?* The purpose of the new technology should be clearly identified by the organization.
- *Will it do what we think it can do?* The new automation/technology needs to function up to the expectations of the organization.
- *Do we need it?* The new automation/technology should be clearly advantageous for the organization to incorporate it and not simply technology for technology's sake.
- *What is the cost-benefit ratio or return on investment?* There should be a clear advantage in terms of cost benefit and return on investment (ROI). For example, an investment of $100,000 in technology that generates an additional profit of $40,000 for a year would have a return on investment or an annualized ROI of 40 percent. If this rate continues over time, the initial investment would be recouped in 2.5 years.
- *Is it affordable?* To answer this question, the organization's strategic plan and capital budget should be consulted.
- *What is its expected longevity?* Technology requires continuous updating and soon becomes obsolete; therefore, one must take a realistic approach when considering how long the technology will last.
- *What kind of support will be needed? What is the cost of these services?* It is important for the potential client to inquire about the type and cost of support services the vendor has to offer.

- *What kind of regular maintenance will be needed?* The cost of regular maintenance and how often it is needed are important considerations when implementing new automation/technology.
- *Will staff and patients accept this change?* If staff members do not accept this change in technology, they will not want to use it. Training programs can help to overcome this barrier.
- *Is the system adaptable?* For example, can the capacity of the system be increased as needed?

Many organizations realize that they do not have adequate time to build their own systems to address organizational needs. These organizations therefore must go through a technology selection process. The decision to partner with IS companies should be taken very seriously. *Due diligence* is the term given the process where purchasers assure themselves of the benefits of the technology and the vendor's financial stability. Whenever a new technology is being considered, it is recommended that organizations determine where they are going with a proposed change before they begin a selection process. In this way, the technology will be selected based on its ability to help achieve organizational goals. Technology is a tool that should be adapted to organizations rather than the reverse (see Chapters 3 and 4 on planning).

Security and HIPAA Compliance Considerations

A survey conducted by the Medical Records Institute in 2002 on health care practitioners' concerns with the implementation of mobile technology devices and applications cited security/confidentiality when sending or receiving information and the lack of Health Information Portability and Accountability Act (HIPAA) compliance as primary concerns by 50 and 34 percent of respondents, respectively. Confidentiality and security of information against unauthorized access must be HIPAA-compliant. A number of systems are available that can help a pharmacy organization to remain in compliance with HIPAA regulations. Pharmacists are required by law to use reasonable methods to ensure that protected health information remains confidential. From a technology standpoint, firewalls, which usually are delivered as combinations of hardware and software, should be used to protect computer systems from undesirable access. Firewalls do this by requiring users to be authenticated in their level of allowable access to the system. A firewall may allow public access to a limited set of information while restricting any access to patient information unless an authorized user with an appropriate password from a known location is making the attempt.

Technology that digitally captures patient signatures, encryption software, and telecommunication all may be necessary to protect the privacy of patients and the security of pharmacy data. Pharmacists also must ensure that affiliated businesses are using proper procedures to protect any information they handle on behalf of the pharmacy. Even transactions necessary for the business functions of a pharmacy must be secure to protect patient identity.

Documentation Is a Must!

In pharmacy, it is often said, "If it isn't documented, it didn't happen." With this in mind, it is easy to understand the importance of a system that is conducive to and promotes documentation. There is a need to build or select systems in which documentation is offered as a by-product of the transactions performed by professionals. Ideally, the system should anticipate and prepopulate documentation forms. Documentation is an absolute must in any well-designed information system, and therefore, a system should not even be considered unless it promotes efficient documentation.

The Vendor as a Selection Criterion

When selecting from a choice of software products, the director of pharmacy should consider the products' vendors. The company's good reputation and its ability to provide referrals from former and existing clients are essential. Installation planning should be suitable for the organization's needs yet realistic for the vendor. While the vendor is responsible for system design, much of the installation, education, and training of employees will fall on the shoulders of the pharmacy department.

Acquisition cost of the system itself can be significant, but it represents, in many cases, only a relatively small percent of the total system cost over time. Many factors in addition to the acquisition cost of the system need to be considered, such as the costs of software updates, hardware maintenance, service contracts, and claims processing (Lewis, Albrant, and Hagel, 2002). Table 6-2 provides a checklist of items that a pharmacy should consider when selecting software and software vendors (Felkey and Fox, 2003b).

Resources to Obtain Necessary Data in the Selection Process

The list of considerations in Table 6-2 is extensive. One can become bogged down in the selection process without a firm grasp of where to seek this information. Directors of pharmacy can employ several resources to

---

Table 6-2. Things to Consider When Selecting Software and Software Vendors

- Identification of vendors being considered
- Evaluation of service offered
- Cost of the system
- Details of installation
- Vendor ability to personalize the technology to meet goals
- Identification of safety and quality assurance features
- Integration with other existing clinical information systems, Internet, managed care, and other existing information systems
- Identification of specialized features that distinguish one system from another
- Appropriate security features (must be HIPPA-compliant)
- Determination of the frequency of system upgrades
- Supplemental equipment needed for the system to function optimally and the cost
- Supplies needed (e.g., special paper, vials, barcoding, labels)
- Provision of employee education and training

obtain the necessary data, such as direct contact with the vendor, contact with current and previous clients of the vendor, evaluation reports on selected technologies, consultants, and the Internet. The Internet can be used to seek feedback on products. Most vendors have information about their product available on the Internet; therefore, research and retrieval are made much easier. If specific information is not included on the Web site, then the vendor can be contacted for further clarification/information. A credible and knowledgeable consultant who specializes in health care technology and, more specifically, in pharmacy technology can offer advantages by doing some of this time-consuming research. The pharmacy manager or director may check with colleagues to see if they have used a consultant and ask them if they would work with that consultant again if given the chance, or consultants may be located via the Internet. Another option would be to visit clients of vendors under consideration to determine if they are satisfied with the vendor's product and service and whether, if given the choice, they would invest with the same vendor again.

■ MAINTENANCE

After the system has been implemented, there is need for ongoing maintenance, and this can often be done by the IS department and the vendor. However, optimization of the technology often depends on the pharmacy department to work with both parties for the technology to be optimized. This is an often underrecognized area and should occur in an ongoing fashion because it is critical to patient safety (Sanborn, 2007).

Maintenance by the Vendor

Regardless of the age or cost of information and hardware systems, all require some form of maintenance. Maintenance involves updating, changing, or improving the existing system. The goal is to continually improve the system's functionality and usability while minimizing the time that it is nonoperational (downtime). Ideally, information systems should require only minor or routinely scheduled maintenance. There are two kinds of maintenance or downtime: scheduled

and unscheduled. *Scheduled downtime* is performed routinely to prevent major system failures that could cause serious interruptions in workflow. Developers of critical systems try to build in levels of redundancy and fail-safe system monitors to reduce unscheduled downtime. *Unscheduled downtime* occurs when a system is not operational and the downtime was not planned.

Most software and hardware companies offer technical support for their products. Technical support usually involves highly trained individuals that update, fix, or change existing hardware and software products. Older programs generally require more expensive and time-consuming modifications and hardware replacements. Newer products continue to improve, and thus maintenance costs should decline (Stair, 1996). Investing money upfront on quality information systems and well-designed programs should pay off in the end.

User-Performed Maintenance and Upkeep

Some maintenance or upkeep will be performed on a routine basis by the vendor and/or IS department. In addition to routine maintenance, including cleaning of equipment and changing of printer toner cartridges, some pharmacy information systems still depend on data cartridges to store valuable data. For example, pharmacists using data cartridges exchange them daily to avoid losing valuable patient-specific data. Loss of data, which includes medication history, allergies, and refill information, may compromise patient safety. There is no way to estimate the time it would take for a pharmacist to reconstruct profiles and gather missing information that would need to be entered manually into an information system.

Systems Integration

The complexity of existing information systems makes system integration difficult. This is further complicated by the general lack of standards in the information technology field. "What is an integrated system?" is a common question in the health care field. Complete integration involves integration from order entry [e.g., computerized physician order entry (CPOE)] to distribution of medication to billing and inventory. An integrated system can consist of a single system or multiple systems that transfer, manipulate, and use information seamlessly across the entire enterprise.

It was reported by the Institute for Safe Medication Practices (ISMP) in 2000 that fewer than 5 percent of physicians were "writing" prescriptions electronically. In a 2000 white paper entitled, "A Call to Action: Eliminate Handwritten Prescriptions within 3 Years," ISMP recommended the use of electronic prescribing by clinician order entry to reduce medication errors (ISMP, 2000). CPOE can help to reduce errors in the delivery and transcribing of orders to the pharmacy where the orders are filled. Order management can be used to control inventory and alert pharmacy staff (and even the patient) of the status of a prescription. For example, some national chain pharmacies have the capability of alerting the patient by phone or e-mail if a prescription is ready or if other action needs to be taken before the prescription can be picked up. The system should also be able to report results, such as the number of prescriptions filled, the revenue generated over a specified time, and medication error reports.

An integral part of the integration process is documentation. The system should support and be conducive to the process of documentation on a patient's electronic medical record. The use of critical pathways and other tools to aid clinical decision support facilitates the use of evidence-based medicine and appropriate therapeutic use of medications. Access to patient-specific data such as drug allergies (e.g., anaphylaxis to penicillins) and laboratory values (e.g., kidney function or liver function) will help to minimize adverse drug reactions and maximize appropriate use of medications. The system should have Internet access or appropriate offline resources available on the organization's intranet to ensure that appropriate clinical literature and drug information resources can be consulted when needed and evidence then can be placed in the electronic medical record (EMR), which is a subset and data contributor to the electronic health record (EHR). The data in the EMR is the legal record of what happened to the patient during his or her encounter with a provider, and the EHR is owned by the patient and can even include patient input and access that spans episodes of care across multiple providers within a community, region, or state (or, in some instances, countries). EHRs are reliant on EMRs being in place, and EMRs will never reach their full potential without interconnected EHRs being in place (Garets and Davis, 2006).

EMRs versus EHRs

The EMR is increasingly a part of the pharmacist's practice in every practice setting.

▪ ACCEPTANCE OF NEW TECHNOLOGY BY EMPLOYEES

Prior to a new system being implemented, careful planning and design must occur. This planning needs to include all relevant potential users of the new technology, including clinicians, staff pharmacists, patients, and other departments that will be affected by the system. Determining the resources necessary for implementation is key to the success of the new system (Sanborn, 2007). No matter what their level of computer skills, employees must see personal advantage to want to use the technology. For instance, they must believe that the technology will provide some benefit to them, such as increased efficiency. Training programs regarding purpose and proper use of new technologies/information systems are critical for gaining acceptance by employees. Implementation of new technologies should be gradual. Tulley (2000) reported that the Davies Program (instrumental in the study of computer-based patient records) identified response time, reliability, and ease of use as critical technology requirements for end users. Thus pharmacy managers/directors must be adept at managing change, allowing input from employees in the selection and implementation of new technologies. They must be empathic to employee concerns about switching technologies yet firm about the need to do so. Managers must train employees properly on the use of the new technology and allow some transition time between the preexisting and new technology.

OFFLINE, ONLINE, INTRANET, INTERNET, WEB PRESENCE, EXTRANET, AND E-COMMERCE

Internet

Enhancements to pharmacy practice made possible by the Internet can be expressed in terms of the three C's: content, communication, and commerce (Felkey and Fox, 2001). In the widely known book, *Internet for Dummies,* the Internet is defined as "all of the computers in the world talking to all of the other computers in the world" (Levine, Bauroudi, and Levine, 1996). Use of the Internet for health care purposes is growing exponentially, with well over 200 countries connected globally.

Internet Content

Thousands of Web sites are available to assist health care professionals in providing drug information useful in pharmaceutical care. One source reported that by the end of 2002, almost 93 million Americans (which equals about 80 percent of adult Internet users) had used the Internet to look for health information (Fox and Fallows, 2003). Owing to the fact that anyone (regardless of educational background or credentials) can post a Web site, the reliability and validity of health care information on the Internet vary widely. Hence pharmacists must have skills to evaluate the usefulness, accuracy, and quality of the information available. Table 6-3 identifies characteristics of credible, reliable information and appropriate criteria for evaluating the quality of Internet sites, respectively.

Many medical and pharmacy information resources can be accessed efficiently via the Internet (including information that can be used at the point of care), such as practice guidelines, tertiary references, and governmental/regulatory information. High-quality graphics are plentiful on the Internet and can benefit pharmacists in both patient education and preparation of presentations. Using multimedia resources with patients should improve their retention and

---

Table 6-3. **Things to Consider When Evaluating the Credibility of Internet Web Sites**

- *Ownership of the site.* Can help to determine if there may be a potential commercial bias.
- *Authors of the material.* Can help to determine credibility of information. This information should be readily available, commonly contained in the "About Us" section of the site. Sites having a qualified staff generally make it known because it is to their advantage to state their credentials and establish credibility with the user.
- *Review process.* Gives the user an idea of how meticulous the site is about its postings. It is preferable that site uses a peer-review process. For example, each document that is posted on the Web site goes through an editorial process of equally qualified persons, or peers (peer review).
- *Last update on each page clearly defined.* This will give the user an idea of how current the information is on the page.
- *Believable claims.* If it is not believable or cannot be validated by a reliable and credible source, the user should beware. As the old saying goes, "If it sounds too good to be true, it probably is."
- *Support for the information found.* If no other source confirms the information found on the site, the site may not be accurate.
- *Referencing of the information.* A good indicator for support of the information is the use of proper referencing on the Web site.

Source: Health on the Net Foundation Web site, www.hon.ch/; accessed on May 19, 2007.

comprehension of health education content. For example, a McGraw-Hill collection of over 150 video-based explanations of common conditions can illustrate visually what is actually happening physiologically during a disease process. Leaflets that contain illustrations and tell patients in a customized manner can equip them to be successful in their treatment regimens.

Internet Communication

E-mail has changed the way in which we communicate drastically. Many people now prefer to communicate via e-mail than by telephone or regular mail. Some patients e-mail questions to their health care providers and access information on consumer-oriented Web sites. E-mail communication may have the potential to improve compliance to medications. For example, some pharmacies provide reminders via e-mail when a chronic medication refill is almost due and a reminder when the prescription is filled and ready for pickup. The cost to send this kind of message is negligible, and the results can be positive both therapeutically and financially. Education can be provided on chronic disease states specific to the individual by electronic newsletters produced by the organization as an attempt at patient education. It is now possible to e-mail, phone, access the Internet, fax, and have pager capabilities all in one device. Videoconferencing can enable pharmacists to communicate with other colleagues and patients at a reasonably economical cost.

One problem with the use of e-mail is its potential lack of security. Employers legally own the e-mail that is delivered to their systems for use by employees. Many information technology (IT) departments routinely monitor e-mail traffic that could contain confidential information. If a pharmacist were to e-mail a patient at work to inform him or her that a refill medication was due, that patient's confidentiality could be compromised. Alternatively, if patients were told that new information is posted on their pharmacy's Web page, a browser would give them access to their confidential information behind a secure firewall, which could protect that information from unauthorized access.

Regulation and quality control of content on the Internet have been difficult, but some organizations have developed criteria for developing health Web sites. A Swiss organization called the Health On the Net (HON) Foundation has provided guidance in setting ethical standards for Web site developers. The mission of the HON Foundation is to guide consumers and health care practitioners to useful and reliable information regarding health and medications. The foundation has a "HON Code of Conduct" ("HONcode") for medical and health Web sites. This includes a set of eight principles that a site must possess before the HON emblem may be displayed on the Web site and a "SiteChecker" to help users determine whether a Web site is following the principles of the HONcode. Table 6-4 displays the ethical principles established by the HON Foundation for Internet-based health information. If the Web site meets criteria from a review process and is granted permission by the HON Foundation, it may display the HON logo.

Internet Commerce

An increasing number of pharmacies are switching to Internet-based prescription claims processing. Pharmacies are discovering that processing prescriptions over the Internet is both quicker and less expensive than dial-up or manual claims processing. E-commerce offers unlimited opportunity for pharmacies to increase visibility, and this opens a new avenue for additional sales. Independent pharmacies can offer personalized services via the Web, whereas chain pharmacies can increase efficiency by allowing online refills and housing a drug information database on their Web sites with consumer access. It is important for pharmacists to recognize that as they incorporate e-commerce into their practices, they must be cognizant of maintaining a personal relationship with their patients. The Internet may be best used by corporate chain pharmacies to refer patients to a bricks-and-mortar (physical) pharmacy when appropriate (Felkey and Fox, 2001a).

The National Association of Boards of Pharmacy (NABP) has recognized the special needs and problems that Internet pharmacy has created. In the spring of 1999, the Verified Internet Pharmacy Practice Sites

Table 6-4. HONcode's Ethical Principles for Internet-Based Health Information

1. *Authoritative.* Indicate the qualifications of the authors. Any medical or health advice provided and hosted on this site will only be given by medically trained and qualified professionals unless a clear statement is made that a piece of advice offered is from a non medically qualified individual or organization.
2. *Complementarity.* Information should support, not replace, the doctor–patient relationship. The information provided on this site is designed to support, not replace, the relationship that exists between a patient/site visitor and his or her existing physician.
3. *Privacy.* Respect the privacy and confidentiality of personal data submitted to the site by the visitor. Confidentiality of data relating to individual patients and visitors to a medical/health Web site, including their identity, is respected by this Web site. The Web site owners undertake to honor or exceed the legal requirements of medical/health information privacy that apply in the country and state where the Web site and mirror sites are located.
4. *Attribution.* Cite the source(s) of published information, date, and medical and health pages. Where appropriate, information contained on this site will be supported by clear references to source data and, where possible, have specific HTML links to those data. The date when a clinical page was last modified will be clearly displayed (e.g., at the bottom of the page).
5. *Justifiability.* Site must back up claims relating to benefits and performance. Any claims relating to the benefits/performance of a specific treatment, commercial product, or service will be supported by appropriate, balanced evidence in the manner outlined above in principle 4.
6. *Transparency.* Accessible presentation, accurate e-mail contact. The designers of this Web site will seek to provide information in the clearest possible manner and provide contact addresses for visitors who seek further information or support. The Webmaster will display his or her e-mail address clearly throughout the Web site.
7. *Financial disclosure.* Identify funding sources. Support for this Web site will be clearly identified, including the identities of commercial and noncommercial organisations that have contributed funding, services, or material for the site.
8. *Advertising policy.* Clearly distinguish advertising from editorial content. If advertising is a source of funding, it will be clearly stated. A brief description of the advertising policy adopted by the Web site owners will be displayed on the site. Advertising and other promotional material will be presented to viewers in a manner and context that facilitate differentiation between it and the original material created by the institution operating the site.

Source: Health on the Net Foundation, www.hon.ch/HONcode/Conduct.html.

(VIPPS) Program was unveiled in response to public concern over the safety of Internet pharmacy sites. VIPPS is a certification that is earned after a pharmacy complies with licensing and inspection requirements of its state and of each state in which it provides goods and services to patients. Pharmacies that have earned the VIPPS seal have demonstrated that they are in compliance with standards on protection of patient privacy, security and authentication of prescription orders, quality assurance, and the provision of consultation between patients and pharmacists. Sites that are certified by VIPPS bear a hyperlink seal.

Intranets

Another source of information that employees of health care organizations commonly have access to is intranets. Often an organization's intranet has Internet access but is firewalled so that its computers cannot be reached directly by anyone outside the organization. This can be achieved by requiring an identification password for access to a Web site. Intranets can provide a rich environment for sharing ideas and receiving consultation from peers and for the efficient sharing of resources. Extranets, on the other hand, while similar to intranets and accessible by the Internet, require access authorization and typically are used to connect a pharmacy with its business partners, such as drug wholesalers. The Web site may be accessed for support in ordering and tracking a pharmacy's order. Patient identifying information often is unavailable for access by business partners and other stakeholders. Yet another source of information is offline references that may be stored on the internal capacity of the computer (Felkey and Fox, 2003b).

■ AUTOMATION AND ROBOTICS

Several key factors drive the need for automation. A national shortage of pharmacists in the face of ever-increasing prescription volumes is one major impetus. Another is the profound need to reduce the incidence of medication errors. Still another is the opportunity created by automation to enhance the role of pharmacists in patient care. Finally, consumers' demand for speed and convenience further enhances the attractiveness of automation in pharmacy operations (Lewis, Albrant, and Hagel, 2002). Technology has the ability to accelerate the movement of pharmacists from the traditional dispensing focus to that of a patient-centered role.

In order for this to happen, pharmacists must be knowledgeable about automated technologies to determine their appropriate management and to incorporate them into their practices. As these technologies become more common, pharmacists will be forced to expand their knowledge of technology and automation. The white paper on automation in pharmacy identifies important skills necessary for pharmacists to acquire: (1) how to operate automated pharmacy systems to produce desired outcomes, (2) how to recognize if a system failure occurs, (3) how to address a failure correctly so that patient safety is protected, and (4) how to get failures corrected quickly (Barker et al., 1998). For pharmacists to obtain these skills, an education and training program for employees that use automation should be developed and evaluated periodically for efficacy. Core objectives of the training must include the purpose and capabilities of the system, minimum competency required by operators, and how system failures can occur. There should also be a plan in place for when system failure occurs, and it should be rehearsed periodically (Barker et al., 1998).

Automation can reduce medication errors if it is implemented properly because it reduces the number of manual functions necessary to complete a task, thus reducing the chance for mistakes. Automation has helped to reduce the time that pharmacists spend preparing, labeling, and packaging medications, and this time can be reallocated to pharmaceutical care activities (Lewis, Albrant, and Hagel, 2002).

Another advantage of automation is inventory control. It is more efficient and accurate than manually completing this task and can result in reduced inventory costs. Automation can capture charges more efficiently and accurately than can be performed manually. It improves the billing process by detailing when medications are used, who dispenses or administers them, and who receives them (Lewis, Albrant, and Hagel, 2002). Automated inventory control can perform a number of functions, including monitoring inventory and automatic reordering when inventory reaches a quantity that can be preset by the pharmacy.

■ SURESCRIPTS

SureScripts was founded in 2001 by the National Association of Chain Drug Stores (NACDS) and the National Community Pharmacists Association (NCPA) their mission is to improve the quality, safety, and efficiency of the overall prescribing process. The Pharmacy Health Information Exchange operated by SureScripts is the largest network to link electronic communications between pharmacies and physicians, allowing the electronic exchange of prescription information. The pharmacy population that it focuses on is community or retail pharmacies (www.surescripts.com/).

COMPUTERIZED PHYSICIAN/PROVIDER ORDER ENTRY (CPOE)

Computerized physician/provider order entry (CPOE) is defined as the computer system that allows direct entry of medical orders by the physician or person with appropriate licensure and privileges to do so. Directly entering orders into a computer has the benefit of reducing errors by minimizing the errors caused by handwritten orders, but even a greater benefit is realized when the combination of CPOE and clinical decision-support tools is implemented together.

Implementation of CPOE is being encouraged increasingly as an important solution to the challenge of reducing medical errors and improving health care quality and efficiency. But use of CPOE is not yet widespread in part because it has a reputation for being difficult to implement successfully.

CPOE.org is a Web site that presents the results of research by the Physician Order Entry Team (POET) at Oregon Health & Science University. The team is funded by a grant from the National Library of Medicine to study success factors for implementing CPOE. This Web site also provides access to a collection of resources and links regarding CPOE (www.ohsu.edu/academic/dmice/research/cpoe/index.php).

TELEHEALTH

Telehealth is a recent innovation that brings care directly to the patient, allowing health care practitioners to provide services from remote locations (Felkey and Fox, 2001b). Telehealth employs telecommunications and information technology. It is an umbrella concept under which telemedicine, telenursing, and telepharmacy fall. It combines practices, products, and services that make it possible to deliver health care and information to any location.

TELEPHARMACY

The NABP defines *telepharmacy* as "the provision of pharmaceutical care through the use of telecommunications and information technologies to patients at a distance" (National Association of Boards of Pharmacy, 2000). For example, one of the most basic forms of telepharmacy is a pharmacy Web site that can be expanded and developed to offer patient care functions. A basic pharmacy Web site may include information that lists hours of operation, location and directions, and specialized services available. This basic setup then can be expanded to offer patient care such as an e-mail request for a refill or more advanced functions such as an "Ask the Pharmacist" service. Even the most basic Web presence provides the potential to expand a customer base by way of increased visibility. Options and services can be added based on the level of commitment that the organization has toward telepharmacy. A high-level option that has significant potential in pharmacy is videoconferencing. By connecting with patients in remote areas, videoconferencing may afford pharmacists the opportunity to enhance outcomes and possibly obtain reimbursement for providing care. ScriptPro is an innovator in this capacity and has developed a videoconferencing system that allows a pharmacist in one location to counsel and dispense a prescription to a patient in a different location.

Pharmacists must demonstrate the importance of their role as medication experts who identify, resolve, and prevent drug-related problems through this medium (Felkey and Fox, 2001b). If a pharmacist wishes to implement counseling by teleconferencing, basic equipment can be purchased for as little as a few hundred dollars; however, more advanced, cutting-edge technology may cost tens of thousands of dollars.

REVISITING THE CASE—MAKING LIFE EASIER

Jennifer's situation would be so much easier if the systems were integrated and information could be pre-populated in the appropriate fields. Why is it not possible that when the drug is entered, it is also subtracted automatically from the pharmacy inventory? The appropriate patient should be charged automatically for the drug. Laboratory information should be sent automatically to Jennifer, who then simply could verify the orders to be sent to the laboratory, and nursing could be notified to draw the appropriate levels. Finally, the EMR should reflect what was done for documentation purposes. This documentation should occur as a by-product of her taking care of the patient. If this were happening, Jennifer could spend more time providing education to physicians on appropriate drug utilization, providing patient care, and having the kind of impact on patient outcomes that she intended when she chose pharmacy as a career and this particular site as her first professional position.

CONCLUSION

The fundamental role of technology is to enhance the work of human beings. In pharmacy, technology will be one of the factors that will greatly assist motivated pharmacists in transitioning their practices from a product to a patient focus. Pharmacists should be able to deploy technology at the point of care that will increase efficiency and reduce medication errors. To accomplish this, it is critical that they be accepting and knowledgeable of the latest innovations. They should also bear in mind that all technologies have limitations. Such technologies as computerized physician order entry and electronic health records will continue to improve in accuracy and efficiency, and fully automated systems will become the norm in future pharmacy operations. Pharmacists can and should take a leadership role by incorporating technology into their practices (Rough, 2001). Integral to this process is identification of needs, selection of vendors that can serve those needs, and proper implementation. Pharmacy directors and pharmacy departments must carefully plan their decision to invest in and select appropriate technologies, as well as ongoing maintenance and optimization.

QUESTIONS FOR FURTHER DISCUSSION

1. How might the use of technology continue to affect the practice of pharmacy in the future?
2. What will be the impact on the quality and cost of health care when quality data are readily available at patient bedsides?
3. How might a pharmacist keep pace with technological advances in the practice of pharmacy?
4. Describe the use of technology at your current workplace. How has this technology enabled the pharmacy to operate more effectively? Is the technology managed appropriately? What could be done to manage it more appropriately?

REFERENCES

Arndt KA. 1992. Information excess in medicine: Overview, relevance to dermatology, and strategies for coping. *Arch Dermatol* 128:1249.

Barker KN, Felkey BG, Flynn EA, Carper JL. 1998. White paper on automation in pharmacy. *Consultant Pharmacist* 13:256; available at www.ascp.com; accessed on June 10, 2004.

CPOE.org Physician Order Entry Team (POET) at Oregon Health & Science University. Available at: www.ohsu.edu/academic/dmice/research/cpoe/index.php; accessed on May 1, 2007.

Clark T, McBride J, Zinn T. 1999. Achieving a computer system's benefits. *Hosp Pharm* 34:534.

Enders SJ, Enders JM, Holstad SG. 2002. Drug-information software for Palm operating system personal digital assistants: Breadth, clinical dependability, and ease of use. *Pharmotherapy* 22:1036.

Felkey BG. 1997. Implementing a clinical information system in a managed care setting: Building the clinical workstation: Software for the health-system pharmacist. *Am J Health-Syst Pharm* 52:1505.

Felkey BG, Fox BI. 2001a. Telehealth for pharmacy care. In *Pharmacotherapy Self-Assessment Program*, 4th ed, book 2, p. 117. Kansas City, MO: American College of Clinical Pharmacy.

Felkey BG, Fox BI. 2001b. How do you spell relief? Automation! *Computer Talk* July–August:38.

Felkey BG, Fox BI. 2003a. Informatics: The integration of technology into pharmaceutical care. In Rovers JP, Currie JD, Hagel HP, et al (eds), *Pharmaceutical Care,* 2nd ed., pp. 283–292. Bethesda, MD: ASHP.

Felkey BG, Fox BI. 2003b. Computer software for clinical pharmacy services. In DiPiro J (ed), *Encyclopedia of Clinical Pharmacy,* p. 214. New York: Marcel Dekker.

First Data Bank Web site, www. firstdatabank.com; accessed on May 19, 2007.

Fox S, Fallows D. 2003. Internet health resources: Health searches and e-mail have become more commonplace, but there is room for improvement in searches and overall Internet access. Pew Internet and American Life Project; available at www.pewinternet.org/reports/pdfs/PIP_Health_Report_July_2003.pdf; accessed on June 10, 2004.

Garets D, Davis M. 2006. Electronic medical records vs. electronic health records: Yes, there is a difference, white paper, HIMSS Analytics, Chicago, www. himssanalytics.org.

Health on the Net Foundation Web site, www.hon.ch; accessed on May 19, 2007.

Institute for Safe Medication Practices. 2000. White paper: A call to action: Eliminate handwritten prescriptions within 3 years. Minneapolis: ISMP; available at www. ismp.org; accessed on May 19, 2007.

Kemper DW, Mettler M. 2002. *Information Therapy,* p. 116. Boise, ID: Healthwise.

Levine JR, Bauroudi C, Levine ML. 1996. *The Internet for Dummies.* San Mateo, CA: IDG Books Worldwide.

Lewis RK, Albrant DH, Hagel HP. 2002. Developing the infrastructure for patient care. In *Managing the Patient-Centered Pharmacy,* p. 66. Washington, DC: American Pharmaceutical Association.

Lowe HJ, Barnett GO. 1994. Understanding and using the medical subject headings (MeSH) vocabulary to perform literature searches. *JAMA* 271:1103.

Malone PM, Mosdell KW, Kier KL, Stanovich JE. 2001. *Drug Information: A Guide for Pharmacists,* 2d ed., p. 108. New York: McGraw-Hill.

Medication Errors Rank as a Top Patient Worry in Hospitals, Health Systems, ASHP Patient Concerns Survey Research Report, September 1999; available at www.ashp.org; accessed on December 27, 2002.

National Association of Boards of Pharmacy. 2000. VIPPS Web site, www.nabp.net; accessed on June 8, 2004.

Pedersen CA, Schneider PJ, Scheckelhoff DJ. 2006. ASHP national survey of pharmacy practice in hospital settings: Dispensing and administration—2005. *Am J Health-Syst Pharm* 63:327.

Rough SS. 2001. The pharmacist-technology interface: Current and future implications for the practice of pharmacy. In *Pharmacotherapy Self-Assessment Program,* 4th ed., book 2, p. 85. Kansas City, MO: American College of Clinical Pharmacy.

Sanborn M. 2007. Developing a pharmacy information system infrastructure. *Hosp Pharm* 42:470.

Stair RM. 1996. *Principles of Information Systems: A Managerial Approach,* 2d ed. Danvers, MA: Boyd and Fraser.

SureScripts Web site, www.surescripts.com; accessed on May 1, 2007.

Tulley M. 2000. The impact of information technology on the performance of clinical pharmacy services. *J Clin Pharm Ther* 25:243.

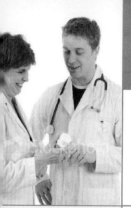

7

ENSURING QUALITY IN PHARMACY OPERATIONS

Terri L. Warholak

About the Author: Dr. Warholak earned a B.S. in pharmacy and an M.S. and Ph.D. in pharmacy administration from Purdue University. Her professional experience encompasses practice in both hospital and community pharmacies, including 5 years as a commissioned officer in the U.S. Public Health Service (Indian Health Service). In addition, she completed a short tour of duty with the Food and Drug Administration (FDA). Since joining the faculty at Midwestern University Chicago College of Pharmacy in 2001, Dr. Warholak's research has focused on medication error reduction. In 2003, she was recognized as a winner of the American Association of Colleges of Pharmacy Council of Faculties Innovations in Teaching Competition for her efforts in a course entitled, "Quality Assurance and Effective Pharmacy Practice."

▓ LEARNING OBJECTIVES

After completing this chapter, students should be able to

1. Discuss the importance of quality in pharmacy practice.
2. Describe how quality is measured in pharmacy practice.
3. Justify the use of successful quality practices employed by other industries in pharmacy practice.
4. Explain the differences between quality assurance, quality control, and continuous quality improvement.
5. List three methods for ensuring quality in pharmacy practice.
6. Outline the steps necessary for a successful continuous quality improvement plan.
7. Prioritize areas/functions most suitable for conducting a quality analysis.
8. Identify sources for additional information about quality assessment and improvement.

SCENARIO

It happened again last night. One of the television newsmagazines aired an exposé on pharmacy errors during prime time. As soon as she saw the advertisement for the program, Anita had that sinking feeling in her stomach. Anita has been employed as a chain community pharmacy technician for the past 3 years during pharmacy school. Recent months have witnessed several dispensing errors made by pharmacists at her store that she has found out about. Luckily, no patients were seriously hurt as a result, but they could have been.

Anita arrived 10 minutes early for work the next morning. The first thing she saw when entering the store was the harried manner in which her boss, pharmacist Pat, was rushing around looking for something, and three of the phone lines were ringing simultaneously. When he saw her, Pat said, "Anita! I'm so glad you are here. We've got a problem, and we need to act fast. Patients started calling an hour ago. They are calling in response to that news show last night on pharmacy errors. Did you see it? Anyway, the patients want to know how they can be sure they are getting the right medications. I remember the district manager asking us to implement the corporate CQI program, but I can't remember where I put the manual—not that I understand it anyway." Pat heaved a sigh, looked at Anita, and said, "You've learned about improving quality in school, right? Can you please help?" Anita knew that it was going to be quite a challenging day.

CHAPTER QUESTIONS

1. How is *quality* defined within the context of pharmacy practice?
2. Define *health care quality* in layperson's terms.
3. How can the need for quality improvement be justified to decision makers?
4. How can quality be measured?
5. What can pharmacy organizations learn from other industries concerning quality?
6. List the steps of a continuous quality improvement (CQI) model.

7. List four practical CQI suggestions for the pharmacist.

WHAT IS QUALITY?

Quality may appear to be a nebulous term. We know what quality is when we see it, but the definition is often subjective. In fact, there are quite a few definitions of quality. For example, *Webster's Dictionary* defines *quality* as a "degree of excellence" (Merriam-Webster, 2003). While this definition provides a framework for quality in general, it is also helpful to examine the definitions of quality specific to health care.

The U.S. Office of Technology Assessment has defined the *quality of medical care* as "evaluation of the performance of medical providers according to the degree to which the process of care increases the probability of outcomes desired by patients and reduces the probability of undesired outcomes, given the state of medical knowledge" (Congress of the United States, Office of Technology Assessment, 1988).

The Institute of Medicine (IOM), in a report entitled, "Medicare: A Strategy for Quality Assurance," stated that "quality of care is the degree to which health services for individuals and populations increase the likelihood of desired health outcomes and are consistent with current professional knowledge" (Lohr, 1990a), whereas Ovretveit (1992) simply states, "A quality health service/system gives patients what they want and need."

An amalgamation of these definitions may provide the best explanation of the concept of quality in health care. Each provides additional insight into quality, what we can expect from quality, and how quality can be perceived. Webster's definition supports the idea that quality is a continuum of excellence or the lack thereof. From the Office of Technology Assessment definition it can be said that in medical care, quality can be measured and used to evaluate the care delivered by health care providers. This definition also implies that the care offered to patients should increase the probability of positive outcomes (e.g., getting rid of an infection) and decrease negative outcomes of care (e.g., death). The care offered to patients should be the most current. The IOM definition is similar but a little more straightforward. The Ovretveit definition incorporates judgments by the end users of medical care to define quality. While this broadened perspective has merit, patients may not be the best judges of the quality of medical care because even though they may know what they *want* from medical care, they may not have well-defined notions of what they *need* from medical care. Thus it is up to the medical provider to offer quality care to benefit the patient even when the patient does not know what he or she needs. While this may appear paternalistic, it seems reasonable that any person who is not an expert in a field may not know all the best alternatives.

So what is quality in pharmacy practice? Extrapolating from the preceding discussion, it can be said that quality in pharmacy practice

- Represents a degree of excellence
- Increases the probability of positive outcomes
- Decreases the probability of negative outcomes
- Corresponds with current medical knowledge
- Offers the patient what he or she wants
- Provides the patient with what he or she needs

Understanding these aspects of quality will help Anita and Pat explain pharmacy quality to patients and will serve as the basis for pharmacy improvement.

▪ HOW IS QUALITY MEASURED?

Historically, pharmacy practice quality has been measured by assessing its structure, process, and outcomes (Donabedian, 1969, 1992). Simply put, for a good or service,

- *Structure* refers to the raw materials needed for production.
- *Process* is the method or procedure used.
- *Outcomes* are the end result.

Each of the preceding (i.e., structure, process, and outcomes) has been used to measure quality. Traditionally, quality in pharmacy practice has been measured by structure and process methods. This relies on a premise that a quality outcome is not possible without appropriate structure or process. Moreover, it is much simpler and less controversial to measure structure and process than it is to measure outcomes. Recently, however, outcomes quality measurement has become more prevalent.

In the realm of pharmacy, the raw materials or structure necessary for quality care are many and varied. Examples include number of pharmacists per shift, counter space, pharmacist credentials or licensing, pharmacy square footage, medication reference books, medication stock, and counseling facilities.

Because pharmacists are responsible for all phases of medication use, processes in the pharmacy can refer to any phase of the medication use process (e.g., prescribing, dispensing, administering, or monitoring). Examples of process measures include, but are not limited to, adherence to clinical guidelines or pathways, percent of prescriptions assessed for appropriateness, and percent of patients counseled.

Outcomes are the driving force behind medication therapy management, which has pharmacists participating in patient education, medication review, and disease-state management. Through such activities, pharmacists have been able to improve patient care by (1) increasing patients' control of their medical conditions (Clifford et al., 2005; Cranor et al., 2003; Garrett and Bluml, 2005; Kiel and McCord, 2005; Leal and Herrier, 2004; Ragucci et al., 2005; Sadik et al., 2005; Scott et al., 2006; Schnipper et al., 2006; Sookaneknun et al., 2004) and (2) decreasing use of health care resources (Cordina et al., 2001; Dedden et al., 1997; Garrett and Bluml, 2005; Rupp et al., 1997), (3) increasing patients' knowledge of their conditions, treatments, and medications (Mangiapane et al., 2005; Schulz et al., 2001), (4) increasing adherence to and persistence with medication regimens (Krass et al., 2005; Lee et al., 2006; Mangiapane et al., 2005; Sookaneknun et al., 2004; Vrijens et al., 2006), (5) increasing patients' satisfaction with their care

(Cranor et al., 2003; Garrett and Bluml, 2005; Weinberger et al., 2002), (6) saving payers money (Cranor et al., 2003; Fertleman et al., 2005; Garrett and Bluml, 2005; Ragucci et al., 2005), and (7) improving patients' quality of life (Cordina et al., 2001; Mangiapane et al., 2005; Rupp et al., 1997; Sadik et al., 2005; Scott et al., 2006; Schulz et al., 2001).

Pharmacists' ability to identify, resolve, and prevent medication-related problems, as well as take responsibility in disease-state management, is well documented (Bluml et al., 2000; Cranor et al., 2003; Fertleman et al., 2005; Hansen et al., 2006; Nolan, 2000; Schnipper et al. 2006). Thus outcomes describe the ultimate goal of the care or therapy and answer the question, "What are we trying to accomplish?"

There are different ways to look at outcomes. One method, the ECHO model, purports three basic types of outcomes: economic, clinical, and humanistic (Kozma et al., 1993). Economic outcomes include direct costs and consequences, both medical and nonmedical, and indirect costs and consequences. For example, when assessing outcomes from a patient perspective, a medication copayment would be a direct medication cost, whereas gas money to pick up the medication from the pharmacy would represent a nonmedical direct cost. Lost wages from missed work could be regarded as an indirect cost.

Clinical outcomes measures can include morbidity and mortality, event rates, and symptom resolution (Ovretveit, 2001). These measures are a direct measure of quality but may be difficult to assess, especially in pharmacy, where their onset could be years following a treatment or intervention (Chassin and Galvin, 1998; Shane and Gouveia, 2000). In these cases, indicators or markers can be used to assess outcomes. These indicators can be condition-specific (e.g., HgA1c) or procedure-specific (e.g., rate of postoperative infection after hip surgery) or address an important issue of patient care. For example, blood pressure may be used as a marker to assess susceptibility to stroke because it is not practical, safe, or ethical to wait and measure the occurrence of stroke.

Humanistic outcomes include measures of the "human" aspects of care. Specific types of humanistic outcomes include patient satisfaction and health-related quality of life (HRQoL). For example, a survey concerning patient satisfaction with pharmaceutical care services could be used to assess humanistic outcomes for patients receiving these services. Alternatively, a QoL assessment may be useful to assess the impact medication therapy has on the patient's life as a whole.

Measuring outcomes can seem to be a daunting task. This may have been why Anita's boss, pharmacist Pat (in the scenario), did not implement the corporate CQI program as recommended by his district manager. Thus the remainder of this chapter will present these concepts in an easy-to-understand manner and will include simple implementation tips.

WHAT CAN PHARMACY LEARN FROM OTHER INDUSTRIES?

Health care traditionally has lagged behind other industries in quality improvement. It has been suggested that medicine should follow the lead of the airline and other industries by using quality management to decrease unnecessary variation and improve quality (Leape, 1994). An IOM report supported this contention when the authors suggested that the American health care system can improve the quality of care by borrowing techniques used in other industries to standardize processes (Kohn, 2000). Many of these techniques are based on systems theory.

Systems theory, developed by von Bertalanffy (1968), has been used in engineering, medicine, and education (Nagel, 1988; Sheridan, 1988). A systems approach involves defining the purpose and performance expectations of the system, examining the characteristics of the input, considering alternative mechanisms for achieving the stated goals, implementing the system, and adjusting the system based on feedback (Park, 1997; Sheridan, 1988). Basically, a systems approach allows for inspection of the interaction between every component of a system, thus expanding the more traditional approach of looking at individual components independently (Rasmussen et al., 1994; Sheridan, 1988).

Airlines, aircraft manufacturers, and the Federal Aviation Authority (FAA) have turned to a systems view of quality improvement termed *human factors principles* (Boeing, 1993; Edkins, 1998; FAA, 1993; Leape et al., 1998a). The human factors view of quality focuses on the relationship between quality problems and the system in which they occur (Rasmussen et al., 1994). "Human factors principles are concepts about the design of work that take advantage of the strengths and weakness of the human mind and compensate for its limitations" (Leape et al., 1998a). Human factors principles include (1) reducing reliance on memory, (2) simplifying and standardizing, (3) using protocols and checklists, (4) using mechanisms to physically prevent error (constraints and forcing functions), (5) improving access to information, (6) decreasing reliance on vigilance, (7) differentiating, and (8) implementing automation (Kohn, 2000; Leape et al., 1998a).

Human factors principles can be used to improve quality (Kohn, 2000; Leape et al., 1998b). For example, instruments, checklists, and decision support can help users to avoid reliance on memory (Boeing, 1993; Leape, 1994; Leape et al., 1998a). In pharmacy practice, decreased reliance on memory can be accomplished by using decision-support systems. Most community pharmacies now use in-store computer systems to assist with Omnibus Budget Reconciliation Act of 1990 (OBRA 90)-mandated prospective drug utilization review (DUR). However, decision-support systems should be used wisely because they are not intended to supplant the pharmacist's clinical decision-making skills (Leape et al., 1998a; Nolan, 2000).

Standardization is thought to be one of the most powerful tools for improving quality (Leape et al., 1998c). If a person does something the same way every time, the chances that he or she will perform the activity incorrectly are greatly reduced (Leape et al., 1998c). Industry has long known that quality and variation are inversely related; quality improves as variation is reduced (Deming, 1986). In pharmacy, standardization is the simplest, most broadly applicable, and most effective method for quality improvement (Leape et al., 1998c). In fact, the move to standardization has created the impetus for critical pathways that focus not only on error prevention but also on opti-

mization of outcomes, cost reduction, and satisfaction (Clearinghouse, 2000; American Pharmacists Association, 2003). These decision-support systems can also be used to decrease reliance on vigilance through alerting the pharmacist of potential problems.

Another mechanism for decreasing reliance on memory and reducing variation is the use of protocols and checklists. Protocols and checklists serve as reminders of critical tasks, especially when an omission can have serious consequences, and are often recommended as mechanisms for increasing quality (Boeing, 1993). Policies and protocols decrease confusion, thus improving overall dispensing quality (Agency for Healthcare Research and Quality, 2001). A constraint that "prevents further action until some condition is met" (Leape et al., 1998a) can also be written into protocols to provide a quality check in a system. For example, protocols usually preclude prescriptions from being dispensed until they are approved by the pharmacist's final check.

Improving access to information leads to improved quality (Abelson and Levi, 1985; Weinstein and Fineberg, 1980). One study indicated that pharmacists make more appropriate prospective DUR decisions when they have access to more complete patient information, such as medication profiles, allergy information, patient age, and diagnosis (Warholak-Juarez et al., 2000). Therefore, medication orders should not be processed without the pharmacist considering these and similar pieces of information.

Moreover, improved quality produces a corresponding increase in productivity because less rework is needed and less waste is produced (Deming, 1986). "Improvement of quality transfers waste of man-hours and machine time into the manufacture of good products and better service" (Deming, 1986). When extrapolated to pharmacy practice, it can be predicted that quality improvements will produce desired clinical outcomes such as improved QoL in addition to positive humanistic outcomes such as greater customer satisfaction. Improved customer satisfaction can help to make the workplace more pleasant and may produce a corresponding increase in employee satisfaction. This ultimately may lead to the pharmacy having a competitive edge and an image as a provider of high-quality pharmaceutical care and may allow the business to recruit and maintain the most highly qualified and desired personnel. These are some strategies Anita (in the scenario) may want to tell her boss about.

METHODS FOR ENSURING QUALITY IN PHARMACY PRACTICE

Quality Assurance

Quality assurance (QA) has been defined as "the systematic monitoring and evaluation of the various aspects of a project, service, or facility to ensure that standards of quality are being met" (Merriam-Webster, 2003). Basically, a check is performed to ensure that a good or service meets a certain quality standard. Problems are addressed after they occur (Godwin and Sanborn, 1995).

Quality Control

Quality control (QC), as defined by *Webster's Dictionary*, is "an aggregate of activities (as design analysis and inspection for defects) designed to ensure adequate quality" (Merriam-Webster, 2003). Quality control improves product or service design to improve the level of quality; it can be thought of as defect prevention.

Continuous Quality Improvement

Continuous quality improvement (CQI) is "a philosophy of continual improvement of the processes associated with providing a good or service that meets or exceeds customer expectations" (Shortell et al., 1998). CQI, which was first employed in the manufacturing field, was introduced into health care by Berwick and Leape (1999). [CQI has been referred to as *quality improvement process, total quality management,* and *total quality control* (Lohr, 1990b).]

CQI introduced two important ideas that transcend QA and QC. First, CQI represents a total systems perspective concerning quality; all workers within the health care system are interconnected (Godwin and Sanborn, 1995). When examined from a systems per-

spective, every action of the health care professional is performed to benefit the patient (Shortell et al., 1998). Therefore, all actions must be planned to improve care and should not focus on correcting individual mistakes after the fact (Godwin and Sanborn, 1995; Shortell et al., 1998). Thus quality problems are not examined (or blamed) on an individual level (Blumenthal and Kilo, 1998). CQI promotes identification of the cause of problems via "fact-based management and scientific methodology, which make it culturally compatible with the values of health care professionals" (Shortell et al., 1998, p. 605). It is likely to achieve optimal benefit when used on a systematic, organization-wide level (Shortell et al., 1998).

Second, CQI demands that the quality improvement process is continuous or never-ending (Blumenthal and Kilo, 1998). Improvement occurs by integrating information concerning quality into the cyclic redesign and improvement of care (Godwin and Sanborn, 1995). The changes can be quick and on a small scale but should be occurring constantly. In this manner, CQI empowers health care providers to improve quality on a daily basis (Shortell et al., 1998).

At this point it may seem as if CQI is "all about looking for things that are/could be wrong." However, CQI is much more than that. It is a systematic process for continuously improving the quality of every aspect of a pharmacy practice setting from patient care to managerial responsiveness. In this manner, CQI is a much more positive process than QA or QC because the focus is on constantly making things better for all who work in and have contact with the practice. CQI is a method for constantly striving for improvement in every facet, every portion of the medication use system. The pharmacy that uses CQI to constantly improve its structure, processes, and outcomes will achieve positive reinforcement from satisfied, well-cared-for patients and employees alike.

One challenge to implementing CQI in pharmacy is a paucity of examples in the literature. Moreover, existing published reports seldom involve rigorous scientific investigation. Regardless, quality improvement has been used to develop (Godley et al., 2001; Jackevicius, 2002; Jones and Como, 2003; LaPointe et al.,

2002), implement (Rischer and Bertolone-Childress, 1998), revise (Matanin and Cutrell, 1994), and improve compliance with clinical guidelines (Bevenour et al., 2002; Chaikledkaew et al., 2002; Roberts et al., 2002) and to increase overall quality (Goff et al., 2002; Griffey and Bohan 2006; Gomez et al., 2001; Jain et al. 2006; Jensen et al., 2002; Moffett et al., 2006; Weeks et al., 2001). Quality improvement processes have been used to monitor medication errors (Braithwaite et al., 2004; Newland et al., 2001) and to improve prescription writing (Meyer, 2000). They have been used to support a culture of improvement (Karow, 2002; Krogstad et al., 2005), decrease medication errors (Briggs et al., 2002; Farber et al., 2002; Hritz et al., 2002; Rozich et al., 2003), implement new technology (Gambone and Broder, 2007; Karow, 2002), and decrease adverse drug events (ADEs) (Weeks et al., 2001). Along these same lines, quality improvement techniques have been used to implement and improve pharmacy services (Wieland et al., 1998) and improve pharmacist interventions (Zimmerman et al., 1997).

For the most part, quality improvement techniques have been used in institutional settings, but they are becoming more commonplace in ambulatory (Jensen et al., 2002) and managed-care pharmacy settings (Godley et al., 2001; Goff et al., 2002; Roberts et al., 2002). This was evidenced in the scenario; Pat's district manager is a believer in CQI and has asked Pat to implement a system in his pharmacy.

■ A CQI IMPROVEMENT MODEL

Many CQI models exist. Examples of specific models include the plan, do, check, and act (PDCA) model and the find, organize, clarify, understand, select, plan, do, check, and act (FOCUS-PDCA) model and six sigma (Lazarus and Butler, 2001; Lazarus and Stamps, 2002). Most models include elements that reflect the following core concepts: (1) plan, (2) design, (3) measure, (4) assess, and (5) improve (Coe, 1998a).

CQI has been described as a practical application of the scientific method (Blumenthal and Kilo, 1998).

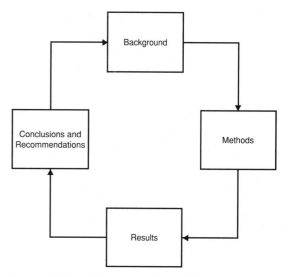

Figure 7-1. The CQI measurement cycle.

Planning in both processes is similar. In this manner, one can think of the steps in the CQI cycle as parallel to the sections of a scientific article: background, methods, results, conclusions, and recommendations. Considering CQI in this manner diminishes the need to memorize additional terminology. See Fig. 7-1 for a flowchart representation of the process.

The steps to CQI discussed in this chapter are included in the CQI Cycle Checklist and Planning Worksheets in Appendices 7A and 7B, respectively. The CQI Cycle Checklist includes an abbreviated list of the actions needed for a successful CQI cycle. The Planning Worksheets are more detailed forms to assist in CQI cycle implementation. Worksheet 1 is intended for use during the first team meeting, Worksheet 2 should be used for second meeting through completion of data collection, and Worksheet 3 begins with data analysis and guides the user through the remainder of the CQI cycle. Therefore, there is no need to memorize the CQI cycle steps—just sit back and read about the concepts presented.

Recruiting the CQI Team

The planning phase of quality improvement is essential. The first step in developing a cohesive plan is to assemble an expert panel. This panel should be inter-disciplinary and should include representatives of those who will be included in or affected by the quality plan. The team should also include subject matter experts, decision makers, and front-line personnel. In a community pharmacy, the entire pharmacy staff should be invited to participate. This will stress the importance of the quality process and help to get staff support for the quality improvement project. It is important to note that while buy-in will be increased by inviting staff participation and opinions, this effect will be lost quickly if staff members do not perceive that their participation is beneficial.

CQI Cycle Background

Focus Selection

The CQI cycle begins with the selection of a quality improvement focus. Selection may be based on mandate (either from within or from an outside source), or the choice may be left to the team. If the team is given the latitude to choose, one of several processes may be used to facilitate this decision. The team could brainstorm possible areas for study. In this case, all team members should provide ideas freely, and each idea should be recorded. Ideas then may be ranked, and team consensus can be used for system selection. Examples of systems that have been shown to provide quality improvement opportunities in health care settings include identifying and measuring the incidence of medication errors, implementing methods to reduce medication errors, measuring medication filling time, analyzing satisfaction with pharmacy services, evaluating the effect of pharmacists' interventions, analyzing adherence to requirements for documentation, documenting the incidence of medication allergy, auditing patient-controlled analgesia pumps, assessing patient-specific medication errors in cart filling, and analyzing hypertension control and guidelines compliance.

Alternatively, processes such as failure mode and effects analysis or root cause analysis can be used to identify systems ripe for quality improvement activities. Failure mode and effects analysis is a prospective procedure used to identify areas for quality improvement before they become a problem (Cohen et al., 1994; DeRosier et al., 2002; NCPS, 2001). Once pos-sible areas are identified, the investigators decide if the results will be tolerable or intolerable (Cohen et al., 1994).

Root cause analysis is a systematic process used to identify the exact or root cause of a problem (Coe, 1998b). It is used after a quality problem has been discovered (a retrospective procedure) to prevent recurrence (Coe, 1998c; NCPS, 2001). The process begins with "triage questions" that help the team decide what issues (e.g., staff training, competency, human factors, equipment, and information) could have contributed to the quality problem (Gosbee and Anderson, 2003). Once these questions are answered, more detailed, specific questions are considered in order to identify ways to improve systems to reduce the chance of it recurring. The investigators create an action plan for implementing system improvements and improvements evaluation (Anonymous, 2002; Bagian et al., 2001). A more detailed account of these two processes is included in Table 7-1.

Focus Description

After the focus for quality improvement has been chosen, it is important to make sure that it is clear to each team member. This can be accomplished by providing a detailed description of the area chosen for study, the setting in which the focus occurs, the portion of the medication use process affected, and baseline data, if applicable.

Flowcharts that explicitly represent all portions of the process can be helpful for system description. Flowcharts use standard symbols that represent all process steps (represented as rectangles), as well as decision points (represented by diamond shapes) and the direction of progression from one subprocess to the other (Coe, 1998a). Flowcharts are also useful because they can help the team to recognize if the process chosen is too broad (i.e., represented by an unwieldy flowchart). An example of a flowchart is given in Fig. 7-1.

Focus Importance

Next, the team should state why the focus is important. The selected focus should be important to the organization and have the potential to lead to improvement. It should be considered high priority, high volume, high cost, or high risk. For example, a community pharmacy

Table 7-1.   Two Tools for Identifying Quality Improvement Priority Areas

Prospective: Failure Mode and Effects Analysis (FMEA)

The Veterans Administration National Center for Patient Safety (NCPS) has translated this industrial and engineering procedure for health care. The NCPS has termed its adaptation *healthcare failure mode effects analysis* (HFMEA), and it offers live and videoconference training courses on use (DeRosier et al., 2002). Before doing FMEA, obtain a copy of the video course and/or articles and worksheets that have been developed as a process guide (available from NCPS at www.patientsafety.gov/pubs.html#cogaids). HCFMEA can be performed for general processes (e.g., use of medications on the night shift) or for specific medications. Steps include

Step 1: Define the scope or topic to be studied.

Step 2: Assemble a multidisciplinary team that includes a subject matter expert.

Step 3: Describe and narrow the focus.

Step 4: Conduct a hazard analysis.

Step 5: Select necessary actions and outcome measures and assign activities to specific persons and dates for follow-up.

Retrospective: Root Cause Analysis (RCA)

A comprehensive "flip card" root cause analysis guide is also available from NCPS (see Web site as listed above). This card set walks the pharmacist through every step of a comprehensive root cause evaluation of a quality problem. For example, the cards begin with triage questions such as

- Was the error a criminal act?
- Was it a violation (intentional) or an error?
- Were human factors an issue?
- Was staff training or competency an issue?
- Was equipment involved?
- Was information lacking/misinterpreted?
- Was communication an issue?
- Were policies/procedures/rules an issue?
- Did a protective barrier fail?

Once these questions are answered, the user is led to more detailed questions that address the specific situation. These more detailed questions cover areas such as human factors, communication, training, fatigue, scheduling, environment, equipment, rules, policy, procedure, or barriers to quality.

may choose to focus on prescription order-entry error if anecdotal evidence suggests that this may be an error-prone step in its dispensing process.

Literature Review

Relate the focus to the literature by investigating what is known and not known about similar situations. This step can save the team an enormous amount of time

in the long run. A brief literature search will help the team to discover techniques, interventions, and other tools that have been successful in improving quality in similar situations.

Goals

Once the focus (i.e., process or problem) is chosen, the team should *determine the overall goal* (Leape et al.,

1998d). Common overall goals include (1) discovery, (2) frequency estimation, and (3) measuring a change (Leape et al., 1998d). For example, after a pharmacy's CQI team has decided that it wants to focus on prescription order-entry error, team members must then decide *what* they want to know about it. They may decide that since this is their first CQI cycle, they will focus on frequency estimation of the problem. This will serve as baseline data for the assessment of improvements.

The overall goal can be used to *choose specific goals for the cycle* (Leape et al., 1998d). To accomplish this, the team must decide if it will assess structure, process, outcome, or a combination of these as measures of quality. The degree of the desired effect may also be stated in the goal. For example, if a process or outcome measure is chosen, an intervention may be assessed using the following formula to express a goal: An x percent reduction in y over z, where $x =$ number, $y =$ process/outcome, and $z =$ time.

Note that it is important to assess the practicality of the specific goal. The CQI team should examine the specific goal carefully to determine whether it is realistic. If the goal is not realistic, then it may need to be scaled back (Leape et al., 1998d). Choosing something reasonable for the first CQI cycle will provide the team with experience, improve its chances for success, and thus bolster team members' confidence for the next cycle.

CQI Cycle Methods

Intervention

Interventions discovered through a literature review should be included on a list of possible interventions. These may include quality improvement techniques such as reducing reliance on memory, simplifying, standardizing, or automating processes.

Process and Outcomes Measured

Next, the CQI team must determine how progress will be measured (Leape et al., 1998d). Team members should list process and/or outcome measures necessary to determine if the goals were met. Usually, a mix of process and outcome measures is recommended (Leape

---

Table 7-2. Health Care Process and Outcome Measurement Resources

Need help selecting a measure?

Many process and outcome measures exist, so there may be no need to develop one of your own. Measure selection can be expedited by examining the core critical literature, soliciting expert opinion, or using recognized guidelines such as those from JCAHO, HEDIS, or Healthy People 2010.

Other resources include the National Quality Measures Clearinghouse (NQMC). NQMC provides information on health care quality measures and measure sets and includes a glossary of terms and information on how to select, use, apply, and interpret a measure. Available at www.qualitymeasures.ahrq.gov. Ready-to-use quality tools can be accessed via www.qualitytools.ahrq.gov/.

---

et al., 1998d). Many measures have been developed, so keep the following in mind: Do not invent a new measure if a good one exists; measure what is important—not easy; and do not measure things you cannot change or interpret (Ovretveit, 2001). See Table 7-2 for additional resources on selecting and developing measures.

Data-Collection Procedures

If the required data are not already being collected, the CQI team should devise a plan to collect the appropriate data. The team can choose from several different data-collection methods (Leape et al., 1998d). One option is using an inspection point. This entails checking the process at a certain point such as a "will call" prescription review or the pharmacist's final check of filled prescription. Another option for data collection is a focus group. A focus group can be used to bring workers or patients together to gather ideas and opinions concerning a structure, process, or outcome. If this method is used, opinions should be gathered from people with various perspectives. Monitoring for markers is another option. A *marker* is a predetermined sign that further investigation is necessary. For example, the use of a fast-acting antihistamine in an inpatient situation may be a sign that an adverse drug reaction has occurred. Therefore, the collection of additional data is warranted. Patient chart review is also an option for retrospective data collection. Observation (e.g., watching a process) and spontaneous reports (e.g., having the pharmacist or some health professional record every time a certain activity happens) are also popular options for prospective data gathering.

Data-Analysis Plan

The planned statistical analysis should be thought out in detail to make sure that all necessary information will be gathered. It can be frustrating and time-consuming to gather forgotten data at a moment's notice. This seems self-evident but is a mistake that many people make.

CQI Cycle Results

Analyze Data

Most often descriptive statistics (e.g., mean, median, and percentages) can be used for data analysis. Some analyses can be performed simply by plotting data onto charts or graphs. Charts and graphs can help the team to determine patterns and trends and monitor performance (Coe, 1998a). A run chart, which displays trends over time (e.g., number of medication errors per month), can be used to determine if a quality problem has a common cause or a special variation (e.g., seasonal variation) (Coe, 1998a). A scatter plot (e.g., a plot of two variables) can be used to determine the relationship between the variables (Coe, 1998a). A histogram (e.g., a bar graph of how many times certain events occurred) can be used to determine where efforts should be focused (Coe, 1998a).

For more sophisticated analysis or hypothesis testing, outside assistance may be required. If there is not a statistician on the CQI team, it may be beneficial to refer to statistics books to make sure that the chosen analysis is appropriate. Asking for outside help is also an option; the team should not hesitate to call the local college of pharmacy for a referral.

CQI Cycle Conclusions, Implications, and Recommendations

The final section in the process is describing the conclusions, implications, and recommendations that the team reached after examining the results. Since this is the "bottom line" of the process, it is important that this section be understandable to those outside the CQI team. This section should concisely explain the conclusions and detail the actions that need to take place. The CQI process is iterative; thus the team's recommendations for *this CQI cycle* and for the *next CQI cycle* must be included (Leape et al., 1998c). This will be good news to pharmacist Pat. Because CQI is a continuous improvement process, an understanding of the iterative nature of the process will take the pressure off him to "fix" all pharmacy system problems at once.

ACCREDITATION/ COMPLIANCE WITH QUALITY STANDARDS PROMOGULATED BY AGENCIES OR ASSOCIATIONS

Often quality improvement activities are necessary for accreditation. Earning accreditation indicates that an organization has met predefined standards. The accreditation process provides a framework to help organizations focus on providing safe, high-quality service and requires that the organization demonstrate to outside reviewers its commitment to continuous improvement (Ovretveit, 2001).

The Joint Commission

The Joint Commission is a nonprofit organization founded in 1951 by the American Medical Association and the American College of Surgeons (O'Malley, 1997). The Joint Commission was established to "continuously improve the safety and quality of health care provided to the public through the provision of health care accreditation and related services that support performance improvement in health care organizations"

(Joint Commission Web site). The Joint Commission's focus is organization-wide (O'Malley, 1997).

The Joint Commission survey process is largely process-oriented but gradually is moving toward more of an outcomes measurement model. This shift has been demonstrated by introduction of the ORYX initiative. ORYX, which began in 1997, was designed to "integrate outcomes and other performance measurement data into the accreditation process" (Joint Commission Web site). The intent is to provide organizations with information they can use to improve patient care" (Anonymous, 2003c). Although Joint Commission compliance is voluntary, many organizations view it as mandatory (O'Malley, 1997). Not obtaining Joint Commission accreditation can adversely affect an organization's prestige and reimbursement status (Coe, 1998c; O'Malley, 1997). Key dimensions of performance evaluation include efficacy, appropriateness, availability, timeliness, effectiveness, continuity, safety, efficiency, respect, and caring (Coe, 1998a).

National Committee for Quality Assurance

The National Committee for Quality Assurance (NCQA) is a nonprofit organization established in 1979 by a managed-care trade association in response to a perceived need to provide standardized quality measurement and reporting (NCQA, 2003). The NCQA reviews and accredits all types of managed health care organizations (NCQA, 2007). The NCQA survey is largely process-oriented (O'Malley, 1997).

Quality Measurement

While health care accreditation organizations have existed for quite a while, quality data were not readily available to the general public until recently. These quality measurements (sometimes called "report cards") make health care quality indicators readily available to the public. This encourages health care organizations to compete on the basis of quality and creates markets where quality, not just cost containment, is rewarded (Blumenthal and Kilo, 1998; O'Malley, 1997).

HEDIS

The Health Plan Employer Data and Information Set (HEDIS) is a health care report card created by NCQA. HEDIS standardizes health plan performance data and disseminates this information so that plans can be compared (O'Malley, 1997). This allows health care purchasers and consumers to make informed choices (O'Malley, 1997). HEDIS's performance domains include effectiveness of care, access and availability of care, health plan stability, use of services, cost of care, informed health care choices, satisfaction with the experience of care, and health plan descriptive information.

Leapfrog Group

The Leapfrog Group was formed by a coalition of Fortune 500 companies and leading health care purchase organizations (Leapfrog, 2003). The Leapfrog Group was developed to create a market that rewards quality, not just the lowest-cost provider, by providing quality information to consumers (Leapfrog, 2003). While Leapfrog measures are currently process-oriented, future revisions may include additional outcome measures (Lovern, 2001).

Deciphering Quality Measures

Quality measures such as those just mentioned are developed for consumer use. However, many patients have difficulty understanding these measures and reports well enough to use them for rational health care decision making. Patients and health care providers can get assistance from a U.S. government Web site called *TalkingQuality.gov*. TalkingQuality.gov was developed to help patients understand the concept of health care quality and to give practical suggestions for choosing health care coverage and providers (Anonymous, 2003b). These may be good resources for Anita, Pat, and their patients.

The Future

Since establishment of the Joint Commission, the scope of health care organizations that are eligible for accreditation has widened from hospitals to encompass health systems and now even pharmacy benefit managers (URAC, 2006). In some countries, such as Australia, pharmacies are accredited (Pharmacy Guild of Australia, 2007). It is probable that community pharmacies in the United States someday may be eligible for similar accreditation (if not through the Joint Commission, then through some other accrediting body). Groups such as the Pharmacy Quality Alliance (PQA) have begun to develop pharmacy-specific quality indicators that may serve as the basis for such accreditation (Reynolds, 2007).

In the future, the accreditation process may become more focused on outcomes measurement. Eventually, health care report cards may be more accessible and easy to understand, thus helping to produce a market for quality. Some discussion of adjusting co-payments to encourage patients to use providers that meet the standards purchasers have set has already occurred (Lovern, 2001). In some cases, pharmacy quality improvement may be mandated by state and local governments. For example, a new law in the state of Arizona requires that every pharmacy participate in a CQI program (Arizona Revised Statutes, 2007).

So what does this mean for pharmacy practice? More pharmacists must understand continuous quality improvement and be able to develop, implement, and measure the outcomes of such a plan. This could provide an opportunity for a community pharmacy report card (quality measurement) system on which pharmacies can compete on the basis of quality. Such a system may provide a great opportunity for pharmacies to advertise quality outcomes to payers and patients. If such a system is successful, quality could drive patient choices and payer decisions. Ultimately, the pharmacies with the highest quality may get more market share or obtain higher reimbursement rates for certain services.

ENSURING QUALITY: PRACTICAL SUGGESTIONS FOR THE PHARMACIST

There are several things that pharmacists can do to improve quality. First, they can try to promote a "systems view" culture within the organization (Hume, 1999). Systems changes should be implemented only when the organization is ready for change and has capable leadership that supports a systems view of "no finger pointing"(Shortell et al., 1994). Everyone in the organization should be informed of and invited to participate in any quality systems changes. Personnel evaluations (i.e., performance appraisals) should comprise a quality improvement component so that employees are rewarded for their efforts in such matters (Shortell et al., 1994).

Second, there should be a focus on high-leverage, important systems changes (Hume, 1999; Shortell et al., 1994). For medication safety, this could be on high-alert medications (e.g., fast movers, narrow-therapeutic-index medications, and medications that are available in multiple strengths), high-risk populations (e.g., pediatrics or geriatrics), or problem processes (e.g., medication order entry). Significant opportunities for improvement can be gleaned from an analysis of intervention data, medication incident reports, patient comments, or employee feedback (Johnson et al., 2002; Rogers, 1997).

Third, small changes should be implemented in quick cycles (Hume, 1999). The quality improvement team should be given the opportunity to learn about quality by attempting small changes at first. It may be too frustrating for them to take on a large project for the first cycle. Team members should be allowed to experience a success and see how much improvement can be made with a relatively small change; then their enthusiasm will redouble.

Fourth, the team should implement interventions that have worked elsewhere (Hume, 1999). This improves the likelihood of success and reduces the amount of effort required in the process. It is worth noting that the most successful interventions changed systems, not people (Nolan, 2000; van Bokhoven et al., 2003).

If a pharmacy organization does not want to develop its own CQI plan, help is available. Pharmacy Quality Commitment (PQC) has developed the Sentinel System for community pharmacies. This system, which incorporates best practices, risk-management techniques, and systematic procedures to increase quality, is ready to use and is available from the National

Alliance of State Pharmacy Associations at www.pqc.net.

REVISITING THE SCENARIO

Anita had anticipated that Pat would ask her for help. She took a few deep breaths and pulled her management textbook out of her book bag. "Maybe I can help," she thought to herself. She was by no means an expert, but thanks to her pharmacy school training on quality improvement, she knew enough to get started and where to find more information.

CONCLUSION

Quality is an essential component of competent, professional pharmacy practice. Increasing quality can have many beneficial effects on any practice, such as minimizing rework and increasing productivity. Many quality improvement changes are simple and can be implemented quickly but may have a large impact on the quality of patient care.

Health care quality finally has achieved a position of "high visibility on the national agenda," and the pharmacist has been recognized as a key player in this process (Kusserow, 1990). Thus pharmacists will be called on increasingly to ensure quality in all portions of the medication use system.

QUESTIONS FOR FURTHER DISCUSSION

Anita has begun to address quality in her pharmacy practice setting.

1. What other steps should she take?
2. How can a quality improvement plan be sustained continuously?
3. How can the pharmacy use the quality improvement plan for marketing?
4. Where can the pharmacist or pharmacy student go for additional information about quality improvement?

ACKNOWLEDGMENT

I would like to thank Dr. Tom Reutzel for his guidance and support in helping to write this chapter.

REFERENCES

Abelson RP, Levi A. 1985. Decision making and decision theory. In *Handbook of Social Psychology*, p. 231. New York: Random House.

Anonymous. 2002. *Root Cause Analysis*. Washington, DC: VA National Center for Patient Safety.

Anonymous. 2003a. *FACCT: Foundation for Accountability*. Portland, OR: FACCT.

Anonymous. 2003b. *The Big Picture*. Talkingquality.gov.

Anonymous. 2003c. *Performance Measures in Health Care*. Washington, DC: Joint Commission on Accreditation of Healthcare Organizations.

Anonymous. 2003d. The virtues of independent double checks: They really are worth your time. *ISMP Medical Safety Alert*; available at www.ismp.org/msarticle/timeprint.html; accessed on March 02, 2003.

Agency for Healthcare Research and Quality (AHRQ). 2001. *Medical Errors: The Scope of the Problem*. Rockville, MD, AHRQ.

American Pharmacists Association (APhA). 2003. *American Pharmacists Association Catalogue*. Washington, DC: APhA.

Arizona Revised Statutes. 2007. Amending Title 32, Chapter 18, Article 3, Arizona Revised Statutes, by adding 32-1973, relating to the state board of pharmacy.

Bagian JP, Lee C, Gosbee J, et al. 2001. Developing and deploying a patient safety program in a large health care delivery system: You can't fix what you don't know about. *Joint Comm J Qual Improv* 27:522.

Berwick DM, Leape LL. 1999. Reducing errors in medicine. *Br Med J* 319:137.

Bevenour K, Karsch A, Keyack RL, et al. 2002. Meperidine restriction program at a community hospital. ASHP Midyear Clinical Meeting, Atlanta, GA.

Blumenthal D, Kilo CM. 1998. A report card on continuous quality improvement. *Milbank Q* 76:625.

Bluml BM, McKenney JM, Cziraki MJ, et al. 2000. Pharmaceutical care services and results in project ImPACT: Hyperlipidemia. *J Am Pharm Assoc* 40:157.

Boeing. 1993. *Accident Prevention Strategies: Removing Links in the Accident Chain*. Seattle: Boeing Commercial Airplane Group.

Braithwaite RS, DeVita MA, Mahidhara R, et al. 2004. Use of medical emergency team (MET) responses to detect medical errors. *Qual Saf Health Care* **13**:255–9.

Briggs FE, Mark LK, Faris RJ, et al. 2002. Innovative solutions to a missing dose problem. American Society of Health System Pharmacy Summer Meeting, Baltimore, MD.

Campbell JR, Tierney WM, 1989. Information management in clinical prevention. *Primary Care* 16:251.

Carey RG, Teeters JL. 1995. CQI case study: Reducing medication errors. *Joint Comm J Qual Improv* 21:232.

Chaikledkaew U, Hopefl AW, Chen S, et al. 2002. Hospital compliance with JCAHO core measured for patients with heart failure (HF). ASHP Midyear Clinical Meeting, Atlanta, GA.

Chassin MR, Galvin RW. 1998. The urgent need to improve health care quality. Institute of Medicine National Roundtable on health care quality. *JAMA* 280:1000–5

Clearinghouse NG. 2000. Evidence-based clinical practice guidelines. Agency for Healthcare Research and Quality; available at www.qualitymeasures.ahrq.gov/.

Clifford RM, Davis WA, Batty KT, et al. 2005. Effect of a pharmaceutical care program on vascular risk factors in type 2 diabetes: The Fremantle diabetes study. *Diabetes Care* **28**:771–6.

Coe CP. 1998a. An overview of the Joint Commission's improving organizational performance standards. In *Preparing the Pharmacy for a Joint Commission Survey,* p. 189. Bethesda, MD: ASHP.

Coe CP. 1998b. Overview of the Joint Commission's Sentinel Event Policy. In *Preparing the Pharmacy for a Joint Commission Survey,* p. 200. Bethesda, MD: ASHP.

Coe CP. 1998c. Joint Commission on Accreditation of Healthcare Organizations. In *Preparing the Pharmacy for a Joint Commission Survey,* p. 1. Bethesda, MD: ASHP.

Cohen MR, Senders J, Davis NM. 1994. Failure mode and effects analysis: A novel approach to avoiding dangerous medication errors and accidents. *Hosp Pharm* 29:319.

Congress of the United States, Office of Technology Assessment. 1988. *The Quality of Medical Care: Information for Consumers,* p. x. Washington, DC: U.S. Government Printing Office.

Cordina M, McElnay JC, Hughes CM. 2001. Assessment of a community pharmacy-based program for patients with asthma. *Pharmacotherapy* 21:1196–203.

Cranor CW, Bunting BA, Christensen DB, 2003. The Asheville Project: Long-term clinical and economic out-comes of a community pharmacy diabetes care program. *J Am Pharm Assoc* 43:173.

Dedden P, Chang B, Nagel D, 1997. Pharmacy-managed program for home treatment of deep vein thrombosis with enoxaparin. *Am J Health-Syst Pharm* 54:1968.

Deming WE. 1986. *Out of the Crisis.* Cambridge, MA: Massachusetts Institute of Technology, Center for Advanced Engineering Study.

DeRosier J, Stalhandske E, Bagian JP, et al. 2002. Using health care failure mode and effect analysis: The VA National Center for Patient Safety's prospective risk analysis system. *Joint Comm J Qual Improv* 28:248.

Donabedian A. 1969. Quality of care: Problems of measurement: II. Some issues in evaluating the quality of nursing care. *Am J Public Health Nations Health* 59:1833.

Donabedian A. 1991. Quality assurance: Structure, process, and outcome. *Nurs Stand* 7:4.

Edkins GD. 1998. The INDICATE safety program: Evaluation of a method to proactively improve airline safety performance. *Saf Sci* 30:275.

Farber MS, Palwlicki KS, Tims PM, et al. 2002. Proactive root cause analysis in a multi-hospital system. ASHP Summer Meeting, Baltimore, MD.

Federal Aviation Authority (FAA). 1993. *Human Factor Policy.* Washington, DC: U.S. Department of Transportation.

Fertleman M, Barnett N, Patel T, 2005. Improving medication management for patients: The effect of a pharmacist on post-admission ward rounds. *Qual Saf Health Care* **14**:207–11.

Gambone JC, Broder MS. 2007. Embedding quality improvement and patient safety: The UCLA value analysis experience. *Best Pract Res Clin Obstet Gynaecol* **21**:581–592.

Garrett DG, Bluml BM. 2005. Patient self-management program for diabetes: First-year clinical, humanistic, and economic outcomes. *J Am Pharm Assoc* 45:130–7.

Godley P, Pham H, Rohack J, et al. 2001. Opportunities for improving the quality of hypertension care in a managed care setting. *Am J Health-Syst Pharm* 58:1728.

Godwin HN, Sanborn MD. 1995. Total quality management in hospital pharmacy. *Am Pharm* NS35:51.

Goff DC Jr, Gu L, Cantley LK, et al. 2002. Enhancing the quality of care for patients with coronary heart disease: The design and baseline results of the hastening the effective application of research through technology (HEART) trial. *Am J Manag Care* 8:1069.

Goldspiel BR, DeChristoforo R, Daniels, CE S, 2000. A continuous-improvement approach for reducing the number of chemotherapy-related medication errors. *Am J Health-Syst Pharm* 57:S4.

Gomez E, Sutton SS, Olyaei A, et al. 2001. Multicenter evaluation of risk factors for aspergillosis in patients treated with lipoid amphotericin B products: Outcomes, utilization parameters, and benchmarking. *Am J Health-Syst Pharm* 36:2.

Gosbee J, Anderson T. 2003. Human factors engineering design demonstrations can enlighten your RCA team. *Qual Saf Health Care* 12:119.

Griffey RT, Bohan JS. 2006. Healthcare provider complaints to the emergency department: A preliminary report on a new quality improvement instrument. *Qual Saf Health Care* 15:344–6.

Hansen LB, Fernald D, Akaya-Guerra R, et al. 2006. Pharmacy clarification of prescriptions ordered in primary care: A report from the Applied Strategies for Improving Patient Safety (ASIPS) collaborative. *J Am Board Fam Med* 19:24–30.

Hepler CD, Strand LM. 1990. Opportunities and responsibilities in pharmaceutical care. *Am J Hosp Pharm* 47:533.

Hritz RW, Everly JL, Care SA, 2002. Medication error identification is a key to prevention: A performance improvement approach. *J Healthcare Qual* 24:10.

Hume M. 1999. Changing hospital culture, systems reduces drug errors. *Exec Solutions Healthcare Manag* 2:1.

Jackevicius C. 2002. Quality improvement initiative for pharmacist-assisted warfarin dosing: Implementation and evaluation of a new protocol. *Can J Hosp Pharm* 55:105.

Jain M, Miller L, Belt D, et al. 2006. Decline in ICU adverse events, nosocomial infections and cost through a quality improvement initiative focusing on teamwork and culture change. *Qual Saf Health Care* 15:235–9.

Jensen MK, Fiscella RG, Lewis T, 2002. Successfully enhancing patient outcomes through quality improvement processes: Experience using an infectious reporting database at an ambulatory eye clinic. ASHP Midyear Clinical Meeting, Atlanta, GA.

Johnson ST, Brown GC, Shea KM, 2002. Reengineering a pharmacist intervention program. *Am J Health-Syst Pharm* 59:916.

Joint Commission on Accreditation of Healthcare Organizations. 2006. Facts about the Joint Commission on Healthcare Organizations; available at www.jcaho.org/about1US/index.htm; accessed on August 6, 2004.

Jones TA, Como JA. 2003. Assessment of medication errors that involved drug allergies at a university hospital. *Pharmacotherapy* 23:855.

Karow HS. 2002. Creating a culture of medication administration safety: Laying the foundation for computerized provider order entry. *Joint Comm J Qual Improv* 28:396.

Kiel PJ, McCord AD. 2005. Pharmacist impact on clinical outcomes in a diabetes disease management program via collaborative practice. *Ann Pharmacother* 39:1828–32.

Kohn L. 2000. To err is human: An interview with the Institute of Medicine's Linda Kohn. *Joint Comm J Qual Improv* 26:227.

Kozma CM, Reeder CE, Schultz RM, 1993. Economic, clinical and humanistic outcomes: A planning model for pharmacoeconomic research. *Clin Ther* 15:1121.

Krass I, Taylor SJ, Smith C, et al. 2005. Impact on mediation use and adherence of Australian pharmacists' diabetes care services. *J Am Pharm Assoc* 45:33–40.

Krogstad U, Hofoss D, et al. 2005. Hospital quality improvement in context: A multilevel analysis of staff job evaluations. *Qual Saf Health Care* 14:438–42.

Kusserow RP. 1990. *The Clinical Role of the Community Pharmacist.* Washington, DC: Department of Health and Human Services.

LaPointe DR, Arnold AD, Eichelberger WJ, 2002. Quality improvement projects to enhance safety and efficacy of gentamicin in a neonatal intensive care unit. ASHP Midyear Clinical Meeting, Atlanta, GA.

Lazarus IR, Butler K. 2001. The promise of six sigma, part 1. *Manag Healthcare Exec* 10:22.

Lazarus IR, Stamps B. 2002. The promise of six sigma, part 2. *Manag Healthcare Exec* 1:27.

Leal S, Herrier RN, Glover JJ, Felix A. 2004. Improving quality of care in diabetes through a comprehensive pharmacist-based disease management program. *Diabetes Care* 27:2983–4.

Leape LL. 1994. Error in medicine. *JAMA* 272:1851.

Leape LL, Kabcenell A, Berwick DM, et al. 1998a. Change concepts for reducing adverse drug events. In *Reducing Adverse Drug Events: Breakthrough Series Guide,* p. 49. Boston: Institute for Healthcare Improvement.

Leape LL, Kabcenell A, Berwick DM, et al. 1998b. The challenge. In *Reducing Adverse Drug Events: Breakthrough Series Guide,* p. xiv. Boston: Institute for Healthcare Improvement.

Leape LL, Kabcenell A, Berwick DM, et al. 1998c. Achieving breakthrough improvement in reducing adverse drug events. In *Reducing Adverse Drug Events: Breakthrough Series Guide,* p. 79. Boston: Institute for Healthcare Improvement.

Leape LL, Kabcenell A, Berwick DM, et al. 1998d. A step-by-step guide to reducing adverse drug events. In *Reducing Adverse Drug Events: Breakthrough Series Guide,* p. 13. Boston: Institute for Healthcare Improvement.

Leape LL, Kabcenell A, Berwick DM, et al. 1998e. *A Model for Accelerating Improvement in Reducing Adverse Drug Events: Breakthrough Series Guide,* p. 1. Boston: Institute for Healthcare Improvement.

Leapfrog. 2002. Leapfrog Group jumps at chance to give consumers health care info. *Healthcare Benchmarks* 9:25.

Leapfrog. 2003. *The Leapfrog Group for Patient Safety: Rewarding Higher Standards.* The Leapfrog Group; available at www.leapfroggroup.org/about.htm; accessed on 23 May 2003.

Lee JK, Grace KA, Taylor AJ, 2006. Effect of a pharmacy care program on medication adherence and persistence, blood pressure, and low-density lipoprotein cholesterol: A randomized, controlled trial (see Comment). *JAMA* 296:2563–71.

Lohr KE. 1990a. Health, health care, and quality of care. In *Medicare: A Strategy for Quality Assurance,* p. 19. Washington, DC: National Academy Press.

Lohr KE. 1990b. Concepts of assessing, assuring, and improving quality. In *Medicare: A Strategy for Quality Assurance,* p. 45. Washington, DC: National Academy Press.

Lovern E. 2001. Minding hospitals' business: Purchasing coalition pushes hospitals to improve patient safety through process measures, but industry says standards are too expensive. *Mod Healthcare* 31:30.

Mangiapane S, Schulz M, et al. 2005. Community pharmacy-based pharmaceutical care for asthma patients. *Ann Pharmacother* 39:1817–22.

Matanin D, Cutrell D. 1994. A continuous quality improvement program for phenytoin IV. *Hosp Formul* 29:212.

National Committee for Quality Assurance (NCQA). 2007. Accreditation, certification and recognition; available at http://web.ncqa.org/tabid/58/Defalt.aspx; accessed on June 25, 2007.

Merriam-Webster. 2003. *Merriam-Webster Dictionary.* Springfield, MA: Merriam-Webster.

Moffett BS, Parham AL, Candilla CD, et al. 2006. Oral anticoagulation in a pediatric hospital: Impact of a quality improvement initiative on warfarin management strategies. *Qual Saf Health Care* 15:240–3.

Meyer TA. 2000. Improving the quality of the order-writing process for inpatient orders and outpatient prescriptions. *Am J Health-Syst Pharm* 57:S18.

Nagel DC. 1988. Human error in aviation operations. In Nagel DC (ed), *Human Factors in Aviation,* p. 263. New York: Academic Press.

National Center for Patient Safety (NCPS). 2001a. Healthcare failure mode and effect analysis. In *Strategies for Leadership.* Ann Arbor, MI: Department of Veterans Affairs, National Center for Patient Safety.

National Center for Patient Safety (NCPS). 2001b. Safety assessment code and triage card training CD-ROM. *Strategies for Leadership: A Toolkit for Improving Patient Safety.* Washington, DC: Department of Veterans Affairs, National Center for Patient Safety.

National Center for Patient Safety (NCPS). 2001c. *NCPS Triage Cards for Root Cause Analysis.* Washington, DC: Department of Veterans Affairs, National Center for Patient Safety, 2001.

National Committee for Quality Assurance (NCQA). 2003. *NCQA Overview.* Washington, DC: NCQA.

Newland S, Golembiewski JA, Green CR, et al. 2001. Continuous quality improvement approach to reducing hydromorphone PCA programming errors. *Am J Health-Syst Pharm* 36:710.

Nolan TW. 2000. System changes to improve patient safety. *Br Med J* 320:771.

O'Malley C. 1997. Quality measurement for health systems: Accreditation and report cards. *Am J Health-Syst Pharm* 54:1528.

Ovretveit J. 1992. *Health Service Quality.* Oxford, England: Blackwell Scientific.

Ovretveit J. 2001. Quality evaluation and indicator comparison in health care. *Int J Health Plan Manag* 16:229.

Park KS. 1997. Human error. In Salvendy G (ed), *Handbook of Human Factors and Ergonomics,* p. 150. New York: Wiley- Interscience.

Pharmacy Guild of Australia. 2006. Quality Care Pharmacy Program; available at www.guild.org.au/qcpp/; accessed on June 25, 2007.

Ragucci KR, Fermo JD, Wessell AM, et al. 2005. Effectiveness of pharmacist-administered diabetes mellitus education and management services. *Pharmacotherapy* 25:1809–16.

Rasmussen J, Pejtersen AM, Goodstein LP, 1994. *Cognitive Systems Engineering.* New York: Wiley.

Reynolds B. 2007. PQA continues work of improving patient safety, care. *Pharmacy Today* June: 40.

Rischer JB, Bertolone-Childress S. 1998. Implementation of the AHCPR clinical practice guideline on the management of cancer pain. *J Pharm Care Pain Sympt Control* 6:79.

Roberts K, Cockerham TR, Waugh WJ, 2002. An innovative approach to managing depression: Focus on HEDIS standards. *J Healthcare Qual* 24:11.

Rogers B. 1997. Preventing medication errors. *Healthplan* 38:27.

Rozich JD, Haraden CR, Resar RK, 2003. Adverse drug event trigger tool: A practical methodology for measuring medication related harm. *Qual Saf Health Care* 12:194.

Rupp MT, McCallian DJ, Sheth KK, 1997. Developing and marketing a community pharmacy-based asthma management program. *J Am Pharm Assoc* NS37:694.

Sadik A, Yousif M, McElnay JC, 2005. Pharmaceutical care of patients with heart failure. *Br J Clin Pharmacol* 60:183–93.

Schnipper JL, Kirwin JL, Cotugno MC, et al. 2006. Role of pharmacist counseling in preventing adverse drug events after hospitalization. *Arch Intern Med* 166:565–71.

Schulz M, Verheyen F, Muhlig S, et al. 2001. Pharmaceutical care services for asthma patients: A controlled intervention study. *J Clin Pharmacol* 41:668–76.

Scott DM, Boyd ST, Stephan M, et al. 2006. Outcomes of pharmacist-managed diabetes care services in a community health center. *Am J Health-Syst Pharm* 63:2116–22.

Shane R, Gouveia WA. 2000. Developing a strategic plan for quality in pharmacy practice. *Am J Health-Syst Pharm* 57:470.

Sheridan TB. 1988. The system perspective. In Nagel DC (ed), *Human Factors in Aviation,* p. 27. New York: Academic Press.

Shortell SM, Bennett CL, Byck GR, 1998. Assessing the impact of continuous quality improvement on clinical practice: What it will take to accelerate progress. *Milbank Q* 76:593.

Shortell SM, O'Brien JL, Hughes EF, et al. 1994. Assessing the progress of TQM in U.S. hospitals: Findings from two studies. *Q Lett Healthcare Lead* 6:14.

Sookaneknun P, Richards RM, Sanguansermsri J, et al. 2004. Pharmacist involvement in primary care improves hypertensive patient clinical outcomes. *Ann Pharmacother* 38:2023–8.

URAC. 2007. Pharmacy Benefit Management; available at www.urac.org/programs/pbm.aspx; accessed on June 26, 2007.

van Bokhoven MA, Kok G, Vander Weijden T, 2003. Designing a quality improvement intervention: A systematic approach. *Qual Saf Health Care* 12:215.

Vrijens B, Belmans A, Matthys K, et al. 2006. Effect of intervention through a pharmaceutical care program on patient adherence with prescribed once-daily atorvastatin. *Pharmacoepidemiol Drug Saf* 15:115–21.

von Bertalanffy L. 1968. *General Systems Theory: Foundations, Development, Application.* New York: George Braziller.

Warholak-Juarez T, Rupp MT, Salazar TA, et al. 2000. Effect of patient information on the quality of pharmacists' drug use review decisions. *J Am Pharm Assoc* 40:500.

Weeks WB, Mills PD, Dittus RS, et al. 2001. Using an improvement model to reduce adverse drug events in VA facilities. *Joint Comm J Qual Improv* 27:243.

Weinberger M, Murray MD, Marrero DG, et al. 2002. Effectiveness of pharmacist care for patients with reactive airways disease: A randomized, controlled trial (see Comment). *JAMA* 288:1594–602.

Weinstein MC, Fineberg HV. 1980. *Clinical Decision Analysis.* Philadelphia: Saunders.

Wieland KA, Ewy GA, Wise M, 1998. Quality assessment and improvement in a university-based anticoagulation management service. *Pharm Pract Manag Q* 18:56.

Zimmerman CR, Smolarek RT, Stevenson JG, 1997. Peer review and continuous quality improvement of pharmacists' clinical interventions. *Am J Health-Syst Pharm* 54:1722.

▪ APPENDIX 7A. CQI CYCLE CHECKLIST

Cycle Background

Focus description
Should describe practice setting, the portion of the medication use process where the focus occurs, and baseline data (if possible).

Focus importance
State why the focus is important.

Literature review
Relate the focus to the literature.

Goal
Global and specific goals should be clearly stated and relate to the focus described in background.

Cycle Methods

Intervention
Describe and justify the intervention made (if any) for this cycle.

Processes and outcomes measured
Describe and justify the processes and outcomes measured (should relate to goal).

Data-collection procedures
Measurement methods should be clearly described and appropriate.

Data analysis
Planned statistical analysis should be clearly described and appropriate.

Cycle measurement

Cycle results

Sample description
Type and size of sample should be clearly described.

Results presented
Results should be reported for each stated goal. Result presentation should include graphs and/or charts.

Cycle Conclusions and Recommendations

Conclusions
Describe the conclusions your team came to after examining the data.

Implications
Describe why these results are important and what actions need to take place.

Recommendations
Recommendations for additional CQI cycles in this area.

APPENDIX 7B. CQI PLANNING WORKSHEETS FOR A REASEARCH PROJECT

Research Planning Worksheet 1

Date of meeting: _____

Name and contact information of each team member present:

1. _____   2. _____
3. _____   4. _____
5. _____   6. _____

Introduction

1. Brainstorm possible areas of study (list here)._____
_____

2. Rank and select an area of focus from the list above.

3. Provide a detailed description of the area chosen for study.

*Area or
project:*_____

*Setting:*_____

_____*Portion of the medication use process involved:*
_____

*Baseline data (if
available):*_____

4. State why the proposed project is important.

_____

_____

5. Relate the proposed project to the literature.

_____

_____

6. State the global goal of the project [*Hint:* Some options may include (1) discovery, (2) frequency estimation, and (3) measure of a change or a combination.] *Note:* Goal should relate to project stated in 3 above.

_____

_____

7. State the specific goal(s) of the project.

_____

_____

Methods

8. List possible interventions (some options may include reduce reliance on memory, simplify, standardize, use constraints or forcing functions, use protocols of checklists, improve access to information, decrease reliance on vigilance, reduce handoffs, differentiate, or automate).

9. Select best intervention to accomplish goals (listed in 7 above).

10. List process and/or outcome measures necessary to determine if goals were met.

11. Determine what data are all ready being collected and what measures exist.

12. Plan data collection methods [*Hint:* May choose from (1) inspection points, (2) focus groups, (3) monitoring for markers, (4) chart review, (5) observation, and (6) spontaneous report.]

13. Plan statistical analysis. Make sure you will collect all information needed.

14. Break the project into steps and detail practical considerations.

Step	Who	What	Where	When	How

15. Sketch preliminary timeline for project.

Timeline											
	Week										
Step	**1**	**2**	**3**	**4**	**5**	**6**	**7**	**8**	**9**	**10**

16. List challenges to be addressed before the next meeting

_____
_____
_____

17. Assign a responsible party to address each challenge listed above.

Challenge	Person Responsible	Due Date
1.		
2.		
3.		

18. Set date for next team meeting._____

Research Planning Worksheet 2

Date of meeting: _____

Name and contact information of each team member present:

1. _____   2. _____

3. _____   4. _____

5. _____   6. _____

Introduction/Methods Revision

1. Review materials from last meeting.
2. Review progress made.
3. Indicate plan changes, if needed.

_____

_____

_____

4. Add additional steps and detail practical considerations, if needed:

Step	Who	What	Where	When	How

5. Discuss challenges solved during this report period.

Challenge	How It Was Solved	Lesson Learned

6. List challenges to be addressed before the next meeting.

1. _____

2. _____

3. _____

4. _____

7. Assign a responsible party to address each challenge listed above.

Challenge	Person Responsible	Due Date
1.		
2.		
3.		
4.		
5.		
6.		
7.		

8. Update the timeline for project.

Timeline											
	Week										
Step	1	2	3	4	5	6	7	8	9	10

9. Set date for next team meeting._____

_____

_____

Note: This worksheet can be used for several team meetings. Proceed to Worksheet 3 when data are collected.

Research Planning Worksheet 3

Date of meeting: _____

Name and contact information of each team member present:

1. _____   2. _____
3. _____   4. _____
5. _____   6. _____

Measurement

1. Just do it!

Results

2. Analyze data.
3. Describe sample type and size.

_____

4. Describe a result for each specific goal.

_____

Conclusions and Recommendations

5. Describe conclusions the group reached after examining the results.

_____

6. Why are these results important, and what actions need to take place?

_____

7. What are the team's recommendations for this project?

_____

8. What are the team's recommendations for the next project?

_____

SECTION III

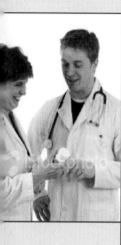

MANAGING PEOPLE

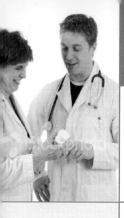

8

ORGANIZATIONAL STRUCTURE AND BEHAVIOR

Caroline A. Gaither

About the Author: Dr. Gaither is Associate Professor and Director of Graduate Studies, Department of Clinical, Social and Administrative Sciences, College of Pharmacy, University of Michigan. She received a B.S. in pharmacy from the University of Toledo and an M.S. and Ph.D. in pharmacy administration from Purdue University. Her teaching interests include the health care workforce, professionalism, career management, work-related attitudes and behaviors, interpersonal communication, and ethics. Her research interests include understanding and improving the work life of pharmacists, specifically focusing on individual-level (organizational and professional commitment, job satisfaction, job stress, role conflict, turnover, and gender and race/ethnicity effects) and organizational-level (culture and empowerment) factors. She also examines the psychosocial aspects of patient decision making and was recently inducted as a Fellow of the American Pharmacists Association.

▪ LEARNING OBJECTIVES

After completing this chapter, students should be able to

1. Discuss the field of organizational behavior and its development over time.
2. Describe the basic components of traditional and newer organization forms.
3. Compare and contrast different elements of formal and informal organizational structure.
4. Discuss the basic incompatibilities between organizational and professional models of structure.
5. Identify influences on pharmacists' job satisfaction, organizational commitment, job stress, and job turnover intention and organizational identification and how they affect organizational behavior and performance.
6. Describe the role of emotions in organizational behavior.
7. Describe different leadership theories and how they can be applied to pharmacy practice.

125

▓ SCENARIO

Joe Smart, a newly hired pharmacy intern, just completed his first week at the ambulatory pharmacy at State University Health System. Having worked previously in an independent community pharmacy, he wanted to get some hospital experience before graduation. Now he is not so sure. He really liked working with the customers that came into Sam's Pharmacy, but frequently he and the pharmacist who worked there were so busy that neither had much time to do anything other than dispense prescriptions. His first week at the ambulatory pharmacy also was quite busy. There were many more people working here than at Sam's. He was overwhelmed by it all. During orientation, he received a copy of the policy and procedure manual that detailed the health system's mission and organizational chart. He was very impressed with all this but could not figure out why it was important to know about the rest of the organization. He was going to be a pharmacist and, as such, was only interested in things that pertained to the pharmacy. He also could not understand why the pharmacy staff was so uptight. At his old job, Sam, the owner, would always notice if an employee was distressed or unhappy about something. Sam had an "open door" policy and was always ready to talk. Joe only saw his new boss, the director of the ambulatory pharmacy, once, and that was at orientation. The pharmacists he worked with were very concerned with showing him the tasks he needed to complete and not much else. Joe began to wonder if this was what it would be like to work for a large health system. He remembered that in his management class, the professor talked about working for large organizations, but he did not pay much attention. Joe thought that it was the responsibility of the manager to make sure that things ran smoothly and that he did not need to be concerned with details unrelated to patients' drug therapy. Anyway, he was new and thought that maybe he should give the place more time. In the back of his mind, however, he had this nagging feeling that things could be better, but he just did not know how to get there.

▓ CHAPTER QUESTIONS

1. What is organizational behavior, and how has it developed over time?
2. Why do pharmacists need to understand how an organization works?
3. What is some basic terminology used to describe organizations?
4. What is the typical organizational structure among common employers of pharmacists? How do newer organizational structures differ from more traditional ones?
5. What factors should be taken into consideration when designing the most appropriate organizational structure?
6. How does a professional work within a bureaucratic organization?
7. What are some of the typical organizational attitudes and behaviors of pharmacists?
8. What are some ways in which a leader is different from a manager?
9. What types of leaders do pharmacy organizations need?

▓ WHAT IS ORGANIZATIONAL BEHAVIOR?

An *organization* can be defined as a group of individuals working to reach some common goal. Organizations can be very small in numbers of personnel (fewer than 3) or very large (more than 5,000). Personnel can include staff (e.g., ward clerk, cashier, technician, pharmacist, nurse, or physician) and management and administrators (e.g., owner, president, vice president, manager, director, or supervisor). Both staff and administrators are important to the overall functioning of any organization. It is not enough for pharmacists to understand only the technical and professional aspects of their job (i.e., dispensing, monitoring, and counseling); they also must understand how the organizations for which they work function and how the people within them work. This is something that

Joe Smart has yet to figure out on his own. An examination of certain tenets in the field of organizational behavior will provide valuable insight into this area.

Organizational behavior is the systematic and scientific analysis of individuals, groups, and organizations; its purpose is to understand, predict, and affect human behavior to improve the performance of individuals, which ultimately affects the functioning and success of the organizations in which they work (Tosi, Rizzo, and Carroll, 1994). To be effective, managers must be able to understand why people in their organizations behave in certain ways. This allows them to take corrective action if problems arise. Managers also must be able to predict how employees will react to new technologies and changes in the marketplace (e.g., implementation of robotics in a pharmacy department or moving from a drug-product orientation to a people orientation). Organizations exert control over their employees through rewards or sanctions to encourage fulfillment of organizational goals and objectives.

Organizational behavior draws on a number of different behavioral science disciplines. Psychology, sociology, social psychology, anthropology, and political science all provide insights into how best to organize work (Robbins, 2005). Psychology allows us to understand individual behavior and focuses on such aspects as motivation, job satisfaction, attitude measurement, and work design. Sociology contributes by helping us to understand how individuals fulfill their roles within a larger system through organizational structures, behavioral norms, and bureaucracies. Social psychology focuses on the influence of individuals on one another and helps us to understand communication patterns, attitude change, and group functioning. Anthropology provides understanding of the environment in which the organization functions. Political science provides insight into organizational politics and informal organizational structures that greatly influence the functioning of an organization.

Understanding the functioning of organizations was not so important when the profession of pharmacy began. As noted in a Chapter 1, most pharma-

cists started out as apprentices of apothecaries, from whom they learned the practice of pharmacy, and then went on to become practitioners who owned their own pharmacies and trained other apprentices. As the roles of the pharmacist have changed over time, so has their training and places of employment. Currently, a doctor of pharmacy degree requires 6 or more years of formal education. Unlike in the past, today most employers of pharmacists are large organizations. These organizations can be chain pharmacies (several stores under one owner or publicly traded on the stock market); integrated health systems that incorporate inpatient and outpatient pharmacies, ambulatory care clinics, and managed-care and mail-order operations; and even pharmaceutical manufacturers.

Other professions are following a similar trend, wherein their practitioners are transitioning from employers to employees. Very few graduates of medical or law school operate independent practices immediately after graduation (Stoeckle and Stanley, 1992; Williams et al., 2002). Many physicians are salaried employees of managed-care organizations, integrated health systems, or group practices. Ownership of an independent community pharmacy or a private medical practice is still a viable employment option for many, but they too will operate in an increasingly complex environment. Understanding how organizations function will enhance health professionals' employment experiences and increase their chances for a rewarding professional career.

Why is this shift from independent practitioner to salaried employee so important? This shift may appear to be in conflict with one of the hallmarks of a professional occupation—autonomy. "The major distinction between a profession and an occupation lies in legitimate organized autonomy—a profession is distinct from other occupations in that it has been given the right to control its work. Professions are deliberately granted autonomy including the exclusive right to determine who can do the work and how it should be done" (Friedson, 1970, p. 73). Given that pharmacy and medicine are professional occupations, the status of practitioners as employees could result in conflict between the professional and the employing organization. In many cases, professionals' primary allegiance is to their work or patients and not to their employer. These practitioners also share a desire to exert at least some control over their work environments. If this desire is not met, job dissatisfaction and stress can result (Williams et al., 2002). Even as an intern, Joe Smart is questioning the autonomy afforded the pharmacists at State University Health System. His initial frustration, however, may be compounded by a lack of knowledge of how operations and communication channels differ in a large organization compared with a much smaller one.

This chapter will help you to gain a greater understanding of how organizations function by introducing basic organizational behavior principles, describing the structure of organizations, discussing the roles of employees within organizations, examining specific pharmacist organizational behaviors, and elaborating on the concept of leadership.

ORGANIZATIONAL PRINCIPLES

Chapter 3 discussed strategic planning and the development of mission statements and organizational goals and objectives. To understand an organization requires knowledge of its purpose or reason for being. Organizations do not function in isolation. They are created to meet some need in the external environment. As shown in Fig. 8-1, at the center of any organization is a set of values that form the reason for existence, the philosophy, and the purpose of the organization (Jones, 1981). Articulations of these values often are represented as the goals of the organization. Some organizations will lose focus if the goals they set are at odds with the core

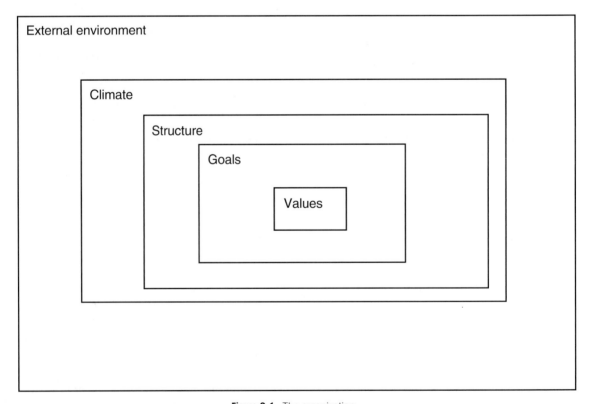

Figure 8-1. The organization.

values of the organization. In order to make the goals of the organization a reality, a structure must be put in place to make the organization operational. Typically, the structure includes such concepts as reporting relationships, communication patterns, decision-making procedures, responsibility/accountability, norms, and reward structures.

Structure produces the climate or the psychological atmosphere of the organization (Jones, 1981). The climate of an organization consists of such factors as the amount of trust, the levels of morale, and the support employees experience (Gibb, 1978). Organizational climate is often confused with organizational culture (Schein, 1985). *Organizational culture* is defined as the system of shared meaning held by members that distinguishes one organization from another (Robbins, 2005). *Culture* refers to the understandings and beliefs regarding how "things are done around here" (Schein, 1985). Once the culture is in place, practices within the organization act to maintain it by exposing employees to a set of similar experiences (Harrison and Carroll, 1991). The very specific and methodical training that Joe Smart is receiving is somewhat a reflection of the organization's culture.

Climate is affected by the organization's culture. A strong culture is characterized by the organizations' core values being both intensely held and widely accepted (Weiner, 1988). A weak culture is characterized by just the opposite—vagueness, ambiguity, and inconsistency. A strong culture will have a greater effect on the climate than a weak one because the high degree of sharedness and intensity creates an internal climate of high behavioral control (Robbins, 2005). Problems in the climate can be traced back to problems in the organization's culture and structure. When improvements in the climate are needed, some managers may only monitor employees' overall job satisfaction and stress levels. While it is important to do this, managers also should determine if there are problems with communication patterns, reward structures, and decision-making procedures within the organization and focus on problem solving in these areas. Has the organization stayed true to its values? If not, the shared meaning that employees hold with management will be confused.

Managers are essential in creating the culture, which influences interactions among coworkers and relationships with patients (Fjortoft, 2006). An unhealthy climate can hinder employee productivity and ultimately affect the overall effectiveness of the organization.

Organizations exist in an environment that is constantly in flux. This is particularly the case in health care. Organizations that employ health professionals and the health professionals themselves must be flexible enough to cope with the unexpected (Jones, 1981). Leaders and managers of these organizations must assess the core values of the organization regularly to determine if they are being challenged or if they need revision (Dye, 2000). Assessing an organization's culture will assist in determining how the organization is responding to both its internal and external environments.

Assessing Organizational Culture

A wide range of tools have been developed to assess organizational culture, including techniques ranging from observation, informal interviews, and attending meetings to the administration of carefully developed survey instruments. These instruments are designed to measure and compare the key cultural characteristics of a single organization or a number of different organizations (Scott et al., 2003). An example of such an instrument is the Competing Values Framework (Fig. 8-2) developed by Quinn and Rohrbaugh (1983; Quinn, 1988). Depending on the degree of flexibility or control in the structure of the organization and a focus on either the internal dynamics or external environment, four types of cultures are derived: hierarchical (i.e., internal focus, high control), group (i.e., internal focus, low control), rational (i.e., external focus, high control), and developmental (i.e., external focus, low control). An overemphasis on any of the cultures can result in a dysfunctional organization (Quinn, 1988); therefore, organizations need to embrace some elements of each culture. The most effective organizations embrace the dimensions that are most important and relevant to their goals and values (Cameron and Freeman, 1991).

To determine the type of organizational culture, employees are given an instrument that contains briefs

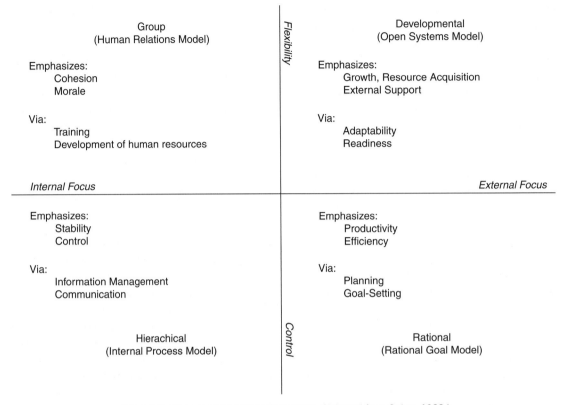

Figure 8-2. The competing values framework. *(Adapted from Quinn, 1988.)*

statements in which they are asked to rate out of 100 points how closely their organization reflects these dimensions. While this instrument has good measurement properties, some question if these four dimensions cover all the complexity that exists in many organizational structures and argue that the only way to really understand all the intricacies of an organization is through qualitative interviews (Scott et al., 2003). Nevertheless, it is a useful framework to understand various components underlying organizational structure.

Organizational Structure

Organizational theorists suggest that the structure of an organization encompasses three major aspects: differentiation (also known as *complexity*), formalization, and centralization (Robbins, 2005). *Differentiation*

refers to the degree to which units are dissimilar. *Formalization* refers to the degree to which jobs in the organization are standardized, and *centralization* refers to extent to which decision making is concentrated at a single point in the organization. Differentiation can occur either horizontally, vertically, or spatially.

Horizontal Differentiation

Horizontal differentiation describes the degree of differentiation based on how many different types of either people or units are included in the organization. Do all the employees of the organization have the same training and education? This is definitely not the case in pharmacy. Many pharmacy organizations focus not only on providing pharmacy services but also on merchandising non pharmacy-related items. If all personnel had the same training, managing the organization would be easier because everyone would have a similar orientation. Since this is not the case in pharmacy, coordinating the work among people in the different units can be more difficult. Horizontal differentiation can also take the form of multiownership of a variety of related industries. A health system can own several hospitals, long-term care facilities, and a managed-care business (Sahney, 1996).

Vertical Differentiation

Vertical differentiation refers to the depth of the organizational hierarchy. One key feature of an organization is the chain of command, or the number of levels between the owner or president of the organization and the staff. Vertical differentiation typically is represented by what is known as an *organizational chart.*

An organizational chart depicts the reporting relationships and the hierarchy of authority in an organization. An example of a typical organizational chart is given in Fig. 8-3. Authority usually flows from top to bottom, with those at the bottom of the chart holding the least authority. *Authority* is the rights given to a certain position in an organization to give orders and the expectation that those orders are carried out. Along with these rights, the responsibility for making sure work is completed is accepted. The solid lines represent direct reporting relationships important to the overall objectives of the organization (line authority). Line-authority positions include vice presidents, directors, managers, supervisors, and staff. The dashed lines represent advisory positions that supplement and support the line-authority positions (staff authority). Examples of staff-authority positions include chief personnel officer or vice president of personnel, finance, legal, real estate, information systems, etc. The degree of staff authority varies with the size of the organization. The smaller the size, the fewer are the number of positions needed to support the line authority. Many independent community pharmacies started out this way. One person (the owner) was responsible for numerous activities. As pharmacies grew and expanded, owners hired individuals to supervise different areas or functions of the store. As owners branched out into running additional stores at various locations, more

personnel were needed to run the day-to-day operations of the organization.

If an organization represents a for-profit company (i.e., portions or shares of the company are sold on the stock exchange), the top position in the organization belongs to the stockholders. Typically, stockholders do not have a say in day-to-day operations but are very concerned about the profitability of the company and will sell their stock if earnings are not up to par. If the company is a not-for-profit organization, the top level will not be stockholders but may represent a board of directors or trustees who oversee the entire operation. This group is also not involved in day-to-day operations but will meet periodically to either review or make important decisions regarding the entire company. The next level represents the chief executive officer (CEO) or president. If the organization is an independent community pharmacy, the owner will occupy the top position in the organizational chart. Depending on the size of the company, a chief operations officer (COO) or the owner of the independent pharmacy will run the day-to-day operations of the organization. If the company is national or international, regional officers responsible for the operations in different areas of the country may assist this person. Under these officers are usually department directors or district managers. Departments in a health system can include nursing, medicine, quality assurance, managed care, long-term care, etc. Each of these departments will have managers or supervisors who oversee staff who carry out the day-to-day responsibilities. Examples of specific pharmacy organizational charts are presented in Chapters 33 and 34.

Spatial Differentiation

Spatial differentiation is the degree to which the location of an organization's units is in one place or spread across several locations. An independent community pharmacy may have only one location that has all operations in one place. A large health system or chain pharmacy operation can have multiple units spread across a city, state, or entire regions of the country. Spatial differentiation can also occur when different

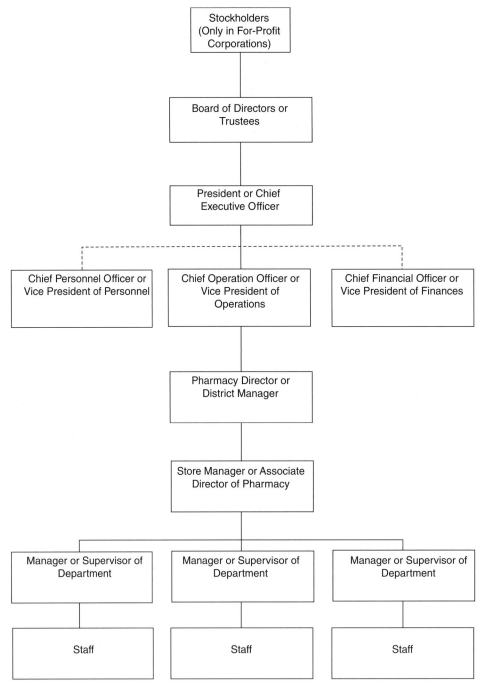

Figure 8-3. The organizational chart.

departments are located in different areas. A pharmaceutical manufacturer may have all its research and development departments in one city or state and the sales and marketing divisions in other areas of the country or the world. As organizations spatially differentiate, more coordination between these units is necessary. Spatial differentiation is also related to the amount of horizontal and vertical differentiation. The more complex the organization, the greater is the extent each of these will exist.

Formalization

Formalization can include the presence of rules (the degree to which the behavior of organizational members is subject to organizational control), procedural specifications (the extent to which organization members must follow organizationally defined techniques in dealing with situations they encounter), technical competence (the extent to which organizationally defined "universal" standards are used in the personnel selection and advancement process), and impersonality (the extent to which both organization members and outsiders are treated without regard to individual qualities)(Hall, 1968). If a job is highly formalized, the employee has little discretion with regard to when and how the job is completed. Standardization grew out of beliefs held by early organizational behaviorists who suggested that in order to make work more efficient, error should be reduced (Taylor, 1911). One way to do this was to standardize procedures to reduce errors and increase efficiency. As noted in Fig. 8-2, hierarchical and rational organizational cultures have high degrees of control usually through formalization and the standardization of procedures.

The degree of formalization can vary considerably within and between organizations (Robbins, 2005). Organizational charts depict different positions and/or units in an organization and formal lines of authority and decision making. This is one type of formalization. Another type is related to performance of the work. Some pharmacies require all pharmacy personnel to punch a time clock at the beginning and ending of a shift; others do not have such a requirement. Positions that make up the organization can have very detailed job descriptions that inform employees what they can and cannot do, whereas other organizations are less formal and do not have written job descriptions. Or if they do, the descriptions are very vague. Individuals who are higher in the organization will have less formal job descriptions than those lower in the company. Some jobs also lend themselves to more or less formalization. The legal requirements of drug procurement and dispensing are highly formalized, but the individualized services that pharmaceutical care requires leave much discretion to the individual pharmacist.

Centralization

Centralization refers to the extent to which decision making is concentrated at a single point in the organization. *Decision making* and *authority* in this context refer to the rights inherent to the position that one holds in the organization. Usually the very top levels of management make most of the policy decisions in a centralized organization. More recently, the trend has been to decentralize decision making and move it down in the organization to lower levels of management and/or even to staff-level employees. Problems with this approach arise when employees are responsible for achieving goals without the authority to make policies or gather the needed resources. Group and developmental organizational cultures have structures that allow for more flexibility in decision making.

Centralization sometimes is confused with spatial differentiation. A hospital pharmacy that has satellite pharmacies located throughout the hospital is often referred to as being "decentralized." However, it is decentralized in location only if decision making concerning the satellites still rests at one centralized point in the organization. Other organizational structure principles include division of labor, span of control, unity of command, and departmentalization.

Division of Labor

Division of labor divides work tasks into specific parts. This can be seen in pharmacy when there is a separation of pharmacists into those who only participate in dispensing functions and those who only participate in clinical functions. Even within clinical functions, pharmacists can specialize in a particular field (e.g., geriatrics, pediatrics, or disease states). This should result in more efficient use of the specialized skills of the individual. A negative consequence of the division of labor is that the professional may become very narrow in his or her abilities, and the job could become routine. Some suggest that enlarging rather than narrowing the scope of some jobs leads to greater productivity by using employees with interchangeable skills (Robbins, 2005). This can be seen in the health system setting, where pharmacists provide both traditional staffing functions on certain shifts and patient care (clinical) functions on others.

Unity of Command

Unity of command is the concept that an individual reports to only one supervisor, to whom he or she is responsible. As pharmacy organizations have tried to decentralize, employees may have more than one person to whom they are reporting. A structure that makes the most of this concept is called a *matrix organization*. A matrix organization integrates the activities of different specialists while maintaining specialized organizational departments (Tosi, Rizzo, and Carroll, 1994). Usually this takes the form of different specialists across several departments working in teams on specific projects. This type of structure works well in environments that are continually changing and in need of innovation. It also works well where project work is the norm, and people are required to get together in interdisciplinary terms (La Monica, 1994).

Pharmaceutical manufacturers and cross-disciplinary teams in health systems (e.g., nurses, physicians, pharmacists, and social workers) are particularly well suited for this endeavor. This allows for diversity of ideas and for the best possible solution to emerge. On the negative side, there is little evidence that employees prefer reporting to more than one supervisor, and confusion as to who is responsible for what can develop (Tosi, Rizzo, and Carroll, 1994).

Span of Control

Span of control refers to how many people a manager effectively controls. In pharmacies, we can see a wide variation in the number of individuals a pharmacist supervises. One pharmacist can supervise only one or two technicians in the pharmacy (in some states, there are legal regulations in this area), or the pharmacist can manage the entire store, including nonpharmacy personnel. Recently, there has been a push to increase the span of control of managers owing to a number of drawbacks to small spans of control: They are expensive because they add layers of management, complicate vertical communication by slowing down decision making, and discourage employee autonomy because of the close supervision by management. It is also felt that highly trained employees do not need as much direct supervision (Robbins, 2005). Some individuals find it quite discomforting to have someone always looking over their shoulder, but others may prefer to have someone who can respond quickly to problems when they arise.

Departmentalization

Departmentalization refers to grouping individuals according to specific tasks. For example, persons responsible for purchasing, distributing, and managing drug products could constitute a department. One of the advantages of having departments is that the individuals in a department share a common vocabulary and training and expertise. This should increase efficiency and effectiveness of the unit. Given the increased complexities of health care and pharmacy in particular, some organizations are requiring that members work across departments so that a diversity of ideas and expertise is given to specific tasks. This team approach helps to supplement the functioning of individual departments and allows for better communication between different areas.

Newer Approaches to Organizational Design

The idea that the best structure for an organization depends on the nature of the environment in which the organization operates is called the *contingency approach* to organizational design (Greenburg and Baron, 2003). In this approach, based on the work of Mintzberg (1983), there are five organizational forms: A *simple structure* is one in which a single person runs the entire organization. An independent community pharmacy would be an example of this structure. This type of organization is quite flexible and can respond to the environment quite quickly, but it is also quite risky because the success or failure of the business depends on one or two individuals. A *machine bureaucracy* is a highly complex formal environment with clear lines of authority. This type of organization is highly efficient in performing standardized tasks but may be dehumanizing and boring for employees. A chain or mail-order pharmacy may be like this depending on the degree of structure and formalization that exists in the organization. On the other hand, a *professional bureaucracy* is one in which much of the day-to-day decision making is vested in the professionals who carry out most of the work. In this type of structure, there are many rules and regulations that may inhibit creativity. An example of this type of structure would be found in a health system pharmacy. The positive side of this structure is that it allows professionals to practice those skills for which they are best qualified. On the negative side, these professionals may become overly narrow, which may lead to errors and potential conflicts between employees as a result of not seeing the "big picture." A *divisional structure* is one that consists of a set of autonomous units coordinated by a central headquarters. In this design, divisional managers have a lot of control, which allows upper-level management to focus on the "big picture." A negative side of this structure is high duplication of effort. A college or school of pharmacy that is structured around the various disciplines of the pharmaceutical sciences is an example of this structure. A fifth structure is called an "adhocracy." An "adhocracy" is very informal in nature. There is very little formalization and centralization. Most of the work is done in teams. An example of this structure may be found in the research and development department of a pharmaceutical company. This type of design fosters innovation but can be highly inefficient and has the greatest potential for disruptive conflict.

One of the newest forms of organizational structure is the *boundaryless organization*. In this type of organization, the chains of command are eliminated, the spans of control are unlimited, and departments are replaced by empowered teams (Greenburg and Baron, 2003). This type of organization is highly flexible and can respond quickly to the external environment. One form of the boundaryless organization is the virtual organization (Robbins, 2005). A *virtual* (also called *modular* or *networked*) *organization* is one that has a small core of individuals, and major organizational functions are outsourced to others. There are no departments in this type of organization, and all decisions are made centrally. An example of one aspect of this model in community pharmacy would be where all refill prescriptions are sent to a central location to be filled and then returned to the community pharmacy for distribution to patients or where technology is used to verify prescriptions while pharmacists are located at an off-site location.

Informal Organizational Structure

Alongside the formal organizational structure, an informal structure exists. The informal system has great influence in shaping individual behavior. Communication within the organization is one area that the informal structure affects. Formal communication patterns exist in the form of meetings, memos, and reports. Informal communication patterns ("the grapevine") can take the form of rumors, gossip, and speculation. The grapevine can be positive in that it allows formal communication to be translated into language that employees understand. In addition, it can provide feedback to the manager about pending problems in the organization. When employees feel frustrated at centralized decision making and their level of input, the grapevine can be a useful source of information. Informal ways of influencing decision making can also emerge through the formation of alliances and favoritism.

Organizational norms and accountability can be influenced by these informal means. *Norms* are explicit rules of conduct that govern such things as employee dress and punctuality in reporting for work. Informal norms can develop through peer-influence systems (i.e., if most pharmacists stay until all the prescription orders are processed, then someone who does not will be looked on unfavorably by peers). The *accountability* system considers ways to measure the achievement of organizational goals. This is usually accomplished through performance reviews (see Chapter 10).

Administrators and managers must monitor their treatment of employees continually to discern problems in the organization. Understanding and managing both the formal and informal structures of the organization are important for effective functioning and improved employee performance.

PROFESSIONALS IN BUREAUCRATIC ORGANIZATIONS

As noted previously, many organizations can be described as following the bureaucratic model of structure (characterized by control, hierarchy of authority, the presence of rules, and impersonality). While most pharmacists are employees of these organizations, they have been socialized through formal education and mentorship to value expertise, self-determination, and care to individual patients. This can be referred to as the *professional model.* Other aspects of this model include the use of professional associations as a major referent with regard to conduct and behavior, a sense of calling to the field (the dedication of the professional to work and the feeling that the practitioner would do the work even if few extrinsic reward were available), and autonomy (the feeling that the practitioner ought to be able to make decisions without external pressures from clients, those who are not members of the profession, or the employer)(Hall, 1968).

In recent years, the professional value system of health care has been challenged by escalating costs and the call for reform (Dye, 2000). Cost is particularly an issue for pharmacy because the cost of prescription drugs continues to escalate, and securing payment for nondispensing services (e.g., patient counseling and drug therapy monitoring) continues to be a struggle. One way in which health care organizations have responded to the need for change is to become more corporate or bureaucratic in values. The *corporate model* values the collective needs of its customers (not individual patients) both now and in the future and works to ensure institutional survival through measures of fiscal responsibility and operating efficiency (Stoeckle

and Stanley, 1992). The professional values the care of individual patients and their present health needs, which leads to a focus on trust-building behaviors such as eliciting personal concerns and exercising technical competence. The professional responds to authority based on expertise, whereas the organization's authority is found in hierarchical positions. Allegiances of the professional outside the organization (professional associations) could conflict with organizational norms. The formalization and standardization found in organizations can stifle initiative and discourage creativity and risk taking. There are some positive aspects to the organizational model. A highly developed division of labor and technical competence should be related to a high degree of professionalism because professionals are considered experts. Accountability and responsibility are important to the professional as well as to the corporation.

Students and pharmacists need to articulate their value system and search for employers that allow them to express this value system. Research suggests that the day-to-day experiences pharmacists have with their employing organization can influence how they view the entire profession of pharmacy (Gaither and Mason, 1992). Employers that exhibit a commitment to professional ideals and supportive management, in addition to their own organizational goals, are ones to consider. Organizations that allow pharmacists' expectations to be met find increased commitment to the organization (organizational commitment) (Gaither, 1999). Increased commitment to the profession also increases organizational commitment (Gaither 1998a; Gaither and Mason, 1992; Gaither et al., 2008). Support from management and administrators is positively related to organizational commitment for pharmacists working for pharmaceutical manufacturers (Kong, Wertheimer, and McGhan, 1992). Supervisor support increased commitment to both the profession and the employer for pharmacists working in community or hospital settings (Kong, 1995). Pharmacists who believe that the call for pharmaceutical care would have a positive effect on pharmacy were more committed to their employer and to pharmacy as a career.

It can be concluded that pharmacists' responses to organizational demands can have important implications for their professional values. This behooves students and pharmacists alike to work for and with organizations that facilitate fulfillment of their expectations. If the values of the organization are not in line with the values of the health profession, negative personal and organizational behaviors will occur.

PHARMACISTS' ORGANIZATIONAL BEHAVIORS

Examining pharmacists' work-related attitudes and behaviors is important if an organization wants to improve the positive and decrease or minimize the negative actions of employees. Increased absenteeism, tardiness, and counterproductive behaviors such as not completing work in a timely manner or theft will decrease organizational productivity and performance significantly. This has the economic consequence of decreasing the profitability of the organization (Barnett and Kimberlin, 1984). An unhappy coworker also can make the work environment unpleasant for other workers. The entire day seems longer and more stressful. Negative organizational attitudes also can compromise patient care. An unhappy or dissatisfied pharmacist may be less motivated to keep skills and knowledge levels current. Job dissatisfaction also has been found to be associated with an increased risk of medication errors (Bond and Raehl, 2001). The physical and mental health of the pharmacist also can suffer owing to the stress of working in an unappealing pharmacy environment with a heavy workload (Kreling et al., 2006). Studies of pharmacists' organizational behaviors have focused on a variety of work-related attitudes and behaviors. The most common are job satisfaction, organizational commitment, job stress, and job turnover.

Job Satisfaction

Job satisfaction can be defined either as an emotional response (the pleasurable or positive emotional state resulting from the appraisal of one's job or job experiences)(Locke, 1976) or as a comparison between expectations and the perceived reality of the job as a whole (Bacharach, Bamberger, and Conley, 1991). Each individual brings a set of expectations to a job. Research in pharmacy suggests that how closely the job meets expectations, performing more clinical or nondistributive work activities, higher levels of autonomy, good environmental conditions (i.e., better work schedules, less workload, and less stress), professional commitment, and working in an independent pharmacy environment are strong predictors of job satisfaction (Cox and Fitzpatrick, 1999; Gaither, 1999; Gaither et al., 2008; Hardigan et al., 2001; Lerkiatbundit, 2000; Mott et al., 2004; Olsen and Lawson, 1996; Reuppell et al., 2003). Being younger, male, in a staff position, working full-time, high role stress (i.e., role ambiguity, role strain, or role overload), and negative interpersonal interactions with either coworkers, management, or patients (Gaither et al., 2008; McHugh, 1999; Mott et al., 2004; Prince, Engle, and Laird, 2003; Stewart and Smith, 1987) are factors associated with less satisfaction. In a study of physicians, an organizational emphasis on quality of care enhanced job satisfaction (Williams et al., 2002). The same should be true for pharmacists. Enhanced job satisfaction leads to more positive feelings toward the employing organization (organizational commitment) (Gaither et al., 2008).

Organizational Commitment

Organizational commitment has been defined both as an emotional attachment (affective organizational commitment) (Allen and Meyer, 1990) and as accepting the organization's goals and values, putting forth effort, and wanting to maintain membership (Mowday, Steers, and Porter, 1979). Organizational commitment is important because it is related to reduced job turnover intention for pharmacists (Gaither et al., 2008; Kahaleh and Gaither, 2005). Organizational commitment is enhanced when health care professionals receive appropriate compensation and benefits (Gaither and Mason, 1992; Gaither et al., 2008) and have access to important organizational information, resources to perform the job, opportunities for advancement within the organization, and organizational support (structural empowerment) (Kahaleh and Gaither, 2005). This enhancement holds true regardless of practice setting (Kahaleh and Gaither, 2007). Psychological empowerment (i.e., finding meaning, feeling competent, and having independence and influence in a job) positively influences commitment for independent community pharmacists (Kahaleh and Gaither, 2007). High job demands (stress) and unpleasant interpersonal interactions decrease affective organizational commitment for hospital pharmacists (Gaither and Nadkarni, 2005).

Job Stress

Role stress in the form of role conflict, role ambiguity, role overload, and work-home conflict increases job stress (Gaither, 1998b; Gaither et al., 2008). Job dissatisfaction is also associated with increased job stress (Wolfgang and Wolfgang, 1992). Stress that continues to be ignored can lead to a phenomenon known as *burnout*. Burnout is thought to develop through a series of stages, and if caught at anytime, it can be reversed. See Chapter 13 for ways to manage job stress and burnout.

Job Turnover

Job turnover is one of most pressing concerns of organizations. The decreased productivity from voluntary turnover is very costly to an organization because less experienced workers must be used to replace the more experienced workers who leave. Advertising, recruiting, and training a replacement employee for someone who has left can be costly not only in monetary terms but also in terms of lost productivity owing to the time spent bringing the new employee up to speed. In a time of shortage of available employees, it is important to retain existing employees. Actual job turnover rates of pharmacists have been estimated to be between 14 and 23 percent per year (Gaither, 1998a; Paavola, 1990; Stewart, Smith, and Grussing, 1987). In an interview of chain pharmacists who recently left their employers, the main reasons pharmacists gave for leaving were related to working conditions: inflexible and long working hours and inadequate support personnel (Schulz and Baldwin, 1990). Other reasons for leaving an organization relate to job dissatisfaction, role stress, and culture and climate factors (Gaither, 1998a; Gaither et al., 2007, 2008; Mott, 2000). Personal variables such as number of children (more), race (whites less), age (older more or less), education (e.g., having an advanced degree), and having a major life event (e.g., getting married, getting divorced, or death in family) also can result in job turnover intention (Gaither et al., 2007, 2008; McHugh, 1999). Market conditions such as the number of jobs available are important because this may make it easier to leave one job for another.

As with burnout, job turnover is viewed as a process in which an individual will first think about leaving, search for job alternatives, form an intention to leave, and then actually leave. Therefore, it can be influenced at various stages. Managers may not be able to control all the factors related to job turnover (e.g., major life events or market conditions), but they should be on the lookout for ways in which the organization can foster commitment, improve job satisfaction, and decrease role stress. A place to start would be with the structure of the organization. Looking for problems in the amount of decision-making ability given to pharmacists, the tasks/workload assigned, the reward structure, and communication between management and staff is a good way to determine areas that need improvement. Another factor that may be particularly important for professional employees such as pharmacists is organizational identification.

Organizational identification is defined as the perception of oneness with or belongingness to a group/organization (Ashforth and Mael, 1989). To identify with an organization implies that one sees oneself as a personal representative of the organization and feels that the organization's successes and failures are one's own. Fostering organizational identification may be a very important way to shape health professionals' organizational behavior because outside influences (e.g., professional associations, colleagues, or patients) are important in the formation and maintenance of professional behavior (Dukerich, Golden, and Shortell, 2002).

The more strongly employees identify with an organization, the more likely they are to engage in citizenship behaviors related specifically to the organization (e.g., courtesy, conscientiousness, sportsmanship, civic virtue, and altruism)(Konovsky and Pugh, 1994). These behaviors are actions that typically are not captured in the normal reward structure of the organization. A recent study of community pharmacists found that participation in pharmaceutical care activities was associated with greater organizational identification (O'Neill and Gaither, 2007). Higher levels of organizational identification were related to lower job turnover intention. Additionally, the way in which an employee believes the organization is viewed by outsiders has a direct impact on both organizational identification and job turnover intention; the more positive the image, the greater is identification. Joe Smart may want to ask some of the patients and even the doctors and nurses who come into the ambulatory care pharmacy how they view the pharmacy and the services it provides. If these "outsiders" have a negative view of the pharmacy, it may be contributing to the tense atmosphere in the pharmacy. This brings us to an emerging area in pharmacists' organizational behaviors: emotions.

Emotions

Emotions are intense feelings that are directed at someone or something (Greenburg and Baron, 2003). Emotions are sometimes confused with moods, which are pervasive emotions not directed at any particular person or object (Fiske and Taylor, 1991). Moods have been shown to be related to withdrawal behaviors such as absenteeism and turnover (Pelled, Eisenhardt, and Xin, 1999). Health care organizations put more emotional demands on employees and patients than many other organizations, yet very little is known about what these demands are and the strategies people use to deal with their emotions (Ovretveit, 2001). One study in pharmacy found that the emotional expression of anger, defensiveness, or disgust is related to job dissatisfaction and depression, whereas the expression of

resentfulness and disappointment is related to emotional exhaustion, a major component of job burnout (Abunassar and Gaither, 2000).

Health care demands both the suppression and expression of emotion and skills to know and manage feelings appropriately (Ovretveit, 2001). Emotional regulation in the workplace has been termed *emotional labor* and is particularly important to health care professionals. Emotional labor is defined as expressing organizationally desired emotions during service transactions (Hochschild, 1983). The difference between the emotions that an individual expresses and those he or she actually feels can be the basis of emotional exhaustion.

Individuals who have the ability to take another's perspective or to know what another is feeling (empathic concern) or who generally express or feel positive emotions (positive affect) will have less of a need to expend emotional labor (Zammuner and Galli, 2005). It is also suggested that persons who are more emotionally mature (or possess greater emotional intelligence) will experience greater job satisfaction than those who do not. The pharmacists in the scenario's ambulatory care pharmacy may be expending in high levels of emotional labor. The pharmacy director may want to explore training for pharmacists to enhance their empathic behaviors, which also may decrease their emotional labor and possibly enhance emotional intelligence. The concept of emotional intelligence also has been linked to another important influence on the organizational behavior of employees: the leadership abilities of those in management or administrative positions.

■ LEADERSHIP BEHAVIOR

In an era of increasing corporatization of health care, securing the welfare of patients requires that health professionals participate in the creation of optimal frameworks to deliver care (Stoeckle and Stanley, 1992). No longer should the individual pharmacist say, "I am not the manager or administrator, so I have no role in determining how the pharmacy is structured or organized." Without highly competent and aggressive leadership, the provision of pharmaceutical care and other new roles advocated by the pharmacy profession could be usurped by other health professionals, corporate entities, or technologies (O'Neil, 2002). This will require the development of leadership abilities in all pharmacists.

Management versus Leadership

Leadership can be thought of as getting a group of people to move toward a particular vision or ideal. Leadership is concerned with change and with motivating employees to move toward a shared vision. *Management,* on the other hand, is concerned with handling the complexities involved in running an organization (i.e., planning, control, evaluation, and financial analysis) (Kotter, 1990). Given this distinction, a manager or an administrator may not necessarily be a leader. She may be more concerned with the day-to-day functioning of the organization. The manager may give little thought to the overall goals of the organization and how her department/pharmacy fits into the overall scheme. In addition, managers may not give much thought to the future and to developing a shared vision with employees as to where the organization should be moving. A good manager should also be a leader because one needs to be concerned with the present situation but have an eye on the future. The future should include not only the tasks and activities in which the organization engages but also the development of motivation and future leadership in the staff. This motivation and energy are essential to facilitate the transformation of pharmacy from drug procurement and dispensing into the provision of pharmaceutical care.

■ THEORIES OF LEADERSHIP

Trait Theories

Much of the early research on leadership focused on identifying personality traits that could distinguish leaders from nonleaders. Intelligence, self-confidence, a high energy level, and technical knowledge about the task at hand are positively correlated with leadership abilities (Robbins, 2005). The problem with the search for traits of leaders is that it implies that leaders are

born and not made. Individuals without these traits could never be leaders. It also ignores the influence and needs of the employees one is trying to lead. Trait theories focus more on leaders and less on followers. Research findings in this area have been inconsistent. Some studies found that one trait was related to leadership ability, whereas another study found that it was not related (Stodgill, 1948; Yukl, 1989).

Recent research suggests that traits do make a difference when categorized into five basic personality characteristics (Judge et al., 2002): *extroversion*—one's comfort level with relationships; *agreeableness*—an individual's propensity to defer to others; *conscientiousness*—how reliable a person is; *emotional stability*—a person's ability to withstand stress; and *openness to experience*—an individual's range of interests and fascination with novelty (Robbins, 2005). High energy and self-confidence can be categorized under extroversion and emotional stability. The other main drawback with the trait approach is that it does a better job of predicting who may emerge as a leader than determining what constitutes effective leadership. This has led contemporary researchers to take a behavioral approach to leadership and to focus on the preferred behavioral styles that good leaders demonstrate.

Behavioral Theories

Researchers have observed three very basic leadership styles: autocratic, democratic, and laissez-faire. *Autocratic leaders* make all the decisions and allow for no or very little input from the employees. *Democratic leaders* consult with their subordinates and allow them some input in the decision-making process. *Laissez-faire leaders* allow employees complete autonomy. In such an approach, employees set their own goals and work toward them with no direction from management. Let's say a pharmacy manager would like to implement a disease management program in the pharmacy. An autocratic leader would just inform the employees of the change in approach and then assign the tasks necessary to implement the program. A democratic leader would present the idea to the employees and ask for their input about the appropriateness of the idea and take into consideration their ideas on how to implement the program. Finally, a laissez-faire leader would not mention the idea unless the employees came to him with it. The leader then would allow the employees to develop the entire program and implement the plan. It has been found that all three styles of leadership behavior can be appropriate depending on the situation (La Monica, 1994). These findings led to researchers to begin examining the components of leadership behavior and the determination of appropriate behavior for the specific situation.

Situational or Contingency-Based Theories

These leadership theories are based on three basic dimensions: task and relationship orientation and follower readiness (Hersey and Blanchard, 1988). *Task orientation* refers to the extent to which a leader engages in one-way communication by defining the roles of individuals and members of the group by explaining (telling or showing or both) what each subordinate is to do, as well as when, where, how much, and by when specific tasks are to be accomplished. This dimension also includes the extent to which the leader defines the structure of the organization (i.e., chain of command, channels of communication, etc.) and specifies ways of getting jobs accomplished. *Relationship orientation* refers to the extent to which the leader engages in two-way communication, provides socioemotional support, and uses facilitative versus directive efforts of bringing about group change. This component takes into account the establishment of effective interpersonal relationships between the leader and the group based on trust. The third component consists of *follower readiness* or *maturity*. In this case, maturity is related the group's or individual's willingness or ability to accept responsibility for a task and the possession of the necessary training or experience to perform the task. As in the example given earlier, a group of pharmacists may be quite willing to develop a disease management program but may be inexperienced at implementing such a program.

Each of these dimensions can be located on a continuum that is divided into four quadrants (Waller, Smith, and Warnock, 1989). Fig. 8-4 illustrates these quadrants.

1. *High task/low relationship.* The leader determines the roles and goals of the group and closely supervises the task. Communication is one way and usually flows from the leader to the followers. This style, also known as *telling,* is most appropriate when followers are unable/unwilling or insecure (R1).
2. *High task/high relationship.* The leader still closely supervises the task but will also explain why decisions are made. The leader may alter the plan given the followers' reactions. This style, also known as *selling,* is most appropriate when followers are unable but more willing or secure (R2).
3. *High relationship/low task.* In this case the leader is more concerned about process and how the group works together to accomplish the task rather than the task itself. In this style, also called *participative* or *supportive,* the leader still may define the problem but supports the group's efforts at accomplishing the task. Followers in this case are able but unwilling or insecure (R3).
4. *Low task/low relationship.* The leader turns over all decisions and responsibility for task accomplishment, goal attainment, and implementation to followers. The leader may be available for consultation but usually maintains a low profile. In this case, also called *delegation,* followers are very able, willing, and secure (R4).

It is the leader's job to determine the readiness of the group and then apply the appropriate leadership style to the situation.

A final component of this model is *leader effectiveness* (La Monica, 1994). A leader's influence over an individual or group can be either successful or unsuccessful. When a leader's behavior fails to influence an individual or group to achieve a specified goal, then the leader must reevaluate what occurred and redesign a strategy for goal accomplishment. Even when a goal is accomplished, a leader's influence still can range from very effective to ineffective depending on how followers feel about the leader's behavior. If a leader knows the personal strengths of her followers and assigns goals or tasks with them in mind, this can make goal accomplishment quite rewarding for the followers. On the

High

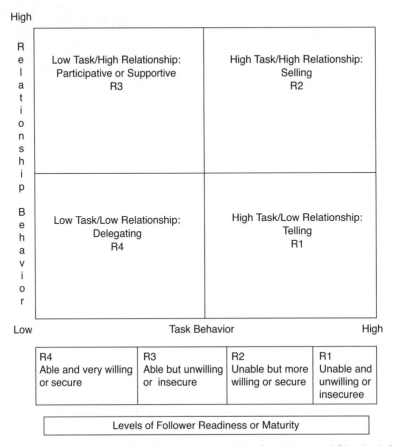

Low Task/High Relationship: Participative or Supportive R3	High Task/High Relationship: Selling R2
Low Task/Low Relationship: Delegating R4	High Task/Low Relationship: Telling R1

Relationship Behavior

Low   Task Behavior   High

R4 Able and very willing or secure	R3 Able but unwilling or insecure	R2 Unable but more willing or secure	R1 Unable and unwilling or insecuree

Levels of Follower Readiness or Maturity

Figure 8-4. Situational leadership theory. *(Adapted with permission from Hersey and Blanchard, 1988.)*

other hand, if the followers feel coerced to accomplish by a leader who uses positional power, close supervision, and rewards and punishments, the followers may be very unhappy and carry negative feelings toward the leader. Leadership effectiveness is very important because effective leadership will lead to followers who are motivated and goal-oriented even when the leader is not present. Ineffective leadership will lead to followers who often will relax the drive to accomplish when the leader is absent.

A study of pharmacists who worked in community settings or for national and state pharmacy associations found that the most common leadership style was selling (high task/high relationship), and the next most common was participation (low task/high rela-

tionship) (Ibrahim and Wertherimer, 1998; Ibrahim et al., 1997). About 26 percent of the pharmacists did not have a dominant style. Not surprisingly, most pharmacists scored in the low (community pharmacists) to moderate (association executives) range in their ability to adapt their style to the needs of their subordinates (leadership effectiveness). These results suggest that while pharmacists possess a dominant leadership style, there is room for improvement in terms of learning to respond and modify their style to best fit the needs and motivational levels of their staff.

Leader-Member Exchange Theory

Another theory related to the leader-follower relationship is the leader-member exchange (LMX) theory

(Green and Uhl-Bien, 1995). This theory suggests that leaders establish special relationships with a small group of followers early on in the tenure of the leader. These individuals make up the leader's in-group, whereas others are considered part of the out-group. It is unclear how these relationships form, but most likely they result from the followers either having similar personality characteristics to the leader or exceptional abilities to perform the job. The in-group gets special attention from the leader and tends to have higher job satisfaction and lower job turnover intention than members of the out-group (Robbins, 2005). These findings suggest that leaders need to pay attention to the nature of their relationships with followers because these relationships can greatly affect employee morale (Greenberg and Baron, 2003).

Leader-Participation Model

One of the more recent additions to contingency-based leadership theories relates leadership behavior and participation in decision making (Vroom and Yetton, 1973). This model assumes five behaviors that may be feasible given a particular situation. These behaviors are (1) you solve the problem yourself using the information you have available at the time, (2) you obtain the necessary information from subordinates and then decide on a solution yourself, (3) you share the problem with relevant subordinates individually, getting their ideas and suggestions without bringing them together as a group, and then you make the decision, (4) you share the problem with your subordinates as a group and collectively obtain their ideas and suggestions, and then you make the decision that may or may not reflect your subordinates' influence, and (5) you share the problem with the group and together you generate and evaluate alternatives and attempt to reach consensus on a solution. The leader-participation model then uses a series of eight yes-no questions to determine how much participation should be used. Questions include:

- Do I have enough information to make a high-quality decision?

- If the decision were accepted, would it make a difference which course of action was adopted?
- Do subordinates have sufficient additional information to result in a high-quality decision?
- Do I know exactly what information is needed, who possesses it, and how to collect it?
- Is acceptance of the decision by subordinates critical to effective implementation?
- If I were to make the decision by myself, is it certain that my subordinates would accept it?
- Can subordinates be trusted to base solutions on organizational considerations?
- Is conflict among subordinates likely in the preferred solution?

These questions allow the leader to determine which of the five behaviors is most appropriate. Results from research on this model suggest that leaders should consider the use of participatory methods when the quality of the decision is important, when it is crucial that subordinates accept the decision and it is unlikely that they will if they do not take part in it, and when subordinates can be trusted to pay attention to the goals of the group rather than simply their own preferences (Robbins, 2005). A more recent update of this model adds several more yes-no questions to consider regarding time constraints that limit subordinate participation, costs of bringing subordinates together, minimizing the time needed to make the decision, and the importance of developing subordinates' decision-making skills (Vroom and Jago, 1988).

This approach may be fruitful in pharmacy because new leadership models of organizing health care have been proposed. Governance models that focus on shared decision making between management and health care professions offer a way to combine both professional and organizational concerns (Young, 2002). The management style of leaders in an era of change is one that has a high regard for people and production and emphasizes shared responsibility, involvement, commitment, and mutual support (Williams, 1986). The most productive and motivated staff members are those who have strong relationships with others with whom or for whom they work (Abramowitz, 2001).

Transactional versus Transformational Leadership

Most of the theories presented in this chapter are considered transactional in nature. In other words, they are largely oriented toward accomplishing the task at hand and maintaining good relations with those working with the leader by exchanging promises of rewards for performance (Dessler, 1998). A newer approach to leadership takes a transformational approach. Transformational leaders make subordinates more conscious of the importance and value of their task outcomes and provide followers with a vision and motivation to go beyond self-interest for the good of the organization (Osland et al., 2001). This focus on task outcomes is a major shift in the health care arena because much of the focus of health care has been on the process of care (DeYoung, 2005). It is suggested that health care organizations need both transactional (for control and efficiency) and transformational (for innovation) leadership. A recent survey of health system pharmacists indicated that pharmacists did possess both transactional and transformational characteristics, but few were interested in becoming the director of pharmacy (Abraham, 2006). This suggests that more research is needed as to why this type of leadership is unattractive to pharmacists and what can be done to remedy this situation. More information on leadership theories can be found in Chapter 14.

There is always the question of whether leadership is really necessary. As mentioned earlier, advocating for patients and the fulfillment of new roles for pharmacists will require that all pharmacists demonstrate leadership behaviors. Such factors as ability, intrinsic motivation, the nature of technology, and the structure of the organization can affect the performance and satisfaction of its members. By the time pharmacists graduate from school, they possess the basic task knowledge to practice pharmacy. Pharmacists may also try to maintain good working relationships with patients and management because of professional values. These factors can substitute for effective leadership. Goals will be met regardless of what the leader or manager does or does not do. But managers and leaders need to recognize that by no means will motivated pharmacists continue to be motivated and energized in working environments that are negative and highly stressful. It is important for leaders to develop a shared vision with individual units in their organizations and support and empower employees to move toward that vision. It is an effective leader who conducts self-diagnoses and is aware of his or her blind spots or weaknesses and actively seeks ways to address them.

One final note regards the increasing diversity in health care organizations regarding not only the type of personnel working together (i.e., physicians, nurses, pharmacists, technicians, and assistants) but also in the demographic characteristics of these workers (i.e., gender, race/ethnicity, and age). Leaders must be able to effectively manage this diversity to maximize individual performance. An approach that links diversity to the actual work performed and values it for what it adds to the organization leads to an environment in which the benefits of diversity can be maximized (Ely and Thomas, 2001). Pharmacy employers should begin to open dialogues with employees to explore these possibilities (see Chapter 12).

■ REVISITING THE SCENARIO

Joe Smart knew that something was wrong with the internal environment of the ambulatory care pharmacy. What he probably noticed was a lack of leadership on the part of the pharmacy director and how the pharmacists were very task-oriented in their behavior. It may be that the employees of the pharmacy do not feel like a part of the health system organization and are feeling frustrated by a lack of recognition by others. It seems as though not a lot of time has been spent building relationships within or outside the department. Since Joe is the newest employee of the pharmacy, he is a bit hesitant to get involved, but he may be the perfect person to inquire about the values and goals of the ambulatory care pharmacy and how the pharmacy is structured to meet these goals. This would be a perfect time to examine the climate in the pharmacy to find out why the employees are dissatisfied. Although Joe does not have a leadership position in the organization, he should think about what he could do to improve the environment of the pharmacy. It is everyone's responsibility to make sure that health care is being delivered in the best manner possible, and unhappy staff members probably are not doing their best. Joe also could work on building relationships with others on the staff. This may help the employees talk about what is going on at the pharmacy. With the help of more experienced employees, Joe could bring these matters to the attention of the pharmacy director. By taking a proactive stance, Joe is developing leadership skills that will serve him throughout his career.

CONCLUSION

An understanding of organizational behavior is needed by pharmacists to function productively in an organizational environment. Looking for employers who facilitate professional goals is necessary for the continued development of new roles for pharmacists. It is important that health care professionals do not stay away from participating in organizational governance. It is a part of their professional responsibility to ensure that health care is delivered appropriately to patients. Leadership ability can greatly influence pharmacists' attitudes and behaviors. Without a clear and shared vision between management and staff, innovative practices will be difficult to implement.

QUESTIONS FOR FURTHER DISCUSSION

1. Why did the focus of organizational behavior change over time?
2. Given that organizations are trying to empower employees at all levels, are organizational charts still necessary? Why or why not?
3. How important is division of labor, span of control, unity of command, departmentalization, and other structural aspects in pharmacy today? Do you see more or less of these structures in pharmacy orga-

nizations? What new organizational forms do you see developing in the future?
4. What are some ways in which professionals respond to organizational demands? Are these appropriate? What are other ways of responding?
5. What role do values play in an organization?
6. Why is it important for pharmacists and employing organizations to monitor organizational behaviors?
7. What role does emotion have in a health care organization? How might we better understand its importance?
8. What are some key features of leadership? Is it important for pharmacists to develop leadership skills? How will you develop your leadership abilities?

REFERENCES

Abraham D. 2006. Pharmacy leadership crisis: Is it the people or the job? Paper presented at American Society of Health-System Pharmacists Midyear Clinical Meeting, Anaheim, CA.

Abramowitz PW. 2001. Nurturing relationships: An essential ingredient of leadership. *Am J Health-Syst Pharm* 58:479.

Abunassar SM, Gaither CA. 2000. The effects of cognitive appraisals and coping strategies on job satisfaction, commitment and burnout levels in hospital pharmacists. Paper presented at the 147th Annual Meeting of the American Pharmaceutical Association, Washington, DC.

Allen NJ, Meyer JP. 1990. The measurement and antecedents of affective, continuance and normative commitment to the organization. *J Occup Psychol* 63:1.

Ashforth BE, Mael FA. 1989. Social identity theory and the organization. *Acad Manag Rev* 14:20.

Bacharach SB, Bamberger P, Conley S. 1991. Work-home conflict among nurses and engineers: Mediating the impact of role stress on burnout and satisfaction at work. *J Org Behav* 12:39.

Barnett CW, Kimberlin CL. 1984. Job and career satisfaction in pharmacy. *J Soc Admin Pharm* 2:1.

Bond CA, Raehl CL. 2001. Pharmacists' assessment of dispensing errors: Risk factors, practice sites, professional functions and satisfaction. *Pharmacotherapy* 21:614.

Cameron KS, Freeman S. 1991. Culture, congruence, strength and type: Relationship to effectiveness. *Res Organ Change Dev* 5:23.

Cox ER, Fitzpatrick V. 1999. Pharmacists' job satisfaction and perceived utilization of skills. *Am J Health-Syst Pharm* 56:1733.

Dessler G. 1998. *Management: Leading People and Organizations in the 21st Century,* 1st ed. Upper Saddle River, NJ: Prentice-Hall.

DeYoung R. 2005. Contemporary leadership theories. In Borkowski N (ed), *Organizational Behavior in Health Care.* Sudbury, MA: Jones and Bartlett.

Dukerich JM, Golden BR, Shortell SM. 2002. Beauty is in the eye of the beholder: The impact of organizational identification, identity, and image on the cooperative behaviors of physicians. *Admin Sci Q* 47:507.

Dye CF. 2000. *Leadership in Healthcare: Values at the Top.* Chicago: Health Administration Press.

Ely RJ, Thomas DA. 2001. Cultural diversity at work: The effects of diversity perspectives on work group processes and outcomes. *Admin Sci Q* 46:229.

Fjortoft N. 2006. Identifying caring behaviors of pharmacists through observations and interviews. *J Am Pharm Assoc* 46:582.

Fiske ST, Taylor SE. 1991. *Social Cognition.* New York: McGraw-Hill.

Freidson E. 1970. *Profession of Medicine: A Study of the Sociology of Applied Knowledge,* p. 73. New York: Dodd, Mead.

Gaither CA. 1998a. The predictive validity of work/career-related attitudes and intentions on pharmacists' turnover behavior. *J Pharm Market Manag* 12:3.

Gaither CA. 1998b. An investigation of pharmacists' role stress and the work/non-work interface. *J Soc Admin Pharm* 15:92.

Gaither CA. 1999. Career commitment: A mediator of the effects of job stress on pharmacists' work-related attitudes. *J Am Pharm Assoc* 39:353.

Gaither CA, Mason HL. 1992. A model of pharmacists' career commitment, organizational commitment and career and job withdrawal intentions. *J Soc Admin Pharm* 9:75.

Gaither CA, Nadkarni A. 2005. The effects of interpersonal interactions and environmental conditions on hospital pharmacists' work environments. Paper presented at the American Association of Colleges of Pharmacy Annual Meeting, Cincinnati, OH.

Gaither CA, Nadkarni A, Mott DA, et al. 2007. Should I stay or should I go? The influence of individual and or-ganizational factors on pharmacists' future work plans. *J Am Pharm Assoc* 47:165.

Gaither CA, Kahaleh AA, Doucette WR, et al. 2008. A modified model of pharmacists' job stress: The role of organizational, extra-role and individual factors on work-related outcomes. *Res Soc Admin Pharm* 4:231.

Gibb JR. 1978. *Trust: A New View of Personal and Organizational Development.* Los Angeles: Guild of Tutors Press.

Green GB, Uhl-Bien M. 1995. Relationship-based approach to leadership: Development of leader-member exchange (LMX) theory of leadership over 25 years: Applying a multi-domain perspective. *Leadership Q* 6:219.

Greenberg J, Baron RA. 2003. *Behavior in Organizations,* 8th ed. Upper Saddle River, NJ: Prentice-Hall.

Hall RH. 1968. Professionalization and bureaucratization. *Am Sociol Rev* 33:92.

Hardigan PC, Lai LL, Carvajal MJ. 2001. The influence of positive and negative affectivity on reported job satisfaction among practicing pharmacists. *J Pharm Market Manag* 13:57.

Harrison JR, Carroll GR. 1991. Keeping the faith: A model of cultural transmission in formal organizations. *Admin Sci Q* 36:552.

Hersey P, Blanchard KH. 1988. *Management of Organizational Behavior: Utilizing Human Resources.* Englewood Cliffs, NJ: Prentice-Hall.

Hochschild A. 1983. *The Managed Heart: Commercialization of Human Feeling.* Berkeley: University of California Press.

Ibrahim MIM, Wertheimer AI. 1998. Management leadership styles of effectiveness of community pharmacists: A descriptive analysis. *J Soc Admin Pharm* 15:57.

Ibrahim MIM, Wertheimer AI, Myers MJ, et al. 1997. Leadership styles and effectiveness: Pharmacists in associations vs. pharmacists in community settings. *J Pharm Market Manag* 12:23.

Jones JE. 1981. The organizational universe. In Jones JE, Pfeiffer JW (eds), *The 1981 Annual Handbook for Group Facilitators.* San Diego: Pfeiffer and Company.

Judge TA, Bono JE, Ilies R, Gerhardt MW. 2002. Personality and leadership: A qualitative and quantitative review. *J Appl Psychol* 87:765.

Kahaleh AA, Gaither CA. 2007. The effects of work setting on pharmacists' empowerment and organizational behaviors. *Res Soc Admin Pharm* 3:199.

Kahaleh AA, Gaither CA. 2005. Effects of empowerment on pharmacists' organizational behaviors. *J Am Pharm Assoc* 45:700.

Kong SX. 2005. Predictors of organizational and career commitment among Illinois pharmacists. *Am J Health-Syst Pharm* 52:2005.

Kong SX, Wertheimer AI, McGhan WF. 1992. Role stress, organizational commitment, and turnover intention among pharmaceutical scientists: A multivariate analysis. *J Soc Admin Pharm* 9:59.

Konovsky MA, Pugh SD. 1994. Citizenship behavior and social exchange. *Acad Manag J* 37:656.

Kotter JP. 1990. What leaders really do? *Harvard Business Rev* 68:103.

Kreling DH, Doucette WR, Mott DA, et al. 2006. Community pharmacists' work environments: Evidence from the 2004 national pharmacist workforce study. *J Am Pharm Assoc* 46:331.

La Monica EL. 1994. *Management in Health Care: A Theoretical and Experiential Approach.* New York: Macmillan.

Lazarus HL, Duncan WJ. 1994. Restructuring pharmacy departments for survival. *Am J Hosp Pharm* 51: 2827.

Lerkiatbundit S. 2000. Predictors of job satisfaction in pharmacists. *J Soc Admin Pharm* 17:45.

Locke EA. 1976. The nature and causes of job satisfaction. In Dunnette M (ed), *Handbook of Industrial and Organizational Psychology.* Chicago: Rand McNally.

McHugh PP. 1999. Pharmacists attitudes regarding quality of worklife. *J Am Pharm Assoc* 39:667.

Mintzberg H. 1983. *Structures in Fives: Designing Effective Organizations.* Englewood Cliffs, NJ: Prentice-Hall.

Mott DA. 2000. Pharmacist job turnover, length of service, and reasons for leaving, 1983–1997. *Am J Health-Syst Pharm* 57:975.

Mott DA, Doucette WR, Gaither CA, et al. 2004. Pharmacists' attitudes toward worklife: Results from the 2000 national pharmacist workforce survey. *J Am Pharm Assoc* 44:326.

Mowday RT, Steers RM, Porter LW. 1979. The measurement of organizational commitment. *J Voc Behav* 14:224.

O'Neil E. 2002. The need for leadership in a changing health care landscape. *Pharmacotherapy* 20:891.

O'Neill JL, Gaither CA. 2007. Investigating the relationship between the practice of pharmaceutical care, construed external image, organizational identification and job turnover intention of community pharmacists. *Res Soc Admin Pharm* 3:438.

Olson DA, Lawson KA. 1996. Relationship between hospital pharmacists' job satisfaction and involvement in clinical activities. *Am J Health-Syst Pharm* 53:281.

Osland J, Kolb D, Rubin I. 2001. *Organizational Behavior: An Experiential Approach,* 7th ed. Upper Saddle River, NJ: Prentice-Hall.

Ovretveit J. 2001. Organizational behavior research in health care: An overview. In Ashburner L (ed), *Organisational Behavior and Organisational Studies in Health Care.* Basingstoke, Hampshire, UK: Palgrave.

Paavola FG. 1990. Trends in advertisements as an indicator of pharmacy workforce demands. *Am J Hosp Pharm* 47:2064.

Pierpaoli PG, Hethcox JM. 1992. Pharmaceutical care: New management and leadership imperatives. *Top Hosp Pharm Manag* 12:1.

Pelled LH, Eisenhardt KM, Xin KR. 1999. Exploring the black box: An analysis of work group diversity, conflict and performance. *Admin Sci Q* 44:1.

Prince M, Engle R, Laird K. 2003. A model of job performance, job satisfaction and life satisfaction among sales and sales support employees at a pharmaceutical company. *J Pharm Market Manag* 16:59.

Quinn RE. 1988. *Beyond Rational Management.* San Francisco: Jossey-Bass.

Quinn RE, Rohrbaugh J. 1983. A spatial model of effectiveness criteria: Toward a competing values approach to organizational analysis. *Manag Sci* 29:363.

Robbins SP. 2005. *Essentials of Organizational Behavior,* 8th ed. Upper Saddle River, NJ: Pearson Prentice-Hall.

Reuppel R, Scheider D, Lawton GC. 2003. Initiative for improving pharmacist satisfaction with work schedules. *Am J Health-Syst Pharm* 60:1991.

Sahney VK. 1996. Integrated health care systems: Current status and future outlook. *Am J Health-Syst Pharm* 53:54S.

Schein EH. 1985. *Organizational Culture and Leadership.* San Francisco, Jossey-Bass.

Schulz RM, Baldwin HJ: 1990. Chain pharmacist turnover. *J Soc Admin Pharm* 7:26.

Scott T, Mannion R, Davies H, et al. 2003. *Health Performance and Organizational Culture.* Abingdon, Oxon, UK: Radcliffe Medical Press.

Stewart JE, Smith SN. 1987. Work expectations and organizational attachment of hospital pharmacists. *Am J Hosp Pharm* 44:1105.

Stewart JE, Smith SN, Grussing PG. 1987. Factors influencing the rate of job turnover among hospital pharmacists. *Am J Hosp Pharm* 43:1936.

Stoeckle JD, Stanley JR. 1992. The corporate organization of hospital work: Balancing professional and administrative responsibilities. *Ann Intern Med* 116:407.

Stodgill RM. 1948. Personal factors associated with leadership: A survey of the literature. *J Psychol* 25:35.

Taylor FW. 1911. *Principles of Scientific Management.* New York: Harper.

Tosi HL, Rizzo JR, Carroll SJ. 1994. *Managing Organizational Behavior.* Cambridge, MA: Blackwell.

Vroom VH, Jago AG. 1988. *The New Leadership: Managing Participation in Organizations.* Upper Saddle River, NJ: Prentice-Hall.

Vroom V, Yetton P. 1973. *Leadership and Decision-Making.* Pittsburgh: University of Pittsburgh Press.

Waller DJ, Smith SR, Warnock JT. 1989. Situational theory of leadership. *Am J Hosp Pharm* 46:2336.

Weiner Y. 1988. Forms of value systems: A focus on organizational effectiveness and cultural change and maintenance. *Acad Manag Rev* 13:536.

Williams ES, Konard TR, Linzer M, et al. 2002. Physician, practice, and patient characteristics related to primary care physician physical and mental health: Results from the physician worklife study. *Health Serv Res* 37:121.

Williams RG. 1986, Achieving excellence. *Am J Hosp Pharm* 43:617.

Wolfgang AP, Wolfgang CF. 1992. Hospital pharmacy directors' perceptions of job stress in staff pharmacists. *Am J Hosp Pharm* 49:1955.

Young D. 2002. Shared governance builds leaders, aids patient care. *Am J Health-Syst Pharm* 59:2277.

Yukl G. 1989. Managerial leadership: A review of theory and research. *J Manag* 15:251.

Zammuner VL, Galli C. 2005. The relationship with patients: "Emotional labor" and its correlates in hospital employees. In Hartel CEJ, Serbe WJ, Ashkanasy NM (eds), *Emotions in Organizational Behavior.* Mahwah, NJ: Lawrence Erlbaum Associates.

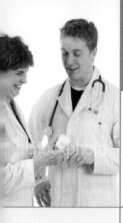

HUMAN RESOURCES MANAGEMENT FUNCTIONS

David A. Holdford

About the Author: Dr. Holdford is Associate Professor at Virginia Commonwealth University (MCV campus) School of Pharmacy in Richmond. He completed a B.S. in pharmacy at University of Illinois in Chicago, an M.S. in pharmacy administration at The Ohio State University, and a Ph.D. in pharmacy administration at the University of South Carolina. At Virginia Commonwealth University, Dr. Holdford teaches professional and graduate students about pharmaceutical marketing, pharmacy management, pharmacy benefits management, and pharmacoeconomics. His current research interests focus on assessing the value of pharmaceuticals and the role of marketing in health care. He is the author of the textbook, *Marketing for Pharmacists,* 2d ed., from American Pharmacist Association Publications.

▓ LEARNING OBJECTIVES

After completing this chapter, students should be able to

1. Explain the importance of human resources management in providing high-quality pharmacist services.
2. Describe the role of the Civil Rights Act of 1964 in managing human resources.
3. Identify critical steps in the recruitment and selection of employees.
4. Compare and contrast job orientation, training, and development.
5. Discuss the roles of motivation and rewards in employee performance feedback.
6. List the steps involved in progressive discipline.

▓ SCENARIO

Scot Phinney has just accepted a position as pharmacy director for a 200-bed community hospital in a fast-growing suburb of a southern city. Scot has a doctor of pharmacy degree and 3 years of work experience as staff pharmacist at another hospital across town. Scot's responsibility in his new position is to take care of the operations of the inpatient pharmacy department and an ambulatory care pharmacy. He is responsible for supervising approximately 20 full- and part-time employees on the day and evening shifts.

After just 1 month on the job, Scot is faced with several personnel problems. Three pharmacists have left the department recently for other jobs. Many of the remaining pharmacists and technicians have expressed dissatisfaction with their jobs by complaining constantly about the smallest problems. Two frequent comments made by employees are "It's not my job" and "I don't get paid enough for this." Some of the discontent has even led to serious arguments. Two times in the last week Scot had to break up shouting matches between employees. In addition to their complaining, the pharmacists show little initiative and appear to be only going through the motions of their jobs. Technicians are not supervised properly and are allowed to disappear from the department for extended periods. To top it off, nursing administration has filed several formal complaints regarding rude behavior and poor service by pharmacy personnel.

The tenures of pharmacists and technicians in their positions range from 5 to 20 years, making Scot the only newcomer to the department. Prior to Scot's arrival, the pharmacy director, a man who retired recently after 20 years of service to the hospital, gave minimal feedback or guidance to employees. The former pharmacy director avoided confrontations, so he typically let personnel problems simmer until they got out of control. Without much guidance from their director, pharmacy employees developed bad work habits and unprofessional behaviors. Scot would like to turn things around in the pharmacy department but is not sure where to begin.

CHAPTER QUESTIONS

1. How might poor human resources management in pharmacies cause (a) job stress and burnout, (b) medication dispensing errors, and (c) pharmacist shortages?

2. Describe basic human resources tasks. What are key elements associated with each?
3. Why are job descriptions and performance standards important in human resources management?
4. Why is human resources management a crucial element of a pharmacy's image in the eyes of its patients?

HUMAN RESOURCES MANAGEMENT AND PHARMACY PRACTICE

The scenario depicts an all too common situation in health care organizations, in which employees lack direction and guidance in their jobs. As a result, the quality and quantity of work suffers, and the work environment becomes intolerable. Without human resources management, even professionals such as pharmacists can lose direction.

The practice of pharmacy management consists of a wide range of complex tasks that involve either managing people or managing nonhuman resources such as property and information. Managing nonhuman resources consists of such activities as inventory control, computer systems design and maintenance, and financial management. This chapter deals with managing people. Managing people, known by the formal name of *human resources management* (HRM), is an essential duty for any pharmacist who must interact with or supervise others. HRM is important because it can make the difference between a smoothly running pharmacy and a dysfunctional, unsuccessful one.

Human resources management (HRM) is defined as the process of achieving organizational objectives through the management of people. Tasks associated with HRM include recruiting, hiring, training, developing, and firing employees. When these tasks are done well, pharmacy employees know their responsibilities and receive sufficient feedback to meet them successfully. When these tasks are done poorly, pharmacy employees are given little or inconsistent direction in their tasks and often are frustrated in their jobs.

HRM is critical to the pharmacy profession because many pharmacists and pharmacy employees probably are capable of much higher performance levels than they are providing currently. The negative consequences of this lost performance can be substantial to both pharmacists and their patients.

Many problems in the pharmacy profession result at least partially from the fact that pharmacists often are poorly managed and led. For example, overwork and stress occur often because pharmacy personnel waste time and effort in their jobs owing to unclear directives from management, poor teamwork, insufficient training, inadequate feedback about productivity and quality of work performance, and conflicts between people. If this wasted effort could be rechanneled into productive activities, then the burden and stress of overwork could be relieved. It can also be argued that many medication errors result from poor personnel management. A manager may contribute to medication errors by emphasizing quantity of work over quality of work. Medication errors may occur when poorly managed pharmacists are permitted to develop poor dispensing habits, provide inadequate supervision of technicians, or maintain incomplete medical documentation. Poorly managed technicians contribute to medical errors when they are permitted to develop bad work habits or do not communicate with pharmacists. If personnel were supported by better HRM practices, fewer errors likely would result, and lives might be saved.

This chapter discusses the recruitment, selection, training, disciplining, and termination of pharmacy employees. It describes the steps involved in HRM and some of the constraints placed on managers. It also offers recommendations to pharmacists for practicing more effective personnel management.

■ LAWS AND REGULATIONS INFLUENCING HRM

The HRM process is influenced by laws and regulations passed by local, state, and federal governments. These laws and regulations were put in place to protect workers from certain employer practices and biases. The Federal Civil Rights Act of 1964 is the primary piece of legislation affecting HRM practices (Donnelly, Gibson, and Ivancevich, 1995). The act and subse-

quent amendments to the act prohibit discrimination in employment hiring, promotion, compensation, and treatment of protected employee groups. Protected groups are those who might be discriminated against based on their gender, race, age, religion, sexual preference, height, weight, arrest record, national origin, financial status, military record, or disability. Laws that amend or supplement the act include (Donnelly, Gibson, and Ivancevich, 1995):

- *Title VII of the Civil Rights Act of 1991.* This amendment to the original 1964 act prohibits discrimination on the basis of race and places the burden of proof on the employer.
- *Age Discrimination Act of 1967.* This act protects employees 40 years of age and older from discrimination.
- *Americans with Disabilities Act of 1990 (ADA).* The ADA prohibits employer discrimination against qualified individuals who are labeled as "disabled." It requires employers to make reasonable accommodations for disabled employees to permit access to their jobs.
- *Family and Medical Leave Act of 1993 (FMLA).* FMLA requires employers of 50 or more employees to guarantee employees 12 weeks of unpaid leave each year for special family duties such as childbirth, adoption of children, illness of family member, or personal illness.

The Equal Employment Opportunity Commission (EEOC) was created in 1972 with an amendment to the Civil Rights Act. The EEOC was given the authority to monitor discrimination and file lawsuits to correct discriminatory practices in the workplace. This amendment was also responsible for *affirmative action,* an activist approach to correcting discrimination. Affirmative action pressures employers to actively recruit and give preference to minorities in order to correct previous prejudice in employment. Although highly controversial, affirmative action is practiced commonly in business.

Every process of HRM is influenced in some way by EEOC oversight. Hiring practices require that diversity in the workplace be considered. Interviewing is constrained by limits on questions that may be legally asked of job candidates. Disciplining employees requires that certain procedures be followed and documentation kept that ensures that discrimination does not occur on the job. Although some managers may chafe at the restrictions, federal employment laws act primarily to enforce what any good manager should already be doing, for example, developing fair and explicit HRM procedures.

In addition to the Civil Rights Act, other laws and regulations affect the management of human resources. For instance, the Occupational Safety and Health Act of 1970 established the U.S. Occupational Safety and Health Administration (OSHA) to develop and enforce workplace standards designed to prevent work-related injuries, illnesses, and deaths (OSHA, 2007). Of particular relevance to pharmacy are OSHA's ergonomic workplace standards and its rules for preventing exposure to hazardous chemicals and bloodborne pathogens.

▩ RECRUITMENT AND PLACEMENT

Importance of Recruitment and Placement

Recruitment and placement of pharmacy personnel are two of the most important tasks a manager can undertake. If a manager finds and hires competent, self-motivated professionals, issues such as motivation and performance are less of a problem. Good hiring practices also diminish employee dissatisfaction and turnover by matching the right person with the right job.

Pharmacy organizations need to exercise great care in recruitment and placement because each employee represents the organization and the profession. All employees who interact with customers help to determine the image they have of your organization. In fact, pharmacy clerks, technicians, and pharmacists are more likely to determine a pharmacy's image than any advertising or promotional events (Holdford, 2003).

Pharmacy employees can also be a source of competitive advantage in the marketplace. A good phar-

macist can generate significant revenue for a firm by maintaining a loyal patient base and drawing others from competitors. In addition, satisfied patients are more likely to recommend a pharmacy to friends and family and purchase greater quantities of merchandise.

Choosing the wrong employee for a position can be quite expensive. If that employee leaves after a short time, the employer must bear the cost of recruiting, selecting, and training a replacement. It has been estimated to cost businesses, in general, from $1,000 to $2,000 to replace service workers and from $4,000 to $8,000 to replace professionals (Reynoso and Moores, 1995; Weinberg and Brushley, 1997). Including the money lost from lowered productivity and lost business, the cost of losing established professionals and managers can rise to as much as $100,000 (Fitz-Enz, 1997). Table 9-1 shows some of the costs that might be seen with the loss of a pharmacist.

Hiring problem employees can also be expensive. Hiring employees who are unproductive or have personal problems can be a nightmare for managers. Many of these employees are able to keep their jobs by riding the line between minimal acceptability and termination. Even problem employees who eventually are terminated can sow conflict within an organization, reduce job enjoyment, increase workplace tension, hinder teamwork, and cause a host of other problems. Problem employees also can take up significant managerial time in counseling, dispute mediation, and oversight. Therefore, it is essential that pharmacy managers do all they can to choose the right employees.

Recruiting

Recruiting consists of all activities associated with attracting qualified candidates to fill job vacancies. The purpose of recruiting is to attract the most qualified candidates to interview for vacant job positions. Recruiting is easier when employers are proactive in their recruitment efforts. Proactive recruitment occurs when employers (1) continually recruit and network, (2) maintain a pleasant work environment where people want to be employed, and (3) establish a positive image in the minds of potential recruits.

Table 9-1.   Negative Consequences Associated with Losing a Pharmacist

- The pharmacy may have to reduce store hours until a replacement can be found.
- Patients may go to competitors.
- The remaining pharmacists and employees have to cover the responsibilities of the missing pharmacist. This can increase employee stress and lead to more overtime costs to the pharmacy.
- The employer incurs costs to replace the pharmacist. The employer may pay to advertise the position in newspaper want ads or professional journals. Salary costs are spent on personnel involved in related clerical and interviewing tasks.
- Personnel need to be freed up from normal responsibilities to train newly hired pharmacists.
- The new pharmacist may spend up to 1 year or more before becoming 100 percent productive to the employer. Productivity is reduced while the pharmacist learns job details such as the location of drugs, computer system procedures, and proper handling of insurance forms.

Source: Used with permission from Holdford, 2003, p 70.

Proactive recruiting of pharmacy employees should be a continuous activity that takes place regardless of whether a position is open or not. Well-run pharmacies continually develop contacts with potential employees who can be approached once an opening occurs. Contacts can be developed at professional meetings and social gatherings or through work. A pharmacy employer can also cultivate potential employees by hiring pharmacy students for part-time work and mentoring pharmacy students in advanced-practice experiences (i.e., clerkships).

Proactive recruiters also recognize that it is easier to find candidates the more desirable the job, so they attempt to build a desirable work environment. These employers try to improve conditions such as employee rewards and recognition, inclusion of employee input into work decisions, benefits, and quality of daily work life. Employers who treat employees well have fewer problems with job turnover because employees do not want to leave. When vacancies occur, they are filled quickly and with less effort because potential employees seek them out. In many cases want ads are unnecessary because applicants apply as a result of word-of-mouth recommendations from current employees.

Employers who are successful in offering the most desirable jobs often develop a reputation as *employers of choice*. Employers of choice have a positive image in the community and can pick and choose among the best candidates for positions. For example, Ukrops is a small grocery chain in central Virginia that employs pharmacists. The company has been twice voted to be one of *Fortune Magazine's* "Top Employers" (Tkaczyk et al., 2003). The company's annual voluntary job turnover rate is under 10 percent for its 5,500 employees. Thus there is strong competition for the limited number of job openings that arise, permitting the company to select the most qualified applicants from a ready supply of excellent candidates

In addition to word-of-mouth recommendations, advertisements are a common way of recruiting pharmacy employees. The first step in advertising is deciding how big of a net to cast for potential employees. Will local advertising bring in sufficient numbers of qualified candidates, or should advertising be regional or national? The answer to this question will be influenced by issues of reach and cost; that is, the more people reached by the ads, the greater is the cost. If local advertising is chosen, then advertisements can be placed in hometown newspapers or state professional journals. For regional or national advertisements, employers can use national newspapers (e.g., *New York Times*), national professional journals (e.g., *Journal of the American Pharmacists Association*), or Internet job Web sites (e.g., www.careerbuilder.com). The decision on where to advertise depends partly on the amount budgeted for advertising the position. The organization must consider the cost-effectiveness of the various advertising media. It has to determine whether there are enough sufficiently qualified persons in the local area to justify local advertising. If so, then local advertising probably is more cost-effective, especially because qualified candidates from distant areas would be reimbursed for travel for the interview. Another consideration is targeting an appropriate demographic. For example, if an organization is seeking a pharmacist with considerable years of experience for a management position, it need not advertise in a newspaper or magazine that targets teenagers. On the other hand, if an organization consistently recruits for a large number of positions, it should be conscious about trying to reach populations diverse in age, gender, and race/ethnicity.

After choosing the advertising medium, an advertisement is written. When writing any advertisement, it is important to keep it simple. It should not make false promises and should not use hyperbolic rhetoric or technical jargon. It should only capture the eye of qualified candidates and persuade them to contact the pharmacy.

Placement

Placement refers to candidate application, screening, interviewing, selection, and hiring processes. In many organizations, pharmacists are assisted in this process by corporate personnel offices. Personnel offices offer valuable assistance in advertising positions, managing applications and paperwork, screening candidates, advising about legal and policy questions, checking references, and extending job offers. They free pharmacy personnel to develop criteria for selecting employees, to interview qualified candidates, and to make the final choice.

It is important to emphasize, however, that pharmacists need to monitor and influence the personnel office's performance in the placement process. One reason is that personnel employees do not understand as well as pharmacists the requirements of pharmacy practice. They may emphasize different knowledge and capabilities than pharmacists. A second reason is that the personnel office does not have to suffer as much from the consequences of a bad employee choice. Pharmacy personnel will bear the brunt of a bad employee selection. Therefore, it is incumbent on pharmacists to

maintain as much control over the process as necessary to ensure a good choice.

Application

One of the first steps in hiring is for a candidate to fill out a job application. Job applications serve two purposes. The first is to help screen unqualified candidates. Applications can identify whether candidates have the necessary training, degrees, and experience for the job. The second purpose of applications is to provide background about the candidate for the interview.

Screening

Once they have submitted an application, applicants are screened to see if they meet the requirements of the job. Screening is a process that attempts to weed out unqualified applicants from the pool of potential candidates. Common screening criteria include lack of job qualifications (e.g., license, degree, residency, or experience), poorly completed applications (e.g., misspelling, missing information, or sloppy writing), and negative applicant history (e.g., felony conviction, lying on the application, or frequent changes in employment).

Screening criteria are developed from job analyses. Job analyses are systematic reviews of the requirements of a job (Donnelly, Gibson, and Ivancevich, 1995). Job analyses attempt to identify some of the following aspects of a job:

- Behaviors, tasks, and outcomes required of the employee on the job
- Skills, capabilities, and knowledge required
- Physical requirements
- Required information, technology, and resources
- Expected interpersonal relationships
- Budget and managerial responsibilities

The job analysis provides useful information for both employees and managers. For managers, information from the job analysis is used in writing job descriptions, interviewing job candidates, screening candidates, and setting performance criteria. For employees, information from the job analysis tells employees how work is to be done and the outcomes expected.

Interviewing

When qualified candidates are identified, interviews are scheduled. Qualified candidates normally are ranked according to desirability, with the top-ranked candidates receiving initial invitations to interview. If a candidate is not chosen from the first round of applicant interviews, a second round is scheduled, drawing from the remaining pool of applicants.

Preparation for an interview is as important for the interviewer as it is for the candidate. The following is a suggested list of interview preparation steps:

* *Send information about the position to the candidate.* It is helpful to provide candidates with specific information about the job description and standards for performance to help them prepare for the interview.
* *Identify interview objectives.* It is important to ask yourself what you want to achieve with the interviews. For example, if you have acute, immediate needs, you may only consider candidates who are available immediately. However, if your interest is long term, you may be willing to wait for an excellent candidate to graduate from pharmacy school or complete a commitment made to another employer.
* *Review the position description and performance standards.* The position description and performance standards will form the basis of your interview questions. Examples of a position description and performance standards are provided in Table 9-2.
* *Develop a list of interview questions.* Pay particular attention to assessing the requirements of the job specified in the performance standards.
* *Study the applications and résumés.* Look for accomplishments and credentials on which you want the candidate to expand. Also note frequent job changes, gaps in employment, demotions, inconsistencies in history, or incomplete information on references about which you want to learn more.
* *Schedule a quiet, uninterrupted interview.* It shows disrespect to the candidate if you permit interruptions and distractions from giving your full attention to the interview.
* Alert coworkers whom you want the candidate to meet so that they can schedule a time to meet.

Most interviews follow a relatively predictable number of steps. The first step consists of introductory small talk designed to put the candidate at ease. Rather than jumping immediately into the questioning, a few minutes may be spent developing some rapport with the candidate. After the small talk, interview questions are posed of the candidate. When the questioning phase is finished, the interviewer describes and promotes the job to the candidate. At this point, candidates typically ask questions of the interviewer about the job. At the end of the interview, applicants either meet with other interviewers or are given a tour of the facilities.

Interviews can be conducted in several different ways. The *traditional interview* attempts to engage candidates in a general discussion about themselves. A common question from a traditional interview might be, "Tell me a little about yourself" or "What are your strengths and weaknesses?" *Situation* (or *role-play*) interviews direct applicants to describe how they would handle a difficult imaginary situation. For example, "You are the pharmacy manager, and one of your employees has just told you that another worker is stealing merchandise. What would you do?" Situation interviews assess candidates' problem-solving capabilities and communication. *Stress interviews* attempt to replace the polite conversation seen in traditional interviews with a deliberate attempt by the interviewer to unnerve the candidate with blunt questions (e.g., "Why would a woman like you want to work here?"), interruptions, and persistent pursuit of a subject. It attempts to discern candidate preparation and ability to handle stress. *Behavioral interviews* try to evaluate an applicant's past behavior, experience, and initiative by asking for specifics about past events and the candidate's role in those events. Classic behavioral questions start with "Give me an example when you . . . " or "Describe your worst . . . ." Behavioral interviewing is based on the assumption that past behavior best predicts future behavior. In many cases interviewers employ more than one style in an interview. Other tools used by some employers to select candidates are standardized personality and skills tests. Their use stems from a belief that persons with certain personality traits (e.g., one who employs a particular leadership style) may be best

Table 9-2.	Sample Job Description and Performance Standards for a Hospital Pharmacist

Description

Responsible for safe distribution and drug administration for patient care, supervising technicians, order entry, drug monitoring, and providing drug information to nurses and physicians.

Qualifications

Bachelor's degree (5-year program) or advanced pharmacy degree (Pharm.D. or M.S.) from an accredited college of pharmacy, hospital pharmacy experience preferred, licensure or eligibility for licensure.

Performance Standards

Dispensing	Dispenses medications in accordance to all state and federal laws
Clinical skills and professional judgment	Integrates clinical, procedural, and distributive judgments using acceptable standards of practice to achieve positive patient outcomes.
Productivity	Prioritizes work to ensure that all tasks are completed in a timely manner.
Service	Fosters favorable relations between hospital personnel, patients, coworkers, families, visitors, and physicians. Accepts chain of command, supervision, and constructive criticism.
Written documentation and communication	Follows all state and federal laws, regulatory agency rules, and hospital policies and procedures regarding written documentation. Consistently, clearly, and concisely communicates oral and written information to all hospital personnel, physicians, and patients.
Technical supervision	Provides oversight and feedback to pharmacy technicians that ensures quality care and adherence to departmental policies and procedures.
Attendance and punctuality	Meets all hospital policies regarding attendance and punctuality.

suited for a position or may fit best within a company's culture. Similarly, a person may have to demonstrate one or more particular abilities on a skills test to minimally qualify for a job. The use of standardized tests has limitations, and thus such tests may not be used to a great extent in health care.

Most interviewers have limited experience and are prone to common interview mistakes (Umiker, 1998). One is lack of preparation. Managers who are very busy with immediate problems may be tempted to skimp on interview preparation. However, that savings of time is not a bargain if it leads to a bad hire. Another typical mistake occurs when the interviewer does most of the talking and does not give the candidate an opportunity to speak. It is hard to learn much about a candidate when the interviewer is talking. In other situations, interviewers treat the interview as an inquisition designed to squeeze the candidate into revealing his or her flaws. Although this may reveal some insights about the candidate, it is also likely to drive the candidate to another employer. Finally, some interviewers assume that the candidate wants the position, so no attempt is made to sell its benefits. Any of these mistakes can result in either losing a desirable candidate or choosing the wrong one.

Selecting Candidates

During the interview process, it is important to keep good notes about each candidate. This is essential for keeping details about candidates organized and for

Table 9-3. Interview Mistakes That May Immediately Exclude a Job Candidate from Consideration

- Arriving late
- Dressing inappropriately
- Poor body language
- Arrogance
- Self-serving questions
- Ignorance about the hiring organization and job itself
- Irritating speech patterns, such as not speaking clearly or an overreliance on slang words
- Failing to answer questions asked

Source: Used with permission from Medley, 1984.

documenting the selection process in case any claims of discrimination should occur. It is better to save note taking until immediately after the interview to avoid distracting the candidate during the interview. It is also helpful to develop an interview checklist to structure interview notes. Table 9-3 lists several interview mistakes candidates make frequently that can exclude them immediately from further consideration (Medley, 1984).

The final choice of the interviewer often comes down to how well a candidate can address the following questions:

- *Can this person do the basic job?* This addresses the ability of the candidate to contribute to the organization's performance. For instance, a good clinical pharmacist who has little dispensing experience may not be chosen for a position in a community pharmacy setting. Although good clinical skills may be helpful in a community position, basic dispensing capabilities are essential.
- *How well do the candidate's skills and capabilities mesh with the organization's needs?* Sometimes the best employee for a position does not have the greatest credentials or the most talent. In many circumstances, the best employee is the one who can fill skill de-

ficiencies in the organization and complement the talents of other employees.

- *Will the candidate make my job easier?* Everyone has some self-interest in the selection of a candidate. Successful applicants often highlight how they will be able to solve problems of individuals and the organization.
- *Would I want to work with this person?* This question deals with the rapport between the applicant and the interviewer. If the rapport is good, the chances of selection are enhanced significantly.

Hiring

In most cases, a candidate cannot be hired until the personnel department completes a reference check. If everything is found to be acceptable, a compensation package is put together, and an offer is extended. Once again, it is important that the pharmacy department be involved in the process to ensure that an offer is not mishandled. For example, if an uncompetitive compensation package is put together for the candidate, pharmacy personnel may need to argue for a better one. Once an applicant accepts a position, the hard part of HRM begins.

Hiring is just the first step in the HRM process. Once hired, employees must be given the training and feedback necessary to do their jobs. There are many reasons why employees may not perform their tasks as they should. Table 9-4 gives a list of them (Fournies, 1999). A quick scan of the list indicates that employees either do not know (1) what they are supposed to do or (2) how to do it and/or (3) they benefit from not doing it. Managers must communicate to employees what is expected of them, train them to do it, and provide feedback about how well they are doing and how they might improve. The remainder of this chapter addresses how employees can achieve these goals.

TRAINING AND DEVELOPMENT

Training

A manager's job is to help staff members succeed at their jobs. One key task in employee success is training.

Table 9-4.	Reasons Why Employees Do Not Always Do What They Are Supposed to Do

- They don't know what they are supposed to do.
- They don't know why they should do it.
- They don't know how to do it.
- They think something else is more important.
- There are no positive consequences for them doing it.
- There are no negative consequences for them not doing it.
- They are rewarded for not doing it.
- They are punished for doing what they are supposed to do.
- They are not and will never be capable to perform as desired.
- They have personal problems that get in the way.

Source: Used with permission from Fournies, 1999.

The purpose of training is to help employees meet the changing demands of their jobs. Training benefits both the organization and the employee. For the organization, it improves the quality and quantity of work provided by each employee. For the employee, it can make the job more interesting and meaningful and lead to greater morale and sense of accomplishment (Holdford, 2003). Excellent pharmacy service organizations invest in the training and development of their employees.

Training and development serve different purposes. *Training* is meant to improve employee performance with current tasks and jobs, whereas *development* prepares employees for new responsibilities and positions. Therefore, training is essential for meeting current needs, and development is an investment in future needs.

Training comes in two primary forms: orientation and job training. The purpose of *orientation training* is to welcome new employees, present a positive first impression, provide information that will permit them to settle into their new responsibilities, and establish early expectations of performance and behav-

ior (Umiker, 1998). It also involves familiarizing new hires with the company's/department's mission, goals, cultural norms, and expectations. Examples of things covered in orientation training include coworker introductions, a tour of the facilities, discussion of employee benefits, review of departmental policies and procedures, discussion of performance objectives for the job, description of behavioral expectations, demonstration of the computer system, and special organizational training (e.g., HIPAA, sexual harassment, and discrimination). It is a good idea to develop a checklist that covers all orientation topics to ensure that nothing is overlooked.

Job training helps current employees learn new information and skills to do their jobs and refresh capabilities that may have diminished over time. Although pharmacists are highly trained professionals, the changing nature of medical and business practice requires continual training throughout their careers. Job training is a responsibility of both the individual and the organization. For example, a pharmacist might attend a continuing-education program offered by a pharmacy school to fill a perceived gap in knowledge about a disease state and its treatment. Alternatively, a pharmacist may be asked by an employer to receive on-the-job training in customer-service methods to fulfill a perceived employer need. Job training can be used to develop habits (e.g., time management), knowledge (e.g., new drug treatments), skills (e.g., blood pressure monitoring), procedures (e.g., handling drug insurance claims), and policies (e.g., sexual harassment).

Pharmacy organizations formally or informally may employ a type of training called *job rotation* (also known as *cross-training*). Job rotation is designed to give an individual broad experience through exposure to different areas of the organization. In a hospital pharmacy, for example, newly hired technicians can be trained in filling carts, outpatient dispensing, intravenous admixture preparation, inventory management, billing and crediting, and working in one or more satellite pharmacy units. Such training would diversify technicians' skills, allowing them to work in any number of areas should one be short-staffed, and may help to improve their self-esteem and sense of contribution to the organization (see Chapter 12 on skill variety and task significance).

Development

Development requires a long-term focus by preparing for future needs of the individual or organization. Professional development typically consists of answering the following questions: (1) What is my present situation? (2) Where do I want to be? (3) What skills, knowledge, and training do I need to get where I want to be?

Development differs from training in that it requires a greater intensity of education and instruction. Whereas job training might be met sufficiently with continuing-education programs, on-the-job instruction, and short courses, professional development may require formal education and structured experiences such as college courses, multiday seminars and certificate programs, residencies, or fellowships.

■ PERFORMANCE FEEDBACK

Types of Performance Feedback

While training and development prepare employees for current and future jobs, performance feedback communicates how well they are doing in their jobs and how they can improve. Managers commonly provide employee feedback in three ways. The first and most important is the *day-to-day feedback* provided on the job. This refers to the verbal and visual messages provided daily to employees through conversations, body language, and behaviors. Daily communication is the most effective performance feedback because it is immediate and often. Other forms of managerial feedback are provided less frequently and often long after the behavior occurred. The following is a list of suggestions for providing useful daily feedback to employees:

- *Practice management-by-walking-around (MBWA).* This management approach consists of getting out the office or from behind the desk and interacting with employees. It is hard to provide feedback to individuals without frequent personal contact.

- *When practicing MBWA, listen more than talk.* The purpose of MBWA is to learn what is happening within the organization and to solicit input and advice from others. That information is then acted on to improve the organization and the work of employees.

- *Focus on the positive.* Encourage people by catching them doing something right, *not* catching them doing something wrong. Employees get enough negative feedback. Surprise them with positive comments specific to an action that you want them to continue doing, for example, "I liked how you went out of your way to listen to the concerns of that patient and find exactly the right solution for her needs."

- *Take notes.* When people make suggestions or you make promises, write them down. Provide a deadline for getting back to them about any documented issue. Then keep your promise to get back to them by that deadline.

- *Make individuals see your presence as helpful.* Try not to waste peoples' time, interrupt their work, nitpick, complicate things, or do anything that makes their day-to-day job more difficult. The purpose of MBWA is to assist and support employees, not to criticize and inspect their work.

A second form of feedback comes through the employees' *annual* (or *semiannual*) *performance reviews.* Annual performance reviews act as long-term planning sessions where managers help employees to review their previous progress, identify successes and areas that need improvement, and establish goals and objectives for the next year (Umiker, 1998). Annual performance reviews augment and summarize feedback provided by managers on a day-to-day basis. Annual performance reviews are discussed in greater detail in Chapter 10.

The final form of managerial feedback comes from reviews scheduled ad hoc in response to certain particularly good or bad performances. Good *ad hoc performance reviews* are designed to provide recognition for outstanding performance and may be accompanied by some award or gift. Bad ad hoc reviews are designed to address unacceptable employee behavior or performance immediately. These negative ad hoc reviews are part of a process called *progressive discipline.*

Progressive Discipline

Progressive discipline is defined as a series of acts taken by management in response to unacceptable performance by employees. The role of progressive discipline is to escalate the consequences of poor employee performance incrementally with a goal of improving that behavior. Responses by management to undesirable behavior become progressively severe until the employee either improves, resigns, or is terminated from the position. Although punitive in nature, the purpose of progressive discipline is not to punish. Rather, the aim is to make explicit to an employee the consequences of unsatisfactory behavior in order to encourage improved behavior. Indeed, improved behavior is always the preferred outcome, never the loss of an employee through resignation or termination. Progressive discipline may be initiated in response to employee behaviors such as discourtesy to customers or coworkers, tardiness, absenteeism, unsatisfactory work performance, and violation of departmental policies. Progressive discipline usually consists of the following steps: verbal warning, written warning, suspension, and termination.

Verbal Warning

A *verbal warning* is a formal oral reprimand about the consequences of failing to perform as expected. A manager might verbally warn a technician that she is performing below expectations in regard to tardiness and that if performance is not improved, further disciplinary action may be warranted. Verbal warnings are relatively common and often the only action needed to correct unacceptable employee performance.

Written Warning

If an employee does not respond to a verbal warning, a more formal written warning is issued. A *written warning* is the first formal step in progressive discipline that may result in eventual discharge of the employee. It differs from verbal warnings, which are relatively informal acts that only require the manager to note the time and place of the reprimand and what

was discussed. A written warning is a legal document that can end up as evidence in a court case. If an employee is discharged and any disciplinary step is handled inappropriately, the employer can be sued successfully for financial damages by the employee. Therefore, written warnings should be crafted carefully with help from superiors and the human resources department.

The written warning should describe the unacceptable behavior clearly, previous warnings, specific expectations of future behavior to be achieved by a precise deadline, and the consequences of not meeting expectations. For example, "You were verbally warned about tardiness on January 16 of this year. You have continued to be tardy at a rate above that specified in your performance standards. If you are late for work more than twice within the next month, you will be suspended for one day without pay." As shown by this example, it is essential for a manager to keep good records of previous warnings because they will be used as the basis for potential written warnings.

Suspension

Suspensions are punitive actions meant to demonstrate the seriousness of a situation. Sometimes written warnings do not result in improved employee performance and need to be backed up by actions. Suspensions are meant to act as a final warning that current behavior is unacceptable. Like written warnings, they must be crafted carefully to include previous warnings, requirements for future actions, and consequences for not improving behavior (e.g., termination).

■ TERMINATION OF EMPLOYEES

Some managers are hesitant to terminate employees because it can be a difficult circumstance for all involved. For the terminated employee, it can have a tremendous impact on self-esteem, reputation, and personal finances. For the manager, it can be an emotionally charged event that results in an unpleasant confrontation. It also can lead to legal action for the business and individual manager. Therefore, some managers avoid dealing with such situations by insisting wrongly that laws and rules make it impossible to fire anyone.

However, if employees are provided clear performance standards and the procedures for progressive discipline are observed, firing bad employees usually is not difficult procedurally. This means that every step leading up to the termination must be appropriate and documented.

Procedures for terminating employees differ depending on the circumstances. For newly hired employees who are on probation (i.e., a trial period for assessing new employees), the process of progressive discipline ordinarily does not need to be followed. The employee can be terminated at any time during the probationary period if it is clear that the employee will not succeed in the job. The steps of verbal warning, written warning, and suspension are not necessary before termination. The same is true for employees who commit acts that can lead to immediate termination, such as fighting on the job, drug or alcohol use at work, stealing, vandalism, or periods of absence without notice.

For employees who do not fall into the preceding categories, termination should not come as a surprise. Following progressive discipline procedures should give employees explicit expectations of what is going to occur when performance is not improved. Many employees will resign before being terminated. Employees who do not resign are asked to attend a termination meeting.

Prior to the termination meeting, the manager must be certain that all the following statements are true:

- The employee is not being terminated for anything but poor job performance or breaking major rules (e.g., theft or fighting).
- The reason for termination can be stated in measurable, factual terms.
- The employee has been given specific feedback regarding the performance deficiency in measurable, factual terms.
- The organization's policies and procedures regarding discipline have been observed and actions documented.

- The employee has been given ample opportunity to correct the poor performance.
- Employee treatment is consistent with similar situations of employee performance.
- The personnel department has been kept informed throughout the disciplinary process and is currently aware of plans to terminate the employee. If there is no personnel department with whom to confer, a lawyer should be consulted.

Most businesses have a procedure for terminating employees, so the manager simply follows that procedure. Most termination procedures require that a witness be present during the meeting to verify conversations and actions.

The primary goal of the termination meeting is to terminate the employee compassionately and in a manner that maintains the employee's dignity and self-respect. This is better achieved by being direct and to the point by stating something such as, "You have not achieved the performance objectives specified in our last meeting, so we have decided to terminate you from your position."

The employee may respond in multiple ways (e.g., anger, tears), but your response should be neutral. You should not argue with or criticize the employee or engage in any negotiations. It is essential to state that this decision is final. Let the employee vent any frustrations, but do not permit abusive or violent behavior. Be ready to discuss a severance package or direct the person to the human resources department, and then end the meeting.

Since an employee may be upset and not thinking very clearly after termination, it is useful to offer recommendations on what he or she should do next. For instance, the employer may tell the employee that he does not need to complete his shift and that his belongings will be packed and left for him to pick up the following day at some designated place.

After termination, several final steps need to be concluded. Documentation of final actions should be completed and filed. All people involved should be reminded about the confidentiality of discussions and actions. Finally, the manager should reflect on how the process went and what changes may be necessary to prevent further terminations.

REVISITING THE SCENARIO—TACKLING HUMAN RELATIONS

Scot Phinney's problems in the scenario revolve around HRM. There appear to be three related problems: (1) There are three pharmacist position vacancies that need to be filled, (2) employee morale is low, and (3) current employee productivity and behavior are unacceptable. Scot has identified several specific employee behaviors that hinder the performance of the pharmacy, including frequent arguments, excessive complaints, pharmacists not supervising technicians, and rude behavior and poor service to nursing. He has decided to focus on these problems first.

Scot's first step should be to examine the current job and performance descriptions of the employees to see if they address the problem behaviors described. If they do, then he can use them to illustrate that specific behaviors are documented as unacceptable. If job descriptions and performance standards do not address problem behaviors, then they need to be updated. With clearly defined duties and performance standards for all employees, Scot can start a dialogue with employees about expected behavior using specific examples. For instance, if a pharmacist states that it is not her job to supervise technicians, Scot can review the performance standards that relate to her supervisory duties. Scot needs to communicate clear expectations of employees and provide feedback in day-to-day discussions, annual reviews, and disciplinary actions.

Scot should realize that changing entrenched employees is a long process, so he should be patient and persistent. Some employees may not accept his efforts immediately and may refuse to alter their conduct. Scot will have to apply pressure through progressive discipline to encourage them to change or find a new employer. If he is consistent and fair, most employees will go along with and even embrace the changes. With successful change, employee morale should also increase and the turnover rate slow down.

CONCLUSION

Good HRM is an important requirement for providing excellent pharmacy services. Pharmacy personnel who are well managed are more likely to be satisfied in their jobs, effective, and productive. Good HRM in health care fields enhances the likelihood that patients will be better served and achieve better health outcomes. Any pharmacist who is serious about serving patients and the profession needs to be committed to good HRM.

QUESTIONS FOR FURTHER DISCUSSION

1. What are the potential advantages and limitations of affirmative action to a pharmacy organization?
2. What knowledge and skills are employers looking for in pharmacists?
3. What questions might an interviewer ask of a candidate for the job described in Table 9-2?
4. Which interview method do you think is most effective? Least effective? Why?
5. When should the job search process for pharmacist jobs start for pharmacy students? What actions should be taken?
6. How effective would you be at terminating an employee for poor job performance? Why or why not?
7. Think about your last job search and employment. Rate your employer's performance in the areas of
   a. Recruitment and selection
   b. Interviewing
   c. Orientation and training
   d. Performance feedback
8. What type of performance feedback have you received from previous employers? Describe a specific example in which an employer did a particularly good or bad job of providing feedback.

REFERENCES

Donnelly JH, Gibson JL, Ivancevich JM. 1995. Human resource management. In *Fundamentals of Management*, Vol 13, p. 444. Chicago: Irwin.

Fitz-Enz J. 1997. It's costly to lose good employees. *Workforce* 76:51.

Fournies FF. 1999. *Why Employees Don't Do What They're Supposed to Do and What to Do About It.* New York: McGraw-Hill.

Holdford DA. 2003. *Marketing for Pharmacists.* Washington, DC: American Pharmaceutical Association.

Occupational Safety & Health Administration (OSHA), U.S. Department of Labor. 2007. Available at www.osha.gov/; accessed on August 15, 2007.

Medley HA. 1984. *Sweaty Palms: The Neglected Art of Being Interviewed.* Berkley, CA: Ten Speed Press.

Reynoso J, Moores B. 1995. Towards the measurement of internal service quality. *Int J Serv Ind Manag* 6:64.

Tkaczyk T, Harrington A, Moskowitz M, Levering R. 2003. The 100 best companies to work for in America. *Fortune* 147:127.

Umiker W. 1998. *Management Skills for the New Health Care Superviser.* Gaithersburg, MD: Aspen Publishers.

Weinberg CR, Brushley CD. 1997. Stop the job hop! *Chief Executive* 122:44.

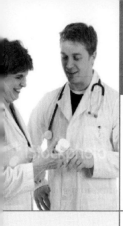

10

PERFORMANCE APPRAISAL SYSTEMS

Shane P. Desselle

About the Author: Dr. Desselle is Professor, Associate Dean for Tulsa Programs, and Chair, Department of Pharmacy: Clinical and Administrative Sciences—Tulsa at the University of Oklahoma College of Pharmacy. Dr. Desselle received a B.S. in pharmacy and a Ph.D. in pharmacy administration from the University of Louisiana at Monroe. He has practice experience in both community and hospital pharmacy settings. Dr. Desselle teaches courses in American health care systems, health care economics, social and behavioral aspects of pharmacy practice, and research methods. His research interests include performance appraisal systems in pharmacy, quality of work life among pharmacy technicians, direct-to-consumer prescription drug advertising, Web-based pharmacy services, and pharmacy benefit design. Dr. Desselle won Duquesne University School of Pharmacy's President's Award for Teaching in 2003 and President's Award for Scholarship in 2004 and was recognized for his contributions to pharmacy by being named a Fellow of the American Pharmacists Association in 2006.

▬ LEARNING OBJECTIVES

After completing this chapter, readers should be able to

1. Discuss the rationale behind the implementation of a systematic performance appraisal system.
2. Discuss the difficulties in implementing a performance appraisal system within a pharmacy organization.
3. Identify various types of performance appraisal processes and evaluate the strengths and weaknesses of each type.
4. Discuss issues of validity and reliability within the context of evaluating a performance appraisal system.
5. Describe how to conduct a performance appraisal interview and how to handle disagreements that may arise during or subsequent to the interview.
6. Discuss the linkage of performance appraisal results with the proper allocation of organizational rewards.

■ SCENARIO

"What?" asked Marcus Green, emphatically. "You've got to be kidding! That's just not fair. I've been here for 3½ years, and I've received only one raise—and that may as well have been nothing. Why did she get another raise? She's probably making more money than I am, and she's only been here for a little more than 1 year." With a look of consternation, Marcus lowers his voice and asks his colleagues at the lunch table, "Where did you hear this from, anyway? Ah, never mind. I don't want to discuss it any further," Marcus chimed as he finished scarfing up the remainder of his lunch and left the table in a huff.

Marcus's fellow pharmacy technicians at Community Hospital were equally upset that Susan Klecko allegedly had received another raise, but they were not sure that they had done the right thing by telling Marcus about it. Marcus, having worked at Community Hospital for nearly 4 years, generally was regarded as the "best tech" in the pharmacy. He filled orders twice as rapidly as anyone else, always showed up on time, and came to work on short notice when others called in sick, even though he was perhaps a bit more prone to making a dispensing error and was well known for being a "hothead." Susan, on the other hand, seemed to be the "boss's pet." Indeed, she was regarded as a very pleasant person who got along with everyone, especially the director, Cynthia Broedl, with whom she shared an appreciation for poetry and theater.

Marcus continued to stew over his plight throughout the afternoon. He didn't really *feel* like looking for another job, making phone calls, filling out forms, and going on interviews, but he also did not understand why other technicians seemed to be rewarded at Community Hospital pharmacy more frequently with raises than he did. He wondered just what about his performance was not up to par. He did not recall being formally evaluated in over 2 years, when he and Ms Broedl had a few words on his suggestion that he often had to "pick up the slack" for pharmacists "not doing their jobs." Meanwhile, Terrence Whitfield, the assistant director, appeared in Cynthia's office to discuss his relief that the apparent exodus of staff oc-

curring over the previous few months appeared to be over.

■ CHAPTER QUESTIONS

1. What is a performance appraisal system? What does formal appraisal have to do with employee motivation, productivity, and turnover?
2. What is the difference between absolute, relative, and goal-oriented systems for appraising employee performance?
3. What kinds of appraisals typically are performed in pharmacy environments? How might these appraisal systems be improved?
4. How are formal performance appraisal mechanisms implemented? What are some strategies to maximize the effectiveness of the appraisal interview?
5. How should performance appraisals be linked to the allocation of organizational rewards? What are some innovative reward strategies that can be used to optimize employee satisfaction and productivity?
6. What is the difference between formal and informal performance feedback? Why is frequent and regular informal feedback so important? What are some methods to provide informal feedback?

■ WHAT ARE PERFORMANCE APPRAISALS?

Virtually every practitioner and many students reading this text have either participated in or know of a discussion similar to the one taking place at the beginning of the scenario. Pharmacists and pharmacy support staff typically are hardworking, honest people who want the best for their patients. However, they are made of the same fabric as everyone else and desire equitable treatment and fair compensation for their work.

The scenario begs the question of precisely what qualities signify a "good" technician. Are promptness, dedication, and hard work the attributes most revered by management, or are they collegiality and amicability? What is more important—the quantity or the quality of the work performed? The scenario raises some additional concerns. Do certain employees get preferential treatment because they have things in common with those in management positions? How do other employees in the pharmacy feel about the way they are being treated and compensated by their employer? Why have so many employees left the pharmacy at Community Hospital of late? Do the director and assistant director know how Marcus feels and that he is contemplating quitting as well? What do the pharmacists at Community Hospital think about the situation?

As humans, we are concerned primarily with the interests of ourselves, our family, and our closest loved ones. Each person's concern for self, manifesting within the cornucopia of personalities that exist among us, practically ensures occasional discontent among employees. And discontent, coupled with the consistency of life changes (e.g., birth of a new family member, sickness, death, or new opportunities) guarantees some level of turnover within all organizations that is beyond the control of management. The lack of a well-planned, well-executed, and equitable performance appraisal system as a major source of discontent, however, *is* well within management's control.

Strictly defined, a *performance appraisal* is a formal assessment of how well employees are performing their jobs, but it is much more than that. It is a way of formally communicating the organization's mission and goals, a foundation on which to establish informal channels of communication, a method on which to base organizational rewards, and a tool to improve the performance of each and every employee within the organization. Unfortunately, performance appraisal is a frequently neglected function. Managers have cited performance appraisals (also known as *performance reviews*) as their least favorite activity (Campbell and Barron, 1982). Constructing, implementing, and monitoring a performance appraisal system presents many formidable challenges. This chapter first will examine more closely why formal performance appraisals are so critical to a pharmacy organization. It then will offer some insights into the various formal appraisal methods available, offering advantages and disadvantages of each type. The state of performance appraisals in pharmacy then will be highlighted, including some exemplary methods from the literature. This proceeds into a discussion of how to conduct the performance appraisal and make accurate, reliable judgments about the employees being evaluated. The chapter concludes with information on how to link employee performance with organizational rewards and how to provide informal feedback to motivate employees when they are not being evaluated formally.

■ THE RATIONALE FOR A FORMAL PERFORMANCE APPRAISAL SYSTEM

As Chapters 8 and 9 pointed out, human resources are among a pharmacy's most valuable assets. Employee wages can account for one of the pharmacy's greater operating expenditures (see Chapter 15). Employees, however, should not be viewed as a cost but as an essential asset for organizational success. The ramifications of executing a good performance appraisal system extend to most human resources decisions. Table 10-1 summarizes some important points about the need for performance appraisals.

Legal

Performance appraisals are necessary to document employees' progress toward achieving goals and heeding the advice of management on how to improve performance. Documentation is necessary to demonstrate fairness in promotion and termination (discharge) practices. Title VII of the Civil Service Reform Act ushered in heightened concern regarding appraisal issues (Martin and Bartol, 1991). Title VII is a federal statute that applies to and sets forth constitutionally protected classes as they pertain to employment, including religion, national origin, race or color, and gender (Blackwell et al., 1996). An employee can initiate a Title VII claim based on disparate treatment, disparate impact, or retaliation (see Chapter 12). As such, the claimant would have to demonstrate that a hiring, promotion, or discharge had a significant adverse impact on a member of a protected class. Should a pharmacy be accused of any one of these, there are a limited number of defenses,

Table 10-1.	Rationale for Implementing Effective Performance Appraisals

Legal
- Title VII of the Civil Service Reform Act
- Age Discrimination in Employment Act

Communicative
- Ensures understanding of performance expectations by managers and staff
- Provides a formal means for employees to voice concerns and make suggestions for system improvement
- Indicates management's commitment to open dialogue and fairness

Productivity of labor
- Provides direction to employees on how to improve
- Establishes an environment conducive to self-motivation
- Assists employees with career planning
- Promotes satisfaction and elicits commitment of employees
- Mitigates turnover

Equity in rewards
- Provides a means for accurate and equitable distribution of organizational rewards
- Provides recognition for past service
- Helps to establish support for terminating "problem" or underachieving employees

Other managerial functions
- Supplies evidence to review organizational and systems problems
- Provides data on recruitment and selection procedures
- Identifies deficiencies in orientation and training programs

Financial position
- Assists in reducing operating costs
- Avoids costly litigation
- Reduces replacements costs

most notably the *bona fide occupational qualification* (BFOQ). With the BFOQ, the pharmacy must demonstrate that the employee claimant could not perform essential job duties safely and effectively. Having implemented a formal performance appraisal system, the pharmacy possesses critical documentation that an employee's performance was lacking and that the employee was provided adequate warning that failure to improve would result in certain consequences (e.g., termination/discharge, failure to obtain a promotion or pay increase, etc.).

Communicative

An employee typically will come to know what is expected of him or her during the performance appraisal process. These expectations may or may not have been communicated adequately during the hiring, training, or informal feedback processes. The performance appraisal process affords management the opportunity to inform employees of the importance of their roles and responsibilities to the organization and how their performance will be measured, thus mitigating the possibility of *role stress* among employees (Eulburg, Wekley, and Bhagat, 1988). Role stress typically is viewed as having two components: role ambiguity and role conflict. *Role ambiguity* exists when an employee is unsure about his or her responsibilities. *Role conflict* is the simultaneous occurrence of two or more role expectations (Kong, Wertheimer, and McGhan, 1992). The prevalence of role conflict and role ambiguity has been widely studied in pharmacy (Desselle and Tipton, 2001; Kong, 1995; Smith, Branecker, and Pence, 1985). It is not difficult to envision their occurrence. In a hospital pharmacy, for example, technicians may appear to be in perpetual turmoil over who maintains responsibility for cleaning the laminar flow hood, delivering medications to the floors, and filling stat orders. In a community pharmacy, conflicting roles for pharmacists may involve demands from management to increase prescription volume while spending more time counseling each patient.

If it becomes apparent to a manager that productivity among the entire staff is suffering, information can be gathered during the performance appraisal process that could lead to constructive changes in non-personnel aspects of the business (e.g., workflow design). In any event, the dialogue emanating from the appraisal process provides data *for* managers as well as data to employees *from* managers.

Performance appraisals have been used increasingly to communicate and inculcate an organization's values to employees. An appraisal system can be designed to reflect a company's mission by incorporating performance criteria deemed important to the organization (Park and Huber, 2007). These criteria may be written as specific competencies among employees needed to transform an organization's entire approach to its business (Kalb et al., 2006). Many pharmacy organizations stress a need to improve the medication use process and reduce medication errors as part of their culture. As such, they are incorporating these values into their performance appraisal systems (Schneider, 1999).

Productivity of Labor

A principal reason for conducting appraisals is to enhance performance. During the appraisal process, employees should be provided with feedback on their strengths and areas of performance that require improvement. Suggestions for improvement may be in reference to general areas of competence or to very specific roles or functions. This feedback, coupled with other components of the appraisal (e.g., equitable distribution in rewards and career planning), provides specific goals that an employee may strive to attain in the future. It is said that managers cannot motivate employees but rather can establish an environment conducive to self-motivation (Umiker, 1998, p. 133). Thus a supervisor cannot force or trick employees into being good performers. A well-planned performance appraisal can make employees aware of what they have to do to be judged as good performers and leaves it up to them to strive and achieve those goals.

The feedback and open dialogue present in performance appraisals are valuable to the career planning process. Career planning helps employees to formulate personal goals and evaluate strategies for integrating their goals with the goals of the organization. This is important because very few people work in the same jobs their entire career, often changing jobs within one organization and/or changing organizations. When these changes are poorly conceived, both the individual and the organization suffer (Griffin, 1996, p. 403). Career planning informs employees that they are valued enough by management to be considered in the organization's long-range plans. Career planning increasingly has been suggested for use among pharmacy technicians (Desselle and Holmes, 2007) and pharmacists (Gaither et al., 2007). Chapter 12 provides additional detail on career planning.

Employees are more likely to be satisfied with their jobs if they have directed feedback and specific goals for which to aim. It has been shown that satisfaction with the performance appraisal process itself is very closely linked to overall job satisfaction (Blau, 1999), which precedes commitment to the employer (Gaither and Mason, 1992a) and avoids costly turnover (Gaither and Mason, 1992b). A high level of turnover often leaves an organization temporarily short staffed, which creates even more stress for current employees. It also results in management having to invest inordinate amounts of time in recruiting, selecting, and training new employees rather than engaging in activities more productive to the organization.

Equity in Rewards

One of the key factors in providing an environment conducive to self-motivation is to distribute rewards equitably. The allocation of rewards (e.g., promotions and salary increases) cannot be arbitrary or even be perceived as arbitrary by staff, as might be the case with Marcus Green in the scenario. Evidence suggests that employees in service organizations, such as pharmacies, who have equitable performance appraisal and reward systems treat customers more fairly (Bowen, Gilliland, and Folger, 1999).

Many performance appraisal systems allow the manager to either rate employees on a given set of attributes or rank them in comparison with other employees with similar jobs. The quantification of performance into a score or ranking creates a foundation from which to base rewards. The culmination of a series of performance appraisals taken over several years can be used as support for recognizing top performers with extraordinary rewards (such as a gift, plaque, or reimbursement for travel to a conference) that exceed annual merit increases.

OTHER HUMAN RESOURCES MANAGEMENT (HRM) FUNCTIONS

The performance appraisal process inherently generates a considerable amount of data for managers. Poor performance of a group or an entire unit of personnel may be indicative of poor direction from an immediate supervisor or a lack of adequate resources for employees to perform their jobs. If not stemming from an organizational or systems problem, deficiencies among a significant number of employees could indicate that management has been ineffective in recruiting and selecting employees or perhaps in orientation and training, particularly if the underachieving employees are new hires (see Chapter 9).

Financial Position

Enhanced productivity translates into efficiency and the reduction of labor costs. For example, Community Pharmacy A may be able to dispense 200 prescriptions per day on average with 10 fewer employee hours worked per week than Community Pharmacy B without any excess stress or burden. The 10 fewer hours is less costly to Pharmacy A and thus enhances profitability. Additionally, having well-constructed performance appraisals can save an organization a significant amount of money by avoiding damage awards from litigation brought on by employees in the types of wrongful termination suits described previously. Finally, if the performance appraisal system is effective in holding turnover to a minimum, this saves the organization money that would have been dedicated to recruiting and training new employees.

TYPES OF PERFORMANCE APPRAISALS

A number of performance appraisal systems are in use. These systems are summarized in Table 10-2. Performance appraisal methods typically are categorized into three broad types: absolute, relative, and outcome-oriented (Segal, 1992).

Absolute Systems

Absolute systems require the rater to indicate whether or not the employee is meeting a set of predetermined criteria for performance. This usually involves the use of a scale or index. Absolute systems are the most commonly employed of the three types of performance appraisal methods (Byars and Rue, 2000, p. 277). The main advantage that absolute systems have over other types of appraisal methods is the feedback that is derived inherently from the process. Allowing employees to see how they are evaluated among criteria deemed important by management enables them to learn about their strengths and the areas in which they will require improvement.

There are two types of absolute systems that do *not* employ any sort of scaling procedure. One is the *essay method*, in which the rater responds to a series of brief open-ended questions concerning the employee's performance, such as, "What are the employee's strengths?" and "How does this employee get along with coworkers?" By allowing the rater to include what he or she thinks is most valuable, the data can be richer than those obtained from the use of scales. However, it is more difficult to translate these data into numeric quantities for the purpose of allocating rewards and communicating organizational goals. Additionally, differences among raters in their detail and writing abilities can subject the process to charges of bias. A second method, the *critical-incident appraisal,* may mitigate some concerns over subjectivity because it requires that the rater keep a written record of significant incidents (both positive and negative) as they occur. These incidents provide a basis for the evaluation. The data are still subject to interpretation, however, and maintaining such detailed records can be cumbersome.

Table 10-2. Performance Appraisals and Their Advantages and Disadvantages

System	Brief Description	Advantages	Disadvantages
Relative			
Alternation ranking	Rater selects most and least valued employee from remaining pools of employees	Eliminates leniency and central tendency	Limited feedback, perceptions of bias
Paired comparisons	Each employee is compared with every other employee one at a time on each criterion	May appear to be less subjective than alternation ranking	Limited feedback
Forced distribution	Rater categorizes employees into one of three groups according to how well they meet expectations	Eliminates leniency and central tendency	Limited feedback, skewing
Absolute			
Essay	Rater prepares a written statement describing the employee's strengths and weaknesses	May provide rich data	Differences across raters, lack of objectivity
Critical incident	Rater maintains a record of incidents indicative of both positive and negative behaviors of the employee	Derived from documented data	Burdensome and subject to interpretation
Checklist	Rater answers with a yes or a no a series of questions about the employee's behavior	Easy to complete, indicative of specific behaviors	Less precision
Graphic rating	Rater indicates various employee traits and behaviors on a scale	Often based on trait measures	Leniency, central tendency, use of traits
Behaviorally anchored rating scales	Rater employs highly descriptive scales to indicate employee's tendency to demonstrate desirable behaviors	Quantitative, conducive to supplying feedback	Central tendency, burdensome
360° feedback	Employees rate themselves, and comparisons are made with ratings by various stakeholders	Multiple points of view, facilitates reflection	Very time-consuming, subject to role conflict
Forced choice	Rater ranks a set of statements describing the employee's performance	Mitigates bias	Irksome to raters, feedback is challenging
Outcome-oriented			
Management by objectives	Rater establishes goals for the employee to achieve during the next period, and employee is evaluated on his or her success	Highly participatory and incentive-driven	Employees evaluated by different standards
Work standards approach	Rater sets a standard or an expected level of output and compares each employee's performance to the standard	Evaluation is more standardized	Standards may be viewed as unfair

Employees who do a "steady" job may complain that this type of evaluation fails to capture their strongest suit.

The *checklist* is one of three types of summated rating scale methods. In a summated rating scale, a rater indicates the employee's level of performance on a list of criteria. The ratings assigned to each criterion are then summed to provide a total score for the employee. With the checklist, the rater simply answers a set of yes/no questions concerning whether or not the employee exhibited certain characteristics. The employee receives a point when the rater assigns an affirmative response to a desirable characteristic or a negative response to an undesirable characteristic. While indicative of specific behaviors and easy for the rater to complete, the checklist ignores levels of performance along each performance criterion. Thus it is less precise and does not generate as much feedback as other summated scale methods.

The *graphic rating* appraisal, on the other hand, has the rater assess the employee's level of performance on a scale, usually from one to five or one to seven. Some graphic rating scales may include written descriptions along with the numerical ranges. An example of such is given in Table 10-3.

Although it has the advantage of lending greater precision and feedback, the graphic rating appraisal, like many absolute systems, is prone to rater biases. One is *central tendency*, which occurs when the rater appraises everyone at or near the median of the scale or rates everyone similarly for fear of causing angst or feelings of injustice among employees. With *leniency*, the rater not only judges each employee similarly but also rates each on the high end of the performance scale. Some graphic rating appraisals may consist mostly of traits as criteria rather than particular performance indicants. While traits may manifest into certain behaviors, they are innately part of every person's character. To this end, managers should avoid evaluating an employee on characteristics such as appearance, knowledge, or friendliness without specifying how this translates into actual performance. The *halo effect* occurs when a rater allows a single prominent characteristic of an employee to influence his or her judgment on each

separate item in the appraisal. For example, a technician who is very friendly may be rated more highly on performance than someone not as outwardly amicable despite the latter outperforming the technician on other aspects of the job. While the halo effect can be problematic for any type of appraisal system, it can be especially problematic when traits are used in a graphic rating scale.

The *behavior-anchored rating scale* (BARS) method of performance appraisal is designed more specifically to assess behaviors necessary for successful performance. Most BARS methods use the term *job dimension* to mean those broad categories of duties and responsibilities that make up a job, requiring development of unique scales for each dimension. Managers often develop BARS in collaboration with employees well versed in the job. An example of how a BARS may look for a community pharmacy technician in dealing with customers is illustrated in Table 10-4. The BARS system lends itself to providing quality feedback, particularly if supplemented with qualitative comments on how to improve. A drawback is the time and effort required to develop an effective BARS appraisal.

More common to larger organizations than retail or institutional pharmacies, *360-degree feedback,* also known as *multirater assessment,* involves the use of a summated rating scale or brief closed-ended questions requiring the employee to rate himself or herself and compare these ratings with those afforded to him or her by managers, peers, customers, suppliers, and/or colleagues on a similar instrument. This mitigates an employee's concern that one particular rater may be biased against him or her and certainly engenders a degree of reflection by any employee who receives feedback from so many points of view. Moreover, managers are relieved from being the exclusive "heavies" in evaluating performance because they learn from other evaluators in the process (Anonymous, 2001). Aside from the time it takes to gather and collate all these data, another disadvantage from the employee's point of view is the role conflict that may arise owing to differing demands placed by various stakeholders in the process. This problem is further exacerbated when there is a lack of interrater reliability among evaluators,

Table 10-3. Sample Items on a Graphic Rating Scale Evaluation Form

Quantity of work—the amount of work an employee does in a workday

Does not meet minimum requirements	Does just enough to get by	Volume of work is satisfactory	Very industrious, does more than is required	Has a superior work production record

Dependability—the ability to do required jobs well with a minimum of supervision

Requires close supervision; is unreliable	Sometimes requires prompting	Usually completes necessary tasks with reasonable promptness	Requires little supervision; is reliable	Requires absolute minimum of supervision

Job knowledge—information an employee sbould have on work duties for satisfactory job performance

Is poorly informed about work duties	Lacks knowledge of some phases of job	Is moderately informed; can answer most questions about the job	Understands all phases of job	Has complete mastery of all phases of job

Attendance—faithfulness in coming to work daily and conforming to work hours

Is often absent without good excuse or frequently reports for work late, or both	Is lax in attendance, or reporting for work on time, or both	Is usually present and on time	Is very prompt, regular in attendance	Is always regular and prompt; volunteers for overtime when needed

Accuracy—the correctness of work duties performed

Makes frequent errors	Careless, often makes errors	Usually accurate, makes only average number of mistakes	Requires little supervision; is exact and precise most of the time	Requires absolute minimum of supervision; is almost always accurate

Source: Byars and Rue, 2000, p. 283; reprinted with permission.

Table 10-4. Example of a Behaviorally Anchored Rating Scale for "Providing Customer Service" in a Community Pharmacy

Scale	Values	Anchors
1	Poor	Does not interact well with customers, who frequently complain about the employee; employee instigates conflict with customers
2	Below average	Courtesy is inconsistent; is not responsive to customer needs
3	Average	Is polite and friendly with customers but lacks creativity in meeting customer needs
4	Above average	Is polite, friendly, and professional in dealing with customers; is adept at meeting customer needs and strives to improve in this area
5	Excellent	Has managed to develop a bond with customers, who anticipate coming to the pharmacy and interacting with this employee; is innovative in creating ways to satisfy customers

as is often the case in many organizations (Valle and Bozeman, 2002).

Another type of absolute method that seeks to mitigate bias or perceptions of bias is *forced-choice rating*. Forced-choice rating is also more common in larger organizations with a formal human resources department. With this method, the rater is presented with a set of statements that describe potentially how the employee might be performing on the job and ranks each statement on how well it describes that employee's behavior. The weights and scoring, known and performed by the human resources department, are unknown to the rater. An example is given in Table 10-5.

Relative Systems

Rather than requiring the rater to evaluate employees on a predetermined set of characteristics or standards, relative systems require the manager to make comparisons among employees. Relative systems have an advantage over absolute systems in that central tendency and leniency effects are minimized. The likelihood of the halo effect occurring is also reduced. The fact that employees are pitted against one another, so to speak, makes it easier to base organizational rewards on merit.

Relative systems have a very significant drawback, however, in that they are not conducive to generating substantive feedback to employees. If, for example, an employee is rated below two-thirds of his or her col-

leagues on overall performance, what does this mean to the employee? What behaviors are being demonstrated that resulted in this ranking? What behaviors could be demonstrated that would result in improved performance and a higher ranking during the next evaluation? This adds to the manager's challenge of establishing an environment for employee self-motivation.

Table 10-5. Sample Set of Statements in a Forced-Choice Rating Scale

Instructions: Rank the following statements according to how they describe the manner in which this employee carries out duties and responsibilities. Rank 1 should be given to the most descriptive and rank 5 to the least descriptive. No ties are allowed.

Rank	Description
	Is easy to get acquainted with
	Places great emphasis on people
	Refuses to accept criticism
	Thinks generally in terms of money
	Makes decisions quickly

Source: Byars and Rue, 2000, p. 283; reprinted with permission.

Three types of relative performance appraisal systems are used. One is called *alternation ranking,* a method in which the rater chooses the most and least valuable persons from a list of employees with similar jobs. Both names are crossed off, and then the procedure is repeated until every employee on the list has been ranked. With its ability to eliminate central tendency and leniency and with its ease of implementation, alternation ranking may appear appealing. However, aside from its failure to generate feedback, the halo effect could come into play. Moreover, employees may be concerned with the potential for bias and inaccuracy by the evaluator, especially when criteria for performance have not been delineated clearly.

The method of *paired comparisons* has the rater comparing each employee against every other employee, one by one, on either specific aspects of performance or overall performance. During each comparison, the rater places a checkmark by the name of the employee who was considered to have performed better. The employee with the most checkmarks is considered to be the best performer. While more precise and perhaps seemingly less ambiguous to employees, paired comparisons still may fail to generate substantive feedback and are more burdensome to implement that other relative systems.

The *forced distribution* method requires the rater to compare the performance of employees and place a certain percentage of them into various groupings. It assumes that the performance level in a group of employees will be distributed according to a bell-shaped, or normal, distribution curve. While lending itself well to the allocation of organizational rewards, levels of actual performance may be skewed by forcing their distribution into a bell-shaped curve, ignoring the possibility that perhaps most or all employees are performing well or performing poorly. Forced distribution, as well as other relative systems, may fail to demonstrate system deficiencies that can be improved by management.

Outcome-Oriented Systems

Where absolute and relative systems focus on behaviors, outcome-oriented systems are concerned with evaluating end results. These systems involve setting quantifiable goals for the succeeding period, to be followed with a performance review at its conclusion. Outcome-oriented systems can be used to generate feedback, but equity issues arise because rewards are allocated according to how well goals are met, and employees with similar jobs may receive substantially different sets of goals and expectations for performance. Because these systems are used more frequently for persons in autonomous positions (e.g., attorneys, college professors, and clinical pharmacists), flexibility has to be built in to allow for contingencies that resulted in an employee changing his or her goals or not being able to meet them. On the other hand, an employee always can come up with excuses as to why certain goals were not met.

The most commonly employed type of outcome-oriented system is *management by objectives* (MBO), also known as *results management, performance management,* and *work planning and review.* The MBO process typically consists of six steps (Byars and Rue, 2000, p. 277):

1. Establishing clear and precisely defined statements of objectives for the work to be done by an employee.
2. Developing an action plan indicating how these objectives will be accomplished.
3. Allowing the employee to implement the action plan.
4. Measuring objective achievement.
5. Taking corrective action when necessary.
6. Establishing new objectives for the future.

The establishment of objectives is critical to the success of MBO. The objectives must be challenging but attainable. They should be expressed in terms that are objective and measurable and should be written in clear, concise, unambiguous language. Table 10-6 presents examples of how some poorly stated objectives for pharmacists might be better stated. It is important that the objectives be derived through collaboration and consent of the employee. In this respect, the objectives and action plan can serve as a basis for regular discussions between the manager and the employee.

Table 10-6.	Examples of How to Improve Work Objectives in Pharmacy

Poor:

To maximize the number of prescriptions dispensed

Better:

To increase the average daily prescription volume by 10 percent at the end of the year

Poor:

To make as few dispensing errors as possible

Better:

To commit no dispensing errors that result in an untoward event during the next 6 months

Poor:

To get all medications up to the floors more quickly

Better:

To get unit dose medications to the floors within 30 minutes after the order arrives to the pharmacy

Poor:

To make sure that nurses are happy with the clinical services you provide

Better:

To achieve a mean score of at least 80 out of 100 on a survey measuring nurses' satisfaction with the clinical services provided

A concern of MBO is the potential incongruence among the goals and objectives of employees with similar jobs, especially when it comes to allocating organizational rewards. While this can be overcome to some degree by basing the rewards on the outcomes themselves, use of another method, the *work standards approach,* can further mitigate the problem. The work standards approach is a form of goal setting in which each employee is compared with some sort of standard or an expected level of output. In other words, the objectives are the same or similar for each employee in the group. Without as much input from each employee, however, the standards established may be viewed as unfair, and employees may not have as much incentive to strive to attain them.

■ SPECIAL CONSIDERATIONS FOR APPRAISAL SYSTEMS IN PHARMACY

A community pharmacy is typically a for-profit organization that must be concerned with its financial position to remain solvent over the long term. Community pharmacies must also conduct their business in an ethical manner. Moreover, it can hardly be argued that pharmacists and support personnel must practice altruism, putting patients ahead of personal motives (Wolfgang, 1989). Like any organization, a pharmacy will be more likely to achieve its goals when its employees derive gratification from performing their jobs (Etzioni, 1964). The pharmacy profession has experienced numerous environmental changes that affect the work experiences of pharmacy personnel. These include higher prescription volumes, greater complexity in third-party reimbursement, increasing professional emphasis on pharmaceutical care, and implementation of automated dispensing technologies (Alvarez, 1997). These trends behoove pharmacy managers to take special care in developing effective performance appraisal systems. One first has to determine whether a similar performance appraisal should exist among technicians and pharmacists working within the same organization. Certain similarities in the jobs of pharmacists and support personnel exist. Additionally, there are certain values (e.g., dependability, dedication, and altruism) that the organization may want to assess in all its employees regardless of their position or status. There are, however, certain aspects of pharmacists' jobs and those of support personnel that may call for alternative systems or at least different components of a similar system. Most notable of these is the level of autonomy and responsibility they share.

Considerations for Support Personnel

A pharmacy organization's effectiveness often is limited to the productivity of its technicians and other support personnel. Pharmacy technicians, for example, are now beginning to take responsibility for more functions, including drug preparation, order entry, and managing technology (Collins, 1999). The profession has recognized the need for thorough job descriptions, training manuals, equitable pay, and productivity-monitoring systems among pharmacy support personnel (Desselle, 2005), yet the literature has little to offer in the way of devising performance appraisal systems. One study found that relatively few community pharmacies engage in routine performance monitoring of support personnel (Desselle, Vaughan, and Faria, 2002). In the same study, a method predicated on a study of the "scope of pharmacy practice" (Muenzen, Greenberg, and Murer, 1999) was suggested. It involved the use of 20 practice functions each with a different weight (for importance) combined with a BARS-type scale to produce a highly quantitative measure. The 20 practice functions and weights are provided in Table 10-7. A similar method can be used to derive a performance appraisal system for technicians working in alternative settings.

Considerations for Pharmacists

Evaluating pharmacist performance may be more challenging than evaluating technician performance because of pharmacists' greater levels of autonomy and responsibility. This may be further compounded by the presence of the disparate roles various pharmacists may play within the organization. It may be fruitful to gather information from customers, or patients, when evaluating pharmacists for the services they provide. This may be accomplished through informal feedback, surveys, or even critical-incidents appraisal, as described previously. While it is beyond the scope of this chapter to describe them in detail, a few types of performance appraisal systems have been suggested for pharmacists, particularly those whose responsibilities are more clinical in nature (Segal, 1992; Schumock et al., 1990).

▓ THE PERFORMANCE APPRAISAL INTERVIEW

Regardless of the type of system selected, the written appraisal should be accompanied by a formal interview of the employee. It is during the interview that the results of the written appraisal are discussed. The success of the performance appraisal hinges significantly on the interview. If the manager is mindful of taking a few pre-cautionary steps and follows some helpful guidelines, most appraisal interviews will come off without a hitch.

Preparing the Employee for the Interview

An appointment should be made with the employee well in advance, at least 3 to 4 weeks. The employee should be provided with a copy of the position description and corresponding performance standards, a copy of the evaluation form used in the appraisal process, a copy of the report of the previous formal review, departmental/organizational objectives for the current and subsequent year, and instructions on how to prepare for the meeting. The employee may be instructed to prepare comments on how well objectives set during the last review were met and to prepare a list of new objectives. The employee may also be asked to discuss what he or she considers his or her most valuable contribution to the organization to be since the last review, barriers to his or her achieving current goals, and what the organization or manager can do to facilitate his or her progress (Umiker, 1998, p. 155). In some organizations, employees are asked to complete a self-evaluation on an instrument similar to the one used by the employer. This may help to identify gaps in perceptions of effectiveness in certain areas and reinforce strengths and limitations in others.

Planning for the Interview

The manager should enter the interview well informed of prior appraisals and be intimately familiar with the responsibilities of the employee's job. The manager should also have appropriate documentation and evidence to support claims of the employee's performance, particularly in areas of deficiency but also in areas of strength. To prepare for the interview, the manager should have answered the following questions (Byars and Rue, 2000, p. 286):

1. What results should the interview achieve?
2. What good contributions is the employee making?
3. Is the employee working up to his or her potential?
4. Is the employee clear about the manager's performance expectations?
5. What strengths does the employee have that can be built on or improved?

Table 10-7.	Community Pharmacy Technicians' Practice Functions and Corresponding Weights
1.	Maintaining inventory I (ordering) 3.79
2.	Maintaining inventory II (receiving goods) 2.25
3.	Maintaining inventory III (other, such as stock appearance and inventory analysis) 3.36
4.	Collecting productivity information 1.63
5.	Participating in quality assurance and quality improvement activities 4.00
6.	Solving problems (of prescribers, customers, and colleagues) 3.80
7.	Billing and accounting 2.00
8.	Customer service activities 4.88
9.	Training other staff members 2.70
10.	Maintaining a positive image 3.93
11.	Being a team player 4.00
12.	Exhibiting a positive attitude 4.75
13.	Maintaining cleanliness 3.00
14.	Receiving and interviewing patients 4.88
15.	Communicating with prescribers 3.72
16.	Assessing prescription orders for completeness and accuracy 3.00
17.	Processing prescription orders 4.00
18.	Filling prescription orders 4.25
19.	Compounding prescription orders 1.00
20.	Appropriately concluding a patient's visit 4.73

Source: Desselle, Vaughan, and Faria, 2002, p. 774; reprinted with permission.

6. Is there any additional training available that can help the employee improve?

Conducting the Interview

The interview should be conducted in the following sequence: (1) review and update the position description and performance standards, (2) discuss the performance ratings assigned to the employee using the prescribed appraisal form, (3) highlight strengths and accomplishments since the previous appraisal, (4) discuss objectives that were not reached since the previous review, and (5) discuss future performance and assist with career planning.

Managers should establish a comfortable, professional atmosphere and maintain a positive tone when conducting the interview. They should be careful not to stereotype or prejudge certain employees. There may be occasions on which the rater simply does not like the person whom he or she is evaluating but must be careful to remain focused on the relevant behaviors and performance. Nonetheless, circumstances will arise in which the manager has to address performance deficiencies with an employee. Some suggestions for addressing these situations are as follows (Umiker, 1998, p. 157):

- Limit criticism to one or two major problems. Do not search for significant problem areas when none exist.
- Reserve critical remarks until after some of the positives have been accentuated.
- Maintain open dialogue with the employee. Offer the employee a chance for self-criticism. Allow the employee to offer reasons why performance was below standard. Allow the employee to suggest ways and an appropriate time frame to expect significant improvement.
- Avoid the use of terms that potentially could be misconstrued, such as *attitude, work ethic, professionalism,* and *weakness.*

Remain firm but supportive. Use assertiveness skills by reinforcing points of agreement, handling disagreements diplomatically, and avoiding defensiveness.

The interview should be concluded with an expression of confidence that the employee will be able to meet the new objectives. The manager should also thank the employee for his or her time spent in the interview and for his or her contributions to the organization.

ENSURING VALID RESULTS FROM THE PERFORMANCE APPRAISAL SYSTEM

A pharmacy manager must carefully consider the advantages and drawbacks of each type of appraisal system. Aside from those specifically designed for pharmacy organizations described in this chapter, the prevailing consensus among employers is that summated rating scales, particularly derivations of BARS methods, are the best systems to employ. Regardless of the type of system selected, managers must be mindful of ensuring that the system is reliable and valid and is helping the organization to achieve its objectives. *Reliability* is another word for consistency, inferring that the system produces similar results in multiple iterations. For example, given a certain employee's level of performance, any rater should view the performance similarly. If a system is unreliable, then it cannot be valid. *Validity* implies that the system is measuring what it purports to measure.

Implementing the System

A primary consideration when implementing a system is how frequently to conduct the formal appraisal. Rating periods usually are annual, either on the employee's anniversary of hire date or during a rating period in which all employees are evaluated, the latter of which is easier to implement (Mohrman, Resnick-West, and Lawler, 1989). Evidence suggests, however, that better results are obtained from more frequent evaluations, such as semiannually or quarterly (Martin and Bartol, 1998). Everyone in the organization should be well informed about the role each person plays in the appraisal process and how the appraisal results are used (Latham and Wexley, 1994).

Monitoring the System

The effectiveness of the appraisal system itself should be monitored. Certain indicators can be helpful, including the quality of performance standards, effective use of appraisal results, tracking of the raters, and elimination of adverse impact. *Quality of performance standards* refers to the standards being specific, challenging, realistic, dynamic, understandable, and consistent with organizational goals. *Use of performance appraisal results* refers to how well these results are tied with rewards and recognition and to what extent the appraisal process has contributed to improved performance among all employees. *Tracking the raters* consists of reviewing the ratings awarded by individual raters and giving them feedback concerning the quality of their ratings, which may be overly stringent, lenient, or biased in some way in comparison with other raters. *Adverse impact* refers to a performance appraisal system whose use results in significantly lower ratings for members of any protected group described previously.

▩ PERFORMANCE AND ORGANIZATIONAL REWARDS

Organizational rewards consist of both intrinsic rewards (those internal to the individual and derived from involvement in the job, such as achievement, feelings of accomplishment, informal recognition, satisfaction, and status) and extrinsic rewards (those controlled and distributed by the organization, such as formal recognition, incentive pay, fringe benefits, and promotions). Proper allocation of both is critical for varied reasons. Recent evidence rejects a popular view that satisfaction leads to performance (Byars and Rue, 2000, p. 303). It does suggest, however, that (1) rewards based on current performance enhance subsequent performance and (2) job dissatisfaction leads to turnover, absenteeism, tardiness, accidents, grievances, and strikes. Research also supports the notion that while extrinsic rewards do not in and of themselves cause satisfaction, perceived deficiencies or inequities can result in dissatisfaction among employees (Barnett and Kimberlin, 1988). A study of pharmacists suggested that percep-

tions of inadequate pay were predictive of their intentions to withdraw from a current job (Gaither and Mason, 1995b).

In addressing employees' base and merit pay, managers must consider internal, external, and individual equity. Internal equity concerns what an employee is being paid for doing a job compared with what other employees in the same organization are being paid to do their jobs. External equity concerns what employees in an organization are being paid compared with employees in other organizations performing similar jobs. Individual equity addresses the rewarding of individual contributions and is related closely to linking pay with performance. Internal equity and external equity are factors considered more in determining base wage and fringe benefits, or those rewards are based merely on employment and seniority with an organization. Pharmacy managers must ensure that pharmacist and support staff salaries and benefits (e.g., vacation, paid holidays, health insurance, child care, and pension plans) are competitive with those offered in similar pharmacy settings and even other types of pharmacy settings in the region.

Managers also must address individual equity and allocate certain rewards (e.g., pay increases, promotions, and formal recognition) in a manner that corresponds with the right types of behaviors. Such behaviors include but are not limited to working extra hours when required, volunteering for unenviable tasks or assignments, substituting for others willingly, and pleasing customers. More specifically, rewarding behaviors listed and evaluated in the performance appraisal system eliminates ambiguity about what constitutes good performance. Other suggestions for allocating rewards are as follows (Byars and Rue, 2000. pp. 360–361):

- *Consider the presence of performance constraints.* The employee's performance should not be hampered by things beyond his or her control.
- Provide a clear distinction between cost-of-living, seniority, and merit pay increases.
- *Enlist trust among employees.* Similarly, employees should not be misled into thinking that their rewards were based on merit, only to find out later

that the increases were across the board. This could result in distrust and dissatisfaction.

- *Make merit pay substantial.* While operating within the organization's budget, merit pay has to be worthwhile. Employees will not appreciate being evaluated very highly and praised only to see very small pay increases as a result.
- *Be flexible in scheduling rewards.* It is easier to establish a credible pay-for-performance plan if all employees do not receive pay adjustments on the same date.
- *Effectively communicate merit and total pay policy to employees.* Additionally, do not prohibit employees from discussing pay because this may be a violation of the National Labor Relations Act.

There are detractors to using performance appraisals as a means to allocate rewards. It has been suggested that appraisals used in this way create "winners" and "losers," ultimately a zero-sum game for an organization, which should not use systems to make miniscule distinctions in pay adjustments (Kennedy and Dresser, 2001). Monetary rewards are said to work best when completely unanticipated by the employee rather than based on the appraisal feedback. Moreover, while managers' ability to reward with pay is limited, there are no such constraints on other forms of recognition.

■ MOTIVATION AND OTHER REWARDS NOT TIED TO BASE PAY

Chapters 8, 9, and 14 discuss motivation of employees through leadership and support. Support by the manager goes a long way toward keeping employees satisfied. In fact, manager and organizational support has proved to be an effective deterrent to pharmacists' uncertainty about their future in an organization (Desselle and Tipton, 2001) and a buffer against the stress that accompanies work (Kong and Wertheimer, 1994; Lahoz and Mason, 1991). Pharmacy managers also should keep this in mind when dealing with support personnel. Managers may believe that support personnel do not value intrinsic rewards, but this is certainly

not true. Managers should be cognizant of the desire for autonomy and personal growth by all employees.

Giving Praise

Support from managers need not be confined to the formal appraisal period. Informal feedback should be rendered on a consistent basis. Employees should be instructed immediately when they demonstrate behaviors detrimental to the organization or if they are not performing to standards, as long as it is done in a professional manner. For example, the manager should never criticize an employee in the presence of others. Offering praise to an employee for a job well done should be done in public, however, as long as the employee truly deserves such praise, the praise is not overdone, and it is not overly repetitive (Rosendahl, 1993). Managers should also consider following up praise with an official memo and boasting of the employee to colleagues so that it may get back to him or her indirectly.

Other Benefits

Pharmacy managers may consider the use of other strategies to recognize and reward good performers:

- Offer to pay for attendance at a local continuing education program.
- Provide funding for attendance at a national conference.
- Offer to offset the cost of professional recognition and certification processes for pharmacists and technicians.
- Fund membership in a professional association.
- Buy lunch.
- Allow someone to represent you at an important meeting.
- Assign tasks with greater levels of responsibility if the employee is ready to handle them.

■ REVISITING THE SCENARIO

Management may consider the fact that Marcus has made more errors than other technicians to be of greater consequence than his promptness and vigorous effort.

Marcus may contend that a greater frequency of errors is bound to occur as a result of him filling a greater number of medication orders. The technicians may not be clear on who is responsible for certain tasks. Finally, pharmacy staff may be concerned that management plays favorites among the employees. Marcus is confused and frustrated at having seldom been evaluated formally. Has management avoided subsequent appraisals because the last one did not run so smoothly? Has this been the case with other employees as well? None of these questions is necessarily an indictment of management at Community Hospital pharmacy because there is much information not known in the scenario. However, it is certain that all employees at the pharmacy must be evaluated formally at least once a year, informed of behaviors that are viewed as desirable, instructed on how they may improve performance, and shown how various aspects of performance translate into the allocation of organizational rewards.

■ CONCLUSION

Managers often view performance appraisals as an undesirable task, but careful planning and implementation should make them less onerous. Performance appraisals are closely linked to employee motivation, performance, commitment, and turnover. Numerous systems are available, each of which has its strengths and drawbacks. The formal appraisal must be accompanied by frequent and substantive informal feedback. The appraisal interview is key to the success of the appraisal system. The allocation of organizational rewards must be linked closely to the results of the appraisal process.

■ QUESTIONS FOR FURTHER DISCUSSION

1. What types of skills do you think are necessary for selecting and implementing a performance appraisal system? What about for conducting an appraisal interview?
2. How would you feel about having responsibility for determining whether or not an employee will receive merit pay?

3. Has your performance ever been assessed formally at a job? How was that experience? What do you think the manager could have done better when assessing your performance?
4. How would you react if you were told that your performance was not measuring up to the expectations of an organization?
5. Does everyone with similar jobs in a pharmacy deserve the same level of pay raises, or should they be based more on performance?
6. Do you know anyone who has left a job because, in part, of the kinds of issues raised in the chapter scenario?

REFERENCES

Alvarez NA. 1997. Searching for utopia. *J Am Pharm Assoc* 37:632.

Anonymous. 2001. Conducting effective performance appraisals. *Clin Leadership Manage Rev* 15:348.

Barnett CW, Kimberlin CL. 1988. Levels of satisfaction among Florida pharmacists. *J Pharm Market Manag* 2:23.

Blackwell S, Szeinbach S, Garner D, Smith M. 1996. Legal issues in personnel management. *Drug Top* 140:74.

Blau G. 1999. Testing the longitudinal impact of work variables and performance appraisal satisfaction on subsequent overall job satisfaction. *Hum Relat* 52:1099.

Bowen D, Gilliland SW, Folger R. 1999. HRM and service fairness: How being fair with employees spills over to customers. *Organ Dynam* 27:7.

Byars LL, Rue L. 2000. *Human Resource Management*, 6th ed. New York: McGraw-Hill.

Campbell B, Barron C. 1982. How extensively are human resource management practices being utilized by practitioners? *Person Admin* 27:67.

Collins PM. 1999. Pharmacy technician: Valuable asset in today's pharmacy. *Wash Pharm* 41:38.

Desselle SP, Holmes ER. 2007. A structural model of CPhTs' job satisfaction and career commitment. *J Am Pharm Assoc* 47:58.

Desselle SP. 2005. Job turnover intentions among certified pharmacy technicians. *J Am Pharm Assoc* 45:676.

Desselle SP, Tipton DJ. 2001. Factors contributing to the satisfaction and performance ability of community pharmacists: A path model analysis. *J Soc Admin Pharm* 18:15.

Desselle SP, Vaughan M, Faria T. 2002. Creating a performance appraisal template for pharmacy technicians using the method of equal-appearing intervals. *J Am Pharm Assoc* 42:768.

Etzioni A. 1964. *Modern Organizations.* Englewood Cliffs, NJ: Prentice-Hall.

Eulburg JR, Weekley J, Bhahat RS. 1988. Models of stress in organizational research: A meta-theoretical perspective. *Hum Relat* 41:331.

Gaither CA, Mason HL. 1992a. Commitment to the employer: Do pharmacists have it? *Am Pharm* NS32:41.

Gaither CA, Mason HL. 1992b. A model of pharmacists' career commitment, organizational commitment and job withdrawal intentions. *J Soc Admin Pharm* 9:75.

Gaither CA, Nadkarni A, Mott DA, et al. 2007. Should I stay or should I go? The influence of individual and organizational factors on pharmacists' future work plans. *J Am Pharm Assoc* 47:165.

Griffin RW. 1996. *Management,* 5th ed. Boston: Houghton Mifflin.

Kalb KB, Cherry NM, Kauzloric J, et al. 2006. A competency-based approach to public health nursing performance appraisal. *Public Health Nurs* 23:115.

Kennedy PW, Dresser SG. 2001. Appraising and paying for performance: Another look at an age-old problem. *Emp Benefits J* 26:8.

Kong SX. 2005. Predictors of organizational and career commitment among Illinois pharmacists. *Am J Health-Syst Pharm* 52:2005.

Kong SX, Wertheimer AI. 1994. Social support: Concepts, theories, and implications for pharmacy research. *J Pharm Market Manag* 9:63.

Kong SX, Wertheimer AI, McGhan WF. 1992. Role stress, organizational commitment and turnover intention among pharmaceutical scientists: A multivariate analysis. *J Soc Admin Pharm* 9:159.

Lahoz MR, Mason HL. 1991. Reducing pharmacists' stress. *Am Drug* 200:38.

Latham GP, Wexley KM. 1994. *Increasing Productivity Through Performance Appraisal,* 2d ed. Reading, MA: Addison-Wesley.

Martin DC, Bartol KM. 1991. The legal ramifications of performance appraisal: An update. *Employee Relat Law J* 17:257.

Martin DC, Bartol KM. 1998. Performance appraisal: maintaining system effectiveness. *Public Person Manag* 27:223.

Mohrman AM, Resnick-West SM, Lawler EE III. 1989. *Designing Performance Appraisal Systems.* San Francisco: Josey-Bass.

Muenzen PM, Greenberg S, Murer MM. 1999. PTCB task analysis identifies role of certified pharmacy technicians in pharmaceutical care. *J Am Pharm Assoc* 39: 857.

Rosendahl I. 1993. Keeping them happy. *Drug Top* 137: 50.

Park EJ, Huber DL. 2007. Balanced scorecards for performance management. *J Nurs Adm* 37:14.

Schneider PJ. 1999. Creating an environment for improving the medication-use process. *Am J Health-Syst Pharm* 56:1769.

Schumock GT, Leister KA, Edwards D, et al. 1990. Method for evaluating performance of clinical pharmacists. *Am J Hosp Pharm* 47:127.

Segal R. 1992. A framework for evaluating the work of pharmacists. *Top Hosp Pharm Manag* 12:130.

Smith HA, Branecker J, Pence BS. 1985. Role orientation, conflict and satisfaction among pharmacists and students. *J Soc Admin Pharm* 3:19.

Umiker W. 1998. *Management Skills for the New Health Care Supervisor.* Gaithersburg, MD: Aspen.

Valle M, Bozeman DP. 2002. Interrater agreement on employees' job performance: Review and directions. *Psychol Rep* 90:975.

Wolfgang AP. 1989. Challenging students to consider pharmacy's professional status. *Am J Pharm Ed* 53:177.

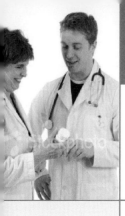

11

CUSTOMER SERVICE

David J. Tipton

About the Author: Dr. Tipton is Associate Professor of Social and Administrative Pharmaceutical Sciences at the Mylan School of Pharmacy at Duquesne University. Dr. Tipton earned an MBA in marketing and a Ph.D. in management from St. Louis University. Prior to obtaining his degree, he practiced pharmacy for 20 years and was an owner/partner in a four-store pharmacy operation. His current research interests focus on customer service, medication errors, and judgment. Dr. Tipton teaches courses at Duquesne University in management, marketing, and customer service.

▪ LEARNING OBJECTIVES

After completing this chapter, students should be able to

1. Identify the distinguishing characteristics of services.
2. Discuss the characteristics of good customer service.
3. Describe the standard for the evaluation of services.
4. Discuss the seven issues in designing services.
5. Describe service strategy.
6. Describe strategies for dealing with service failures and medication errors.
7. Discuss the management of service employees and professionals.

▪ SCENARIO

Entering the pharmacy, Maria Perez remembered the numerous advertisements and commercials touting the expertise, availability, and compassion of the pharmacists at this pharmacy. Maria entered the pharmacy clutching a handful of prescriptions for her aging mother who had just been discharged from the hospital following a heart attack. Maria anticipated that she would be taking care of her mother in her home for the next several weeks and would be responsible for her mother's medications.

Fighting her way down aisles clogged with boxes, Maria made it to the pharmacy and was greeted by a 19-year-old clerk. The clerk was chewing gum and was casually indifferent, instructing Maria to take a seat. Counting the prescriptions yet to be completed, the clerk said that it would take at least an hour, if there were no problems.

Ninety minutes later, Maria was still waiting. In addition, her mother was waiting outside in the car. Insistently and loudly, Maria asked what the problem was. At this point a beleaguered pharmacist walked over. Without calling her by name, the pharmacist said he was very busy, only worked in this store once a month, was having problems with the insurance company, and needed to talk to the doctor. Further, the pharmacist informed Maria that interrupting him by asking questions would only add to the wait.

Finally, 30 minutes later a new technician, not the one who had greeted her, came to the counter with her prescriptions. Maria never saw the pharmacist again but remembers signing some book. This is what Maria got: Of the six prescriptions she presented, four were filled and two were not filled, one because the pharmacy was out of the medication and the other because of delays in the doctor callback. Of the four prescriptions filled, two of the names on the prescription bottles did not match the list of names given her by the doctor. Maria left the pharmacy considering the discrepancy in the experience at this pharmacy portrayed on the television and the reality of actually being there.

■ CHAPTER QUESTIONS

1. Based on the scenario, how should the pharmacist have acted?
2. Based on the scenario, how could the problem have been avoided completely?
3. Is telling the truth following a medication error clearly the best policy. Why? Why not?
4. What are some primary considerations in the design of services?
5. How does the treatment of employees relate to their effectiveness in providing services?

6. How should an organization handle media relations in the event of a highly publicized error?

■ INTRODUCTION

An industrialized economy is composed of three principal sectors: extractive (i.e., mining and farming), manufacturing, and service. The services sector can be divided into five subgroups:

- *Business services*—consulting, finance, banking
- *Trade services*—retailing, maintenance and repair
- *Infrastructure services*—communications, transportation
- *Social/personal services*—restaurants, health care
- *Public administration*—education, government

Pharmacy is clearly a service business. As such, an understanding of a service business is beneficial to pharmacists. For pharmacists, the unique characteristics of services make working in that environment challenging, and even more so for pharmacy managers. The first section of this chapter describes the fundamental elements of services, along with the issues related to designing services and the elements of a service strategy. The second section of the chapter focuses on topics of special interest to pharmacists, specifically issues related to service failures and medication errors, dealing with service employees and professionals, and burnout.

■ CHARACTERISTICS OF SERVICES

Services can best be viewed and defined relative to their differences from manufacturing. These differences have implications for how services are marketed and managed. Services are distinguished by the following features:

- *The customer is a participant in the service process.* With rare exceptions, the customer is always present, at least for some part of the process. Although a patient may not be on site when a prescription is filled, there is generally an interaction of some kind between the pharmacist and the patient or the patient's agent.

- *Services are produced and consumed simultaneously.* Services cannot be produced ahead of time and stored in inventory. A filled prescription cannot be put into inventory because it is a custom-designed product for a specific patient.
- *Services are perishable.* A service that is not used is lost forever. An empty airline seat is revenue lost forever, and a pharmacy without patients is an expense without compensating revenue.
- *Service site location is dictated by the consumer.* For convenience and access, the site must be located where consumers are concentrated.
- *Economies of scale are difficult to achieve in services.* While there may be an optimal size for efficiency in a pharmacy, a single pharmacy in a rural county is unlikely to achieve that size.
- *Standardization of services is difficult.* An effective communication with one type of patient may be totally inappropriate for another.
- *Services are labor-intensive.* While the backroom operations of a pharmacy likely will be completely automated some day, the final counseling session always will require human interaction.
- *Output is difficult to measure.* The number of patients seen in a given period obviously can be counted, but assessing the quality of the interaction is problematic (adapted from Fitzsimmons and Fitzsimmons, 1994).

Most important, services are intangible. While there may be a tangible expression of the service, in this case a prescription, the cognitive evaluations and judgment of the pharmacist always will remain intangible. Managing and marketing services is "selling the invisible" (Beckwith, 1997). The task for a pharmacy manager is equal to that faced by a stage manager of a long-running theatrical production—deliver a performance that is professional day after day while the audience changes nightly and the performers come and go.

Given the factors detailed above, pharmacy managers are confronted with the fact that the customer "interferes" with efficient operations and introduces five types of variability to the system, forcing a trade-off between efficient operations and good customer service. Those five types of variability are (1) arrival variability—customers do not want service at times convenient for the company or in a steady, predictable pattern, (2) request variability—customers' desires are not standard, (3) capability variability—customers' own abilities to contribute to the service process vary (e.g., a visually impaired patient who requires training on the use of a nebulizer), (4) effort variability—how much energy will the customer expend to facilitate the service encounter (e.g., will the customer call the doctor ahead of time and provide updated insurance information), and (5) subjective variability—customers vary in their opinion as to what it means to be treated well (Frei, 2006).

■ CUSTOMER SERVICE DEFINED

What exactly is good customer service? Ask 20 people, and you will get 20 different answers: a prompt response to a question, a statement calculated correctly, a friendly reassurance that things will work out, work done on time, a knowledgeable technician at the other end of the line, extra help in negotiating with a third party, and so on. Delivering good customer service requires the following:

- Solving customer problems with no hassle
- Solving customer problems promptly
- Providing people who know what they are doing
- Providing people empowered to solve customer problems
- Treating people with dignity and empathy
- Correcting mistakes when they are made (adapted from Karr and Blohowiak, 1997)

Intuitively, everyone knows and understands what good service is. Everyone has experienced good service and bad. It is as simple as giving the customer what he or she wants, and yet it is difficult. It is doing it consistently time after time.

THE SERVICE ENCOUNTER

The critical point in services is the service encounter. The *service encounter* is the interaction between the service organization, the service provider, and the customer. It is the familiar scene in the pharmacy where the patient drops off and picks up the prescription, as well as being counseled. This interaction has been termed the *moment of truth* in services (Norman, 1984, pp. 8–9). The rise and fall of huge corporations, as well as individual employees' bonuses, can hinge on management of this brief interaction.

SERVICE EMPLOYEES

Service is a full-contact sport. It is people interacting with people in what has been termed a *moment of truth.* Because what happens in that moment of truth cannot be scripted or controlled, the secret to a successful service encounter is an employee empowered to meet the idiosyncratic needs of the consumer. Empowering employees to deliver superior service requires that the organization share with front-line employees (1) information about the organization's performance, (2) rewards based on the organization's performance, (3) knowledge that allows employees to understand and contribute to organizational performance, and (4) power to make decisions that influence organizational direction and performance (Bowen and Lawler, 1992). Nordstrom Department Stores, noted for its outstanding service, empowers its employees in this way: When new employees are hired, Nordstrom provides them with a single-page statement of how to act in dealing with a customer. That statement is: "Rule 1: Use your good judgment in all situations. There will be no additional rules." In other words, employees are given responsibility for their work; in doing so, the organization says, "I trust you." The end result, more often than not, is a satisfied consumer.

The benefits of an empowered employee are these:

- Quicker responses to customer needs during the service encounter

- Quicker responses to dissatisfied consumers during service recovery
- Employees feeling better about their jobs and themselves
- Employees interacting with consumers with more warmth and enthusiasm
- Empowered employees as a source for innovation and improvement (adapted from Bowen and Lawler, 1992)

A second critical element is for the organization to provide its employees with the same type of service that they expect them to deliver to consumers. It is not acceptable for the organization to espouse service commitment to consumers but not to its own employees. Everyone in the organization, from the executive suite to the recently hired, lowest-paid employee, is in the service business. An employee who cannot get problems regarding his or her benefits resolved in a timely and professional manner by the human resources department is likely to provide inferior service to consumers. It is what you do, not what you say, that counts in dealing with service employees. Research has indicated that service industry employees who perceive fair treatment by their employers are more likely to treat customers fairly in return (Bowen, Gilliland, and Folger, 1999).

PROFESSIONALS

Professionals may be even more achievement-oriented than the traditional service employee. They consistently seek new challenges and may demonstrate a propensity toward boredom in their absence. They are interested in personal growth and advancement. An organization that stifles this need hardly can expect its professional service staff to deliver superior customer service. Latent, if not outright open, resentment toward the organization is likely and, by extension, toward the organization's customers. Professionals are interested in meaning. Effort should be directed toward explaining why something should be done, not how it should be done.

STANDARDS FOR EVALUATING SERVICES

Customers evaluate services and the service encounter on five broad dimensions. The five dimensions are

- *Reliability*—the ability to perform the promised service dependably and accurately
- *Responsiveness*—the willingness to help customers and provide prompt service
- *Assurance*—the knowledge and courtesy of employees and their ability to convey trust and confidence
- *Empathy*—the caring, individualized attention provided to customers
- *Tangibles*—the appearance of physical facilities, equipment, personnel, and communication materials (Berry, Parasuraman, and Zeithaml, 1994)

Of these five dimensions, reliability is most highly valued by consumers. Nothing fancy is required; just do what you say you will do.

MEASURING SERVICE QUALITY

Since services are for the most part intangible, customers use a psychological standard to evaluate services and service quality. Customers assess their perceptions of a service relative to their expectations for that service. The expectation the consumer holds for the service becomes the standard. These standards may be completely arbitrary, differ among consumers, and change constantly. If someone is told that the wait for a table in a restaurant is 30 minutes and then is seated in 20 minutes, the service experience is likely to be viewed with satisfaction. Conversely, if the same person is told that the wait is 10 minutes and is seated in the same 20 minutes, the service experience is likely to

be evaluated with displeasure. As with the restaurant, if in arriving at a pharmacy a patient expects that his or her prescription will be ready in 20 minutes and that the pharmacist will take a few moments to explain the medication in a simple, straightforward manner, the degree to which this psychological standard (i.e., personal expectation) is either exceeded or not determines the customer evaluation of the service. What this means is that services are evaluated by the customer on the difference in expectations for the service versus the perception of that service (Parasuraman, Zeithaml, and Berry, 1994). Customer expectations for service arise from the customer's own experiences with that service, other services like it, and the experiences of other customers. In services, quality is defined by the gap between the expectation for the service and the perception of how it was delivered (Fig. 11-1).

Customer expectations for service operate at two levels—desired and adequate. In other words, there is the ideal of what customers expect and the level of service that will satisfy them. Ideally, one would expect every airline flight to arrive and depart precisely on time, the attendants be personally solicitous, and luggage never be lost or damaged. Realistically, the customer personally may find a 15-minute delay, a courteous attendant, and a rare problem with luggage to be acceptable. Any level of service in the gap between ideal and adequate service is characterized as a *zone of tolerance*. The zone of tolerance for acceptable service varies based on the specific service dimension. The zone of tolerance for reliability on the filling of a prescription is exceedingly narrow. More than likely there is no zone of tolerance on this dimension. Conversely, the *zone of acceptance* for the appearance of a pharmacy for many customers is probably quite wide. More than likely, once a minimum standard for cleanliness is met, the customer may care little about how the pharmacy looks (Parasuraman, Berry, and Zeithaml, 1991).

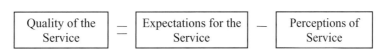

Figure 11-1. Quality-of-service equation.

Recent work has highlighted the impact of emotions on the assessment of service quality. Consumers base their assessment of service quality on a complicated mix of rationality and emotion, with emotion playing a larger role. Quality in manufacturing is often measured using the Six Sigma standard (a one-in-a-million error rate). A quality improvement methodology in services has been developed called *Human Sigma* (Fleming, Coffman, and Harter, 2005). This approach to service quality asks managers not to think like engineers or economists when assessing the service encounter, but to factor emotions into the assessment; to measure the service encounter locally owing to the enormous variation in quality at this level rather than rely on company-wide averages, and to use a single measure of service encounter effectiveness. To improve service quality, the organization must engage in short-term coaching at the local level along with long-term changes in hiring, promotion, and structure. Highlighting the value of the Human Sigma approach is the fact that emotionally engaged customers contribute more to the bottom line than rationally satisfied customers (Fleming, Coffman, and Harter, 2005). Strategically, this infers the necessity for assessing the emotional commitment of customers, even beyond traditional measures of customer loyalty and satisfaction (e.g., overall satisfaction, likelihood to repurchase, and likelihood to recommend). The first measure of emotional commitment is *confidence*—Does the company always deliver on its promises? The second measure is *integrity*—Am I treated the way I deserve to be treated? The third is *pride*—Do I have a sense of positive identification with the company" Fourth, *passion*—Is the company irreplaceable in my life? Passionate customers are rare. The strategic implication of this is that customers are made one at a time, and businesses are built one customer at a time, one human relating to one human—if you will, one heart to one heart.

Customers evaluate the services they receive continuously. There is a constant assessment of expectations versus perception. An organization that cannot consistently deliver a level of service where customer expectations exceed perceptions simply will disappear. Since the customer will evaluate the service encounter whether it is managed or not, it only makes sense that a prudent manager will design, manage, and market his or her service to meet this standard.

DESIGNING SERVICES

In designing services for profit and to exceed customer expectations, a manager ought to consider the following issues:

- *What is our product (service)?* When buying a good or service, consumers purchase a bundle of attributes, both tangible and intangible, aimed at satisfying wants and needs. This bundle of attributes is termed a *consumer benefit package.* In designing the consumer benefit package, the following issues must be addressed: (1) verify that the attributes included in the consumer benefit package are appropriate, (2) evaluate each attribute in terms of importance to the consumer, (3) evaluate each attribute in terms of ability to deliver, (4) maximize consumer satisfaction, and (5) maximize financial return.
- *How will this service be priced? Are our pricing objectives to generate financial returns, capture market share, or meet the competition?* Having determined the pricing objectives, a pricing structure must be decided on. The issues related to a pricing structure include the following: (1) Should a standard list price be charged? (2) Should frequent or large customers get the same base price? (3) Should different prices be charged for different aspects of the service? (4) Does the time of purchase affect the price? (5) Does the price reflect the cost of doing business with a specific customer? (6) Should customers who value the service more highly be charged a higher price? (7) Are there discounts?
- *How will the service be promoted, positioned, and branded?* On what basis can the market be segmented—demographic, geographic, psychographic, or usage variables? Can a market segment be targeted that is identifiable, measurable, and large enough to be profitable, reachable, responsive, and stable? Can a position be found that is singular and simple,

distinguishes one from the competition, and is focused? Finally, is branding the service advisable and affordable?

- *How will the service be delivered?* Where will facilities be located? Is a single site the best choice, or are multiple sites required? Is the Internet a viable option?
- *What will the facility look like—interior, exterior, decor, signage, lighting, etc.? How will the employees be presented?* Appearances, including those of employees, serve to shape first impressions, particularly if little is known about the service; convey trust (particularly if the consumer has no other way to judge quality); convey an image; and provide sensory stimulation to make the experience memorable.
- *What procedures and protocols will be put in place for the delivery of the services?* How will the system function that delivers the service? How will outcomes versus level of inputs be measured? How will quality be measured and reliability maintained? How fast can the service be delivered, the system improved?
- *Who actually will deliver the service? How will they be trained, promoted, and motivated?* A significant issue with professional services is one of compensation. Is compensation based on profitability of work output, profitability of work supervised, client satisfaction as to work output, or contributions to practice development?

These questions reflect the seven P's of service, the four traditional marketing P's of product, price, place, and promotion and three additional P's of service, namely, physical attributes, process, and people. Considering these questions and formulating winning responses are the essence of what managers and pharmacists are required to do to win the service game.

Strategy

A well-designed service offering must fit within a strategic framework. A *strategy* is a long-range plan, a pattern of decisions, in pursuit of a goal. Business strategies develop in one of two ways. One method is intuitive and informal; the other is formal and explicit. Establishing a strategy requires answering the following questions:

(1) Do we fully understand the service business we are in? (2) How can the business be defended against competitors? (3) What is the direction of the industry? and (4) What does the consumer want in this industry? A successful strategy is grounded in the sustainable competitive advantage that a pharmacy possesses. Competitive advantage arises from something you do better than the competition. Winning strategies are the result of strategic thinking. Strategic thinking is characterized by the ability to look at all the obvious factors related to the business with the right perspective while not being influenced by fad or emotion. In pharmacy, one obvious factor is this: There will be plenty of business (number of prescriptions) with ever-declining margins. Another is that pharmaceutical care will succeed only when the consumer wants it and is willing to pay in some fashion, either directly or through higher insurance premiums.

■ SPECIAL TOPICS

When Things Go Wrong: Service Recovery

When delivering a service, no matter how well managed, things inevitably go wrong. This section deals with the issues of what happens when things go wrong in the pharmacy. First, catastrophic prescription errors are considered. Second, noncatastrophic prescription errors and service failures (e.g., technicians are rude, services are delayed, charges are inaccurate, etc.) are discussed. The process of *service recovery*, dealing with and correcting errors and service failures, is critical. As Sir Colin Marshall, chief executive officer (CEO) of British Airways, observes, "The customer doesn't expect everything will go right all the time; the big test is what you do when things go wrong . . . . Occasional service failure is unavoidable." The logic underpinning this discussion is this: Errors are inevitable; dissatisfied customers are not.

Catastrophic Prescription Errors

Despite the best efforts of pharmacists and managers, delivering error-free pharmaceutical services, specifically the distribution of pharmaceuticals, is impossible.

In writing on human error, Senders and Moray (1991, p. 128) conclude: "Human error rates can be reduced to as low a level as desired, at some unknown cost. The occurrence of a particular error at a particular instant, however, cannot absolutely be prevented." Even if the patient suffers no permanent harm, a service failure or mistake in a pharmacy is a significant event. The consequences of a service failure or mistake in a pharmacy include a deterioration of trust in the pharmacist and the system, the spread of negative word-of-mouth advertising, the possibility of legal action, possible board of pharmacy involvement, the erosion of customer patronage, and a diminished level of profit (see Chapters 7, 28, and 30 on minimizing the occurrence of prescription errors).

The Institute of Medicine reports that medication errors result in 7,000 deaths per year (Agency for Healthcare Research and Quality, 2007). *Catastrophic errors* are defined as causing severe damage to a patient that is not easily reversed, for example, an error that results in a 4-day stay in a hospital or worse. A catastrophic medication error affects more that just the victim and the involved practitioners. Those interested in and affected by an error include other workers, management, other consumers/patients, regulators, competitors, the media, suppliers, accrediting bodies, the legal system, and stockholders/investors. These people can be viewed as stakeholders in the pharmacy. In managing the response to a catastrophic medication error, relevant stakeholders need to be identified, the costs and interests of each stakeholder must be protected, total costs should be minimized, and control of the situation should be maintained. The standard for adjudicating these interests is equity of outcomes and procedural fairness. In other words, is each group treated fairly by a process that is responsive and open (Seiders and Berry, 1998)? Following a catastrophic medication error, there will be pressure on managers to favor the bottom line and minimize legal costs. Favoring one group of stakeholders over another is shortsighted, unethical, and bad for business overall.

Most important, involved practitioners and health care organizations must avoid being perceived as the villain. It is one thing to be presented as well-meaning practitioners who simply made a mistake and quite another to be portrayed as malicious or insensitive.

Victims of catastrophic medication errors are due just and equitable compensation for their trouble. The following recommendations are made for responding to the victim and the victim's family following the occurrence of a serious error. First, the victim and family want the truth about what happened. The consumer/ patient demand for this is unequivocal—over 98 percent (Witman, Park, and Hardin, 1996). Next, the victim and family want compensation for the emotional, psychological, and financial costs of the catastrophic medication error. Emotional costs are ameliorated through an apology, the psychological costs through assurances that the system will be fixed, and the patient costs in time, money, and inconvenience through financial settlements.

The Ben Kolb Case: An Example of What to Do

Ben remained in a coma for nearly 24 hours. His parents and older sister remained at his bedside as their fog of denial slowly lifted. The next day they agreed that his ventilator should be removed, and he was declared brain dead. As with the death of Jose Martinez, a lot can be learned by what happened after Ben Kolb died. First, the hospital's risk manager, Doni Haas, had all the syringes and vials used on Ben locked away and then sent to an independent laboratory for analysis. Second, Haas promised Ben's parents that she "was going to find them an answer, if there was one." There was. Tests showed that there had been a mix-up, a mistake, a human error in a system that made that error more likely. Ben Kolb, lab reports showed, was never injected with lidocaine at all. The syringe that was supposed to contain lidocaine actually contained epinephrine in a highly concentrated strength that was intended only for external use. Procedure in the Martin Memorial operating room at the time was for topical epinephrine to be poured into one cup, made of plastic, and lidocaine to be poured into a cup nearby, made of metal. The lidocaine syringe then was filled by placing it in the metal cup. It is a procedure used all over the country, a way of getting a drug from container to operating table. According to Richmond Harman, the hospital's CEO, "It has probably been done 100,000 times in our facility without error." But it is a flawed procedure, the hospital learned. It allows for the possibility that the solution can be poured into or drawn out of the wrong cup. Instead, a cap, called a *spike,* could be put on the vial of lidocaine, allowing the drug to be drawn directly out of the labeled bottle and into a labeled syringe. The elimination of one step eliminates one opportunity for the human factor to get in the way. Haas received the lab results 3 weeks after Ben died. The family had hired an attorney by then, and Haas and McLain drove 2 hours and met with the Kolbs at the law firm od Krupnick, Campbell, Malone, Roselli, Buser, Slama and Hancock. "It was very unusual," said Richard J. Roselli, one of Florida's most successful malpractice lawyers and the president of the Academy of Florida Trial Lawyers. "This is the first occasion where I ever had a hospital step forward, admitting their responsibility and seeking to do everything they can to help the family." A financial settlement was reached by nightfall, but neither side will confirm the amount paid to the Kolbs. After the papers were signed, the family asked for a chance to talk with the doctors at the hospital. The first thing Ben's father, Tim, did when he entered the motion-filled room was to hug his son's surgeon. Then came the torrent of questions, questions that had kept the Kolbs awake at night, questions they might never have been able to ask had the case spent years in court. Was Ben scared when his heart rate started dropping? Was he in pain? How much did he suffer? The doctors explained what the Kolbs did not know, that Ben had been put under general anesthesia long before anything went wrong. "The decisions I made for him were the same I would have made if it were my child," McLain said. Just before the family left, they asked if it would be okay for them to continue to use Martin Memorial for their medical care. "Of course," Haas said, grateful and amazed. Would the hospital promise to spread the word about how Ben died so that the procedure in question could be changed in other places? Haas promised. With that, the Kolb case was closed, but it wasn't over. Tim Kolb still coaches his son's soccer team. The family still

grieves (from "How Can We Save the Next Victim?" by Lisa Belkin, *New York Times Magazine,* June 15, 1997, pp. 63–64).

Media Relations

Catastrophic medication errors, particularly when someone dies, are a newsworthy event. Health care is not immune. Such errors are not likely to remain secret. As a result of the adverse public exposure, reputations will be diminished, with potentially significant consequences for individual practitioners and institutions. The only means available, at least initially, to rehabilitate individual and institutional reputations is an appropriate message and response through the media.

There often is, and most likely always will be, a natural adversarial relationship with the media. In dealing with outside media, the choices are (1) to say nothing at all, (2) to deny or repudiate the charge, (3) to claim no responsibility for the event, (4) to minimize its impact, (5) to admit and ask for forgiveness, and (6) any combination of these (Benoit and Brinson, 1994). There are two audiences for information following a medication error. The first audience is the general public, which wants information about what is going on and how it happened; the focus is on "What if I had to go there?" The second audience consists of the various stakeholders, who, on the other hand, want to know how the crisis will affect their interests and how management is doing. One audience demands openness; the other may require circumspection.

Advice on what to say and how to deal with the media is contradictory. One approach is to tell them nothing and tell it slowly. However, such advice may be costly. Rather than a closed approach, the best way to polish a tarnished reputation through the media is quite simple—be honest, be open, and be first. Disarm the media by telling the bad news first and fast. Establish openness and candor. Not being honest, open, and first puts you on the defensive. In addition, emphasize the good you have done.

Whether to apologize or not is a delicate issue. "Confession is good for the soul, and when you offend someone, even unintentionally, it feels good to say 'I'm sorry.' But when there is a chance you might end up in court, you'd better think twice" (Iacocca, 1984). Rather than an outright apology, ambiguity in announcements is recommended (Sellnow and Ulmer, 1995). Ambiguity is saying something without saying it or saying nothing while saying something. An example of an ambiguous approach is that used by Jack in the Box in 1993 following reported deaths owing to *Escherichia coli*–contaminated hamburgers. The company stated, "Although it is unclear as to the source of an illness linked to undercooked beef, Jack in the Box announced today that it has taken measures to ensure [that] all menu items are prepared in accordance with an advisory issued yesterday by the Washington State Department of Health" (Sellnow and Ulmer, 1995. p. 142).

No one can put a price on a human life nor adequately compensate for the suffering that a catastrophic medication error causes. Nor can one really understand the impact of such an event on a practitioner. What happens can never be undone. What can be done is this: The response can be open, caring, concerned, empathetic, and ethical. It is a test of character. The choice, ultimately, is between taking the high road or taking the expedient path of self-interest. As practitioners involved in the higher moral activity of health care as opposed to pure commerce, it is an obligation. The high road also will be good for business.

As a practical matter, a successful response to a catastrophic medication error proceeds through the following stages:

- *Signal detection.* Catastrophic medication errors should not be a surprise. "Routine" and noncatastrophic errors foreshadow the inevitable.
- *Preparation and prevention.* The best organizations do all they can to prevent catastrophic medication errors while recognizing that they must prepare and plan for their inevitable occurrence.
- *Containment/damage limitation.* The goal of this stage is to limit the immediate damage.
- *Recovery.* This stage involves establishing procedures for short- and long-term business recovery while understanding what the key activities are in serving key stakeholders.

- *Learning.* Reflection and critical examination of what happened aimed at prevention (adapted from Pearson and Mitroff, 1993).

Noncatastrophic Prescription Errors and Service Failures

Occurring frequently in the commerce of pharmaceutical goods and services are noncatastrophic medication errors (i.e., the damage is easily reversible) and service failures (i.e., technicians are rude, billings are late, etc.). The emerging view in service quality and relationship marketing emphasizes the conversion of dissatisfied customers, owing to a service failure or mistake, into satisfied or recovered customers. *Service recovery* is a process, a sequence of events beginning with the recognition of a service failure or mistake, followed by a series of interactions between the aggrieved consumer and the service provider. The process concludes with a decision and the allocation of outcomes. Each sequence of interactions is subject to evaluation by the consumer.

Empirical work on service recovery seeks to identify organizational responses to service failures that effectively ameliorate consumer dissatisfaction. Bell and Zemke (1987) identified five elements for service recovery: apology, urgent reinstatement, empathy, symbolic atonement, and follow-up. Johnston (1995) identified the following elements for service recovery: provision of information about the problem and what is being done, action either in response to the customer or preferably without needing to be asked, the appearance of putting themselves out by the staff, and involvement by the customer in the decision making. In a retail setting, the recommendations for service recovery include discount, correction, manager/employee intervention, correction plus replacement, apology, refund, and store credit (Kelly, Hoffman, and Davis, 1993).

While it would appear intuitive that companies, as a matter of course, would try to correct their mistakes, research indicates that over 17 percent of companies do nothing following a service failure or mistake and that as many as one-third of the service recovery initiatives are unacceptable to the consumer (Kelly, Hoffman, and Davis, 1993). The "paradox of service recovery" is that effective service recovery causes consumers to rate an encounter more favorably than if no problem had occurred in the first place (McCullough and Bharadwaj, 1992). In addition, effective service recovery following a service failure or mistake has been found to have a larger influence on overall satisfaction than the initial service encounter (Spreng, Harrell, and Mackoy, 1995). In addition, effective service recovery has been found to have a significant and positively impact on consumer behavior; specifically, loyalty to the company, propensity to switch, and willingness to pay more, complain to external agents, or complain to employees (Zeithaml, Berry, and Parasuraman, 1996). Finally, research has demonstrated that effective service recovery results in retention of over 70 percent of consumers (Kelly, Hoffman, and Davis, 1993).

Schweikhart and Strasser (1993) pointed out the problems of service recovery in a health care context. Those problems are (1) lack of a strong marketing tradition, (2) the cost and time of implementing programs, (3) lack of organizational and professional readiness for service recovery, (4) the dilemma of who to target, the patient or the family, and (5) understanding what is an appropriate response. These authors summarized the service recovery dilemma in health care when they declared, "It may be possible to waive $50 for automobile repair, but is it possible for a hospital to waive $5,000 for a left inguinal hernia repair?" Despite these impediments, delivering quality service that exceeds customer/patient expectations requires that pharmacists understand the inherent problems and take appropriate steps to respond to the situations caused by catastrophic prescription errors, noncatastrophic prescription errors, and service failures. Although redundant, the point bears repeating: Errors are inevitable; dissatisfied customers are not.

REVISITING THE SCENARIO

Maria Perez experienced service failures from the pharmacy, and her expectations clearly were not met. Some contingencies arise that are beyond the immediate control of the pharmacist. For example, a physician may require contact prior to dispensing a prescribed agent, and said physician or an appropriate agent of the physician may not be able to get back with you very promptly. However, you have direct influence over the kind of service you deliver and the resulting customer perceptions regardless of the situation. The manager of the pharmacy that Maria visited has underestimated the importance of various intangibles to Maria, such as the pharmacy's appearance and the way support personnel greeted her.

CONCLUSION

It is said that great companies treasure the goodwill of each customer as if it were a valuable account. The goal is to deposit into that account, adding more than you take out and paying unexpected dividends. Adding to that account is simple—deliver superior service. Delivering superior service requires designing, managing, and marketing pharmaceutical services in such a manner that results in customer perceptions of the service exceeding their expectations. Will the customer, on leaving the pharmacy, think, "That was a pleasant experience"? Superior service also requires people and professionals who are attuned to the needs of the customer. How does that happen? Make sure that employees are empowered. Treat employees as you would want them to treat your customers. And when things go wrong, as they inevitably will, fix the problem cheerfully and promptly. Compensate people for their costs. Reassure them that it will not happen again. Treat them as you would want to be treated. Is delivering good service on a consistent basis easy? No. Is it rewarding? Yes.

QUESTIONS FOR FURTHER DISCUSSION

1. Describe an incident where you experienced service that was particularly good. What made it so?
2. Describe an incident where you experienced service that was particularly bad. What made it so?
3. What do you believe a typical pharmacy customer values most in a service encounter?

4. Describe an incident at work where you, as an employee, got good service from the company. What made it so? How did this make you feel?

5. Describe an incident at work where you, as an employee, got poor service from the company. What made it so? How did this make you feel?

6. What is the consumer expectation for pharmacy services in an ambulatory setting, long-term care environment, hospice, and hospital? How do they differ?

7. Explain how service in a late-night diner can be rated superior to service in a five-star restaurant.

REFERENCES

Agency for Healthcare Research and Quality. 2007. Medical errors: The scope of the problem. Available at www.ahrq.gov/qual/errback.htm.

Beckwith H. 1997. *Selling the Invisible*. New York: Warner Books.

Bell C, Zemke R. 1987. Service breakdown, the road to recovery. *Manag Rev* October:32.

Benoit W, Brinson S. 1994. Apologies are not enough. *Commun Q* 42:75.

Berry L, Parasuraman A, Zeithaml V. 1994. Improving service quality in America: Lessons learned. *Acad Manag Exec* 8:32.

Bowen DE, Gilliland SW, Folger R. 1999. HRM and service fairness: How being fair with employees spills over to customers. *Organ Dyn* 27:7.

Bowen D, Lawler E III. 1992. The empowerment of service workers: What, why, how, and when. *Sloan Manag Rev* Spring:31.

Fitzsimmons JA, Fitzsimmons MJ. 1994. *Service Management for Competitive Advantage*. New York: McGraw-Hill.

Fleming J, Coffman C, Harter J. 2005. Manage your Human Sigma. *Harvard Business Review* (HBR) July-August:106.

Frei F. 2006. Breaking the tradeoff between efficiency and service. *Harvard Business Review* (HBR) November:93.

Iacocca L. 1984. *Iacocca: An Autobiography*. New York: Bantam Books.

Johnston R. 1995. Service failure and recovery: Impact, attributes, and process. *Adv Ser Market Manag* 4:211.

Karr R, Blohowiak D. 1997. *The Complete Idiot's Guide to Great Customer Service*. New York: Alpha Books.

Kelley S, Hoffman K, Davis M. 1993. A typology of retail failures and recoveries. *J Retail* 69:429.

McCullough M, Bharadwaj S. 1992. The recovery paradox: An examinations of consumer satisfaction in relation to disconfirmation, service quality, and attribution based theories. In Allen C et al. (eds), *Marketing Theory and Applications*. Chicago: American Marketing Association.

Norman R. 1984. *Service Management*. New York: Wiley.

Parasuraman A, Zeithaml V, Berry L. 1994. Reassessment of expectations as a comparison standard in measuring service quality: Implications for further research. *J Market* 58:111.

Parasuraman A, Berry L, Zeithaml V. 1991. Understanding customer expectations for service. *Sloan Manag Rev* Spring:39.

Pearson C, Clair J. 1998. Reframing crisis management. *Acad Manag Rev* 23:59.

Pearson C, Mitroff I. 1993. From crisis prone to crisis prepared: A framework for crisis management. *Acad Manag Exec* 7:48.

Schweikhart S, Strasser S. 1993. Service recovery in health service organizations. *Hosp Health Serv Admin* 1:3.

Seiders K, Berry L. 1998. Service fairness: What it is and why it matters. *Acad Manag Exec* May:8.

Sellnow T, Ulmer R. 1995. Ambiguous argument as advocacy in organizational crisis communication. *Argument Advocacy* 31:138.

Senders J, Moray N. 1991. *Human Error: Cause, Prediction, and Reduction*. Hillsdale, NJ: Lawrence Erlbaum Associates.

Spreng R, Harrell G, Mackoy R. 1995. Service recovery: Impact on satisfaction and intentions. *J Serv Market* 1:15.

Witman A, Park D, Hardin S. 1996. How do patients want physicians to handle mistakes? *Arch Intern Med* 156:2565.

Zeithaml V, Berry L, Parasuraman B. 1996. The behavioral consequences of service quality. *J Market* April:31.

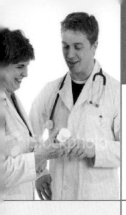

12

CONTEMPORARY WORKPLACE ISSUES

Vincent J. Giannetti

About the Author: Dr. Giannetti is Professor of Social and Administrative Pharmaceutical Sciences at the Mylan School of Pharmacy of Duquesne University. He teaches organizational behavior and health care management part time in the School of Business. Dr. Giannetti is a licensed psychologist in the State of Pennsylvania and has graduate degrees in psychology, public health, and social work. His publications have focused on health care ethics, substance abuse, and behavioral health.

■ LEARNING OBJECTIVES

After completing this chapter, students should be able to

1. Describe the process and implications of providing job enrichment in the workplace.
2. Describe how the unionization of employees and the presence of labor unions affect managerial processes and decision making.
3. Describe fundamental issues in occupational safety.
4. Discuss methods for assisting employees to cope with stress.
5. Identify the requirements for intervening with impaired pharmacists.
6. Identify and discuss developmental and anchor methods for understanding and managing employee careers.
7. Describe legal concepts involved with workplace discrimination.
8. Identify and discuss major provisions of federal legislation that addresses workplace discrimination and equal opportunity.
9. Describe how the issues proffered in this chapter fit within the context of ethical business management.

SCENARIO

Ann Kolawieczki has been working at a local hospital pharmacy for 3 years since graduating from pharmacy school. Ann has become dissatisfied with the routine nature of her job and is beginning to question her career choice. In addition, she has been having some personal problems that have caused her to appear preoccupied and distracted at work. She recently lost her temper with a nurse who requested clarification regarding a medication sent to the floor. She went out after work one evening with some staff members and "appeared to have too much too drink." Her supervisor thought that he detected the faint odor of alcohol on her breath, and shortly after that incident, Ann started to be come to work late and appeared more disorganized in her work. Ann has complained about the behavior of some of the male pharmacy technicians and pharmacists. They have teased her about her drinking the night she went out and have been making what she considers inappropriate remarks.

CHAPTER QUESTIONS

1. How might the work of pharmacists and support personnel be redesigned to reflect modern, patient-centered practice?
2. What types of stresses are caused by the workplace, and how does personal stress affect work?
3. What are the responsibilities of managers in identifying employee personal problems and helping employees obtain the appropriate assistance?
4. How might a lack of career planning be a source of dissatisfaction? How can managers assist employees in developing their careers?
5. What are some of the principal workplace equal opportunity and discrimination issues? How do federal laws relate to a manager's responsibility for ensuring a fair and equitable work environment?
6. How might the presence of a unionized labor force affect the way that human resources management decisions are made by an organization?
7. What are the major issues and requirements when ensuring workplace safety and health?

8. How should basic business ethics govern decision making in pharmacy and health care?

INTRODUCTION

Intervening with Ann in the workplace poses many challenges and requires basic knowledge and skill in human relations and resources. Is Ann's dissatisfaction a function of personal problems, or is the organizational environment a major contributor to her dissatisfaction? Is the nature of work organization and culture responsible for dissatisfaction in the workplace? How can Ann's supervisor approach her work performance, and what are the obligations and responsibilities of the manager to confront Ann about her alcohol consumption? Finally, if a hostile environment exists, what are Ann's options and the manager's responsibilities in addressing the situation?

Proper management of human resources in modern organizations is no simple task. Managing career progression, working within an organization characterized by diversity, and navigating through a host of complex rules and regulations in an increasingly litigious society presents significant challenges to managers. Human resources divisions of companies normally manage these issues and related functions. However, managers must have a basic awareness and knowledge of employee stress, career development, and diversity to manage effectively and mentor. Early identification of problems and challenges and effective monitoring in consultation with human resources are integral parts of the routine functions of management. Employee satisfaction, job-related stress, career progress, and fairness in the workplace are the most significant factors in the overall health and effective functioning of organizations.

JOB ENRICHMENT AND QUALITY OF WORK LIFE

While there have been numerous surveys regarding job satisfaction in pharmacy, the development of the concept of medication therapy management as a new paradigm for education and practice has created a dilemma for pharmacy management. Management of pharmacy services will face unique challenges because of the continuing shift in educational and practice philosophy toward the delivery of value-added services and shared responsibility for therapeutic outcomes. While the concept of pharmacy care was well integrated into education, there has been a considerable lag in its application to the practice setting (Cipolle and Strand, 1998). This lag or dissonance between educational philosophy and practice reality has the potential to cause disillusionment and dissatisfaction with professional practice, particularly as recently graduated pharmacists work their way through career progression. Within this context, enriched job environments, job satisfaction, and career counseling are critical for both pharmacists and the profession. In addition, as the American population continues to become more diverse and universal access to health care becomes a greater possibility, pharmacists will need to manage with a better understanding of cultural diversity.

In many ways, the work of pharmacists continues to be influenced by classical job design theory that emphasizes standardization, segmentation, and overdependence on procedures, rules, and hierarchy. Classical job design correlates well with production jobs that require accuracy, efficiency, and compliance with directives. Tight controls, supervision, and rigidity in rules are favored in order to reduce quality problems (Taylor, 1911). Classical job design is well suited to the dispensing functions of pharmacists. If the primary mission of pharmacy is to get the right medication in the right dose to the right patient, then classical job design best accommodates this mission. However, as "clinically educated" pharmacists enter the market, bringing with them a different set of expectations, a desire for increased professionalism, and a different practice philosophy, enriched job environments will need to be created to address these "higher-order needs" for exercising professional autonomy and judgment. The goodness of fit among education, professional expectations, and practice environments should be the proper focus of pharmacy management. The educational environment has raised expectations for pharmacy care and

medication therapy management (MTM). The practice environment will need to shape demand in the market. The first step in this change process will be redesign of the work environment to create intrinsically enriched situations. The most effective way to market MTM is for the public to both see and learn to value the knowledge-based services that pharmacists can offer. An enriched job environment will facilitate this process, reinforce its importance, and meet the expectations and needs of clinically trained pharmacists.

While high salaries have the potential of maintaining at least short-term commitment to the profession, money does not compensate for professional and job stagnation over time. As pharmacists more fully evolve into "knowledge workers," intrinsic motivating factors will become increasingly important for recruitment and retention. As automation and technicians continue to take over the routine and less judgmental aspects of the work, there is an opportunity to reconsider job redesign for the pharmacist.

Ideally, the best job design for pharmacy would be the alignment of practitioner education and expectations with marketplace realities. Job design plays a role in determining the satisfaction and quality of work life for practitioners. If the education of pharmacists is for a market that does not exist or jobs that do not provide opportunities to exercise education and knowledge, dissatisfaction and career stagnation will result.

Intrinsically motivating jobs and enriched job environments have as their common goals both increased satisfaction and better performance. The job characteristics theory strives to encourage three basic psychological states related to intrinsic motivation: (1) experienced meaningfulness of work, (2) responsibility for outcomes, and (3) knowledge of work outcomes (Hackman et al., 1975). The core job characteristics to accomplish these goals are built into the design of the work. They include *skill variety, task identity, task significance, autonomy,* and *feedback*. These characteristics of enrichment function best with workers who have strong needs for growth, personal accomplishment, self-direction, and learning. The first step in the enrichment process is to define the current job in terms of core characteristics. Jobs then can be redesigned to reflect the critical psychological states necessary for enriched jobs. The following questions can be used as a guide:

1. To what degree does the job require a variety of tasks that demand a greater knowledge and skills for which the employee has been educated? (*Skill variety*)
2. To what degree does the work require performing a complete set of interventions or tasks for which the employee is responsible? (*Task identity*)
3. To what degree are the tasks performed highly significant for the well-being of others and for the organization? (*Task significance*)
4. To what degree can the employee exercise independent judgment in performing the work? (*Autonomy*)
5. To what degree does the work provide feedback about the outcomes of effort independent of supervisors or coworkers? (*Feedback*)

Various practice environments possess differing degrees of enriching characteristics, and the need for highly enriched jobs may vary among pharmacists. The specifics of job redesign will also vary according to practice setting, resources of the organization, and desire for innovation. However, modifying or increasing the amount and frequency of these characteristics will require changes in both the internal and external environments of pharmacy practice. The internal environment must be modified by changing financial incentives. Work reorganization needs to fully recognize the value of knowledge-based service. If prescription volume remains the main driver of pharmacy care and the main source of revenue, then the low-lying fruit of dispensing will crowd out the possibility of enriched jobs. The external environment must be modified to create consumer demand and perceived value added to the health care system as a result of the integration of cognitive services into pharmacy practice.

Front-line managers and supervisors often have limited control over both the internal and external environments of health care delivery. However, if job satisfaction, professionalization, and quality service are to continue and improve in pharmacy, there must be an alignment among ideals, education, and market and practice realities. Managers must see the role of innovation as an integral part of their responsibilities. Lack of attention to job enrichment will inhibit the profession from realizing its full potential and can lead to disillusionment with the profession by both the public and practitioners. As organizations compete to attract and retain quality pharmacists and support personnel, job enrichment and quality of work life will continue to be a factor.

■ UNIONS AND MANAGEMENT

The proportion of workers who are unionized and the strength of their constituent labor unions have ebbed and flowed over the years. When working conditions, pay, and benefits do not meet reasonable employee expectations, the formation of unions is much more likely. The National Labor Relations Board is responsible for overseeing the process of union organization. A union is certified to exclusively represent employees when 50 percent of all employees vote for a union. Closed shops and union shops require membership in a union to work at a specific organization; however, some states have "right to work" laws that override these provisions. A closed shop requires membership in a union to be hired and is considered illegal under the provisions of the National Labor Relations Act. A union shop requires that an individual join a union within a specified amount of time after hiring.

The process of contract administration and grievance procedures can have an impact on the routine duties of managers. The enforcement of contract provisions and fair treatment in the workplace are mediated by grievance procedures. Usually, grievances can be discussed informally with a supervisor; however, if they are not resolved, then union stewards (i.e., official representatives of the union) can become involved with both the grievance and management's response to it. If the situation is not resolved, the grievance can be placed in arbitration for a binding decision. The most frequent grievances are disciplinary actions, discharge, promotions, layoffs, transfers, work assignments, and scheduling (U.S. Mediation and Conciliation Service,

1997). Due process is the key to resolving grievances. Certain criteria can be used as guidelines for arbitration determinations. Managers should adhere to the following criteria in enforcing and resolving problems with employees, thus increasing the probability that arbitration will be resolved in favor of reasonable management decisions (Redecker, 1989):

1. Rules, expectations, and consequences must be communicated and documented.
2. Rules must be applied consistently and violations documented carefully.
3. Discipline must be progressive, with opportunities for the employee to modify behavior.
4. The right to question and appeal must be provided.
5. Mitigating circumstances should be considered.

WORK SAFETY ISSUES

Another issue related to quality of work life is job safety. The Occupational Safety and Health Act created the Occupational Safety and Health Administration (OSHA) and established the federal government's role in promulgating and enforcing safety and health standards for places of employment that engage in interstate commerce. It is the responsibility of every employer to provide a work environment that is free from recognized hazards. Employees have a right to have an inspection of the workplace performed, have dangerous or hazardous substances or situations identified, be properly informed of hazards, have accurate records kept regarding exposure to hazards, and have violations posted at the workplace (Occupational Safety and Health Administration, 2003). Failure to comply with rules and regulations can result in severe fines and other penalties from OSHA.

The National Institute for Occupational Safety and Health (NIOSH) conducts research on criteria for specific functions and occupations. NIOSH publishes numerous safety and health standards related to workplace hazards. There is an entire section of standards devoted to the safety of health care workers. Of particular interest are standards regarding blood-borne pathogens and chemical hazards. These standards require employers to develop exposure plans and implement specific control methods for individual positions, to develop postexposure follow-up plans, and to develop procedures for evaluating situations in which employees have been exposed (National Institute of Occupational Safety and Health, 2003). As with all other workplace issues, simply complying with relevant government regulations is a minimalist approach. Job hazard analysis and periodic safety awareness programs are essential for ensuring a safe workplace. It is essential that managers in large organizations interact regularly with safety staff and risk managers or consultants to ensure the well-being of their employees. Managers of smaller organizations must be familiar with the necessary rules and regulations to ensure compliance with the law and a safe, productive workforce.

JOB STRESS AND EMPLOYEE IMPAIRMENT

Work stress in pharmacy can be exacerbated, precipitated, or made more likely if long-term stagnation is not addressed. As in all other areas of health care, prevention is always preferable to reacting after the problem has become serious. Stress is a function of demands, coping ability, skills, and supports. It can be divided into acute, chronic, mild, and severe and classified according to its source, organizational or personal. A clear or clean separation between personal life and work life cannot be assumed, and many of the personal and family problems employees have affect workplace performance.

Complicating the experience of job stress is personality. Type A personality, sometimes referred to as a *coronary-prone behavioral pattern,* places a person at high risk for stress-related problems (Freidman and Rosenman, 1974). Type A personality is a constellation of personal characteristics including time urgency, hostility, extreme competitiveness, and free-floating anxiety. While many of the characteristics of type A personality seem suited for highly competitive business environments, type A personalities are at higher risk for heart disease and tend to be "sprinters" more prone to burnout than type B personalities, who embody characteristics directly opposite those of type A personalities. Type A personalities can be stress "carriers" and cause stress in organizations. While personality is difficult to change, type A personalities can learn to cope better with life challenges and the work environment through stress management and counseling interventions.

The sources of stress can be varied, including personal, family, work-related, or a combination of all three. When the ability of employees to cope with stress is exceeded by the demands placed on them, employees began to suffer from stress reactions. The first and most obvious stress reaction is a decrease in job performance. Other reactions can include emotional problems such as depression or anxiety, exacerbation or precipitation of physical diseases, and engaging in unhealthful coping strategies such as smoking, overeating, or the misuse of other addictive substances such as drugs and alcohol (Quick and Quick, 1984).

Managers have at their disposal a number of strategies to reduce the effects of stress-related disorders on the workplace. One of the indicators of good management practice is to match the capabilities, talents, and interests of employees with the type and demands of the job. A mismatch of talents, interests, and job demands can contribute significantly to job stress. Managers should also be sufficiently aware of and attentive to employee behavior to be able to observe symptoms of stress reactions. The most natural entrée into a dialogue with employees regarding evidence of stress is through their work performance. Since work normally requires a high degree of attention to detail and investment of cognitive and emotional energy, performance will be affected by a high degree of stress. Typical stress reactions that affect work performance include low frustration tolerance leading to angry outbursts, substandard work product or service owing to lack of concentration and attention to details, and lack of motivation and initiative owing to depression.

While there are sufficient human and ethical reasons to be concerned with the well-being of others, managers have an additional responsibility to identify and address employee stress reactions because high-stress environments lead to high turnover, absenteeism, and poor work performance. Managers who confront employees appropriately regarding declining work performance while maintaining a nonjudgmental and concerned attitude can engage employees in explorations of the reasons and provide appropriate referrals and follow-up for intervention.

Many organizations have confidential employee assistance programs (EAPs) that refer employees for counseling and that train managers in early identification and referral (Smith, 1992). EAPs can be established by contract with independent behavioral health providers. Mental health and substance abuse services usually are "carve-outs" similar to pharmacy services, and EAPs can be integrated into existing health coverage. Through a confidential intake, professionals and supervisors can identify employees with problems, and costs can be stabilized by early identification and referral. In addition, employees who are valuable to a company often can benefit from brief interventions and return to work more productive and committed to the organization.

Referral to a company-sponsored EAP program normally is voluntary; however, managers can suggest a referral based on a history of poor work performance or other work-related problems. Managers can use work performance as a vehicle for discussion of employee problems that are affecting the workplace. Successful resolution of personal problems not only affects the quality of life of employees but also usually contributes to their increased focus on work responsibilities. EAP professionals (e.g., psychiatrists, psychologists, addiction counselors, and clinical social workers) who contract with health plans are licensed and regard the information on assessment and treatment as confidential and subject to Health Insurance Portability and Accountability Act (HIPAA) regulations. Employees can sign releases to share limited information with employers, especially if there is a clear relationship between the personal problem and work performance.

Drug and alcohol problems are personal problems that can affect work performance significantly. Many states have mandatory reporting requirements for pharmacists who have substance abuse problems so that interventions and referrals for treatment and follow-up may be made. Pharmacists and managers have special responsibilities and obligations not to "enable" another's substance abuse through lack of intervention because of the potential harm posed to the public health from an impaired pharmacist. The profession of pharmacy has taken a rehabilitative rather than a punitive stance toward impaired pharmacists. The American Pharmacists Association and many state pharmacy associations have information and programs oriented toward substance abuse in pharmacy that are helpful to managers in developing policies and procedures for substance abuse in the workplace (Giannetti, Galinsky, and Kay, 1990). Pharmacists can be at special risk for substance abuse problems because they have universal access to drugs and may have a false sense of invulnerability owing to their extensive education regarding the mechanisms and effects of drugs. In addition, the tendency to self-medicate among some pharmacists can cause serious difficulty when applied to addictive medications.

The general procedures for managing impaired pharmacists are summarized as follows:

1. Mandatory state board reporting requirements for pharmacists who have substance abuse problems but are not receiving treatment
2. Intervention by an organization usually working with the state board
3. Professional assessment
4. Treatment recommendations
5. After-care counseling and monitoring usually involving Alcoholics Anonymous or Narcotics Anonymous, as well as random drug testing for a defined period
6. Reinstatement to practice contingent on successful completion of treatment

For the program to be effective, all employees should be educated about the issue of substance abuse, with special attention paid to early identification, intervention, and responsibilities of management in ensuring intervention and referral for treatment.

■ MANAGING A DIVERSE WORKFORCE

Another critical management issue germane to the contemporary workplace is the management of an increasingly diverse workforce. Managing diversity requires creating a workplace environment of equality of opportunity and respect for individual differences and capabilities. In its simplest form, equal opportunity and managing a diverse workforce involve the basic ethical imperatives of a commitment to fairness and justice and respect for the basic dignity of all persons. While a culture of respect for differences and acceptance of cultural diversity and a merit system based on fairness are ideal goals for all organizations, managers must at a minimum ensure compliance with laws that require equal treatment.

Ideally, managers will also develop ongoing interventions to orient organizational culture to respect diversity and equality. Compliance with the various laws to ensure equal opportunity in the workplace is a necessary but not sufficient condition for managing diversity in organizations. Training programs that increase awareness of and respect for cultural pluralism and that educate people regarding practices that involve negative stereotyping and negative impact on minorities should be ongoing and institutionalized. Counseling and intervention are necessary when stereotyping and potential discriminatory practices take place. For example, training sessions can identify "flag" words that can be demeaning to certain groups, explain why these words may be offensive, and remove the words from discourse within the organization. Simple choice of language such as addressing grown women as "girls" or telling ethnic jokes that ridicule certain groups can create hostile environments. While there has been a backlash against cultural sensitivity and social competence by labeling these efforts as "political correctness," managers must monitor the environment actively. The results of overconcern may be excessive formalism in the workplace. However, the consequence of lack of concern and intervention can be a negative environment, institutionalized unfairness, and legal action. An organizational culture that has a high degree of awareness of cultural pluralism and provides clear guidelines with managerial monitoring will be able to fully use the diverse talents of all its employees and also avoid the stress and negative publicity of possible regulatory and legal action.

There are a number of benefits to having a diverse workforce, such as a larger talent pool, greater knowledge of broader and diverse markets, and better organizational agility. The ability to recruit and retain a diverse workforce allows organizations to draw on varying perspectives, thus escaping the tunnel vision that often accompanies operating under only one set of cultural assumptions. Second, organizations that are more diverse have a greater probability of addressing the unique needs, preferences, and values of a diverse customer base. Finally, when diverse views and minority viewpoints are present, problem solving and creativity are enhanced by overcoming the problems of "groupthink" in organizations (Carnevale and Stone, 1995).

To manage diversity effectively, managers need to be aware of general concepts of discrimination to prevent and respond to problems arising out of a diverse workforce. Legal theory has identified three basic concepts regarding discrimination: reasonable accommodation, disparate treatment, and disparate impact. These concepts are contained in the application and implications of laws regulating workplace diversity. *Reasonable accommodation* requires making the workplace both accessible and capable of use by individuals with disabilities. *Disparate treatment* means that different treatments and opportunities are afforded to individuals based on race, color, gender, national origin, age, or disability. Finally, *disparate impact* involves neutral employment practices that lack apparent discrimination but exclude a group protected by law from opportunity, manifested as disproportionate representation in the workforce. The critical distinction between treatment and impact is that with disparate impact, intentional discrimination does not need to be present. There are rules based on formulas to determine impact. Disparate impact may exist when employment opportunities for minorities fall below 80 percent of the majority rate (four-fifths rule) or

when the difference between expected and actual rates of hiring or promotion occurs with a greater probability than chance (standard deviation rule) (Noe et al., 2003).

In addition to legal concepts, there are a number of federal laws strictly prohibiting job discrimination (Lindeman and Grossman, 1986). Title VII of the Civil Rights Act of 1964 prohibits employment discrimination based on race, color, religion, sex, or national origin. The Equal Pay Act of 1963 protects men and women from gender-based wage discrimination. For individuals 40 years of age or older, the Age Discrimination Act of 1967 protects against age as a discrimination factor in employment. In addition, Titles I and V of the Americans with Disabilities Act of 1990 protect qualified individuals with disabilities against employment discrimination in both the private and public sectors (U.S. Equal Employment Opportunity Commission, 2003).

While there are other federal laws addressing employment discrimination, these laws provide the nexus of legislation that protects against discrimination. Discrimination covered by these laws includes the following aspects of employment:

- Hiring and firing
- Compensation, assignment, or classification of employees
- Transfer, promotion, layoff, or recall
- Job advertisements, recruitment, or testing
- Use of company facilities, training, and apprenticeship programs
- Pay, retirement plans, disability leave, fringe benefits, and other conditions of employment

Additionally, the following practices are covered:

- Harassment because of race, religion, color, gender, national origin, disability, or age
- Retaliation for filing or participating in a discrimination charge
- Employment decisions based on stereotypes related to gender, race, age, religion, ethnic group, or individuals with disabilities

- Denying employment because of marriage or association with or participation in worship or schools with individuals of a particular race, religion, national origin, or disability

Employers are required to post notices that are accessible to all employees advising them of their rights under the law.

While federal law, case law, and many local and state laws address the issue of equal opportunity and discrimination in the workplace, there are general guidelines with which all managers should be familiar. The human resources office, along with legal counsel, normally is responsible for implementation and monitoring of compliance with relevant laws. For any specific situation, competent legal advice should be sought. Information regarding complaints can be found on workplace postings, through human resources offices, or through local and national Equal Employment Opportunity Commission (EEOC) offices. All laws enforced by the EEOC, with the exception of equal pay complaints, require that an EEOC complaint be filed before a private lawsuit can be filed in court. There are common situations involving equal employment opportunity with which managers will be confronted and should be able to address.

Sexual harassment in the workplace has been an issue that has received much publicity and can become a problem in organizations if not taken seriously. While sensitivity, fairness, and respect cannot be legislated, and individuals are free to hold any attitudes they wish, the laws and regulations regarding workplace behavior are well specified. For example, any request for sexual favors in the workplace, especially when among unequals, and the creation of a hostile environment through inappropriate pictures or repetitive comments of a sexual nature constitute harassment. The "hostile environment" concept can also apply to race, color, religion, age, disability, and national origin. The accommodation of religious beliefs by an employer is also required unless accommodating those beliefs would cause an undue hardship. The provisions of equal opportunity laws most likely would cover pharmacists having religious objections to certain medical procedures or dispensing medications that violate religious beliefs.

In addition to sexual harassment and accommodation of religious beliefs, equal treatment for individuals with disabilities is a significant issue for the treatment of both employees and customers. The Americans with Disabilities Act provides equal opportunity for persons who are disabled in the workplace. This act prohibits discrimination in all aspects of employment from hiring to firing, similar to practices that are covered by equal opportunity employment laws. Persons are considered disabled if they have either a physical or mental impairment that significantly limits one or more major life activities or have a record of impairment. Also, discrimination against a person who has a relationship with a disabled person is prohibited.

Impairments that significantly limit major life activities include seeing, hearing, speaking, walking, learning, caring for self, and performing manual tasks. People recovering from chronic physical and mental illness would be covered as well as people who have severe disfigurement as a result of a problem. The law defines "qualified individual with a disability" as someone who possesses the education, skill, and experience requirements of a job but who may require "reasonable accommodation" to function in the job because of a disability. Providing accommodation and reasonable access to persons with disabilities is a significant portion of the Americans with Disabilities Act and requires some understanding by management. *Reasonable accommodation* is any modification to the work environment or job that will enable a disabled person to participate in the application process or perform essential work. These accommodations can include

- Job redesign and structuring
- Modifying or providing special equipment
- Providing readers or interpreters
- Modifying training programs or examinations

Reducing standards for performance is not required based on a standard of reasonable accommodation. In addition, employers are not required to make accommodations if they involve undue hardship resulting in significant difficulty and/or expense. In addition, public accommodations, such as community pharmacies, must ensure that people with disabilities are not excluded from access to services because the facilities are inaccessible. Actively excluding any person with a disability from service or having a requirement for service that a person with disability could not fulfill (e.g., a driver's license to cash a check for a visually impaired person) is prohibited.

CAREER PLANNING

In addition to providing a stable, hospitable, and safe working environment, managers can help to ensure quality of work life by assisting employees with their careers, preferably within the organizations in which they are currently employed. Career progression can be a source of fulfillment or frustration as employees pursue job pathways. Employee retention and productivity can be enhanced with proper career planning by managers. While managers can use concepts in career pathway research and counseling to assist employees in choosing the right fit among talents, interests, and job opportunities, the main responsibility for career man-

agement rests with the individual. Companies have an interest in identifying, mentoring, developing, and retaining their employees who hold promise for significant contributions to the organization. However, each individual needs to view his or her career as an important source of both financial and personal rewards and take responsibility for the optimal development of that career.

There are a number of models for organizing and understanding career development and progression. Career development goals vary with general stages of adult development beginning with early-adult transition to the late-adult era. The developmental tasks of establishing an identity, stable value systems, and relationships are correlated with career progression (Levinson et al., 1978). The research on developmental stages has focused on men. The progression, timing, and dominant values of the stages of development among women may vary but still follow similar general patterns (Gallos, 1989). Table 12-1 summarizes the adult stages of development that correlate with career development.

Transition into adulthood usually is characterized by advanced education and exploration of occupation

Table 12-1. Levinson's Stages of Career Development

Age Ranges	Life Stages	Characteristics
17–22	Early adult transition	Transition from adolescence through exploring and experimenting with different roles and career choices mainly through course work and practical experiences
22–28	Entering adulthood	Experimenting with different job settings, stabilizing relationships, and possibly starting a family
28–33	Age 30 transition	Reassessing initial career choices and a sense of exigency to stablize important life choices such as family and relationships
33–40	Settling down	Rapid progress in pursuing occupational goals and focus on career
40–45	Midlife transition	Time of questioning and reevaluation of life and career choices that can be stressful and lead to a focus on redoubling efforts toward career or change in career and values
45–60	Middle adulthood	Directing more focus on developing nonwork interests or reaping the benefits and consolidating the gains of a lifetime of career focus
60 and above	Late adult era	Preparation for retirement, planning possible part-time work

Source: Adapted with permission from Levinson et al., 1978.

through course work and practical experiences. Early adulthood involves experimenting with different job settings and deciding on specific lifestyles and roles, including stabilizing relationships and possibly starting a family. The adult continues through various transitional phases, refocusing efforts and emphases on career, family, and lifestyle. While not everyone mimics this pattern exactly, many follow these career stages of investigation, consolidation, advancement, preservation, and preparing for retirement.

The active management of a career involves providing or attaining developmentally appropriate experiences, education, and training to decide, focus on, and nurture career progression. In addition, maintaining a harmony between personal and family relationships and investment in work goals requires a balancing act throughout the life cycle. Balancing the demands of work with personal life can be a difficult task. Values clarification, compromise, and conflict resolution are processes that need to be engaged in regularly to find the right career mix at the appropriate stage of life.

Along with the developmental approach to career, the career-anchor approach can facilitate the organization of talents, motives, and values into "anchors" that allow the individual to pursue a career pathway that is consistent with both his or her aspirations and capabilities. These career anchors are technical/functional, managerial, security-oriented, autonomy-oriented, and creativity-oriented (Schein, 1975). Persons with a technical/functional anchor tend to enjoy the detail of the work itself and avoid responsibilities that take them away from the day-to-day performance of specific tasks that produce the product or service. In contrast, persons with a management anchor tend to like analyzing and problem solving, seek influence through interpersonal communication, and are emotionally and intellectually able to take responsibility and exercise power. Individuals who value security in work seek jobs and organizations that offer long-term work stability and retirement benefits with clear and predictable career pathways and will sacrifice other opportunities to have security. Autonomy seekers are most concerned with freedom in decision making and a minimum of constraints, whereas individuals who value

creativity seek innovation and invention as the primary motivation in work.

These anchors can be used as guides in managing career pathways in pharmacy. For example, a pharmacist who prefers the technical and functional anchor may seek employment focused on the dispensing and compounding aspects of pharmacy practice in initial career choice and move into nuclear pharmacy, where more technical aspects of pharmacy can be realized. By contrast, pharmacists who seek management careers would develop competency with advanced management degrees while seeking increased responsibility for management across a variety of settings before settling in on a specific organization, such as a pharmaceutical company or managed-care organization to gain specific skills in an industry of interest. Security-oriented individuals may look to government positions such as the U.S. Public Health Service or the military, which offer predicable and stable career progression. If autonomy were a major anchor, becoming a consulting pharmacist or a small business owner or obtaining an academic position would provide a wide range of opportunities for freedom in job expression. Finally, if creativity is a major focus, becoming an entrepreneur and developing new services in disease-state management, specializing in nutrition and herbal medications, or becoming a research scientist to develop new drug products would offer opportunities for creative expression. Of course, the assumption is that aptitude must be correlated with interest and motives. In addition, some careers combine anchors, such as an academic pharmacist with a clinical or research site that can satisfy both autonomy and creativity. Managers should take the time to be aware of employee interests and abilities through frequent interactions and performance appraisals. Appraising, encouraging, and making opportunities available are essential for assisting employees with career progression and fulfillment.

MANAGERIAL (BUSINESS) ETHICS

The unifying issue for this chapter is ethical decision making. An appreciation of the role of ethics in managerial decision making is essential to effective management. The delivery of health care transcends a simple mercantile transaction because it involves issues of quality of life and suffering and death itself. Health care, at its foundation, is a moral enterprise with a long tradition of ideals dating back to the Hippocratic Oath. All health care professions have codes of ethics, and pharmacy in particular defines the pharmacist–patient relationship as a *covenant* (American Pharmaceutical Association, 1984), a term with particular moral overtones.

While there are specific ethical principles that guide patient care ethics for all practitioners (Beauchamp and Childress, 2001), standards and principles that guide managers in their work are less clear. The specific ethical issues raised by pharmacy management are complex and often not always discussed as an integral part of decisions in organizations. Some issues in pharmacy management involve conflicts of interest between the business aspects and the health care orientation of pharmacy. Should community pharmacies sell cigarettes? How does the role of dispensing and prescription volume affect the relative importance of patient counseling and disease-state management in community pharmacy? What is the proper response to medication errors, and how should all stakeholders to the error, including the pharmacist, be treated?

In many respects much of the material in this chapter regarding fair treatment, encouraging diversity, enriching jobs, and assisting persons with managing personal and job-related stress all have an ethical dimension. It is easy to ignore or minimize ethical values when pursuing other technical or economic goals. The role of the manager should be to provide leadership in creating an ethical culture as a context for facilitating decision making (Longenecker, 1985). The first step in this process is assessing the major values that drive the organization. Determining the essential focus of the organization in terms of service and respect for the welfare and dignity of all persons are critical statements regarding the mission of an organization. In this context, it is also important to understand that generating profits is a necessary and core value for organizations. The pursuit of profits is not necessarily inconsistent with other core values. However, when profits trump all other values and "ethical shortcuts" are taken to increase profits, health care organizations lose public trust and subvert their very reason for existence.

Second, the core values of an organization must be "modeled" by managers. Talking about or espousing values without customers, employees. and other stakeholders in the organization experiencing those values will lead rapidly to cynicism regarding ethics.

Third, expecting one set of ethical behaviors while rewarding others inconsistent with ethical values will cause confusion and lack of commitment to ethical behaviors in an organization.

Finally, while there are many good arguments for the intrinsic value of ethical behavior, relating ethical values to both health care and economic outcomes clearly demonstrates the utility of ethics and will reinforce ethical values in an organization. Increasing adherence, reducing health care costs, and preventing litigation owing to failure to warn all can be practical outcomes of a patient consultation and service orientation.

One of the most critical ethical issues in pharmacy practice is the relative importance of patient counseling and disease management in community pharmacy. The Omnibus Budget Reconciliation Act of 1990 (OBRA 1990) and many state boards of pharmacy have now instituted offer-to-counsel regulations. Legal mandates are necessary but not sufficient conditions for patient counseling. The values of an organization must support patient counseling, and these values must be integrated into the evaluation and reward system of pharmacy. Informed consent is a "gold standard" in health care ethics, and depriving patients of informed consent by not assessing and counseling regarding risks and benefits of medication taking could be viewed as unethical practice (Resnik, Ranelli, and Resnik, 2000). In some cases, it could also lead to litigation. Ensuring proper workflow, staffing patterns, and reasonable workload and working to make patient consultation cost-effective are also expanded ethical obligations of managers. If managers do not organize the environment and encourage a patient-oriented culture, no amount of clinical training and exhortation by academic institutions will suffice.

■ REVISITING THE SCENARIO

This chapter focused on a wide range of contemporary workplace issues, discussing management concepts in relationship to facilitating quality of work life, including safety, unionization, equal opportunity, stress management, and career planning. These responsibilities for the manager can be the most difficult yet most rewarding aspects of their jobs. Referring to the case of Ann Kolawieczki in the scenario, it is important to note that managers must be able to establish basic trust in relationships with employees by demonstrating concern and respect for their points of view and fairness in judgment regarding work issues. They must also take seriously their responsibility to enforce standards and hold people responsible for actions in the workplace. Focusing on Ann's work performance, the manager in the scenario can attempt to offer Ann the opportunity to explore personal issues that may be affecting her work. Demonstrating an accepting attitude and providing explanations of the types of assistance available to her may motivate Ann to seek assistance. Of course, if there is significant evidence of a substance abuse problem affecting patient safety, then the manager does have an obligation to require an assessment. Further, the manager should investigate the nature and circumstances of remarks made to Ann and address the situation with her and other employees to make them aware of the relevant laws and culture of no tolerance of behavior that can be construed as offensive.

■ QUESTIONS FOR FURTHER DISCUSSION

1. What would you do as a manager to ensure an optimal work environment that encourages the practice of pharmaceutical care?
2. Is the unionization of health care practitioners and technicians a desirable trend? Does it have the potential to improve work conditions? Why or why not?
3. What specific safety issues are relevant to working in a health care and pharmacy environment, and how would you address these issues?
4. What are the most likely consequences if a work environment does not allow opportunities to exercise professional judgment and expertise?
5. How can work and personal stress affect organizations, and what approaches should managers take when confronting these problems?
6. Who has major responsibility for career management? What steps will you take to manage your own career?
7. How can managers remain vigilant regarding workplace discrimination, cultural pluralism, and equal opportunity? How would you handle a situation in which a hostile environment was present at your place of work if you were among the staff being affected? If you were the manager?
8. How prepared are you to engender a culture for ethical decision making and practice in your organization? What challenges and barriers must you face down to accomplish this endeavor?

REFERENCES

American Pharmaceutical Association. 1984. Code of Ethics for Pharmacists. Washington, DC: American Pharmaceutical Association.

Beauchamp TL, Childress JF. 2001. Principles of Biomedical Ethics, 5th ed., New York: Oxford University Press.

Carnevale AP, Stone SC. 1995. *The American Mosaic.* New York: McGraw-Hill.

Cipolle RJ, Strand LM. 1998. *Pharmaceutical Care Practice.* New York: McGraw-Hill.

Friedman M, Rosenman RH. 1974. *Type A Behavior and Your Heart.* New York: Knopf.

Giannetti VJ, Galinsky AM, Kay DH. 1990. Education, assistance and prevention program for chemical dependency problems among pharmacy students. *Am J Pharm Ed* 54:275.

Gallos JV. 1989. Experiencing women's development: Implications for career theory, practice and research. In Arthur BB, Hall DT, Lawrence BS (eds), *Handbook of Career Theory,* p. 110. Cambridge, England: Cambridge University Press.

Hackman JR, Oldham GR, Janson R, Pardy K. 1975. A new strategy for job enrichment. *Calif Manag Rev* 17:57.

Levison DJ. 1978. *The Seasons of a Man's Life.* New York: Knopf.

Lindeman B, Grossman P. 1986. *Employment Discrimination Law.* Washington, DC: BNA Books.

Longenecker JG. 1985. Management priorities and management ethics. *J Bus Ethics* 4:65.

National Institute of Occupational Safety and Health. 2003. Available at www.cdc.gov/niosh; accessed on May 7, 2003.

National Labor Relations Board. 2003. Available at www.nlrb.gov; accessed on May 7, 2003.

Noe RA, Hollenbeck JR, Gerhart B, Wright PM. 2003. *Human Resources Management.* New York: McGraw-Hill.

Occupational Safety and Health Administration. 2003. Available at: www.osha.gov; accessed on May 8, 2003.

Quick JS, Quick JD. 1984. *Organizational Stress and Preventive Management.* New York: McGraw-Hill.

Redecker JR. 1989. *Employee Discipline: Policies and Practice.* Washington, DC: Bureau of National Affairs.

Resnik DB, Ranelli PL, Resnik SP. 2000. The conflict between ethics and business in community pharmacy. *J Bus Ethics* 28:179.

Schein EH. 1975. *Career Dynamics.* Reading, MA: Addison-Wesley.

Smith J. 1992. EAPs evolve into health plan gatekeeper. *Employee Benefit Plan Rev* 46:18.

Taylor FW. 1911. *The Principles of Scientific Management.* New York: Harper & Row.

U.S. Equal Opportunity Commission. 2003. Available at www.eeoc.gov/index.html; accessed on May 7, 2003.

U.S. Mediation and Conciliation Service. 1997. Fifteenth Annual Report. Washington, DC: U.S. Government Printing Office.

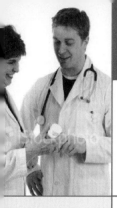

13

TIME MANAGEMENT/ ORGANIZATIONAL SKILLS

Dana P. Hammer

About the Author: Dr. Hammer is the Director of the Bracken Pharmaceutical Care Learning Center and Teaching Certificate Program in Pharmacy Education for the University of Washington School of Pharmacy. Dr. Hammer received a B.S. in pharmacy from Oregon State University, worked in hospital and community independent pharmacies, and then returned to school to earn M.S. and Ph.D. degrees in pharmacy practice education from Purdue University School of Pharmacy. Her teaching responsibilities include an introductory pharmacy practice course, several electives in pharmacy and medical education, and coordination of an advanced compounding elective. Her research involves assessment of students' educational outcomes and professional development. Dr. Hammer serves on the editorial boards of the *Journal of Pharmacy Teaching* and *Research in Social and Administrative Pharmacy* and has won several awards for teaching, innovations in teaching and education, and educational research. She has most recently honed her time management skills working full time while parenting two young children.

■ LEARNING OBJECTIVES

After completing this chapter, students should be able to

1. Determine if they need to improve their time management skills.
2. Critically analyze the choices they make in how they spend their time.
3. Describe common myths or pitfalls with regard to time management.
4. Take action to avoid time management pitfalls.
5. Discuss various theories and approaches to time management.
6. Apply concrete suggestions, through a series of steps, to improve their time management skills.
7. Explain how time management techniques apply to pharmacy practice.
8. Recognize the relationship between poor time management and stress.

▦ SCENARIO

Revisit the Krista Connelly scenario from Chapter 2. It appears as though Krista is a good time manager—she seems to attend all her classes, prepares for classes ahead of time and reviews material with professors, holds down a part-time pharmacy job, and even is able to squeeze in routine home activities and down time with friends and family. Granted, Krista may not be taking very good care of herself with regard to diet, exercise, and sleep, but all in all, she seems to have her act together. One question remains, however, after reading about Krista: When does she study? Perhaps she is one of the "genius" students who doesn't seem to have to study very much but is still able to achieve high grades. Consider a different scenario below.

Tom Chan is also a second-year pharmacy student. Tom describes himself as a busy pharmacy student, although he would not necessarily say that he is stressed out most of the time. Tom tries to get out of bed by 7 a.m. so that he can get to class by 8 a.m., but he often oversleeps and misses his first class. He realizes that he should go to bed earlier, but it seems that the only time he can find to study or maybe watch some TV to unwind is between 10 p.m. and 2 a.m. Tom's normal day consists of attending classes, getting in an hour of basketball, and then heading into work at his pharmacy intern job at a local chain pharmacy. In between classes, he usually hangs out with friends, eats, or attends extracurricular activities and meetings. Tom finds it hard to try to get in any quality study time during the day and usually puts off studying for major exams or completing large assignments until the night before they are due. Because of this, he usually pulls all-nighters once every week or two. During midterm and finals weeks, he sometimes will stay up all night on several occasions. Tom averages B's and C's in school, although he got a D in pharmacology last year and had to repeat the course.

Tom usually works about 20 hours per week to help pay his tuition and other school-related expenses, as well as costs related to his cell phone, cable TV, and Internet subscriptions; car payment and insurance; rent; and other living expenses. He usually manages to have a little left over each month to buy CDs, go to movies, and go out on the town with friends, but he also maintains some credit-card debt from furniture and apartment supplies he bought when he started pharmacy school. The local chain that employs Tom as a pharmacy intern has an intern development program that helps interns to learn chain pharmacy management and administrative skills. At a recent employee annual review, Tom's preceptor shared his disappointment with Tom's tardiness to work, his inability to prioritize work tasks very well, and his lack of desire to want to improve or become engaged in management functions. Tom was discouraged with his preceptor's observations and is not sure what to do.

Do you have classmates like Krista and Tom? Do their lives sound similar to yours? Read on to find out how applying some simple time management and organizational skills can make you a better pharmacy student, better future pharmacist, and a more productive, healthy person.

▦ CHAPTER QUESTIONS

1. How do I know if I need to manage my time better?
2. What can I do to better manage my time?
3. What are some resources I can use to help me better manage my time?
4. What are some of the common pitfalls with regard to time management?
5. How does personal time management relate to time management in pharmacy practice?
6. How can time be better managed in pharmacy practice?
7. How does poor time management affect my stress level?

▦ THE NEED FOR TIME MANAGEMENT AND ORGANIZATIONAL SKILLS

There are 24 hours in a day. Research tells us that for a person to be healthy, roughly 7 to 8 hours of that time should be used for sleeping. That leaves 16 to

17 hours to accomplish everything else we need and want to do in a day: go to school and/or work (usually 3 to 10 hours per day), study (rule of thumb for lecture courses is 2 hours outside class for every 1 hour in class, so let's say approximately 6 hours per day), eat (approximately 1 hour per day), shower and get ready (0.5 to 1 hour per day), exercise (0.5 to 1 hour per day), routine maintenance (e.g., pay bills, pick up room, etc.—1 hour per day), participate in a nonschool or nonwork interests (1 hour per day), relax and have fun (0.5 to 1 hour per day), and spend time with family and/or friends (via face-to-face, e-mail, or phone—0.5 to 1 hour per day). Not all of us participate in all these activities each and every day, but if we did, we are looking at spending anywhere from 14 to 23 hours per day engaged in them. And this estimate doesn't even include time spent on transportation or unexpected events.

Time is one of the most valuable resources we have. Several philosophies have been iterated about time:

- The gift of your time is the most valuable gift you can give.
- If you want to know what people's *real* values are, look at how they spend their time and their money.
- Time is money.
- Time management is *not* about managing time; it is about managing yourself.

Many advances in technology and other areas are all about saving time. Think about computer programs for word processing, spreadsheet creation, and statistical analyses. Think also about personal digital assistants, cell phones, microwaves, airline travel, and overnight mail. All these inventions were created to make our lives easier and to allow us to be more productive and spend the time we save through their use on other activities. It has been written, however, that we can never *save* time—we can only *spend* it—so we must make wise decisions about how we choose to spend our time (Ensman, 1991).

Time management and organizational skills are important both personally and professionally. Poor time management can lead to frustration, stress, and a failure to complete daily tasks or achieve personal and professional goals. We already know that frustration and stress can be physically detrimental. Poor time management can also cause others to lose respect for and faith in us—we may be considered less reliable and dependable, less likely to follow through on commitments, and less responsible. If others feel this way about us, we are less likely to be involved in committed relationships or receive promotions at work. Safety can also be compromised—personal safety, for example, if one is constantly late and so feels compelled to consistently drive over speed limits. Patient safety certainly can be compromised if pharmacists practice in a manner that is hurried, disorganized, and haphazard. Conversely, good time management skills can lead to a higher quality of life for most people because they affect so many aspects of our lives, both personal and professional. The reasons to become a better time/self-manager are painfully obvious and so extremely important that anyone reading this chapter should be motivated immediately to improve their time management skills.

■ COMMON MYTHS/PITFALLS

"I don't have time . . . "

How often do you hear this phrase or utter it yourself? The truth is that we *all* have 24 hours in every day to accomplish what we need and want to do, so saying that you don't have time is actually a lie. The difference is how we *choose* to spend our time. Thus, unless you are in prison or some kind of work camp where you do not make the decisions on how your day is spent, most of us consciously decide how to spend our time. It was your choice to apply to pharmacy school. It is your choice to go to class. It is your choice to study. It is your choice to get a part-time job. It is your choice to read this book. No one is forcing you to do these things. Granted, there may be significant consequences if you do *not* choose to do these things, but the bottom line is that you *choose* how to spend your time. The next time that you feel compelled to say, "I don't have time to _____[fill in the blank]," rephrase it to, "I can't take the time to _____[fill in the blank]." At least that way you will not be lying.

"I'm too busy . . ."

Once again, you *choose* how to spend your time. If you feel that you are too busy to maintain your personal health, achieve your personal and professional goals, or be as successful in all your tasks and responsibilities as you would like to be, then *change your schedule*. Do not take on as many tasks. Find your success limit, and maintain it! Contrary to popular belief, the busier people are, the more productive they are, and the more they accomplish. Think about the last time that you had a week without appointments or without deadlines. How much did you get done? Granted, you may have caught up on some needed rest and relaxation, but you may not have attended to many other items on your to-do list because you were in relaxation mode and were not feeling the subtle pressure of "something needs to be done." Deadlines creep up once again and cause stress when the realization occurs that you do not have as much time to meet that deadline as you would like. It is certainly important to recharge your batteries once in awhile, but the quote "If ever the going seems easy, check to see if you are going downhill" should be heeded. Although it was stated that busy people are more productive, it is not necessarily true to say that *all* busy people are productive. Many folks spend their time working on tasks and activities that could be better handled by others. They may not be able to prioritize their responsibilities very well or may be easily distracted or consistently interrupted. And it is certainly true that some folks are just *too* busy. You know that your plate is too full when your health begins to fail, your personal relationships begin to fail, and you cannot follow through reliably with all your responsibilities. You begin to forget things. You miss meetings and deadlines. You constantly feel stressed out and guilty if you relax at all or "get off task." These are not healthy feelings and can escalate to the point of illness and exhaustion. It is important to find that balance of where you feel like you are able to stay on top of things and are getting things accomplished but not that your schedule is so easy that you are wasting your potential to achieve higher goals.

"My personal time management skills have nothing to do with how I manage time at work."

It is plausible to think this way, however, mostly because we are *proactive* at home (i.e., determine *when* we want to fix dinner, do laundry, pay bills, etc.), whereas pharmacy practice is often *reactive*—we help patients when they ask for it/need it, fill medication orders as they come in, and answer the phone when it rings. These different situations give the impression that personal and professional time management are different. It is possible that a person might be completely organized at home and a train wreck at work, but this is a rare and unusual case. Most people who have a good sense of organization and time allocation know when to say "no" and how to apply those skills at home and at work. We do not usually purposefully apply different criteria for how we manage our time at home and at work; these skills usually are unconscious, routine, habit. The good news is that these skills *can* be learned.

"I need time to focus in order to . . ."

The ability to multitask is an absolute necessity for any pharmacist or pharmacy student. This does *not* mean doing several things simultaneously—if that were the case, you would never get anything fully accomplished, and patient safety certainly would be compromised. What it *does* mean, however, is that it is important that you have the ability to "switch gears" easily and maintain a sharp mind so that you can give your undivided attention for a few moments to the task at hand and then move on to the next task or back to the original task. Rarely will you have full days without any appointments or activities scheduled so that you can spend the entire day on one task.

"I'm a perfectionist . . ."

It is certainly important to do your best and to always "put your best foot forward," but as a pharmacy student or pharmacist with many demands on your time, it is critical that you discern which tasks must be perfect and which can be less than perfect. Dosing and preparation of chemotherapeutic agents, for example, should be as close to perfect as possible—it is crucially important that enough time be spent on these tasks to make sure that they are correct because people's lives are at stake. Revising a term paper five times for a three-credit course, however, does not have such severe consequences, and the time spent in the extra three revisions could have been spent studying for an examination that is worth twice the number of points as the paper. It is okay not to be perfect all the time, unless, of course, the consequence of *not* being perfect is severe. In other words, sometimes we have to "choose our battles" in order to win the time management war.

"They didn't teach time management in my curriculum."

Some pharmacy schools provide regular workshops for students or parts of courses devoted to time management, study skills, stress management, and other pharmacy school and life survival skills. If your school is not one of those, however, this chapter is here to help get you on your way to being a better time manager. Additionally, there are books and articles referred to throughout this chapter that can serve to help you become a successful time manager.

■ THEORIES AND PRACTICES OF TIME MANAGEMENT

In 1675, R. T. wrote a letter to a Mr. R. A. describing "the art of good husbandry, or the improvement of time: being a sure way to get and keep money."[1] In this

---

[1] R. T. The art of good husbandry, or The improvement of time. 1675. A copy of the original reference is available via Microfilm from the University of Michigan, Ann Arbor, MI (1991). Also available at http://eebo.chadwyck.com/search/full_rec?SOURCE=pgthumbs.cfg&ACTION=ByID&ID=99830667&FILE=../session/1210961294_2335&SEARCH SCREEN=CITATIONS&SEARCHCONFIG=var_spell.cfg &DISPLAY=AUTHOR (Accessed on May 16, 2008.)

letter, R. T. discusses several rules for merchants, shopkeepers, "mechanicks," tradesmen, and others to follow in order to use time to their advantage for themselves and families. He describes the loss of a man's time, which includes time spent in taverns, coffeehouses, or alehouses, as "the sole cause of poverty in this city and nation." This citation possibly may be one of the earliest that begins to describe the importance of time management.

Fast forward to the 1950s, where the industrial revolution had long been in place, Americans were enjoying postwar success, and management as a business discipline was evolving. Peter Drucker, well-known business management guru, wrote *The Practice of Management* in 1954, which helped to put the art and education of management on the map. Within his text, he put forth the philosophy and practice of "management by objectives" and described time as "the scarcest resource, and unless it is managed, nothing else can be managed" (as paraphrased in Applebaum and Rohrs, 1981). In a subsequent book, Drucker articulated four suggestions for helping executives to better manage their time (Drucker, 1967, pp. 26–28):

1. Find out exactly how you actually use your time.
2. Determine what does and does not have to be done (and discontinue doing the latter).
3. Delegate work to others who are equally or better qualified than you are.
4. Stop wasting other people's time.

Moving into the 1980s and 1990s, Stephen Covey became a national hero with *The Seven Habits of Highly Effective People* (Covey, 1989). Covey focuses on character development through the practice and internalization of seven habits, two of which relate directly to time management: (1) Begin with the end in mind, and (2) put first things first. Both tenets center on determining what is really important to you and then finding ways to make sure that those goals are achieved. Covey states that the essence of time management is to "organize and execute around priorities." Covey created a time management matrix (Table 13-1) to help us

Table 13-1. Time Management Matrix

	Urgent	Not Urgent
Important	*Quadrant I* *Activities:* Crises, pressing problems, deadline-driven projects	*Quadrant II* *Activities:* Prevention and "principle-centered" activities, relationship building, recognizing new opportunities, planning and recreation
Not important	*Quadrant III* *Activities:* Interruptions, some calls, some mail, some reports, some meetings, proximate and pressing matters, popular activities	*Quadrant IV* *Activities:* Trivia and busy work, some mail, some phone calls, time wasters, pleasant activities

Source: Used with permission from Covey, 1989, p. 151.

to categorize our daily activities and to understand how we can maximize our time by doing so. Covey says that we are the most effective personal managers when we are operating primarily in quadrant II. In the section on putting first things first, he also offers suggestions for long-term organizing, weekly organizing, and how to say no.

Julie Morgenstern describes a more recent approach in her book, *Time Management from the Inside Out* (Morgenstern, 2000). Morgenstern, founder and owner of Julie Morgenstern's Professional Organizers in New York City, draws a comparison between time and space (Table 13-2) and describes each day as "a container, a storage unit that has definite capacity you can reach." Her book walks readers through four phases:

1. *Laying the foundation*—thinking about creating a time management system that works for you.
2. *Analyzing*—defining your personal style, preferences, needs, and goals.
3. *Strategizing*—mapping your ideal schedule and staying on track.
4. *Attacking*—putting your plan into action.

Table 13-2. Comparison of Time and Space

Cluttered Closet	Cluttered Schedule
Limited amount of space	Limited amount of hours
Crammed with more stuff than storage	Crammed with more tasks than time
Items jammed into any available pocket of space in no particular order	Tasks jammed into any available pocket of time in no particular order
Haphazard arrangement makes it difficult to see what you have	Haphazard arrangement makes it difficult to see what you have to do
Inefficient in its use of organizing tools	Inefficient in its use of time management tools

Source: Used with permission from Morgenstern, 2000, p. 11.

Morgenstern's book was featured in a *Pharmacy Student* article entitled, "Yes, You Can Find the Time" (English, 2003). It also contains helpful appendices with lists of time management resources and additional references.

Marilyn Paul, author of *It's Hard to Make a Difference When You Can't Find Your Keys* (Paul, 2003), offers a "seven-step path to becoming truly organized" (Fig. 13-1). She claims that unlike other self-help organizational books, hers takes a more holistic approach and incorporates mental, physical, emotional, and spiritual aspects of one's life into the context of getting organized and thus living a better life. All the books just described offer meaningful and valuable advice related to time management and other life challenges.

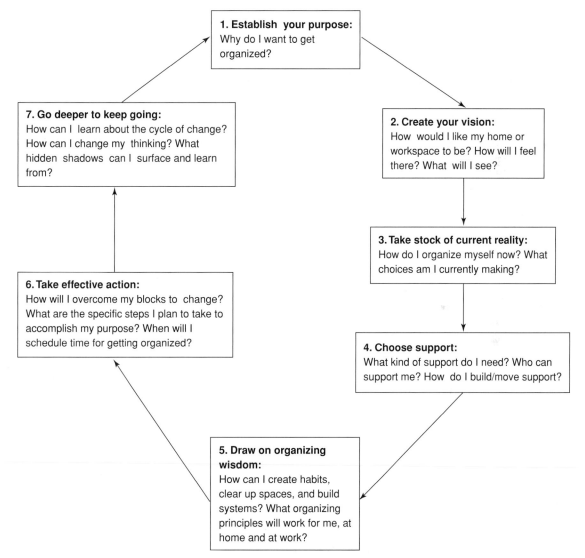

Figure 13-1. Seven-step change cycle. (Data adapted from White SJ. Working efficiently. *Am J Health Sys Pharm.* 2007;64(15): 1587–1591.)

■ *REAL* TIME MANAGEMENT—HOW TO DO IT

The books listed thus far are just a few of the many sources on time management. Some sources focus specifically on the busy professional and go into detail about how to manage meetings, phone calls, interruptions, and other activities that potentially can waste time in a busy professional's day. Other sources address time management as a subset of the "whole" person—personal and professional goals or mission in life, personality, communication style, and other traits because all these affect how we use our time. Although discussions about each of these subjects are beyond the scope of this chapter, this section highlights many of the principles from these references because they apply to all of us, no matter what our full-time job or personal characteristics.

Care has been taken to distill the most common themes from a variety of references that would apply to the busy pharmacy student. The steps/themes involved in practicing better time management are

- Recognize the need for improvement.
- Conduct an honest self-reflection or analysis of how you currently use your time.
- Establish your "mission" and set goals.
- Get organized (sort through tasks, create a master list, schedule tasks, use a system).
- Take action.
- Review, revise, and modify.

These themes are described more fully below along with a variety of helpful tips from many different sources.

Recognize the Need for Improvement

Almost all literature that describes successful behavioral change programs, such as 12-step programs, start at the same point: the recognition that one's behavior needs to change or that a person desires to change his or her behavior. Hopefully, you have decided already that your time management skills could use some improvement. If you have not decided this, then the chances of your being able to improve are much less. If you are in this latter category, then the next section may just convince you that you could benefit from changing some of your current habits.

Conduct an Honest Self-Reflection or Analysis of How You Currently Use Your Time

Conducting a thorough review of how you currently spend your typical day or week can be very helpful in determining how to best proceed with improving your time management. Asking yourself some key questions can also help to identify problem areas and how you should best plan your time based on your personal preferences and style. One of the most useful tools to help you diagnose the areas that could use some improvement is to keep a *time journal*. On a detailed calendar, document how you spend your time in blocks of 15 minutes. The most accurate way to do this would be to keep your calendar with you at all times and document an activity and the time you spent on it each time you change activities. Do this for an entire week, and *be honest*, for example, 75 minutes surfing the Internet for fun, 15 minutes day dreaming, 30 minute power nap, etc. After a week, analyze those areas where you think your time could have been better spent, and evaluate factors that could have contributed to wasting time. For example, Tom Worrall, ambulatory care clinical pharmacy specialist for the Ralph H. Johnson Veterans' Affairs Medical Center in Charleston, South Carolina, explained that as a student he chose to study in the city library instead of the school's library so that he could get more done. "What takes 4 hours at the student center can take 2 hours at the city library because of fewer distractions" (English, 2003). Another author suggests asking a coworker (or significant other or roommate, for that matter) to observe your habits for 1 week and provide some constructive feedback (Wick, 1997). Be sure not to be too hard on yourself—it is important to reward hard work. Vida Farrar, a former graduate student in medicinal chemistry, indicated that "3 to 4 hours of straight studying deserves a 15- to 20-minute break. And the second round gets a half-hour to an hour break" (Dance, 1991).

When conducting the analysis of how you spend your time, Bond (1996, p. 51) suggests asking yourself these questions with regard to each activity:

- Why am I doing this?
- What is the goal?
- Why will I succeed?
- Is what I am doing at this minute moving me toward my objective?
- What will happen if I choose not to do it?

Bond continues with a few general questions about how your time is spent:

- What am I doing that does not really need to be done?
- What am I doing that could be done by someone else?
- What am I doing that could be done more efficiently?
- What do I do that wastes others' time?
- If I do not have time to do it right, do I have time to do it wrong?

Douglass and Douglass (1993) advocate creating a pie chart to visually depict where your time was spent (Fig. 13-2). They also suggest asking yourself 12 questions when reviewing a day in your time log to better determine how well you are managing your time (Douglass and Douglass, 1993, p. 44):

1. What went right today [with regard to spending your time wisely]? What went wrong? Why?
2. What time did I start my top-priority task [assuming that you have identified your top-priority task; see the section on getting organized]? Why? Could I have started earlier in the day?
3. What patterns and habits are apparent from my time log?
4. Did I spend the first hour of my [work] day doing important work?
5. What was the most productive part of my day? Why?
6. What was the least productive part of my day? Why?
7. Who or what caused most interruptions [or what kept you from staying on task]?
8. How might I eliminate or reduce the three biggest time wasters?
9. How much of my time was spent on high-value activity and how much on low-value tasks?
10. Which activities could I spend less time on and still obtain acceptable results?
11. Which activities needed more time today?
12. Which activities could have been delegated? To whom?

While not all these questions are applicable to the typical pharmacy student, many of them do provide good food for thought with regard to self-evaluation of how you use your time.

Morgenstern offers a more thorough approach to analyzing your "personal relationship to time" and suggests that readers complete four miniexercises. The first exercise is to determine "what's working," and the author suggests that you ask yourself 12 questions, including, "No matter how busy I get, I always find time for _____[fill in the blank]," "I never procrastinate about _____[fill in the blank]," and "I have no problem tackling difficult projects when _____[fill in the blank]" (Morgenstern, 2000, p. 47). The second exercise suggests nine questions to ask yourself to determine "what's *not* working," including, "I never have time to _____[fill in the blank]," "I am usually late for _____[fill in the blank]," and "One thing I wish

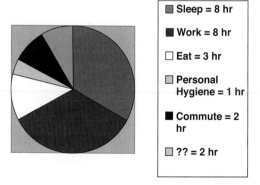

■ Sleep = 8 hr

■ Work = 8 hr

□ Eat = 3 hr

□ Personal Hygiene = 1 hr

■ Commute = 2 hr

□ ?? = 2 hr

Figure 13-2. Example pie chart of a typical day. *(Used with permission from Douglass and Douglass, 1993, p. 154.)*

I could do every day is _____ [fill in the blank]" (p. 51). The third exercise involves identifying your time management preferences. Morgenstern advocates circling each preference in a set of 12 opposites, such as "working independently versus collaboratively," "concentrating in short bursts versus long stretches," and "tight deadlines versus long lead times" (p. 54). The last exercise in her self-analysis, which consists of two parts, helps the reader to identify personal energy cycles and sources. The first part asks the same set of two questions for each period of the day (mornings, afternoons, evenings, and late night): ("Mornings) are the best times for me to _____ [fill in the blank] and the worst time for me to _____ [fill in the blank]." The second part asks you to identify what helps you "recharge" from a potential list of 13 items. Douglass and Douglass also include mini–diagnostic quizzes throughout their entire text to help readers determine their strengths and weaknesses with regard to several areas of time management (Douglass and Douglass, 1993).

Woodhull (1997) suggests that identifying your time management style will help you to better know how to use your unscheduled time, or "white spaces." She states that workaholics often have no white spaces in their schedules, which is unhealthy. She describes the four basic types of time managers:

- "*Leaders* above all value getting the job done and moving forward. . . . Their communication style is direct and succinct. Their motto is 'be brief and be gone.' Say what you have to say in 10 words or less. They are experts at making quick decisions" (Woodhull, 1997, p. 43).
- "*Analytics* value getting tasks done with precision and accuracy. They pay a lot of attention to detail. Their style is systematic. They use facts, logic, and structure. When communicating with them, make sure you tie new ideas to old concepts and make sure you provide a thorough explanation" (Woodhull, 1997, p. 45).
- "*Relaters* believe that getting along with others is the most important thing. Nourishing the primary relationships in their life is of utmost importance to them. They dislike making decisions that affect others. Sometimes they feel overburdened by all the things they have agreed to do for others" (Woodhull, 1997, p. 45).
- *Entertainers.* "Once considered too offbeat for the normal world of work, these types are now the ones who generate new ideas that are keeping companies alive. Unlike the other three types, entertainers do not like having a precise, predictable schedule. Instead, they enjoy a great deal of variety and flexibility" (Woodhull, 1997, p. 46).

If you are unsure of which type of time manager you are, Woodhull (1997, p. 47) offers a quiz you can take to find out. She advocates, however, that better time managers incorporate features of each style in order to be more flexible and adaptable to a variety of situations.

Now that you have thoroughly analyzed your time management style, preferences, and current use of time, you are ready to move on to the next step of becoming an improved time manager.

Establish Your "Mission" and Set Goals

While this step and the diagnostics just described are not necessarily critical to becoming a better time manager, completing them will help you to improve your time management. Setting short- and long-term personal and professional goals *is* critical to help determine priorities and stay focused. Covey (1989) and Douglass and Douglass (1993) each advocate writing your personal mission statement; from this, all your goals and priorities should flow. According to Covey, a personal mission statement is "the most effective way I know to begin with the end in mind" (Covey, 1989, p. 106). Your personal mission statement, or philosophy or creed, "focuses on what you want to be (character) and to do (contributions and achievements) and on the values and principles upon which being and doing are based" (Covey, 1989, p. 106). Covey provides several examples of people's mission statements and guidance on how to write such statements. Douglass and Douglass describe a personal mission statement as focusing "directly on your roles, relationships, and responsibilities . . . where you really figure out who you are and why you are here, . . . carefully consider your relationships with [a higher power, significant other, loved ones], friends, community, employers, and self. What kind of a person do you really want to be? What should the sum total of your life add up to? Write out your rough ideas, then edit and refine them" (Douglass and Douglass, 1993, p. 179). Some authors advocate writing your obituary as a way to help define how you want to be known and what you want to accomplish in your life. Although these ideas may seem a little "pie in the sky," many experts say that without thinking these ideas through and setting goals, many of us will not achieve our potential in our lifetimes. And remember, we only have 24 hours in each day!

Once you have thought through these deeper questions, it is much easier to identify your long- and short-term goals and priorities. Douglass and Douglass (1993, pp. 16–17) describe how to write SMART (*specific, measurable, achievable, realistic, and timed*) goals:

1. *Goals should be specific.* The more specific a goal, the more direction it provides, and the easier it is to measure progress. For example, you may have a goal of studying more, which is stated very broadly. However, if you were to say, "I will increase my study time by 1 hour every day or at least 6 hours a week," this goal is more specific and clearly defined.
2. *Goals should be measurable.* Similar to the preceding comments, it is easier to determine if you are making progress toward your goal if you can somehow try to quantify the specifics in your goal. The preceding example would be easy to quantify if you were keeping track of how your time is spent each day.
3. *Goals should be achievable.* "Goals should make you stretch and grow," but they should not be set so high that they are realistically unachievable. For example, a person may want to be a famous singer, but if that person has no previous musical training or talent, this goal may be unachievable. Goals "should be set at a level at which you are both able and willing to work. In general, your motivation increases as you set your goals higher. But if a goal is so high that you don't believe it can be achieved, you will probably never start."
4. *Goals should be realistic.* Closely related to achievability, goals should be realistic—take into account

available time, resources, and skills. The preceding example illustrates this case well.
5. *Goals should be timed.* You are much more likely to achieve a goal if it has a target date by which it should be accomplished. Assigning target dates for accomplishing goals increases motivation, commitment, and action. Goals without time schedules quickly become daydreams under the pressure of daily affairs. For each step along the way, you should set a realistic target date that can, and should, be adjusted if conditions change.

Douglass and Douglass go onto to describe three additional recommendations to help you achieve your goals: *Goals should be compatible*—because if they are not, working to achieve one goal may prevent you from accomplishing another; *goals should be your own*—otherwise, your motivation to achieve them is much less—you should take ownership of at least *part* of the goal if it is not your own; *goals should be written*—writing helps to clarify goals and makes them more real—our commitment to goals improves if they are written and posted in a place where they can be seen regularly.

If you have a lot of goals, some people find it easier to focus on them if they categorize them into personal versus professional and short versus long term. It is important, however, to keep your goals posted somewhere, perhaps in multiple places, so that you will look at them regularly. The more often you are reminded of your goals, the more likely you are to continue working toward them. Morgenstern (2000, pp. 71–72) tells readers to classify their "big picture" goals into one of six categories: self, family, work, relationships (such as spouse and friends), finances, and community (such as making contributions and getting involved). She goes on to say that it is much easier to determine specific activities and then daily tasks that help to achieve each goal in each category. Often some daily tasks can be used to help achieve more than one goal, such as exercising with a good friend.

With regard to tackling one's goals, Woodhull (1997, p. 221) advocates using the Benjamin Franklin approach—do not try to accomplish all your goals in the same time frame, or you will become overwhelmed and discouraged. Instead, work on one or two at a time. Franklin also believed that it took 21 days for a new behavior to take root and become a routine habit; he would carry a card in his pocket with his goal for at least 21 days to constantly remind him of it.

Get Organized (Sort Through Tasks, Create a Master List, Prioritize and Schedule Tasks, and Use a System)

You have now come to the meat of time management—*getting organized*. Organizing your life and keeping it that way are the absolute best ways to save time and feel good about how you use your time. There are several steps that many authors take readers through when helping them to get organized. First, you need to sort through what you already have. This refers to tangible items such as possessions, papers, e-mail messages, bills, and tasks that need to be accomplished. There are numerous texts and resources to help people get their possessions organized. One need only think about closet-organizing companies and "storables" stores. A complete discussion of these is beyond the scope of this chapter. However, this section will provide you with some tips about organizing some of the other parts of your life that are more difficult: papers, e-mails, computer documents, and tasks that lie before us.

Sort Through Tasks

You probably have heard the statement, "Handle each piece of paper once." This is a very good rule of thumb for most of us that literally means that each time we get a new piece of mail, an assignment handed back, or a memo of some sort, we need to decide how we are going to use that piece of paper and do something with it—file it, recycle it, or read later. This implies that we need to set up a filing system that works for us. Also, it is not bad to have a "read it later" pile as long as you make sure that you *schedule some time* somewhere in your calendar to actually read through the papers. Perhaps this is a task that you can work on once a week. These same ideas apply to e-mail messages and computer documents. Most of us have some sort of computer file system set up on our hard drives that allows us to keep computer documents organized. Similar to handling paper, as you receive new e-mail messages or

computer documents, you need to determine whether to file them, delete them, or read them later. Most e-mail programs allow users to create files in which to store e-mail messages in a place other than one's in-box. Just like paper, however, e-mails and computer files take up space on a server and/or hard drive that has limited capacity. With both paper and computer files, it is important to go through them periodically, say, once or twice a year, to clean them out and make sure that you are not running out of space.

Create a Master List

Organizing and prioritizing your tasks are often more difficult than organizing papers and e-mails. Many authors advocate creating a master list of all the tasks you need to do and then prioritizing and scheduling them. You can create your master list on your computer, on paper, in your planner (different planner options are discussed below), or by other means as long as it is on something that you can refer to regularly and are unlikely to misplace. Some folks have more than one master list, such as a "work list" and a "home list." Whatever system works best for you, the main idea is to document *all* tasks that you need to complete at some time or another. This includes any new tasks that may come your way after reviewing your mail, e-mail, phone calls, and conversations. Make sure that you keep your list(s) in a place that is easily accessible so that you can add to it when the need arises, as well as cross off tasks as you complete them.

Prioritize Tasks

Creating your master list is not too challenging as long as you remember to document everything. The more difficult task is determining how to approach the multitude of tasks on your list. Where do you start? Sometimes it can be overwhelming to think about if you have a variety of tasks that all seem very important. Thankfully, experts in the field have helped us determine how best to prioritize tasks and responsibilities so that we can be most effective and satisfied. Three general approaches in helping you to prioritize tasks are (1) the goal-achievement approach, (2) the deadline approach, and (3) the consequences approach. Using a combination of these three will be help you to prioritize the tasks in your life effectively.

Briefly, the goal-achievement approach advocates prioritizing tasks that you know will directly help you achieve your goals as most important. For example, if one of your goals is to achieve a grade-point average (GPA) of 3.5 or higher, then the task of studying at least 4 hours a day should be high on your priority list. As another example, if you are seeking a certain internship position, then completing the paperwork and other tasks necessary to get hired should be high on your priority list. The deadline approach is relatively self-explanatory—when are your tasks due? Often others provide the deadlines for tasks, for example, assignments, examinations, and birthdays. Using the deadline approach is easy when the deadlines have been set by others as long as you allocate yourself enough time to complete the task. The deadline approach is not as effective, however, when certain tasks have no deadlines or when you have to set a deadline yourself. Regular exercise, for example, is easy to put off because working out does not carry with it a deadline. The deadline approach is also not very effective in helping you to achieve your goals. The consequence approach is somewhat related to the deadline approach and essentially asks the question, "What will happen if this task is not completed or not completed on time?" The more detrimental the consequences, the higher is the priority of the task. For example, if the brakes on your car are beginning to fail, it is extremely important that you get them fixed right away, or the consequences could be fatal. On the other hand, if the penalty for turning in a late assignment is only a loss of 5 points out of 100, then completing that assignment on time may have a lesser priority than getting your brakes fixed. Some people also consider the number and importance of people who would be affected if the task or project were not completed or not completed on time—the higher the number of people or the more "important" they are, the higher is the priority of the task.

There are additional ways to prioritize activities and tasks. Many of them are similar to the goal, deadline, and consequence approaches. Covey (1989, p. 150) tells us that activities in our lives can be classified into four quadrants (see Table 13-1). Two factors that define any activity are how urgent it is and how important it is. *Urgency* refers to activities that require immediate attention, such as a ringing phone. These activities usually are visible, popular or pleasant, easy, and "in front of our noses." Often, however, these activities may be unimportant. They may be important to others but not necessarily to you. Urgent activities require us to be *reactive. Importance,* on the other hand, requires us to be *proactive.* Brushing your teeth is an example. This activity may not be urgent, but it is certainly important, and you must motivate yourself to complete this task regularly.

Covey advocates using his quadrants approach as a way to categorize and prioritize tasks and activities. Go through your master list and try to classify each task as quadrant I, II, III, or IV. How many tasks do you have in each quadrant? For those whose tasks are primarily in quadrant I, Covey explains that this is a crisis-driven, problem-minded approach that leads to stress and burnout. He says that many folks who feel that they are in quadrant I are actually in quadrant III, which can lead to short-term focus, a feeling of lack of control, and continual operation in crisis mode. They may feel like most of their tasks are urgent and important, but usually these impressions are based on the priorities and expectations of others. This is where the consequence approach may be helpful—ask yourself and others exactly what the consequences are if this task is not completed or not completed on time. This will help to determine if certain activities should be in quadrant I or in quadrant III. People whose tasks are primarily in quadrant III or quadrant IV "basically lead irresponsible lives" and often are fired from jobs and are dependent on others for the basics (Covey, 1989, p. 153). Optimally, Covey advocates that most of our tasks and activities should be in quadrant II—activities such as exercising, preparation, and preventative maintenance—these are all very important in helping us to be happy and healthy, but because they frequently do not seem urgent, they do not always get done. The results that come from primarily operating in quadrant II, however, are vision and perspective, balance, discipline, and control, and few crises arise (Covey, 1989, p. 154).

Bond (1996, p. 54) also advocates the "important and urgent" categorization process and describes the categories in this way:

- *Important* and *urgent (priority 1)*. These tasks are yours alone and must be planned into your day. They consist of the most important steps to "completing your priority" (i.e., achieving your goals, avoiding negative consequences). They generally must be done well and immediately.
- *Important* not *urgent (priority 2)*. Importance outweighs urgency. Important things are those which only you can do or which can advance you toward your life goals.
- *Urgent* not *important (priority 3)*. Priority 3 tasks and paperwork are delegated, if possible, or assigned a small time slot and made part of a routine.
- Neither *important* nor *urgent (priority 4)*. Priority 4 tasks get the least, if any, attention and are worked on in spare time or when all other tasks are completed.

Another approach to prioritization is to employ the *Pareto principle*. Commonly known as the "80/20 rule," this principle was first discussed by Italian economist Vilfredo Pareto in the nineteenth century when studying the distribution of wealth in a number of countries. He observed that about 80 percent of the wealth in most countries was controlled by a consistent minority—about 20 percent of the people.[2] This principle suggests that we should focus on those few tasks which produce the most significant results (Petersen and Halstead, 1983). When applied to the "important and urgent" prioritization scheme, the 20 percent of most the fruitful activities fall into quadrant II or priority 2, and it is on these activities that we should focus most of our effort (Douglass and Douglass, 1993, pp. 28–29).

Similar to these approaches is the "big rock" approach. You may have heard the story about the time management seminar speaker who was presenting to a class of business students one day.[3] He had a large

glass jar and proceeded to fill it up with large rocks. He asked the class if the jar was full.

"Yes," the students responded.

He then took a bag of gravel and proceeded to add it to the jar and shake it down—the gravel filled up space among the large rocks in the jar. "Is the jar full?" he asked the class.

"Probably not," replied one student.

"Good!" the speaker responded. Then he added a bag of sand to the jar, which filled up any remaining space among the rocks. "Now?" he asked the class.

"No!" the students emphatically responded.

Then the speaker brought out a pitcher of water and proceeded to pour the entire amount into the jar without causing the jar to overflow. "What's the point of this illustration?" the speaker asked.

One student responded, "The point is, no matter how full your schedule is, if you try really hard, you can always fit some more things in it!"

"No," the speaker replied, "that's not the point. The truth this illustration teaches us is: If you don't put the big rocks in first, you'll never get them in at all." He goes on to explain that the big rocks in our lives are time spent with family and friends, taking care of ourselves, our faith, and time spent on other worthy causes. The sand and water are "fillers" in our lives, and although some quantity is important, if we fill up our jars with these activities first, then we will have no room left for the big rocks.

Lastly, you probably have observed that some of these approaches discussed delegating certain tasks. As you review your master list, especially the tasks that are of lesser priority and importance, ask yourself if any of those tasks could be done by someone else or if someone else could help you with them? Would it be appropriate to enlist the help of a significant other, a roommate, a friend, a family member, or another person to complete a task? This is a very important question to ask so that you can avoid getting bogged down in activities

---

[2] Pareto principle, available at http://en.wikipedia.org/wiki/Pareto_principle (Accessed on May 16, 2008).

[3] In the 1st edition of this text, this reference was an internet reference from Gerald Nash. For subsequent editions,

this same reference could not be found but a similar story was found at http://www.acekayak.com/EarthScience.html (Accessed on May 16, 2008.)

that detract from your higher-priority tasks. One pharmacy student who was active in student organizations described delegation in this way: "You have to ask yourself if an activity suits you personally or your role as a member of an organization. You must ask, 'Is this something I need to do? Is this something the president of a corporation would do, or would someone else benefit from this experience?' Depending on the answer, you delegate. It frees your schedule and gives someone else an opportunity to have some responsibility" (Dance, 1991, p. 12).

Schedule Tasks

This is not without its own set of challenges because it is often difficult to know how much time a particular task will take—especially if it is a task that you have not done before. It is best to take a conservative approach and allow yourself *more* time than you think you will need to complete a task. It is always better to undercommit and overdeliver (e.g., telling your boss that you will have a particular project done by a date later than you actually think it will take for you to complete and then turning the project in early *or* telling a patient that her prescription will be ready in 15 minutes when you are positive that it will only take 5 to 10 minutes) than to overcommit and underdeliver. Convince yourself of the phenomenon that "things always take longer than I think they will" to allow for unexpected interruptions and other unscheduled events. Then, when you finish a task early, you can reward yourself with a break or fun activity that you had not scheduled previously.

Morgenstern (2000, pp. 143–149) advocates timing yourself and then using a mathematical approach to estimating how much time tasks will take. For different activities that you work on at any given time, ask yourself how long you think it will take you to complete the task, and then keep track of how long it actually takes. The more often you do this, the better you will be at accurately estimating the amount of time tasks will take. Morgenstern tells the story of her brother who had 10 weeks to study for his medical board examination. Based on his experience as a medical student, he knew he could effectively study 10 pages of material per day. Since he had 420 pages of

material to review, he calculated that it would take him 7 weeks of going through the material the first time if he studied 6 days per week. This left him with 3 weeks to review any weak areas and also served as a buffer if for some reason he was not able to study 6 days a week for 7 consecutive weeks. This schedule put him at ease and helped him to relax more about the test.

It is also important to break larger tasks into smaller ones with their own deadlines. If you are working on a semester-long research paper for a class, for example, you are much more likely to do a better job and save yourself a lot of stress if you set some deadlines for yourself to complete the paper:

Month 1: Complete literature search and reading about the topic; draft outline of paper.
Month 2: Complete rough draft of paper; turn in to instructor voluntarily for feedback.
Month 3: Revise first draft based on instructor's feedback; turn in final paper.

Breaking down large tasks also makes them seem less daunting and less overwhelming. Setting intermediate deadlines and sticking to them helps you not to procrastinate.

Lastly, it is important to schedule *all* tasks if not on paper at least in your mind; otherwise, they will not get done. Some doctors make weekly appointments with *themselves* to make sure that they can squeeze in some personal or down time without being interrupted by another appointment. This is not to say that you need to be so rigid that you have every activity in your life entered into a master schedule, but at least allocating time for quadrant II activities is vital to make sure that they are accomplished (e.g., family time, working out, and personal time). It is also important to review your schedule and master list several times a week to make sure that you are prepared for tasks that are coming up. Some authors advocate doing this each night before going to bed.

Use a System

You have the tasks on your master list prioritized and scheduled—but how are you going to keep track of all this? Many people have found that the busier they are and the more tasks they need to complete, the more they rely on some sort of planner system to stay organized. There are a wide variety of daily, weekly, monthly, and yearly planning systems available. While a comprehensive discussion of such systems is beyond the scope of this chapter, several approaches are described that you may find useful:

- *Paper calendar.* Many people use a simple portable calendar on which they can document scheduled tasks as well as their master or to-do list. If this system sounds appealing to you, make sure that the squares on the calendar are large enough so that you can legibly write down all your tasks and appointments. You also want to make sure that your master list can be attached easily to the calendar so that you can keep track of unscheduled tasks that need to be completed. The written calendar system has the advantage of allowing you to easily review daily tasks as well as others coming up in the week or month.
- *Paper-based planner/organizer systems.* You may have heard of the Franklin–Covey planner system or the Day Runner system or seen them in stores. These are just two examples of popular paper-based organizing systems that go beyond the traditional calendar. These systems help the user to prioritize and schedule tasks and to keep a detailed calendar, master to-do list, and address book. They allow the user to customize it so that you only include the types of pages you use most. They come with instructions on how to best use their systems in order to get the most out of them.
- *Personal digital assistants (PDAs) and computer programs.* In this technological age, more and more people are opting for digital systems. Many pharmacy students already own PDAs for their ability to store lots of drug information references as well as keep a daily schedule and check e-mail. These systems have the ability to sound an alarm to alert you of an upcoming meeting or event. Another advantage is that they can be backed up to a computer system so that if either system crashes or is lost, you do not

completely lose everything. One challenge of these systems, however, is that it is difficult to look at multiple pages easily. The master list is kept in a different place than the daily schedule, and the weekly schedule may not show up in much detail. Many of the paper-based organizer programs are now available as computer programs. These work well for those who work on a primary computer most of the time, but if you are not able to download the information onto something that you can carry, such programs may not be as useful.

Morgenstern (2000, pp. 109–134) devoted an entire chapter in her book to "selecting a planner that works for you." She mentions that many of us probably have tried to use a particular planner system but then abandoned it for one or more of these three reasons:

1. You did not pick a planner that was right for you.
2. You did not take time to master its features and make it yours.
3. You did not make it the one and only place to record your appointments and to-dos, so you never came to rely on it.

She advocates determining your style and preferences first (refer to the earlier section of this chapter on self-reflection and analysis) and then considering whether you prefer visual/tactile options (such as paper-based calendars and appointment books) or linear/digital options (such as computer programs and PDAs). She also warns that no system is perfect. Whatever your choice, Morgenstern recommends that you customize it, use it to its fullest, and accept its imperfections.

Take Action

You are ready! On paper or computer you are extremely organized and ready to hit the ground running. In order to help you be successful in accomplishing all your well-organized tasks, Douglass and Douglass (1993, pp. 22–23) feel that it is important to review some of the realities of human nature and how we normally spend our time—not all of which are bad. Some highlights from their 21-item list are noted:

1. We do what we like to do before we do what we do not like to do.
2. We tackle what we know how to do faster than we tackle what we do not know how to do.
3. We do activities that we have resources for.
4. We do things that are scheduled before we do non-scheduled things.
5. We respond to the demands of others before we respond to demands from ourselves.
6. We wait until a deadline approaches before we really get moving on projects.

Being aware of some of these patterns can better help you to avoid them and to stay on track in accomplishing your tasks. Always keep the big picture in mind—think of the goals that you want to achieve and how completing a task will help you do that. A great slogan for dieters who are having trouble with self-discipline is "Nothing tastes as good as thin feels." Constant self-motivation is important when you are trying to change your behavior.

Morgenstern (2000, p. 195) says, "Plan your work, and then work your plan." She recommends three actions to help you stay focused and disciplined so that you can overcome bad habits and achieve more each day (p. 196):

1. Minimize interruptions (i.e., unexpected events) and their impact.
2. Conquer procrastination and chronic lateness.
3. Overcome perfectionism.

She goes on to provide helpful suggestions on how to do all these things because they sound much easier than they are (pp. 196–210). In the end, if you are able to "containerize" your activities, you will be able to get your to-dos done and move through your day "feeling energized, optimistic, and satisfied" (p. 195).

General Tips from the Experts
Although many parts of this chapter contain helpful hints to improve your time management skills, you may have missed a few, and they are worth mentioning again:

- Take care of yourself. It is extremely difficult to be productive and successful if you subsist on junk food, get less than 7 hours of sleep per night, or only exercise when you walk from the fridge to the couch.
- Most people do their best work in the morning, so tackle the tough projects at that time.
- Schedule meetings and less intensive activities in the afternoon.
- Check your e-mail and phone messages only twice a day, once in the morning and once in the afternoon or evening.
- Cluster tasks and activities together when possible. For example, if you have a class or meeting in building A, what other tasks or activities can you accomplish that need to be done in or near building A before you trek across campus to building Z?
- Quantity does not equal quality.
- Busy does not equal productive.
- Working harder does not equal working smarter.
- Reward yourself. It gives you something to shoot for and look forward to. Besides, all work and no play make Jack a dull boy!

Douglass and Douglass (1993, pp. 184–186) offer 39 tips for becoming a "top time master." They have even created a poster with these tips that they offer free to anyone who contacts one of the authors (contact information is included in their book). They describe it as "an excellent way to keep reminding yourself to develop good time management habits" (p. 186).

Review/Revise/Modify
Now that you are working on your plan in full swing, it is important periodically to review all the steps that you went through to determine if your system is working well. Are you accomplishing tasks and goals to your satisfaction? Are you feeling less stressed? Do you procrastinate less often? Have your preferences or your style changed in any way? Do you want to try out a new organizational system? Have your goals or priorities changed? What major changes have occurred in your

life to modify your goals and priorities? When you ask yourself these questions, especially the first three, remember to cut yourself a little slack. Real change takes time, and old habits are hard to break. It is okay if you did not follow your plan to a tee. Celebrate your successes, learn from your failures, and keep striving to improve.

Bond created a 43-item questionnaire to help us review our goals and priorities to see if they have changed (Bond, 1996, pp. 89–92). Questions include

- Do you feel as strongly about your priority (goal) as you did when you set it?
- Do you reward yourself for daily or weekly successes?
- Are you adhering to your priority (goal) deadline?
- Do you spread yourself too thin and run out of time?
- Do you review your activities to determine which ones can be shortened, reorganized, or terminated?
- What are the most important factors in your success?

Analyzing your responses to these questions, along with what contributed to or detracted from your success, is an important process to help you make adjustments and corrections. As long as you are making progress toward your goals, *that* is what is most important. Remember, slow and steady wins the race. It is also helpful to remember that as much as we might like to, we will never have complete control over all our time. Douglass and Douglass (1993, p. 147) remind us to recall the Serenity Prayer:

God, grant me the serenity to accept the things I cannot change,

The courage to change those things I can,

And the wisdom to know the difference.

▌ TIME MANAGEMENT IN PHARMACY PRACTICE

So how does all this information about personal time management relate to pharmacy practice? As mentioned earlier, it is unlikely that a person who is extremely disorganized at home will be very organized in his or her work environment, and vice versa. Certainly, however, time management skills in practice depend on

the type of job you have. If you have a position that is more administrative, project-based, or appointment-based, you will have more control over how your time is spent, and you can better use many of the skills described in this chapter. For example, White (1996) wrote a helpful article that describes how pharmacy managers can better control their time. She updated this piece in 2007 and offered several strategies that any pharmacist could use to improve work efficiency (Table 13-3) (White, 2007). In most pharmacy environments, however, we do not get to determine how we spend our time—the nature of the job involves responding to the demand of medication orders and questions from patients, health care providers, and others. Rarely do we have the luxury of planning our daily work activities.

Time management in practice is based on two issues: how organized you are personally at work (e.g., Can you work well in a scattered, chaotic environment, or must you work in a very structured and systematic fashion?) and what the workflow is like in your environment. Most of us have some control over the first issue but not always the second. If you do have some say, however, in yours' and others' duties and how the workflow progresses, there are numerous recommendations about how to improve efficiency and patient

Table 13-3.	General Strategies for Working More Efficiently
Determine the cost of your time	
Understand your responsibilities	
Log your activities	
Plan for productive time	
Avoid time-wasting behavior	
Develop reminders	
Prioritize your goals	
Assign times for your tasks	
Manage e-mail	
Manage clutter	
Manage retrieval of information	
Employ other time savers, such as templates for regular reports	

Source: Used with permission from White, 2007.

safety. A full discussion of these is beyond the scope of this chapter, but a few specific recommendations are shared below.

Mark Jacobs, pharmacist for Shopko Pharmacy in Beloit, Wisconsin, published his thoughts about making more time for patients in the pharmacy in the book *101 Ways to Improve Your Pharmacy Worklife* (as noted in Jacobs, 2002). He suggests six specific tasks for handling the volume of phone calls in practice that can help to improve your professional satisfaction and ability to care for patients (a few of which apply specifically to outpatient and community practices):

1. *Make full use of pharmacy technicians.* If you work with capable technicians, use them as fully as the law will allow. One example is never to answer the phone yourself unless it is a prescribers' line. Jacobs mentions that no other professionals (e.g., doctors, lawyers, etc.) answer their own phones.

2. *Respond to questions on the phone through your pharmacy technicians whenever possible.* This does not mean that you should avoid talking with patients on the phone at all possible costs, but by training your technicians to ask the caller the proper "triage" questions, you can avoid calls where the patient wants to talk to the pharmacist and then goes on to give you a prescription number to refill. Doctors most often respond to patients on the phone through their nurses.

3. *If a patient insists on speaking with a pharmacist, explain that the pharmacist is busy with another patient right now.* Jacobs advocates having the technician take down the patient's name and phone number and the reason for the call so that the pharmacist can prepare for the call prior to calling back, which also saves time.

4. *Find out when and where would be the best time to call the patient back.* Jacobs states that this will help "condition" patients to realize that you are a busy health care professional and that you may not always be available on-demand. Additionally, if they really need help right now, they may be willing to ask the technician.

5. *Gracefully exit the conversation after 2 minutes* "by explaining to the patient that you have time for one more question. They will either ask it or thank you for your time."

6. *Have the technician take down all the information for prescription transfers* (depending on what the law will allow). At the very least, the technician can pull up the prescription on the computer or pull the hard copy before handing the phone to the pharmacist.

For some patients and phone calls, it may not be appropriate to adhere to all these suggestions, but for many calls, these tips can help a busy pharmacist to save time each day. Other efficiencies that many practices are implementing include a variety of dispensing technologies and robotics, automated refill phone lines and Web sites, and reconfiguring technicians' and pharmacists' job descriptions so that technicians perform most technical duties and pharmacists can concentrate on reviewing and monitoring patients' drug therapy, as well as engaging in patient and provider education. All these suggestions can be implemented relatively easily so as to better manage time in the pharmacy. Jeff Rochon, Pharm.D., Director of Pharmacy Care Services for the Washington State Pharmacists Association, reminds us that above all, we must make time to communicate with patients and other health care providers (Rochon, 2003).

▪ STRESS AS A PRIMARY CONSEQUENCE OF POOR TIME MANAGEMENT

Research has shown that individual characteristics related to job stress include balance between work and personal life, a person's outlook on life, the stressfulness of family life, and various aspects of personality (Stress at Work, 1999. The issue of balance, in all aspects of one's life, is the crux of this chapter. Effective use of time management strategies should help to reduce the probability that a person will feel overly stressed.

Interestingly, it has been shown that pharmacy students reported higher stress levels as students than they did as practicing pharmacists (Ortmeier, Wolfgang, and Martin, 1991; Wolfgang and Ortmeier, 1993). Another study indicated that stress among pharmacy students was partially related to "excessive study load"

Table 13-4. Consequences of Job Stress for Pharmacists

- Job dissatisfaction
- Lower commitment to one's organization
- Job turnover (leaving one's job)
- Lower commitment to pharmacy as a career
- Substance abuse potential
- Burnout

Source: Used with permission from Gupchup and Worley, 2005.

(Dutta, 2001). Effective time management strategies with regard to study time certainly could help to reduce these feelings.

Research on consequences of pharmacists' job stress could be informative for students (Table 13-4). It is logical to conclude that what is considered "job stress" for pharmacists could be "school stress" for students or a combination of work and school. Thus, if students feel stressed about school and perhaps their internship, they likely might suffer similar consequences as pharmacists: dissatisfaction with their Pharm.D. program or internship, lower commitment to completing one's degree program or even pharmacy as a career, quitting school or the internship or both, and the potential for substance abuse and burnout.

Thankfully, coworker social support, or the material and emotional support received from one's coworkers, has been shown to buffer the impact of job stress on job dissatisfaction (Wolfgang, 1994). For students, this applies to coworkers and classmates. It is presumed that most pharmacy students probably have a network of friends in their academic class experiencing the same "stress" (at least related to the Pharm.D. program), so a natural buffer exists. How one copes with stress also makes a difference; problem-focused coping strategies, where one attempts to tackle the problems at hand, are most effective in reducing the impact of job stress on job dissatisfaction (Gupchup and Worley-Louis, 2005). Implementing time management strategies could be an example of a problem-focused cop-

ing strategy. Emotionally based coping strategies, such as distancing oneself from the problem or trying to avoid the problem, are unsuccessful (Gupchup and Worley-Louis, 2005). Other strategies to combat stress include meditation and relaxation (e.g., yoga and massage), biofeedback, and physical exercise (Gupchup and Worley-Louis, 2005).

■ REVISITING THE SCENARIO

This chapter has presented a lot of tips and ideas that Tom may heed so that he can improve his time management skills. While Tom may have a routine, he definitely does not have a system. At the very least, Tom must ask himself some important questions and establish some goals and priorities. He may also consider the use of a master list and implement the use of technology such as a PDA to help him focus on the tasks at hand. We certainly would not want to see him lose his job or have to resign from the school of pharmacy.

■ CONCLUSION

The goal of this chapter was to raise awareness about the importance of time management in one's personal and professional lives. Readers should have come away with concrete strategies about how to improve thier skills so that they can achieve their full potential. Remember, time management is not about managing time, it's about managing yourself - and all of us can proabably use at least some improvement so that we can be more effective in all that we do.

■ QUESTIONS FOR FURTHER DISCUSSION

1. After applying the techniques described in this chapter, are you better able to accomplish your goals?
2. Are you healthier? Why or why not?
3. Are you happier? Why or why not?
4. How can you help others to learn and employ these skills?
5. How can these skills help you as a practitioner?

6. What kinds of time management techniques can you employ in your practice to help improve the process of health care delivery?

7. In addition to time management, what strategies would you employ to reduce your stress level?

REFERENCES

Applebaum SH, Rohrs WF. 1981. *Time Management for Health Care Professional.* Rockville, MD: Aspen Systems.

Bond WJ. 1996. *Managing Your Priorities from Start to Success.* Chicago: Irwin Professional.

Covey SR. 1989. *The Seven Habits of Highly Effective People: Restoring the Character Ethic.* New York: Simon & Schuster.

Dance B. 1991. Managing time means managing yourself. *Pharmacy Student* 21:11.

Douglass ME, Douglass DN. 1993. *Manage Your Time and Your Work Yourself: The Updated Edition.* New York: AMACOM.

Drucker PF. 1954. *The Practice of Management.* New York: Harper & Row.

Drucker PF. (1967). *The Effective Executive.* New York, NY: Harper and Row.

Dutta AP. 2001. Measuring and understanding stress in pharmacy students. Published dissertation, Virginia Commonwealth University.

English T. 2003. Yes, you can find the time: Experts present time management for dummies. *Pharmacy Student* 33:16.

Ensman RG. 1991. Time test: How well do you manage time? *Consultant Pharmacist* 6:61.

Gupchup GV, Worley-Louis MM. 2005. Understanding and managing stress among pharmacists. In Desselle S, Zgarrick D (eds), *Pharmacy Management,* pp. 52–62. New York: McGraw-Hill.

Jacobs M. 2002. Time management in the pharmacy: Efficient use of your time will leave more time for your patients. *Washington Pharm* Autumn:17.

Morgenstern J. 2000. *Time Management from the Inside Out: The Foolproof System for Taking Control of Your Schedule—and Your Life.* New York: Holt.

Ortmeier BG, Wolfgang AP, Martin BC. 1991. Career commitment, career plans, and perceived stress: A survey of pharmacy students. *Am J Pharm Ed* 55:138.

Paul MJ. 2003. *It's Hard to Make a Difference When You Can't Find Your Keys: The Seven-Step Path to Becoming Truly Organized.* New York: Viking Books.

Petersen DJ, Halstead EG. 1983. The ABC's of effective time management. *Top Hosp Pharm Manag* 3:47.

Peterson CL. 1999. Stress at Work: A Sociological Perspective. Amityville, NY: Baywood Publishing.

Rochon J. 2003. Developing relationships is an essential aspect of your practice. *Washington Pharm* Summer:9.

White SJ. 1996. High-touch human resource management: Finding the time. *Pharm Pract Manag Q* 15:75.

White SJ. 2007. Working efficiently. *Am J Health-Sys Pharm* 64:1587.

Wick J. 1997. Time management tips. *Consultant Pharmacist* 12:1042.

Wolfgang AP. 1994. Job stress and dissatisfaction: The role of coworker social support and powerlessness. *J Pharm Market Manag* 9:19.

Wolfgang AP, Ortmeier BG. 1993. Career commitment, career plans, and job related stress: A follow-up study of pharmacy students as pharmacists. *Am J Pharm Ed* 57:25.

Woodhull AV. 1997. *The New Time Manager.* Brookfield, VT: Gower.

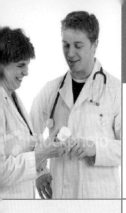

14

LEADERSHIP IN PHARMACY

Virginia (Ginger) G. Scott

About the Author: Dr. Scott is Professor and Director of Continuing Education in the Department of Pharmaceutical Systems and Policy at West Virginia University School of Pharmacy. She received a B.S. in pharmacy from the University of Kentucky, an M.S. in pharmacy administration from Purdue University, and a Ph.D. in social and administrative pharmacy from the University of Minnesota. Her teaching interests include patient health education, outcomes and quality improvement, pharmacoeconomics, and patient-reported outcomes. Her research interests include health services and health outcomes research, specifically patient-reported outcomes and cost-effectiveness of patient care services and drug therapy; educational research on continuing professional development; and examining the relationship between educational programming and the implementation of pharmacy services. She has been involved actively in pharmacy professional organizations, has served in numerous leadership positions on the state and national levels since 1977, and was selected as an Academic Leadership Fellow in 2004.

▨ LEARNING OBJECTIVES

After completing this chapter, students should be able to

1. Define leadership.
2. Identify qualities needed to be an effective leader.
3. Discuss evaluative tools used to identify and develop leadership skills.
4. Discuss how to use your personal strengths to advance an organization.
5. Discuss the development of leadership in others.
6. Describe leadership roles within the profession and community for students and pharmacists.

▓ SCENARIO

Jennifer Leader is a fourth-year pharmacy student who is involved in several student pharmacy organizations at her college of pharmacy. Recently, she was recognized by her peers and inducted into Phi Lambda Sigma, a pharmacy leadership organization that fosters and recognizes student pharmacy leaders. Jennifer's long-term goal is to become a director of pharmacy or a regional manager or to own her own store. Other goals are to be actively involved in local, state, and national pharmacy organizations and to have a leadership position in one of the pharmacy organizations on both the state and national levels. Based on her leadership class in pharmacy school, Jennifer feels that she has a broad understanding of the concepts of leadership and leadership theories. During her rotations to date, she has encountered several leaders who do not exhibit the leadership styles and skills that she was taught in pharmacy school. Thus, she is thinking that she may need additional leadership development to further her self-awareness of her strengths and leadership skills as well as to gain a better understanding on how to interpret the leadership style of others.

▓ CHAPTER QUESTIONS

1. How do you define leadership? What is not leadership?
2. What are some evaluative tools to assess an individual's leadership skills?
3. How do you use your personal strengths to advance the organization and profession?
4. What qualities are needed for effective leadership?
5. How would you develop your employees to be future leaders of the organization?
6. What leadership styles are important in pharmacy?
7. What types of leadership roles should pharmacists and/or pharmacy students assume?

▓ LEADERSHIP

The hallmarks of effective leadership are important from both a personal and an organizational perspec-tive, and the concepts of leadership have intrigued individuals for centuries. A plethora of literature exists related to the meaning of leadership, qualities of an effective leader, leadership styles, leadership theories, the development of a leader, and other dimensions of leadership.

This chapter builds on the leadership theories related to organizational behavior discussed in Chapter 8. Specifically, this chapter will help you to gain a greater understanding of the definitions and concepts of leadership, qualities of an effective leader, leadership theories and styles, how to use your personal strengths to enhance your leadership abilities, developing leadership in others, evaluative tools to identify your personal leadership style, and leadership roles within the profession and community for students and pharmacists.

▓ WHAT IS LEADERSHIP?

Leadership has been described in many ways by many persons, but there exists no universally accepted definition. Carson Dye (2000) confirmed this when he stated, "After all these years . . . no one is able to articulate a comprehensive, absolute definition of leadership." Common to many leadership definitions are the following dimensions: Leadership is inherent (Dye, 2000), a learned skill (Dye, 2000; Giuliani, 2002; Maxwell, 2003), adapting principles to circumstances (Patton, 1999), a process that focuses on making organizational changes (Kotter, 1990), not controlling people (Autry, 2001), a blend of characteristics and talents that individuals can use to develop into a leader (Lombardi, 2001), and attracting the voluntary commitment of followers to reach for common goals (Krieter et al., 1997; Nanus, 1992; Tichy, 1997).

Even though there are many leadership definitions, Komvies, Lucas, and McMahon (1998) noted several basic assumptions about leadership that are incorporated into the preceding definitions. These assumptions are that leadership is a learned behavior, is teachable, occurs at all levels of the organization, does not require a charismatic personality, is a relational process, is culturally influenced, requires followership, involves purposeful change that satisfies collective needs and aspirations, includes the components of effectiveness and ethics, and develops over life.

Leadership is an important concept that transcends all health care professions. The acceptance of this role by all health care professionals is vital to the invention of new technologies and dosage forms, changes in the delivery of health care, enhancement of patient outcomes and quality of life, and success of their specific health care organization. The opportunities for pharmacists to be leaders in their practice setting, the pharmacy profession, and the community are plentiful. Leadership is a critical component for positive change within pharmacy organizations and the profession.

LEADERSHIP THEORIES AND STYLES

Leadership theories help us to understand the leadership style of your immediate boss and other administrators. Understanding leadership theory and leadership styles enables us to identify the personal values and vision that guide the organization's management team. It also provides insight into your employer's expectations of you as an employee.

The leadership theories discussed in Chapter 8 were trait, behavioral (i.e., autocratic, democratic, and laissez-fare), situational or contingency-based, transactional, and transformational. The majority of these theories are transactional in nature; however, transformational leadership is used more often to implement innovation and change within the profession and achievement of organizational goals (Bass, 1985). Building on Chapter 8, other leadership theories or styles used extensively in the health care industry are servant-leadership and strengths-based leadership.

Servant-Leadership

Servant-leadership is a term coined by Robert Greenleaf in 1970, and it has been studied and expanded on by other authors, such as Covey (1998), Autry (2001), and Martin (2002). It is based on the philosophy that an individual's first desire is to serve. Later, the individual makes a conscious decision to lead (Greenleaf, 2002).

Authors have identified many characteristics that are important in the development of servant-leaders. Larry Spear, chief executive officer (CEO) of the Greenleaf Center, identified 10 principles of servant-leadership based on Greenleaf's original writings. These characteristics are listening, empathy, healing, persuasion, awareness, conceptualization, foresight, stewardship, commitment to the growth of people, and building community (Spears, 2003). Autry (2001) noted that servant-leaders have a deeper connection to their work, and the connection transcends power and money. In his writings, he discusses several other characteristics of a servant-leader. These are to be authentic (i.e., the same person in every circumstance), vulnerable (i.e., to realize that you are not in total control but depend on others), accepting (i.e., to focus on ideas presented, not on the person), present (i.e., available, centered, and grounded), and useful (i.e., caring, useful, and creating a meaningful workplace).

Strengths-Based Leadership

Strengths-based leadership is based on the theory of positive psychology. The theory implies that individuals are more effective leaders when they become aware of and understand their unique talents and capitalize on these strengths (Hendricks, 2001). Talents, knowledge, and skills of the individual are the basis for strength-based leadership. Talents are naturally unique to each individual and can be maximized by knowledge and skill development (Buckingham, 2005; Buckingham and Clinton, 2001; Coffman and Gonzalez-Molins, 2002). Research in this area has been conducted by the Gallup University using interviews of great leaders and a Web-based assessment tool to determine the importance of using strength-based leadership in the workplace.

REFRAMING LEADERSHIP

Bolman and Deal (2003) present another concept of leadership style that incorporates the use of *frames* to maximize the success of the organization. Frames are defined as "windows on the world of leadership and management. A good frame makes it easier to know what you are up against and what you can do about it." These authors further noted that "frames [are] like maps; frames are both windows on a territory and tools for navigation. Every tool has distinctive strengths and limitations. The right tool makes the job easier, but the wrong one just gets in the way" (Bolman and Deal, 2003). These frames are an essential part of the leadership process and are labeled *structural, human resources, political,* and *symbolic.* Most leaders will not exhibit strengths in all four frames. The key is for the leader of an organization to surround himself or herself with individuals who have strengths in the other frames to maximize the success of their organization.

Structural leaders do homework; rethink the relationship of structure, strategy, and environment; and focus on implementation. Whereas, human resources leaders believe in people and communicate their beliefs. They are visible, accessible, empower others, and refer to employees as partners or associates. Political leaders clarify what they want and what they can get. They persuade first, negotiate second, and coerce only if necessary. Symbolic leaders lead by example, offer plausible interpretations of experience, communicate a vision, tell stories, and respect and use history. Reframing leadership is a leadership style that will be valuable in assisting future leaders to create new opportunities within their environments.

■ QUALITIES OF EFFECTIVE LEADERS

Recent authors (Ahoy, 2007; Buckingham, 2005, Maxwell, 1995) have identified five hallmark characteristics of effective leaders. These are modeling, mentoring, motivating, monitoring, and multiplying successes (i.e., reproducing future leaders). Leaders must be role models within the organization because employees will model the role they exhibit. They also are mentors by teaching other employees on the workings of the organizations and guiding their employee development. Leaders motivate employees to be responsible for their performance within the organization. Responsible employees assist leaders in helping the organization grow and succeed. The leader must monitor the operations

of the organization on a daily basis to ensure that the organization remains efficient and effective. *Multiplying success* refers to the fact that as individuals are given greater responsibility for and control of their own work, they are more likely to work toward improving the organization. Ahoy (2007) noted other characteristics, such as empowering, guiding, and coaching your employees while delegating responsibility, that are also important characteristics for leading an organization. The W. K. Kellogg Foundation Report (2000) indicated that collaboration between leadership and employees, shared purpose, respect, and a inhanced learning environment also are important to the success of organizations.

Additional qualities frequently mentioned by authors include vision (Ahoy, 2007; Bolman and Deal, 2003), integrity (Maxwell, 1995), communicating a vision effectively (Clifford and Cavanaugh, 1985; Kouzes and Posner, 1987), commitment (Bolman and Deal, 2003; Clifford and Cavanaugh, 1985; Collins, 2001; W. K. Kellogg Foundation Report, 2000), positive attitude (Maxwell, 1995), confidence (Maxwell, 1995), character (Maxwell, 1995), passion (Bolman and Deal, 2003; Clifford and Cavanaugh, 1985; Collins, 2001), (Bolman and Deal, 2003; Kotter 1990; Kouzes and Posner, 1987; Nanus, 1992), honesty (Bolman and Deal, 2003), relationship building (Coleman 2002; Kotter 1990; Kouzes and Posner, 1987; Nanus, 1992), charmisa (Denny, 2002), team spirit (Cureton, 2002), creativity (Dave, 2002), being ethical (Keim, 2002), courage (Haverson, 2002), networking (Malinchak, 2002), self-knowledge (W. K. Kellogg Foundation Report, 2000), authenticity/integrity (W. K. Kellogg Foundation Report, 2000), empathy/understanding of others (W. K. Kellogg Foundation Report, 2000), and competence (W. K. Kellogg Foundation Report, 2000).

After decades of research and thousands of interviews with great leaders, Gallup University research discovered seven challenges, referred to as the "seven demands of leadership" that leaders must meet to maximize their leadership impact on an organizations and critical to their leadership success (Conchie, 2004). These challenges are visioning, mentoring, knowing self, making sense of experience, maximizing values, building a constituency, and challenging experience.

LEADERSHIP DEVELOPMENT

A prevailing myth about leadership is that it is innate or, in other words, something with which you are born. In the definitions of leadership above, many great leaders stated that leadership is a learned behavior (Dye, 2000; Giuliani, 2002; Maxwell, 2003). Maxwell (2003) classified four levels of leadership based on the concept that leadership is a learned behavior. These are the *leading leader,* the *learned leader,* the *latent leader,* and the *limited leader.* Each category is based on the individual's level of leadership and desire to become a leader. The classifications vary along a continuum from being born with leadership qualities (the leading leader) to the leader who has had little or no exposure to leadership (the limited leader). Other characteristics used to classify an individual into a specific category depend on whether the individual has seen leadership modeled, has had leadership training, and has the desire to be a leader. In all four classifications, the only characteristic not acquired is "born with leadership qualities." Thus any individual with the desire to be a leader can develop his or her leadership skills. Mason and Wetherbee (2004) noted two assumptions of leadership development. The first emphasizes the preceding point that leaders can be developed through education and training. The second is that management differs from leadership (Table 14-1) and that managers can be transformed into leaders.

Dye (2000) identified four stages in the growth of leadership. Individuals in stage 1 do not think that leadership is their job, and they resist leadership development (unconscious incompetence). Stage 2 refers to individuals being consciously incompetent or who have the desire to grow and improve but may not realize it until they lose their job. Stage 3 is conscious competence, where individuals are competent but are not seen as strong leaders. They need the opportunity to practice skills and continue learning. Stage 4 refers to unconscious competence and is the ultimate stage of leadership. In this stage, an individ-

Table 14-1. Warren Bennis's 12 Distinctions Between Leaders and Managers

Leaders	Managers
1. Innovate	1. Administer
2. Ask what and why	2. Ask how and when
3. Focus on people	3. Focus on systems
4. Do "the right thing"	4. Do "things right"
5. Develop	5. Maintain
6. Inspire trust	6. Rely on control
7. Long-term perspective	7. Short-term perspective
8. Challenge the status quo	8. Accept the status quo
9. Eye on the horizon	9. Eye on the bottom line
10. Originate	10. Imitate
11. Their own person	11. Emulate the classic good solider
12. Show originality	12. Copy

Source: Bennis, 1989; used with permission.

ual's leadership skills are smooth and happen without hesitation.

A different concept to enhancing leadership effectiveness was presented by Jim Collins (2001) in his book, *Good to Great.* He encouraged the development of a "stop doing" list by business leaders. Collins's rationale for this concept is that leaders lead busy lives with many "to do" lists. By developing a "stop doing" list, leaders can channel their resources into a few focused areas.

Gallup University's "seven demands of leadership" were noted under essential qualities of leadership (Conchie, 2004). To further monitor your leadership and the leadership of your employees, choose two of the seven demands and develop measures to determine their impact on the organization. Review the results of the measures and make changes and modifications to ensure the organization's success. Other resources available from Gallup include an e-learning course that provides concepts of strengths-based theory and the Clifton StrengthsFinder (see "Leadership Evaluative Tools" below)

Maxwell (2003) developed a workbook to correspond to the material presented in his book, *The 21 Irrefutable Laws of Leadership,* to aid in the development of leaders. The workbook provides multiple instruments that individuals can employ for the purpose of identifying strengths related to leadership skills, such as vision, relationship building, coaching, and connectivity. This is a good place to begin to identify your strengths as a leader. The results can be used in the development of a more elaborate leadership development plan. Reliable and valid instruments have been developed to identify an individual's personality style and skills related to the resolutions of conflicts, critical thinking, motivation, and personal strengths.

Strengths-based development at the individual level is a more recent model for leadership development. There are three steps in the development process. First, an individual's talents are identified, and the person is made aware of these talents. Second, the individual begins to integrate these into his or her daily routines, shares with other members of the organization, and identifies ways to maximize his or her strengths. Last, a behavior change occurs as the individual is able to tie his or her successes to his or her themes of talent (Clifton and Harter, 2003). Being cognizant of your own strengths and leadership skills enhances your ability to develop leadership in others.

Developing Leadership in Others

Stanley (2003) stated, "Sometimes it really is easier and less time consuming to do things yourself than to train someone else." But leadership is not always about getting things done "right." Leadership is about getting things done through other people. Covey (1989), in his book, *The 7 Habits of Highly Effective People,* notes that transferring responsibility, or delegation, results in growth for both the individual and the organization. As a leader, you have the responsibility to develop future leaders to ensure the continual success of your organization. Conger (1992) and Conger and Benjamin (1999) identified four types of leadership development

used in corporations. These are skills-building training (e.g., practice exercises for skills, simulations, lectures, and video case studies), intensive feedback programs (e.g., observational exercises, survey and verbal feedback, and fellow colleagues), conceptual approaches (e.g., written and video case studies, lectures on conceptual models, and discussion groups), and personal growth approaches (e.g., teamwork, risk-taking, and personal values exploration). Other types of leadership development used are mentoring, coaching, and profile evaluative instruments.

◼ LEADERSHIP EVALUATIVE TOOLS

Numerous leadership evaluative tools help individuals increase self-awareness, recognize interpersonal communication skills, and identify thinking skills. Some of the most commonly used evaluative tools are the Myers-Briggs Types Indicator (MBTI) (Myers and Briggs, 1988), the Strength Deployment Inventory (SDI) (Scudder, 1996), the Watson-Glaser Critical Thinking Appraisal (WGCTA) (Watson and Glaser, 2000), the Thomas Kilmann Conflict Mode Instrument (TKI) (Kilmann and Kilmann, 1972), 360-degree feedback, and Q12.

Myers-Briggs Type Indicator

The Myers-Briggs Type Indicator (MBTI) personality inventory was developed in the 1940s by Isabel Myers and Katherine Briggs. The instrument was based on Carl Jung's theory of psychological types introduced in 1920. Jung's theory indicates that random behavior variation is due to differences in the way individuals prefer to use their perception and judgment. The instrument identifies an individual's preference for the four dichotomies specified in Jung's theory. These are favorite world (i.e., extroversion or introversion), information (i.e., sensing or intuition), decisions (i.e., thinking or feeling), and structure (i.e., judging or perceiving). Your answers to questions comprising the inventory are used to place you into one of 16 personality types. It is assumed that none of the personality types is "better" or "superior" to others. As such, the purpose of the feedback is to help you to understand and appreciate differences between people (Myers and Briggs, 1988).

Currently, there are two MBTI forms, MBTI Step I and MBTI Step II. MBTI Step I (Form M) consists of 93 questions and is based on preferences, whereas MBTI Step II (Form Q) consists of 144 questions. Feedback from this form provides a broader picture related to communication, decision making, and ability to deal with change and conflict. Research shows that both MBTI forms continue to be valid and reliable. The MBTI, after more than 60 years, continues to be the most popular personality measure for understanding individual differences and helping a person to uncover different methods to use when interacting with other people (Myers and Briggs, 1988). Identification of your personality style is important in interacting with other members of your organization. Feedback from this tool provides tips on interacting with individuals who exhibit a different personality style. By knowing how to interact with individuals with different personality styles, the organization can grow, and conflicts can be avoided.

The Strength Deployment Inventory

The Strength Deployment Inventory (SDI) is based on relationship awareness theory. This theory implies that individual relationships can be improved and/or transformed by a better understanding not only of themselves but also of others through the creation of shared meanings (Noce, 1999, Porter, 1996). The SDI differs from other instruments assessing an individual's behavior in that an individual's motivation value system is also assessed. Values are assessed when things are going well for an individual, as well as when the person faces conflict. The questions are self-scored and worded to measure behaviors and the motivations and values that underlie those behaviors. Some applications of the SDI are conflict management, enhanced awareness of self and others, development of communication and negotiation skills, team building, and leadership development. The SDI is available in three editions: Standard, Component, and Premier. The Standard Edition is the most widely used of the three tools. In the Com-

ponent Edition, the motivational value system can be presented to the individual gradually. For example, instructions for using the tool, definitions, and inventory items can be sent to the individual to view in advance of actual administration of the instrument. The Premier Edition is the most comprehensive of the three editions. Feedback to individuals is based on the measures in the edition administered to the individual. Measures include the portrait of personal strengths, the portrait of overdone strengths, information on the relationship awareness theory, relationship awareness model, strength management card, and expanded conflict information. Each edition also includes instructions for drawing a visual representation of an individual's SDI results (Jones, 1976). This information is important because leaders must build relationships within the organization for the organization to grow and succeed.

The Watson-Glaser Critical Thinking Appraisal

The Watson-Glaser Critical Thinking Appraisal (WGCTA) is the most commonly used tool in business today to assess critical thinking skills. It assesses inference, recognition of assumptions, deduction, interpretation, and evaluation of arguments skills (Watson and Glaser, 2000). The WGCTA has been used extensively in business settings to determine hiring, promotion, and development of individuals for succession planning of a company. It is believed that high-potential performers with good critical thinking skills use sound decision making (Watson and Glaser, 2000).

There are two versions of the WGCTA instrument, the WGCTA-A and WGCTA-B. The original version of the instrument contains 80 questions. A shorter (WGCTA-S) version that takes less time to administer was developed later and consists of only 40 items. Individuals being assessed are asked to evaluate reading passages that include statements, problems, arguments, and interpretations. When completed, a single score is determined for each individual. The score and information related to interpretation of the score are then provided to the individual. Since critical thinking skills are important in all organizations, individuals need to have critical thinking skills or develop this skill to be an effective leader. Since the pharmacy profession requires pharmacists to use critical thinking skills daily, the WGCTA would be an excellent tool to assess an employee's skill in this area.

The Thomas Kilmann Conflict Mode Instrument

The Thomas Kilmann Conflict Mode Instrument (TKI) was developed to assess an individual's preferred mode of five conflict-handling styles. These are avoiding, accommodating, competing, compromising, and collaborating. The TKI instrument consists of 30 items. Individuals are forced to choose between two possible statements that describe their most likely behavior in a given situation. Responses then are transferred to a scoring sheet, and scores are totaled for each of the five modes of conflict resolution. Feedback allows individuals to determine their primary mode of conflict resolution and to identify situations when other modes of conflict resolution might be more effective. This is important in an organizational setting because leaders may be faced with a variety of conflicts that need to be resolved by different techniques.

The StrengthsFinder Profile

The StrengthsFinder Profile was developed by the Gallup Organization (Buckingham and Clifton, 2001) to identify the strengths that an individual possesses. The profile actually measures an individual's themes of talents. Since strengths are a result of talents, knowledge, and skills, a profile of various themes of talents can be developed for an individual (Buckingham and Clifton, 2001). The profile consists of a pair of statements. The responses are then sorted. The feedback lists your five most dominant patterns of behavior. These are referred to as your *signature theme*. Research by Gallup University has identified 34 themes (Table 14-2).

The book, *Now, Discover Your Strengths,* by Buckingham and Clifton (2001), discusses development of the profile and describes each of the signature themes in depth. A second version of the StrengthFinders Profile was released in the fall of 2007. Version 2 can be ac-

Table 14-2.	The 34 Themes of Strengths Finder
Achiever	Futuristic
Activator	Harmony
Adaptability	Ideation
Analytical	Inclusiveness
Arranger	Individualization
Belief	Input
Command	Intellection
Communication	Learner
Competition	Maximizer
Connectedness	Positivity
Context	Relator
Deliberative	Responsibility
Developer	Restorative
Discipline	Self-assurance
Empathy	Significance
Fairness	Strategic
Focus	Woo

Source: Buckingham and Clifton, 2001; used with permission.

cessed by using the personal identification code in the back jacket of the book, *Now, Discover Your Strengths: StrengthFinders Profile 2.0* (Rath, 2007). By knowing their strengths and the strengths of their employees, leaders can assign individuals' responsibilities based on their strengths, resulting in a more effective and successful organization.

360-Degree Feedback

This is a performance appraisal tool focusing on leadership effectiveness, planning, and teamwork (Edwards and Even, 1996). The system or process ultimately helps individuals to be more effective managers and/or leaders by better understanding their overall strengths and weaknesses. There is a self-evaluation and a peer evaluation. Employees (i.e., managers, peers, and staff) provide their perceptions on a broad range of workplace competencies. Participants use a rating scale to respond to the questions in addition to providing written comments. Afterwards, responses for each category of employees (e.g., peers) are collated to ensure anonymity. Feedback is provided on the difference between the self-evaluation and peer evaluation in relation to leadership skills such as listening, goal setting, and planning. The feedback is provided to the leader in a format such that the individual can create a development plan. An advantage of the 360-degree feedback is that it can also be used as a development tool for nonmanagers (DeBare, 1997). Even though nonmanagers have no staff reporting directly to them, feedback from coworkers can be useful in helping them to be more effective in their current position. Second, it serves as a development tool for individuals aspiring to move into a management position. By identifying their strengths and areas for improvement, they can adjust their behaviors or develop new skills to be effective leaders within the organization and excel in their jobs.

Q12

The Q12 was developed by the Gallup Organization (Gallup Organization, 1999; Coffman, 2002) to determine the level of employees' engagement within the organization. The Q12 assesses 12 key dimensions that describe a great workplace (Gallup Organization, 1999). The report from the Q12 instrument identifies how the leader's management style influences the perception of team members and engagement of employees. This information is important to leaders within the organization because disengaged employees are often not productive, which eventually may lead to a decline in the success of the organization.

▓ LEADERSHIP ROLES FOR PHARMACY STUDENTS AND PHARMACISTS

Pharmacists and pharmacy students have unlimited opportunities to become leaders within their individual practice settings; pharmacy professional organizations on the local, state, and national levels; the overall health care profession; and their communities. Within their practice settings, leaders will make changes within their practice setting prior to other pharmacists within their immediate vicinity, such as implementing

medication therapy management (MTM) services or providing new pharmacy service in the hospital. Other professional leadership opportunities include being an officer in local, state, and/or national pharmacy organizations. Community leadership roles involve community organizations such as the Lion's Club and Rotary Club, public health initiatives, and political involvement. Students can be leaders in their student pharmacy organizations by providing services to local community organizations and providing disease-state management services such as blood pressure, cholesterol, and glucose screening to the citizens within their local communities and state. Leadership in each of these areas is important to provide effective patient care, to enhance the quality of life of patients, to advance the profession of pharmacy, to make for a healthier community and for the pharmacist's own self-worth and actualization.

▓ REVISITING THE SCENARIO

Jennifer Leader is a month away from graduation. On her last two rotations, her preceptors have modeled the qualities of an effective leader that Jennifer learned about in pharmacy school. She has talked extensively to both individuals about serving as a mentor when she graduates from pharmacy school. Her preceptors suggested that she be willing to accept a supervisory position in her selected practice setting on graduation. Several types of leadership development were recommended to enhance Jennifer's leadership skills. These include exploring the opportunities to attend a leadership development program with her future employer; becoming active in her local, state, and national organizations for the purpose of networking and building relationships with other pharmacists; identifying who administers the different leadership evaluative tools such as StrengthFinder and Myer-Briggs; and attending a pharmacy leadership program such as the American College of Clinical Pharmacy (ACCP) Academy Leadership and Management Certificate Program, University of California, San Francisco's Leadership Institute, and/or other pharmacy leadership programs. The results from the leadership evaluative instruments will help Jennifer to develop a plan to enhance her leadership skills. This will also be the beginning of a process for her to realize her goal of becoming a pharmacy leader on the state and national levels.

CONCLUSION

Pharmacists have assumed leadership roles in their practice settings, profession, and communities. However, opportunities for pharmacists to assume leadership roles within the health care profession have never been greater. This is occurring as a result of changes in the provision of health care such as medication therapy management and the invention of new technologies. Employers will be seeking pharmacists who can be leaders in this changing environment so that patients will receive the best quality of care. Leadership resources are plentiful, and many tools are available to assist individuals in developing their leadership skills. Resources are available in both print and Web-based format. Other resources include leadership development programs and evaluative tools. Recent evaluative instruments provide feedback on a pharmacist's strengths. Once an individual knows his or her strengths, the information can be used to maximize his or her strengths, resulting in greater successes. Pharmacists are encouraged to use these resources not only for their own leadership development but also to develop leadership skills in others.

QUESTIONS FOR FURTHER DISCUSSION

1. What are the challenges to becoming a leader? What characteristics of an effective leader mentioned in this chapter do you currently possess? How might you acquire or improve on some others?
2. What is the importance of developing insight into your personal leadership style?
3. Why is it important to use evaluative tools in discovering and developing your leadership style?
4. As a leader, how would you implement change within the profession and practice setting?

5. How would you develop leadership in others within your organization?
6. What role should leadership play in your organization?

REFERENCES

ACCP Academy Leadership and Management Certificate Program. 2007. Available at http://academy.accp.com/leader.asp; accessed on December 2, 2007.

Ahoy CK. 2007. *Leadership in Educational Facilities Administration.* Alexandria, VA: Association of Higher Education Facilities Officers.

Autry JA. 2001. *Servant Leadership,* pp. 20–21. Roseville, CA: Prima Publishing.

Axelrod A. 1999. *Patton on Leadership,* p. 31. Paramus, NJ: Prentice-Hall.

Barnes R, Coleman D, Cureton D, et al. 2002. *Let Your Leadership Speak: How to Lead and Be Heard.* Paxton, MA: The Future is Yours to Create! Company.

Bass B. 1985. *Leadership and Performance Beyond Expectations.* New York: Free Press.

Bennis W. 1989. *On Becoming a Leader.* Reading, MA: Addison-Wesley.

Bolman LG, Deal TE. 2003. *Reframing Organizations: Artistry, Choice, and Leadership,* 3d ed. San Francisco: Jossey-Bass.

Buckingham M. 2005. *The One Thing You Need to Know... About Great Managing, Great Leading, and Sustained Individual Success.* New York: Free Press.

Buckingham M, Clifton DO. 2001. *Now, Discover Your Strengths.* New York: Free Press.

Cashman K. 1999. *Leading from the Inside Out: Becoming a Leader for Life.* Provo, UT: Executive Excellence.

Clifton DO, Harter JK. 2003. Strengths investment. In Cameron, JE Dutton, RE Quinn (eds), *Positive Organizational Scholarship.* San Francisco: Berrett-Koehler.

Coffman C, Gonzalez-Molina G. 2002. *Follow This Path.* New York: Warner Books.

Coleman DD. 2002. On relationships. In Barnes R, Coleman D, Cureton D, et al. (eds), *Let Your Leadership Speak: How to Lead and Be Heard.* Paxton, MA: The Future is Yours to Create! Company.

Collins J. 2001. *Good to Great,* pp. 139–140. New York: HarperCollins.

Complete 360-Degree Feedback. 2007 Available at www.custominsight.com/360-degree-feedback/; accessed on November 30, 2007.

Conchie B. 2004. The seven demands of leadership: What separates good leaders from all the rest? *Gallup Manag J,* May 13, 2004.

Conger JA. 1992. *Learning to Lead: The Art of Transforming Managers into Leaders.* San Francisco: Jossey-Bass.

Conger JA, Benjamin B. 1999. *Building Leaders: How Successful Companies Develop the Next Generation.* San Francisco: Jossey-Bass.

Covey SR. 1989. *The 7 Habits of Highly Effective People,* p. 171. New York: Simon and Schuster.

Covey SR. Merrill RA, Jones D. 1998. *The Nature of Leadership.* Salt Lake City, UT: Franklin Covey Co.

Dave L. 2002. On creativity. In Barnes R, Coleman D, Cureton D, et al. (eds), *Let Your Leadership Speak: How to Lead and Be Heard.* Paxton, MA: The Future Is Yours to Create! Company.

DeBare I. 1997. "360 Degrees of Evaluation: More Companies Turning to Full Circle Job Reviews," *San Francisco Chronicle,* May 5,1997.

Denny NH. 2002. On leading with charisma. In Barnes R, Coleman D, Cureton D, et al. (eds), *Let Your Leadership Speak: How to Lead and Be Heard.* Paxton, MA: The Future is Yours to Create! Company.

Dye CF. 2000. *Leadership in Healthcare,* pp. 12, 15. Chicago: Health Administration Press.

Edwards MR, Even AJ. 1996. *360-Degree Feedback: The Powerful New Model for Employee Assessment and Performance Improvement.* New York: American Management Association.

Gallup Organization. 1999. What is a great workplace? The twelve key dimensions that describe a great workplace (part 1). *Gallup Manag J,* March 15, 1999.

Gallup University. 2007. *Demands Leadership.* Available at www.gallup.com/university/1435/Demands-Leadership.aspx; accessed on December 2, 2007.

Gallup University. 2007. *Strengths-Based Leadership Programs.* Available at www.gallup.com/university/1408/StrengthsBased-Leadership-Programs.aspx; accessed on November 30, 2007.

Giuliani RW. 2002. *Leadership,* p. xii. New York: Hyperion.

Greenleaf RK. 2002. *Servant-Leadership.* New York: Paulist Press.

Haverson R. 2002. On leading with courage. In Barnes R, Coleman D, Cureton D, et al. (eds), *Let Your Leadership Speak: How to Lead and Be Heard.* Paxton, MA: The Future is Yours to Create! Company.

Hedricks M. 2001. Play to your strengths: Skills testing and evaluation. *Entrepreneur,* May.

Hodges TD, Clifton DO. 2004. Strengths-based development in practice. In Linley PA, Joseph S (eds), *Positive Psychology in Practice.* Hoboken, NJ: Wiley.

Jones JE. 1976. A review of E. H. Porter's Strength Deployment Inventory. *Group Organ Manag* 1:121–123.

Keim WS. 2002. On becoming an ethical leader In Barnes R, Coleman D, Cureton D, et al. (eds), *Let Your Leadership Speak: How to Lead and Be Heard.* Paxton, MA: The Future is Yours to Create! Company.

Kilmann T, Kilmann RH. 1972. *Thomas Kilmann Conflict Mode Instrument.* Palo Alto, CA: CPP, Inc..

Komives SR, Lucas N, McMahon TR. 1998. *Exploring Leadership: For College Students Who Want to Make a Difference.* San Francisco: Jossey-Bass.

Kotter J. 1990. *Leadership Theories: A Force for Change—How Leadership Differs from Management.* New York: Free Press.

Kouzes JM, Posner BZ. 1987. *The Leadership Challenge,* p. 48. San Francisco: Jossey-Bass.

Kreiter R, Kinicki A. 1997. *Organizational Behavior.* New York: Irwin.

Lombardi V Jr. 2001. *What It Takes to Be #1: Vincent Lombardi on Leadership,* p. 2. New York: McGraw-Hill.

Martin J. 2002. On leading by serving. In Barnes R, Coleman D, Cureton D, et al. (eds), *Let Your Leadership Speak: How to Lead and Be Heard.* Paxton, MA: The Future Is Yours to Create! Company.

Malinchak J. 2002. On masterful networking. In Barnes R, Coleman D, Cureton D, et al. (eds), *Let Your Leadership Speak How to Lead and Be Heard.* Paxton, MA: The Future Is Yours to Create! Company.

Mason FM, Wetherbee LV. 2004. Learning to lead: An analysis of current training programs for library leadership. *Library Trends* 53:187–217.

Maxwell JC. 1988. *The 21 Irrefutable Laws of Leadership: Follow Them and People Will Follow You.* Nashville, TN: Thomas Nelson.

Maxwell JC. 2002 *The 21 Irrefutable Laws of Leadership Workbook.* Nashville, TN: Thomas Nelson.

Maxwell JC. 2003. *Developing the Leader within You.* Nashville, TN: Nelson Business.

Maxwell JC. 1995. *Developing the Leaders Around You in Three Books in One Volume.* Nashville, TN: Nelson Business.

Myer-Briggs. 2007. Available at www.myersbriggs.org/my-mbti-personality-type/mbti-basics; accessed on November 30, 2007.

Myers & Briggs Foundation. 2007. Available at www.myersbriggs.org/my-mbti-personality-type/mbti-basics; accessed on November 30, 2007.

Myers I, Briggs K. 1988. *Myers-Briggs Type Indicator.* Mountain View, CA: CPP, Inc.

Myers IB, McCaulley MH. 1985. *MBTI Manual (A Guide to the Development and Use of the Myers Briggs Type Indicator),* 3d ed. Mountain View, CA: CPP, Inc.

Nanus B. 1992. *Visionary Leadership,* p. 10. San Francisco: Jossey-Bass.

Noce DJD. 1999. Seeing theory in practice: an analysis of empathy in mediation. *Negotiation J* 15:277.

Personal Strengths Publishing. 2007. Available at www.personalstrengths.com/catalog_sdi.htm; accessed on November 30, 2007.

Porter E. 1996. *Relationship Awareness Theory.* Carlsbad, CA: Personal Strengths Publishing.

Rath T. 2007. *Now, Discover Your Strengths: Strength Finder 2.0.* New York: Gallup Press.

Scudder T. 1996. *Strength Deployment Inventory.* Carlsbad, CA: Personal Strengths Publishing.

Spears L. 2003. Introduction: Understanding the growing impact of servant-leadership. In Beazley H, Beggs J, Spears C (eds), *The Servant-Leader Within: A Transformative Path.* Mahwah, NJ: Paulist Press.

Stanley A. 2003. *The Next Generation Leader.* Sisters, OR: Multnomah Publishers.

Strength-Based Leadership Programs. 2007. Available at www.gallup.com/university/1408/StrengthsBased-Leadership-Programs.aspx; accessed on November 30, 2007.

Strength-Based Leadership Programs. 2007. *Demands on Leadership.* Available at www.gallup.com/university/1435/Demands-Leadership.aspx; accessed on November 30, 2007.

StrengthFinder Profile. 2007. Available at www.stregthsfinder.com; accessed on December 2, 2008.

10 Principles of Servant-Leadership. 2007. Available at www.butler.edu/studentlife/hampton/principles.htm; accessed on November 15, 2007.

Tichy N. 1997. *The Leadership Engine,* p. 42. New York: HarperCollins.

USCF Pharmacy Leadership Institute. 2007. Available at www.futurehealth.ucsf.edu/Program/pli/Default.aspx?tabid=235; accessed on December 2, 2007.

Watson G, Glaser E. 2000. *Watson-Glaser Critical Thinking Appraisal.* San Antonia, TX: Harcourt Brace & Co.

W. K. Kellogg Foundation Report. 2000. *Leadership Reconsidered: Engaging in Higher Education in Social Change.* Battle Creek, MI: W. K. Kellogg Foundation.

SECTION IV

MANAGING MONEY

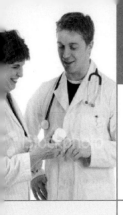

15

FINANCIAL REPORTS

Rashid Mosavin

About the Author: Dr. Mosavin is Chair of the Department of Pharmaceutical Sciences and Associate Professor in the Department of Pharmacotherapy and Outcomes Science at Loma Linda University's School of Pharmacy. Dr. Mosavin received a B.S. in Pharmacy from the University of Kansas, a Ph.D. in Pharmaceutical Sciences from the University of Wisconsin–Madison, and an MBA from the University of Chicago. Dr. Mosavin has experience in pharmaceutical industry, hospital pharmacy, and ambulatory care pharmacy settings. His research interests encompass economic evaluation of health care delivery systems and the role of pharmacists in these systems (especially as it relates to management of chronic diseases by pharmacists). Another key area of his research is analysis of economic gains achieved by health information technology implementation in ambulatory care pharmacy practice.

▮ LEARNING OBJECTIVES

After completing this chapter, students should be able to

1. Compare and contrast the fundamental objectives of a balance sheet and an income statement.
2. Demonstrate the relationship between a balance sheet and an income statement for a given fiscal year.
3. Describe the utility of financial ratios and interpret basic financial ratios used in community pharmacy practice.
4. Describe and integrate the financial information depicted in a balance sheet and an income statement in community pharmacy practice.
5. Define the flow of funds involved in community pharmacy practice, including expenses, prescription adjudication, receipt of payment, and revenue generation.
6. Describe the basic financial reports used in hospital pharmacy practice.

SCENARIO

It was a beautiful summer day when Marco and Diana met at a coffee shop near where they had gone to pharmacy school. It had been just a couple of years since they had graduated, but they had a lot to catch up on. Marco had always wanted to own a community pharmacy but was currently working in a chain community pharmacy to gain experience and save money. Diana had recently finished a cardiology fellowship and had accepted a clinical faculty position at a large teaching hospital. Diana was interested in hospital pharmacy management and was hoping eventually to be given managerial responsibilities in the pharmacy department.

Over the past 2 years, Marco and Diana had begun to gain an appreciation for the need to track the use of money. On a personal level, Marco was beginning to pay off his student loans. Not only was he successfully paying off his loans, he was actually beginning to save some money for his future. While Diana was able to defer payment on her loans during her residency and fellowship, she had to learn to manage her own money wisely given that she earned substantially less during the past 2 years than many of her friends who took pharmacist positions immediately on graduation. Both were beginning to understand that to become a successful hospital pharmacy administrator or independent pharmacy owner, one needs to also understand how money moves through an organization. Just as Marco and Diana have had to carefully track their own finances to meet their personal financial goals, tracking the use and flows of money is an essential element in operating any type of pharmacy. They hoped that if they could understand the flows of money in personal finance, they would be able to learn the financial management principles necessary to succeed as pharmacy administrators.

Marco and Diana decided to meet once a month for the next 3 months. Over the course of these meetings, they planned to learn more about accounting, financial reports, and their uses in pharmacies.

CHAPTER QUESTIONS

1. Why is it essential for pharmacy students to study the fundamentals of financial accounting?

2. Even though they may not be responsible for the organization's financial performance, why is it important for pharmacists to have a basic understanding of the financial reports in their workplace?

3. How do financial reports in hospital pharmacy practice differ in the type and scope of information they contain from the financial reports of a community pharmacy?

4. How would mastering financial reports make a pharmacist a more effective manager?

INTRODUCTION

As mathematics is the language of the physical sciences, accounting is the language of business. The American Institute of Certified Public Accountants (AICPA) defines *accounting* as "a service activity, whose function is to provide quantitative information, primarily financial in nature, about economic entities that is intended to be useful in making economic decisions." Although society may perceive accounting as a mundane task involving the endless juggling of numbers, the truth is that accounting provides the framework for critical decision-making processes essential for the success of any organization. Accounting is the dynamic process by which corporations, small businesses, and even individuals determine and report how they finance their activities and use their money. A major use of accounting is to track the flow of money (cash or credit) between financing and investing activities. Understanding financial reports is essential to understanding the flow of money. Financial reports are prepared based on standard accounting principles. Determining profitability, future growth, and tax liability are examples of the vital functions accounting plays in the day-to-day operations of any type of organization or even at the personal level.

Let's use a simple example to define a few terms fundamental to our understanding of an organization's financial health. If your goal is to operate a taxicab, you need to obtain a car. The car is an *asset*. By definition, assets are things that a business owns that can be used to generate income (e.g., driving paying passengers to their destinations in your cab). Obtaining the money needed to acquire an asset requires *financing*.

Financing for the taxi may come from a combination of personal savings, gifts, a bank loan, or even money borrowed from friends and relatives. These sources of financing can be further classified as *liabilities* (money owed to others) and *owner's equity* (the owner's own funds). Whatever the total amount invested in an asset, it always must equal the amount financed for its acquisition. If you paid $25,000 for the car, the value of your asset is recorded as $25,000. Now let's say that you financed this asset by putting up $10,000 of your own money and getting a $15,000 from your bank. In accounting language, this *investment* in the *asset* ($25,000 for the car) is financed by *owner's equity* (your $10,000) and a *liability* (the $15,000 you owe the bank).

This brings us to the most important rule in accounting, often referred to as the *accounting equation:*

$$Assets = owner's\ equity + liabilities$$

This rule always holds, whether you own a small community pharmacy or a major multinational corporation. Mastering this relatively simple equation will help you to better understand even the most complex financial concepts that arise over the course of your professional career!

▓ REVIEW OF ACCOUNTING PRINCIPLES

Accounting principles are essential tools that can be applied in all areas of pharmacy practice (Stickney, 1999). This is so because any pharmacy, just as any other type of organization, engages in three fundamental activities:

- Obtaining financing
- Making investments
- Conducting a profitable operation

Obtaining Financing

To start a business, one needs to acquire assets. Financing activities to acquire assets involve obtaining funds from owners and creditors (i.e., banks). When owners fund the activities of a corporation, they become shareholders of the corporation. Shareholders have a claim on the company's assets, and their investments in the company are rewarded by either regular distributions from the company to the owners (also known as *dividends*) or by an increase in the value of company's total assets owing to profitable operations.

Creditors, on the other hand, provide funds to the company but do not receive dividends. They require the company to repay the funds with interest over a specified period of time. This period of time can range from days from vendors that supply companies with inventory or raw materials to years from banks that grant long-term loans. There are many other types of financing, the discussion of which is beyond the scope of this chapter. Interested readers can learn more by reading *Investments* (5th edition) by Bodie, Kane, and Marcus (2007) and *Principles of Corporate Finance* (6th edition) by Brealy and Myers (2007).

Making Investments

The types of investments a company makes depend largely on the type of business it is conducting. In pharmacy settings, funds are invested in acquisition of inventory, computer software and hardware, robotics, buildings, and land. Acquiring the resources necessary to employ the appropriate number of pharmacists, pharmacy technicians, and other staff also can be viewed as an investment activity.

Conducting a Profitable Operation

We started this cycle by obtaining financing for our business. We invested those funds to acquire needed assets. Our final step is to engage in operations. Generally, the operating activities of pharmacy settings include purchasing, distribution (i.e., prescription-filling activities), clinical activities, and administration. In many pharmacies, marketing is also a significant operation activity, in that it is required so that others can learn of the goods and services that the pharmacy offers (see Chapters 21 and 22).

▓ THREE ESSENTIAL FINANCIAL STATEMENTS

Most organizations use a number of different financial statements. However, there are three types of financial statements that are essential to the operations of any organization. Before learning about these essential financial statements, though, it is important to define *fiscal year.* The fiscal year is a unit of time—a year as the term implies—that businesses use to record their financial interactions. A fiscal year can start on January 1 and end on December 31, or it can start on any other date and end 1 year later. Businesses (such as retail department stores) that experience heavy sales during the month of December usually begin their fiscal years in March or April. Businesses have to pay their taxes to the Internal Revenue Service (IRS) based on dates set by IRS rules regardless of the calendar dates of their fiscal year. IRS rules on corporate taxes are beyond the scope of this discussion, but readers can learn more by visiting the IRS Web site at www.irs.gov (United States Department of the Treasury, 2007). Click on "business" and then "corporations" to learn more about corporate tax rules and regulations.

The three financial reports that are essential to the operation of any organization are the *balance sheet,* the *income statement,* and the *statement of cash flows* (Table 15-1). Please note that several other types of financial

reports are also generated by organizations that are not discussed in this chapter. A publicly traded organization, that is an organization whose shares are traded on the stock market, is required to file with the Securities and Exchange Commission (SEC) a number of other financial reports. An example of this is Form 10-Q, which reveals the organization's quarterly financial numbers. The methodology used to prepare this and other financial reports is established by the Financial Accounting Standards Board (FASB), a nongovernmental agency dedicated to establishing standards in accounting practice.

For investor protection, Congress passed the Securities Act of 1933 and the Securities Exchange Act of 1934. These acts provided government oversight on U.S. capital to prevent the kind of fraud that had resulted in the 1929 stock market crash. In 1934, Congress established the Securities and Exchange Commission (SEC) to enforce the new laws and to provide stability for U.S. capital markets (United States Securities and Exchange Commission, 2007).

The Balance Sheet

Table 15-2 shows the balance sheet for Whole Health Partners Pharmacies (WHP). The *balance sheet* provides a snapshot of an organization's assets, liabilities, and shareholder equity at any particular point in time. While organizations generally prepare a balance sheet at the end of a fiscal year, they may prepare this statement at any point in time (e.g., at the end of a month or a quarter). As discussed in the introduction, the balance sheet's total assets must equal the total liabilities plus shareholders' equity at all times.

As of November 1, year 0, WHP had not yet started operations. However, WHP had acquired all the assets it needed to begin operations. When we examine WHP's balance sheet after 1 year of operations (year 1), we notice changes in assets, liabilities, and shareholders' equity. WHP's goal, like that of most businesses, is to increase its assets through profitable operations throughout the fiscal year. Assuming that WHP is able to keep its liabilities unchanged, an increase in assets would result in an increase in shareholders' equity, and that will make for one happy pharmacist owner!

Table 15-1.	Three Main Types of Financial Statements
Type	**Use**
Balance sheet	Snapshot of the firm's investments (assets) and how they are financed (liabilities and owner's equity)
Income statement	Connects the beginning and ending balance sheets in any given period by providing the details of operating activities (such as sales and expenses)
Statement of cash flow	Connects the beginning and ending balance sheets by indicating the impact of the company's investments, financing, and operations on cash flows

Table 15-2. Whole Health Partners Balance Sheet

November 1	Year 0 ($)	Year 1 ($)
Assets		
Current assets		
Cash	50,000	100,000
Accounts receivable	0	50,000
Inventories	200,000	300,000
Noncurrent assets		
Building	300,000	300,000
Equipment	50,000	50,000
Total assets	**600,000**	**800,000**
Liabilities		
Current liabilities		
Accounts payable to wholesalers	200,000	170,000
Salaries payable to employees	0	30,000
Noncurrent liabilities		
Bonds payable	100,000	100,000
Total liabilities	**300,000**	**300,000**
Shareholders' equity		
Common stock	300,000	300,000
Retained earnings	0	200,000
Total shareholders' equity	**300,000**	**500,000**
Total liabilities and shareholders' equity	**600,000**	**800,000**

Remember that owner's equity represent the funds that an owner puts up to start the business. WHP's balance sheet indicates that the owners started with $300,000 of their own money. At the end of year 1, the owners have increased this amount by $200,000 to $500,000 owing to profitable operations during year 1. The owners could leave this extra $200,000 of profit to be used in the business (known as *retained earnings*), or they could take some or all of the money to pay themselves (known as *dividends*).

The Income Statement

The balance sheet in Table 15-2 shows the values of assets, liabilities, and shareholders' equity, but because it is only a snapshot, it does not reveal much about what caused these values to change over the course of the year. The balance sheet also does not tell us how income was generated and what types of expenses were incurred during the accounting period.

The *income statement* is a dynamic document that provides information about money coming into an organization (*income*) and money necessary to obtain that income (*expenses*). The difference between income and expenses is commonly referred to as *net income, net profit*, or *earnings*. The income statement tells the reader what happens to an organization over a period of time. While organizations generally create income statements that span their fiscal year, they often create income statements that describe revenues, expenses, and net income over shorter periods of time, such as quarters, months, weeks, or even over a single day.

Table 15-3 shows WHP's income statement for year 1. The income statement shows all the operating activities that resulted in either revenues or expenses.

Table 15-3. Whole Health Partners Income Statement for Year 1 ($)

Revenue	
Sales—prescription	2,000,000
Sales—nonprescription	500,000
Total revenue	**2,500,000**
Expenses	
Cost of goods sold	1,800,000
Administrative expenses	350,000
Income tax expense	50,000
Total expenses	**2,200,000**
Net income	**300,000**

It also shows the net income for year 1. It is important to understand that the terms *net income* and *earnings* are used interchangeably in financial reports. You will note that the net income for year 1 is $300,000. The balance sheet (Table 15-2) shows retained earnings of $200,000. This is the portion of the net income that the owners have reinvested in the business. Where did the rest ($100,000) of the net income go? It was redistributed among owners as dividends (as depicted in Table 15-4). The connection between the net income value from the income statement and retained earnings from the balance sheet is an example of how these two reports are linked. In this particular example, the details of this linkage can be examined by the statement of retained earnings (Table 15-4).

The Statement of Cash Flows

Throughout the fiscal year, the inflows and outflows of cash are recorded in the *statement of cash flows.*

Table 15-4. Whole Health Partners Statement of Retained Earnings for Year 1 ($)

Retained earnings year 0	0
Net income year 1	300,000
Dividends distributed to shareholders	100,000
Retained earnings year 1	200,000

Table 15-5. Whole Health Partners Statement of Cash Flows for Year 1 ($)

Operating	
Revenues providing cash	2,300,000
Expenses using cash	2,110,000
Cash flow from operating	190,000
Investing	
Acquisition of noncurrent assets	40,000
Sales of noncurrent assets	0
Cash from investing	(40,000)
Financing	
Issue of bond	0
Dividends	(100,000)
Cash from financing	(100,000)
Change in cash	50,000
Cash—end of year 0	50,000
Cash—end of year 1	100,000

These recorded values generally fall into three categories: operating, investing, and financing. Table 15-5 shows WHP's statement of cash flows. It is customary in accounting to represent negative values (i.e., cash outflows) in parentheses. By the end of year 1, WHP has increased its cash by $50,000. The last line in the statement of cash flows, indicating the amount of cash available at the end of a fiscal year, is always the same as the amount of cash recorded on the balance sheet for the beginning of the following fiscal year. Once again, you should note the fluid nature of these reports and the degree to which they are linked.

■ FINANCIAL RATIOS

Organizations, investors, creditors, and even individuals use financial ratios to examine an organization's financial performance. Some financial ratios, such as net income/average total assets, provide useful information on the profitability of the organization. Other ratios can be calculated that provide insight into the liquidity of the organization (how much cash is available to pay the bills) or how well the organization is converting its accounts receivable to cash. Data are taken from the balance sheet and income statement for calculating most ratios. Although financial ratios can be used to quantify many aspects of an organization, they should not be used in isolation from other financial reports. In general, financial ratios allow users of financial information to make comparisons between

- A single organization and the entire industry average
- Differences within an organization over time (e.g., months, quarters, years)
- Two or more units with a single organization (e.g., pharmacies within the same chain)
- Two or more organizations with each other (e.g., comparisons between chain pharmacy corporations)

Financial ratio analysis is only as valid as the financial information on which it is based. If the information provided in the financial statements hasn't been independently verified (audited), the results of a financial ratio analysis are not likely to give the reader an accurate assessment of the financial performance of that organization. While financial ratio analysis can provide valuable insight to the performance of any organization, it is important that the users of financial ratios are also mindful of their limitations:

Financial ratios should be compared to a reference point (such as historical values of the same company).

When calculating financial ratios at the end of each quarter, keep in mind seasonal factors that may distort the ratio. Firms use different, accepted accounting methods to prepare their balance sheet and income statement. Therefore, it is imperative to understand how the values used in calculating the ratios were obtained.

Financial ratios are classified according to the information they provide. Table 15-6 provides a list of selected financial ratios used in various pharmacy settings. Different ratios give different pictures of the company's performance and serve different analytical needs. Profitability ratios, liquidity ratios, and turnover ratios are described below. For further discussion of other financial report ratios please refer to Stickney (1999).

Table 15-6. Financial Ratios

Name	Formula
Profitability ratios	
Gross profit margin	(Sales – cost of goods sold)/total sales
Net profit margin	Net income (after tax)/total sales
Return on assets	Net income/average total assets
Return on equity	Net income/average owner's equity
Liquidity ratios	
Current	Current assets/current liabilities
Quick	Quick assets/current liabilities
Turnover ratios	
Inventory turnover	Cost of goods sold/average inventory
Receivables turnover	Credit sales/average account receivable

Profitability Ratios

Since an inherent goal of any business is to be profitable, we can view profitability ratios as measures of overall success in the daily operations of a business. More specifically, profitability ratios provide a method to measure the overall financial success of a company. Examining profitability ratios allows managers to assess the company's level of success in generating profits. The most commonly used profitability ratios are the *gross profit margin* and the *net profit margin*.

$$\text{Gross profit margin} = (\text{sales} - \text{cost of goods sold}) \div \text{total sales}$$

By considering the cost of goods sold, this ratio provides information on the company's ability to generate gross profits. Higher gross profit margin ratios are desirable because they indicate the availability of funds for the company's other expenses.

$$\text{Net profit margin} = \text{net income (after taxes)} \div \text{total sales}$$

Net profit margin indicates the fraction of net profit that is generated for every dollar of sales. As mentioned earlier, as a profitability ratio, it could be used to determine how well the organization manages its operating expenses. It could also be used to compare the performance of two or more pharmacies within a chain or to assess the performance of a pharmacy against industry averages.

$$\text{Return on assets (ROA)} = \text{net income} \div \text{average total assets}$$

This ratio provides information on the company's ability to generate profits using the company's assets. As stated in the introduction, profits can only be generated from the company's assets. Therefore, effective use of assets results in a high ROA ratio.

$$\text{Return on equity (ROE)} = \text{net income} \div \text{average owner's equity}$$

Return on equity, also known as *return on investment* (ROI), is a measure of how well the company can make profits from funds provided by owners or investors. High ROE levels are desirable because investors—similar to companies—are interested in maximizing their profits. ROA and ROE sometimes are used to gauge the manager's performance. All else equal, managers who make better financial decisions are better able to produce higher ROA and ROE ratios for their organizations.

Liquidity Ratios

Liquidity ratios provide information on the business's ability to meet its short-term financial obligations. The most popular liquidity ratios are the *current ratio* and the *quick ratio.*

The *current ratio* is the ratio of current assets to current liabilities.

$$\text{Current ratio} = \text{current assets} \div \text{current liabilities}$$

An organization with a high current ratio is taking fewer risks in meeting its financial obligations. For ex-ample, having a lot of cash in the bank and few debts (*liabilities*) to pay results in a high value for current assets, a low value for liabilities, and therefore a high current ratio. While high current ratio values generally are considered desirable, values greater than 5.0 are considered by some to be too high. This might be a sign of a company that is too conservative, leaving too much of its money in the bank rather than investing it in ways that could help the organization grow (e.g., building new pharmacies or expanding existing services). A low current ratio (<2.0) indicates that the organization has low current assets (especially cash) relative to its current liabilities (often bills that are due in 30 to 60 days). This is not a desirable position for any organization because the inability to pay current liabilities may result in bankruptcy.

An alternative to the current ratio is the *quick ratio* (also known as the *acid test*). For this ratio, *quick assets* are defined as assets that are easily converted to cash. Therefore, inventories and prepaid expenses (such as prepaid rent and insurance policies) are not included in calculating assets. Because the quick ratio considers only assets that are easily converted to cash (and therefore can be used to pay bills, etc.), it provides a better picture of a company's liquidity and its ability to meet its financial obligations.

$$\text{Quick ratio} = (\text{current assets} - \text{inventories} - \text{prepaid expenses}) \div \text{current liabilities}$$

The standard quick ratio that any organization strives to obtain is at least 1.0. Simply put, having a quick ratio of greater than 1.0 means that the organization has more quick assets than it has current liabilities. On the other hand, having a quick ratio of less than 1.0 means that the cash that organization has on hand would not be sufficient to pay all its current liabilities, particularly its short-term bills and other obligations.

Now that we have the definition of current ratio and quick ratio, let's calculate these ratios for WHP (see Table 15-2, year 1). The current ratio at the end of year 1 is $450,000 \div $200,000 = 2.25$, which appears to be acceptable. However, the amount of quick assets on hand at the end of year 1 is only $150,000 (current assets − inventories). The resulting quick ratio is $150,000 \div $200,000 = 0.75$. One concludes from the calculation of these two ratios that WHP has a large inventory ($300,000) and may have difficulty satisfying its short-term debts. A quick ratio of less than 1 is very alarming. This example also illustrates the point that financial ratios should not be considered in isolation because a single ratio rarely will provide a comprehensive picture of the organization's financial health.

Turnover Ratios

Turnover ratios measure the efficiency with which an organization uses its assets. They are also referred to as *efficiency ratios* or *asset utilization ratios*. The two most commonly used turnover ratios are *inventory turnover* and *receivables turnover*.

$$\text{Inventory turnover ratio} = \text{cost of goods sold} \div \text{average inventory (at cost)}$$

The inventory turnover ratio measures how quickly, on average, an organization's inventories are sold. The data for this ratio come from two different financial statements. Cost of goods sold (COGS) is found on the income statement, and the average inventory comes from the balance sheet. Let's assume that a community pharmacy reported COGS of $1,200,000 for a given year and an average inventory of $100,000 over the course of that year. This results in an inventory turnover ratio of 12.0. In other words, the pharmacy is able to sell (and therefore replace) its entire inventory, on average, once a month.

Low inventory turnover ratios (6.0 or below) indicate that the organization's inventory is too large for its operations and that cash that could be better spent elsewhere is tied up in inventory. High inventory turnover ratios are generally desirable because this means that the organization was able to sell and replace its inventory with high efficiency and therefore generate higher revenues and profits. Although a high inventory turnover ratio generally is desirable, it can also result in the loss of sales and profits if the average inventory is kept too

low. Remember that one can achieve a high inventory ratio by keeping a very small inventory. As the denominator value decreases, the ratio will increase, assuming that all else is unchanged. However, the pharmacy will face chronic shortages during its daily operations that may result in patients switching to other pharmacies for better service.

$$\text{Receivables turnover ratio} = \text{credit sales} \div \text{average accounts receivable}$$

This ratio measures how quickly receivables (money owed to the organization by others) are turned into cash. A high receivable turnover ratio shows that the organization can collect its receivables efficiently while keeping the total amount it is owed by others at any given time relatively low. If you divide the receivable turnover ratio by 365, you will have a ratio known as the *average collection period*. The average collection period indicates the number of days (on average) that credit sales remain in accounts receivable before they are collected.

The receivable turnover ratio and the average collection period are particularly important in community pharmacy practice. In the 1950s and 1960s, the majority of expenditures on prescription drugs were paid by patients with cash out of their own pockets. Today, third-party payers [e.g., private insurance, Medicaid, Medicare Prescription Drug Plans (PDPs)] are responsible for paying the vast majority of these expenditures (see Chapter 16). Unlike patients, who pay their copayments at the pharmacy when they pick up their prescriptions, third-party payers often take up to 90 to 120 days before they reimburse the pharmacy for prescriptions dispensed. This lag period increases the accounts receivable and depletes the cash reserves of the pharmacy. This becomes a significant problem for independent pharmacies that do not have large cash reserves to cover their expenses (current liabilities) during this period.

Although community pharmacists pay close attention to the types of third-party payer contracts to ensure that they understand the reimbursement timetables, in many instances they are not able to influence the third-party practices. For example, being a pharmacy provider for Medicaid patients is a profitable business for many pharmacies across the nation. However, the contracted pharmacies have very little influence on reimbursement schedules set by the Centers for Medicaid and Medicare Services (CMS).

FINANCIAL REPORTS IN COMMUNITY PHARMACY PRACTICE

Financial reports used in independent pharmacy practice are very similar to those used in chain community pharmacies. Managers in chain community pharmacies pay attention to the same financial ratios and key indicators on balance sheets and income statements. It was with this knowledge that Marco and Diana decided to spend some time with WHP's owner to gain more insight into the preparation and review of financial reports in community pharmacy practice.

Almost all prescriptions filled in a community pharmacy are paid for through a third-party payer, and nearly all of them are adjudicated online. Table 15-7 shows a section of WHP's Daily Plan Payment report. As depicted in this report, the manager is able to monitor the daily number of prescriptions filled for each plan, the total amount paid by each third-party payer, the total copayments made by patients, and total cost of drug products used to dispense these prescriptions. From this information, the gross margin for each payer can be calculated (as shown in the last column). Daily inspection of this report identifies plans with low reim-

bursement rates. Additionally, when a low gross margin is detected, the manager examines the cost of prescription products dispensed to ensure that the pharmacy has received the best prices from the wholesaler. This is especially true for multisource medications (e.g., generics).

The revenues and expenses from the Daily Plan Payment report are compiled each month and entered into the income statement report (typically by the organization's accountant or bookkeeper, not by the pharmacists themselves). WHP begins its fiscal year on November 1. In addition to the yearly income statement and balance sheet, WHP's accountant prepares a monthly income statement and balance sheet to provide managers with a more precise picture of the financial status of the pharmacy. Before we examine these reports, we have to consider an important point about the preparation of the monthly income statement.

The revenues on the monthly income statement have to be revised once reimbursements have been received from third-party payers. The reason for making adjustments is that most payers make adjustments to each claim and charge the pharmacy administrative fees. Therefore, the actual amount paid to the pharmacy for prescriptions dispensed is almost always lower than the amount indicated on the Daily Plan Payment report. If the manager fails to revise the revenues, the income statement will show artificially inflated revenue. This can have a number of adverse consequences for a pharmacy, including inaccurate financial reports and higher income taxes. In other words, if the revenues are recorded from online adjudications, the pharmacy

Table 15-7. Whole Health Partners Plan Payment Report for Tuesday, January 2, 2007*

Plan ID	Plan Name	Rx's	Rf's	Total Plan Pay ($)	Copay ($)	Cost ($)	Gross Margin, (%)
AETNA	AETNA	10	32	851.03	335.30	1,010.18	15
ANTHEM	ANTHEM	7	2	1,096.65	15.00	1,014.49	9
BLCS-D	Blue Cross-D	93	119	14,155.35	432.16	15,316.89	(5)
CIGNA	CIGNA	31	10	1,290.78	562.12	1,426.73	23

*Only an excerpt of the entire plan is shown.

will pay taxes for revenues it never earned. The pharmacy generally receives the reimbursement check with an Explanation of Benefits (EOB) or Pharmacy Reconciliation Report (PRR) form. This form will show the details of the reimbursement (i.e., beneficiaries' names, prescription numbers, amounts paid for each prescription, and all adjustments and administrative fees deducted). WHP's manager points out that for every $1,000 in third-party reimbursement, the pharmacy may lose $30 to $40 in administrative and other fees. This is a 3 to 4 percent reduction in revenue that should be reconciled on the income statement.

Table 15-8 shows the balance sheet for the last 2 months of WHP's last fiscal year (September and October 2007) and the first month of the next fiscal year (November 2007). After careful examination of the information in Table 15-8, notice that the retained earnings of $825,000 in October is reduced to $798,000 in November. What has caused the retained earnings to drop by $27,000? Did the owners redistribute the funds to themselves as dividends? Table 15-9 depicts the income statement for the last 2 months and the entire 2007 fiscal year. In looking over the yearly income statement (fourth column in Table 15-9), note that WHP recorded a loss of $27,000. In November 2007, the previous year's loss was taken out of the retained earnings. Therefore, the new fiscal year began with $27,000 less in shareholders' equity. Consequently, a reduction in retained earnings on the balance sheet does not provide the reader with concrete evidence of the status of the pharmacy's financial health. Once a change in retained earnings is observed on the balance sheet, one has to further examine the income statement to get a "true" sense of the pharmacy's financial status.

Examining the income statement in Table 15-9, we observe that WHP recorded a significant loss for October 2007. In looking closely at the income and expenses for that month, note that the COGS and total expenses for the month of October are significantly higher than for the previous month. What has caused such a dramatic change in just one month? While there can be many potential reasons for such a change, remember that October is the last month of WHP's fiscal year. Pharmacies often make extra drug purchases and pay more of their expenses before ending their fiscal year. Many managers believe that spending more money at the end of a fiscal year allows them to have more cash throughout the rest of the year to use for financing and investing activities. However, keep in mind that all necessary inventory purchases and other expenses have to take place and be recorded so that the net income for the year is not artificially inflated. This is another reason why it is important to evaluate more than a single income statement or balance sheet when evaluating the financial performance of any organization.

■ FINANCIAL REPORTS IN HOSPITAL PHARMACY PRACTICE

Financial reports used to manage the department of pharmacy in hospitals are often quite different from those used in community pharmacy practice. The budget for a hospital pharmacy department consists primarily of drug costs and labor (i.e., pharmacists, technicians, and administrators) and is a part of the global budget of the entire hospital. Drug costs are generally the larger of the two components, although this varies with the size of the hospital, the size of the pharmacy department, and the types of clinical and administrative services the hospital provides.

The four management principles discussed in Chapter 2 (i.e., plan, organize, lead, and control) are relevant in the financial planning of a hospital's pharmacy department. The financial stability of the department will depend on planning and implementation of financial management programs that span these four principles.

The director of pharmacy is responsible for the creation of policies and procedures to manage expenditures. These include, but are not limited to, group purchasing, utilization review protocols, and cost-effective clinical pharmacy services (Goodwin, 1995). In their efforts to manage expenditures, hospital pharmacy directors are faced with a set of unique challenges unlike those seen in community pharmacy. While all

Table 15-8. Whole Health Partners Balance Sheet

Assets	September 2007 ($)	October 2007 ($)	November 2007 ($)
Current assets			
Petty cash	1,500	1,500	1,500
Cash in bank	105,000	133,000	75,000
Accounts receivable	680,000	658,000	776,000
Allow for doubtful accounts	(16,000)	(16,000)	(16,000)
Inventory—prescription	378,000	441,000	440,000
Inventory—other	17,000	20,000	19,000
Prepaid federal income tax	33,000	44,000	44,000
Prepaid state income tax	16,000	15,000	15,000
Total current assets	1,214,500	1,296,500	1,354,500
Noncurrent assets			
Automobiles	50,000	50,000	50,000
Machinery & equipment	130,000	130,000	130,000
Office equipment	140,000	140,000	140,000
Leasehold improvements	97,000	97,000	97,000
Accumulated depreciation	(308,000)	(310,000)	(313,000)
Total noncurrent assets	109,000	107,000	104,000
Total assets	**1,323,500**	**1,403,500**	**1,458,500**
Liabilities			
Current liabilities			
Accounts payable	223,000	393,000	369,500
Line of credit—Wells Fargo	60,000	55,000	55,000
Payroll taxes payable	0	30,000	0
Sales tax payable	500	500	1,000
Federal income tax pay—current	90,000	0	100,000
State income tax pay—current	25,000	0	35,000
Total current liabilities	398,500	478,500	560,500
Noncurrent liabilities			
Note payable	40,000	40,000	40,000
Loan payable	50,000	50,000	50,000
Total noncurrent liabilities	90,000	90,000	90,000
Total liabilities	**488,500**	**568,500**	**650,500**
Shareholders' equity			
Common stock	10,000	10,000	10,000
Retained earnings	825,000	825,000	798,000
Total shareholders' equity	**835,000**	**835,000**	**808,000**
Total liabilities and shareholders' equity	**1,323,500**	**1,403,500**	**1,458,500**

Table 15-9. Whole Health Partners Income Statement

	September 2007 ($)	October 2007 ($)	Fiscal Year 2007 ($)
Income			
Sales—current prescriptions	702,000	864,000	9,313,000
Sales—taxables	5,000	8,000	80,000
Total income	**707,000**	**872,000**	**9,393,000**
Cost of sales			
Purchases—prescriptions	623,000	920,000	7,600,000
Purchases—other	400	1,000	18,000
Purchases—supplies	0	600	2,000
Total cost of sales	**623,400**	**921,600**	**7,620,000**
Gross profit on sales	**83,600**	**(49,600)**	**1,773,000**
General & administrative expenses			
Advertising	1,400	1,500	25,000
Automobile	2,900	2,900	25,000
Bank charges	0	600	14,000
Billing services	0	4,000	26,000
Benefits	7,000	7,000	82,000
Depreciation	2,000	2,000	26,000
Dues and subscriptions	150	150	500
Interest expense	4,000	3,800	15,000
Insurance—general	400	8,000	50,000
Legal and accounting	1,000	2,500	29,000
Licenses	500	500	6,000
Maintenance and repairs	0	3,500	7,000
Meals and entertainment	1,000	2,400	22,000
Office expense	1,500	6,500	4,500
Office salaries	52,000	52,000	650,000
Officer salaries	19,000	100,000	422,000
Outside services	9,000	12,000	100,000
Postage	400	400	1,500
Pension plan expense	2,400	50,000	54,000
Promotion	400	400	1,500
Rent	8,000	8,000	95,000
Taxes—payroll	3,800	4,900	70,000
Telephone	1,900	2,600	20,000
Travel	0	0	4,000
Utilities	1,100	1,000	10,000
Total general & administrative expenses	**119,850**	**277,150**	**1,800,000**
Net income	**(36,250)**	**(326,750)**	**(27,000)**

pharmacies have experienced large increases in the costs of drug products since the 1990s (often greater than 10 percent per year), unlike community pharmacies, hospitals generally cannot pass on higher drug costs to consumers in the form of higher prices for their goods and services. Medicare and other payers often use prospective payment systems in hospitals (see Chapter 16), in which they are provided with fixed payments based on a patient's diagnosis or the number of lives they agree to provide services for over a given period of time. While community pharmacies generally can improve their profitability by selling more goods and providing more services, hospital pharmacies generally can't "sell" their goods and services because their payers are paying a set amount regardless of how many drugs the hospital dispenses or clinical services it provides. While community pharmacies generally are considered to be *profit centers,* hospital pharmacy departments are considered to be *cost centers* because they don't generate revenue directly and only help to contribute to their hospitals' overall profitability by using drug therapy and clinical pharmacy services to help lower the overall cost of caring for patients. The director of pharmacy manages the performance of this cost center by evaluating complex financial reports that compare actual to budgeted values and the variance between budgeted and actual costs.

The director of pharmacy uses an expense report prepared on a monthly or weekly basis. In this report, all pharmacy department expenses are categorized into at least five major sections. Each expense is also given a unique code so that not only the pharmacy department but also the hospital's central accounting office can access and monitor expenses. The expense report indicates the amount budgeted for each expense, the actual expense incurred, the variance between budgeted and incurred expenses, and the variance percentage. Table 15-10 shows an abbreviated, simplified expense report for the pharmacy department of a large tertiary-care hospital.

An important element of financial cost analysis in the pharmacy department is the development of productivity assessment reports. Most directors of pharmacy prepare a productivity report for each pay period

in which the number of full-time equivalents (FTEs) and the quantity of outputs (such as clinical services provided by pharmacists) are analyzed. These reports are useful because they enable managers to use historical data to create budgets and monitor trends over time.

Finally, the director of pharmacy pays special attention to external financial reports. Professional associations such as the American Hospital Association and the American Society for Health-System Pharmacists publish reports that show the national trends in pharmaceutical expenditures and labor productivity in hospitals (American Hospital Association, 2007; Hoffman et al., 2005). Pharmacy managers can gauge the efficiency of their operations by comparing their financial ratios and other indicators with national averages.

Table 15-11 depicts the hospital's total patient revenues for fiscal year 2007. It also indicates the total expenses for the pharmacy department and the percentage of revenues consumed by the department. Although not shown in this exhibit, a revenue/expense report is generated every month so that the cost center's expenses as a percentage of total revenue can be monitored closely.

CONCLUSION

Familiarity with basic accounting concepts and preparation of financial reports is essential knowledge for every pharmacist. The financial success of any organization depends on proper management of its funds. Those who understand how organizations finance operations, generate revenue, and allocate financial resources will have a easier task understanding many of the factors that affect their success.

QUESTIONS FOR FURTHER DISCUSSION

1. Marco has found two other pharmacists willing to invest in purchasing an existing community pharmacy. This pharmacy has been open for only 2 years and is located in the lobby of an ambulatory-care

Table 15-10. Department of Pharmacy Expense Report: Budgeted versus Actual

	December 2007				Fiscal Year 2007 (January–December)			
	Budget ($)	Actual ($)	Variance ($)	Variance (%)	Budget ($)	Actual ($)	Variance ($)	Variance (%)
Salaries & wages								
502050 Management wages	28,000	28,400	400	+1	300,000	280,000	−20,000	−7
502250 Pharmacists/tech wages	465,000	550,000	−85,000	+18	5,600,000	5,900,000	300,000	5
Supplies								
505600 Pharmaceuticals	2,400,000	2,058,000	342,000	−14	32,500,000	29,500,000	−3,000,000	−9
Repairs & services								
506050 Maintenance	10,000	1,000	−9,000	−90	200,000	50,000	−150,000	−75
Other expenses								
50700 Postage	50	24	−26	−52	600	500	−100	−17
508270 Copy center	500	750	250	+50	10,000	12,000	2,000	+20
Employee benefits								
503050 FICA	45,000	47,000	2,000	+47	500,000	450,000	−50,000	−10
503350 Worker's compensation insurance	20,000	72,000	52,000	+260	200,000	120,000	−80,000	−40
Investment/depreciation								
509460 Department equipment	2,000	2,400	400	+20	23,000	23,000	0	0
Total expense for cost center 8107—Department of Pharmacy	2,970,550	2,759,574	210,976	−7	39,333,600	36,335,500	−2,998,100.00	−8

Table 15-11. Hospital Cost Center Report

Department of Pharmacy—Cost Center 8107 Revenue/Expense Actuals for Fiscal Year 2007	
Inpatient revenue	$210,000,000
Outpatient revenue	$26,000,000
Total patient revenue	**$236,000,000**
Total DOP expenses (see Table 15-10)	$36,335,500
Pharmacy cost center expense as a percent of revenue	15%

clinic affiliated with a 200-bed community hospital. This year the pharmacy is projected to have sales of $2 million.

  a. To prepare for purchasing negotiations, what financial documents should Marco review? Name specific financial indicators that Marco should pay special attention to as he reviews these documents.

  b. Based on the material in this and other chapters in this book, what strategies should Marco employ to increase prescription volume, increase pharmacy revenues, and ensure the pharmacy's long-term success?

2. A few years after Marco and his associates purchase this pharmacy, the director of the affiliated hospital pharmacy retires. Marco announces this news to Diana and encourages her to apply for the position. Diana begins to update her résumé and prepare a letter of intent.

  a. What type of questions should Diana ask during an interview to gain insight into the pharmacy department's financial status? What key financial indicators should hospital administration share with Diana to convince her of the pharmacy department's financial strengths?

  b. Based on the material in this chapter and other chapters in this book, what strategies should Diana employ to ensure the pharmacy department's long-term success?

GLOSSARY

Bond A long-term debt-type of security generally issued by corporations or governments to generate cash. The *coupon rate* is the interest rate paid to the bondholder. The *maturity date* is when the face value of the bond will be paid to the bondholder.

Cost center A unit of an organization for which costs are recorded and analyzed. In general, cost centers add to the overall cost of the organization but contribute to the profits of the organization indirectly. Some examples of cost centers are customer-service centers and research and development departments.

Dividend Distribution of a portion of a company's net income to its shareholders.

Current ratio A liquidity ratio that reflects a company's ability to satisfy its short-term financial obligations.

Quick ratio A liquidity ratio that reflects a company's ability to satisfy its short-term obligations with its most liquid assets.

Inventory turnover A ratio that reflects the number of times in a fiscal year that a pharmacy's inventory is sold and replaced.

Receivables turnover A ratio that reflects a pharmacy's ability to collect its debt and extend credit to its customers.

Gross profit margin Also known as *gross margin,* this represents the amount of money left in a firm once the cost of goods sold is subtracted from revenues. It reflects the company's ability to pay for its other expenses.

Net profit margin A profitability ratio that indicates the fraction of net profit generated for every dollar of sales. It is calculated by dividing net income after taxes by total sales.

Return on assets A profitability ratio reflecting a company's ability to generate net income as a percentage of its total assets.

Return on equity A profitability ratio reflecting a company's ability to generate net income as a percentage of total investments by shareholders.

ACKNOWLEDGMENTS

First and foremost, I am indebted to my administrative assistant, Mr. David Yaeger, for his talented work in the preparation of this manuscript. I would like to thank Dr. Paul Norris, director of pharmacy at Loma Linda University Medical Center, and Dr. Robert Beeman, owner of Beeman Pharmacies in San Bernardino, CA, for their consultations. Finally, I would like to thank Emillie Hanlon and Si Khanh Nguyen, pharmacy students at Loma Linda University, for providing their perspectives and contributions.

REFERENCES

American Hospital Association. 2007. Available at www.aha.org; accessed on November 12, 2007.

Bodie Z, Kane A, Marcus A. 2007. *Investments,* 5th ed. New York: McGraw-Hill.

Brealy R, Myers S. 2007. *Principles of Corporate Finance,* 6th ed. New York: McGraw-Hill/Irwin.

Financial Accounting Standards Board. 2007. Available at www.fasb.org; accessed on November 12, 2007.

Goodwin H. 1995. ASHP guidelines: Minimum standards for pharmacies in hospitals. *Am J Health-Syst Pharm* 52:2212.

Hoffman J, Hontz K, Hunkler R, Shah N. 2005. Projecting future drug expenditures 2005. *Am J Health-Syst Pharm* 62:149.

Stickney C, Weil R. 1999. *Financial Accounting: An Introduction to Concepts, Methods, and Uses,* 9th ed. New York: Harcourt.

United States Department of the Treasury, Internal Revenue Service. 2007. Available at www.irs.gov; accessed on November 12, 2007.

United States Securities and Exchange Commission. 2007. Available at www.sec.gov; accessed on November 12, 2007.

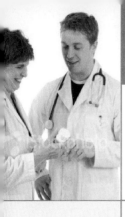

16

THIRD-PARTY PAYER CONSIDERATIONS

Julie M. Urmie

About the Author: Dr. Urmie is an Assistant Professor in the Clinical and Administrative Pharmacy Division at the University of Iowa College of Pharmacy. She received a B.S. in pharmacy from the University of Wisconsin and worked as a community pharmacist prior to returning to the University of Wisconsin for graduate school, where she received an M.S. in pharmacy administration and a Ph.D. in social and administrative sciences in pharmacy. Her teaching interests include insurance and reimbursement in pharmacy, health insurance, the U.S. health care system, and pharmacy management. Her main areas of research are prescription drug insurance and consumer preferences related to health care use.

▧ LEARNING OBJECTIVES

After completing this chapter, students should be able to

1. Discuss the history of third-party reimbursement for prescription drugs and its impact on pharmacy management.
2. Understand the basic principles of third-party reimbursement for prescription drugs and define commonly used reimbursement terminology.
3. Evaluate the financial impact of third-party reimbursement on the pharmacy using an average net profit comparison, a differential analysis, and a pro forma analysis.
4. Identify the broad range of other factors that a pharmacy manager should consider when evaluating a third-party contract.
5. Discuss issues related to third-party reimbursement for prescription drugs.

▧ SCENARIO

Marcie Hawkins, a pharmacist who was promoted recently to pharmacy manager at Good Service Pharmacy, opens her mail and sees that Better Health Insurance has sent a new contract. Better Health is the insurer for about 20 percent of the patients at Good Service Pharmacy, so Marcie is anxious to see what the new reimbursement rates will be. As Marcie reads the new contract, she is dismayed to find that the new Better Health rates are average wholesaler price (AWP) less 20 percent plus a $1.00 dispensing fee. This is a substantial decrease from the previous rate of AWP less 15 percent plus a $2.50 fee, and the new rate is among the lowest of all the third-party rates at Good Service Pharmacy. Marcie knows that signing this contract will decrease the pharmacy's profit margins, and she wonders if she should decline the contract. After all, what signal would she be sending to other insurers and pharmaceutical benefit managers (PBMs) if she accepts this low reimbursement rate? Good Service Pharmacy might become "Poor Service Pharmacy" or even go out of business if all its third-party contracts had such low rates. Then Marcie remembers Mrs. Anderson, a 78-year-old woman with Better Health Insurance who has been coming to Good Service Pharmacy for over 20 years. Marcie has spent many hours over the years talking with Mrs. Anderson about her medications, and she cannot imagine having to tell her that Good Service Pharmacy no longer accepts her insurance. Marcie also worries about the financial impact of losing 20 percent of her patients if she declines the contract. As the pharmacy manager, Marcie knows that it is her responsibility to make a decision about the contract, but as a new manager, she worries about how to make an informed decision that balances the financial needs of the pharmacy with other considerations. Marcie wonders:

1. How much would the change in reimbursement affect the net profit on an average Better Health prescription? Would the pharmacy be losing money on each Better Health prescription it dispenses?
2. Would Good Service Pharmacy be better off financially by accepting or declining the contract? How do you determine whether it is worse to accept a very low reimbursement rate or lose about 20 percent of your prescription volume?
3. What other factors need to be considered? Could the contract be renegotiated? Other than prescriptions, what other goods and services do the pharmacy's Better Health customers purchase? Just how many of the pharmacy's Better Health customers would leave if her pharmacy declines the contract, and how much business (both prescriptions and other goods and services) would they take with them.

4. Good Service Pharmacy will likely lose revenue in the future because it will get less money per prescription if it accepts the contract and will lose customers if it rejects the contract. Are there any ways for the pharmacy to make up the lost revenue? Are there any expenses that could be decreased?

OVERVIEW OF THE IMPACT OF THIRD-PARTY REIMBURSEMENT IN PHARMACY

This scenario is a common occurrence in pharmacies of all sizes and types across the country. Pharmacy managers and owners are forced to make difficult decisions about whether to accept or reject third-party plans; pharmacists and patients deal with the consequences of those decisions. A *third party* is defined as an organization that reimburses a pharmacy or patient for all or part of the patient's prescription drug costs. Since most prescriptions dispensed in pharmacies today are paid for by third parties, it is essential that pharmacy managers and pharmacists understand the effect of third parties on pharmacy operations.

Pharmacies have third-party patients and private-pay patients. Private-pay patients, sometimes referred to as *cash patients*, are people who do not have any health insurance coverage or people who have health insurance that does not cover prescription drugs. From the pharmacy's perspective, patients who pay the pharmacy directly for their prescriptions and later are reimbursed by their insurance company often are indistinguishable from private-pay patients. This type of prescription drug insurance, called *indemnity insurance*, used to be common, but it now has been replaced largely by *service benefit plans*. Under a service benefit plan, the patient may pay the pharmacy a predetermined portion of the prescription cost, but the pharmacy is reimbursed directly by the third party for most of the prescription cost.

Third parties may be public or private. Private third parties typically are insurance companies, although other private entities sometimes pay for a patient's prescriptions. For example, some pharmaceutical manufacturers provide free or discounted prescriptions through an indigent care program. Public third parties are government entities that pay for prescriptions through a government program, for example, Medicaid, Medicare Part D, or a state prescription drug assistance program for the elderly. Medicaid is the program to provide health care for the poor. The program is funded jointly by federal and state governments, with each state determining its own prescription drug reimbursement rates. Medicare, the government program that provides health insurance for the elderly and disabled, implemented a voluntary Medicare Part D outpatient prescription drug benefit in January of 2006. Medicare Part D has had a significant impact on pharmacies because many former private-pay patients now have Part D coverage. Medicare Part D is a mixed public and private third party because the government regulates the benefit, but private third parties deliver the benefit. See Chapter 17 for further description of the new Medicare drug benefit.

Many third parties hire pharmacy benefit managers (PBMs) to provide prescription claims processing and other services. Examples of third parties that hire PBMs are insurance companies, employers, Medicare prescription drug plans, and state Medicaid programs. PBMs establish pharmacy networks as part of their claims management services, so many pharmacy third-party contracts are with PBMs. Examples of other services PBMs provide include rebate negotiation with pharmaceutical manufacturers, drug benefit design, formulary development and management, drug utilization management, and disease-state/case management. Some PBMs also offer mail-order pharmacy services.

The past two decades have been a time of tremendous growth in third-party payment for prescriptions. The percentage of prescription costs reimbursed by a third party increased from 41.0 percent in 1990 to 74.6 percent in 2005 (Fig. 16-1). Most of the growth was in private third-party payment, but there has also been a slight increase in public third-party payment. Although data from 2006 currently are not available, the start of Medicare Part D likely resulted in a significant increase in the percent of third-party payment. The percent of prescriptions paid by third parties is higher than the percent of prescription drug expenditures paid by third parties. In 2006, 24 percent of prescriptions dispensed by independent pharmacies were Medicare Part D prescriptions, 15 percent were Medicaid prescriptions and 52 percent were other third party prescriptions (NCPA-Pfizer Digest, 2007).

This shift toward more third-party payment for prescription drugs has had a significant impact on pharmacy management. Pharmacies determine what price they want to charge private-pay patients, but as will be discussed in more detail later in this chapter, third

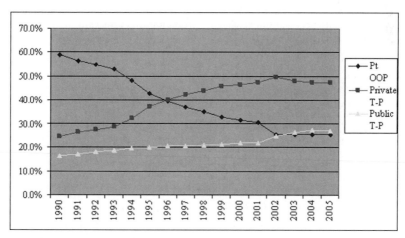

Figure 16-1. U.S. Prescription Drug Expenditures by Source of Payment, 1990–2005. Source: Data were obtained from the Centers for Medicare and Madicaid Service at http:// www.cms.hhs.gov/NationalHealthExpendData/ Note: PT OOP is direct spending by consumers for prescriptions drugs. It includes prescriptions not covered by a third party and patient cost-sharing for third party prescriptions.

parties establish the reimbursement rate that they will pay pharmacies for prescriptions. Pharmacies usually are not allowed to charge more than the established reimbursement rate, so, in practice, prescription drug prices are determined by the third party. This decreases the flexibility that pharmacy owners and managers have to price prescription drugs dispensed at their pharmacies. Owners and managers decide what third-party contracts to accept, but once the contract is accepted, the price is determined by the contract between the pharmacy and third party.

A significant concern in pharmacy is the level of reimbursement specified in these contracts. In 2000, the average third-party reimbursement for a prescription was 15 percent lower than what a patient would pay for the prescription without third-party reimbursement (USDHHS, 2000). This difference may have increased in recent years because third-party payers have continued to decrease their reimbursement rates. There also are substantial differences in reimbursement rates across third-party payers. For example, many state Medicaid programs reimburse at far better rates than private third-party payers.

Insurers and PBMs usually have pharmacy networks in which pharmacies must accept the third party's reimbursement rate in order to participate in the network. Most insurers and PBMs require that patients obtain their prescriptions from a network pharmacy, although some will let patients use nonnetwork pharmacies but require them to pay more for their prescriptions. These incentives for patients to use network pharmacies put considerable pressure on pharmacies to participate in third-party networks. There usually are many pharmacies in an area but just a few major third parties, giving each third party considerable bargaining power over the pharmacies because most pharmacies need to be in a network more than a third party needs any particular pharmacy in its network. However, there is some evidence that bargaining power varies across pharmacies (Brooks, Doucette, and Sorofman, 1999). Large chain pharmacies, as well as pharmacies that serve large geographic areas, are likely to have more bargaining power than single independent pharmacies or pharmacies that compete with many others in a small area. The pharmacy access standards that Medicare requires

for prescription drug plans participating in Part D may increase bargaining power for pharmacies located in areas with no other pharmacies. For example, if there is only one pharmacy in a rural area of Iowa, and the access standards require at least one network pharmacy in that part of Iowa, then that pharmacy should be able to negotiate better reimbursement terms.

Another concern associated with third-party prescriptions is that they generally cost more to dispense than private-pay prescriptions because of the extra steps involved in dispensing a third-party prescription (Carroll, 1991; Huey, Jackson, and Pirl, 1995; Schafermeyer et al., 1992). For third-party prescriptions, the pharmacy staff must verify patient eligibility, submit and reconcile claims, wait for payment, and comply with third-party rules and requirements, such as formularies. Dealing with third-party issues consumes an estimated 20 percent of pharmacy personnel time (NACDS, 1999). Understanding and knowing how to calculate the cost of dispensing prescriptions are important managerial tools that will be discussed in more detail later in this chapter.

Lower third-party reimbursement combined with higher third-party cost of dispensing means that average net profit is lower for third-party prescriptions than for private-pay prescriptions. This implies that pharmacy owners and managers need to evaluate carefully the financial impact of accepting third-party contracts. Tools for this evaluation are discussed later in this chapter. Pharmacy managers also need to consider many nonfinancial factors when making a third-party contract decisions, and these factors will also be discussed in this chapter.

■ THIRD-PARTY REIMBURSEMENT FOR PRESCRIPTION DRUGS

The *reimbursement rate,* or price, for a third-party prescription is based on a reimbursement-rate formula that is specified in the contract between the pharmacy and the third-party payer. The reimbursement-rate formula almost universally consists of two parts: the product cost portion and the dispensing fee. The *product cost portion* is intended to pay the pharmacy for the cost

Table 16-1. Product Cost Terminology

Actual acquisition cost (AAC)	The price that the pharmacy pays the drug wholesaler or manufacturer to obtain the drug product.
Average manufacturer price (AMP)	The average price received by a manufacturer from wholesalers for drugs distributed to the retail class of trade. This price used to be proprietary but the Deficit Reduction Act of 2005 required the Centers for Medicaid & Medicare Services (CMS) make AMPs publically available.
Average wholesaler price (AWP)	A list price for what drug wholesalers charge pharmacies. This is an overestimate of what the wholesaler actually charges the pharmacy.
Estimated acquisition cost (EAC)	The third party's estimate of what the pharmacy pays the drug wholesaler or manufacturer.
Maximum allowable cost (MAC)	The maximum cost that the third party will pay for a multisource drug. This typically is an average of the generic drug price drug from several manufacturers.
Wholesaler acquisition cost (WAC)	A list price for what pharmaceutical manufacturers charge drug wholesalers. This is an overestimate of what manufacturers actually charge wholesalers.

of the drug product, and the *dispensing fee* is intended to cover the cost of dispensing the prescription. The total reimbursement rate (product cost + dispensing fee) should be higher than the costs of obtaining and dispensing the drug to provide some profit to the pharmacy. In reality, most third-party contracts currently provide product reimbursements that are higher than the actual pharmacy cost to obtain the drug but provide dispensing fees that are less than most pharmacy's actual cost of dispensing a prescription. This tendency for higher-than-cost product reimbursements may change as third-party payers such as Medicaid move toward the average manufacturer price (AMP)-based reimbursement described later in the chapter.

Most third-party contracts state that the reimbursement rate for a prescription is the lower of two prices: (1) the price from the reimbursement-rate formula and (2) the usual and customary (U&C) pharmacy price. The U&C price, also referred to as the *cash price,* is the price that the pharmacy would charge a private-pay patient for the prescription.

Understanding the product cost portion of the reimbursement-rate formula requires an understanding of an alphabet soup of acronyms. A list of com-

monly used reimbursement terms, their acronyms, and their definitions is provided in Table 16-1. *Actual acquisition cost* (AAC) is the price that the pharmacy pays to purchase the drug product. Third parties would like to base their reimbursement on AAC but are unable to do so because the AAC is proprietary information that pharmacies do not disclose to third parties. AAC also varies across pharmacies and may change frequently, making it administratively difficult to base reimbursement on AAC. As a result, the product cost portion of the third-party reimbursement rate is an estimate of AAC and is called the *estimated acquisition cost* (EAC).

To establish EAC, most third parties use a standardized drug cost estimate that often is based on *average wholesaler price* (AWP) or *wholesaler acquisition cost* (WAC). Theoretically, AWP is the price that the wholesaler charges to pharmacies, but in reality, AWP is the *list price* rather than the actual price. Just as the sticker price for a car is an overestimate of the price someone actually pays for the car, AWP is an overestimate of the price pharmacies pay for the drug product. A government study found that pharmacies purchase brand-name drug products from the wholesalers at an average rate of AWP less 21.84 percent (OIG, 2001) and generic drugs at an average rate of AWP less 65.93 percent (OIG, 2002). AWPs are published for all drug products, so AWP represents a convenient, standardized basis for determining EAC. Third parties do not know the exact amount of discount that pharmacies receive, but they recognize that pharmacies receive some discount from AWP. As a result, the EAC used by third parties almost always is the AWP less some percentage. The percentage off of AWP has been steadily declining. For example, in the mid-1980s, product reimbursement rates were commonly in the AWP less 5 to 10 percent range, whereas by the mid-1990s, rates often were about AWP less 15 percent (AMCP, 2007). There are anecdotal reports that some Medicare prescription drug plan reimbursement rates in 2006 were around AWP less 20 percent.

Example 1: Reimbursement Formula Using AWP

AWP − 18% + $2.00 dispensing fee

An alternative way for third parties to establish EAC is to use the WAC. WAC used to be the actual price that drug wholesalers paid to pharmaceutical manufactures to purchase drug products and thus was proprietary information that was unavailable to third parties. Over the years, WAC has evolved to become an alternative list price. Wholesalers now purchase drug products at some percent off the WAC, and there are some standardized WAC lists available for use by third parties, although the information may not be as accessible as the AWP. The EAC typically will be the WAC plus a small percentage.

Example 2: Reimbursement Formula Using WAC

WAC + 3% + $2.00 dispensing fee

The EAC for generic drugs sometimes is determined differently from the EAC for brand-name drugs. AWP is a particularly inaccurate estimate of AAC for generic drugs because, as mentioned previously, pharmacies purchase generic drug products at a large discount from AWP. There also often is wide variation in the price for the same generic drug product across different generic manufacturers. One way to handle this problem is to have a separate reimbursement-rate formula for generic drugs that specifies a larger discount from AWP than for brand-name drugs.

An alternative method is to specify a *maximum allowable cost* (MAC) for each generic product. The MAC is an average cost to obtain the generic drug product. The federal government calculates and publishes a list of MACs for selected generic drug products. Some third parties use the federal MAC lists, and some establish their own MAC list. The MAC also may be used for all multisource drugs in some third-party plans. *Multisource drugs* are drug products that have at least one generic equivalent available. In this case, the MAC is the reimbursement level for both the brand-name product and the generic equivalent. The result of this type of MAC policy is that the pharmacy needs to collect the difference between the MAC and the brand-name cost from the patient if the patient requests the brand-name product.

The Deficit Reduction Act of 2005 monolated a change to an *average manufacturer price* (AMP)-based reimbursement for their multisource MAC list. AMP is defined as the average price received by a manufacturer from wholesalers for drugs distributed to the retail class of trade. The *retail class of trade* refers to entities that purchase drugs for sale to the general public. Under the final government rules on AMP, this retail class includes chain pharmacies, independent pharmacies, and mail-order pharmacies but excludes other entities such as long-term care facilities and PBMs. The change from AWP- to AMP-based generic reimbursement in the Medicaid program is expected to significantly reduce pharmacy reimbursement for generic prescription drugs dispensed under Medicaid. It is possible that other third parties also will switch to AMP-based reimbursement in the future, a trend that requires close attention by the pharmacy profession.

As mentioned previously, the dispensing fee is intended to cover the cost of dispensing a prescription. In actuality, determination of the dispensing fee is rather arbitrary, and the amount of the fee usually is lower than the actual cost of dispensing. For example, a 2007 study reported that the average cost of dispensing per prescription was $10.50 (Thornton, 2007), but dispensing fees often are in the $0.50 to $6 range, with the higher fees usually occurring in state Medicaid programs. In some cases, a higher dispensing fee will be paid for selected types of drug products (e.g., generic drugs or drugs that are on the third party's formulary). Some third parties also may pay a "bonus" dispensing fee or other incentive if the pharmacy meets specified performance goals (e.g., a targeted generic dispensing rate or formulary compliance rate). For example, assume that a third party pays a $0.50 bonus dispensing fee if the generic dispensing rate at the pharmacy for the quarter is 55 percent. If the pharmacy dispenses 6,000 of that third party's prescriptions for one quarter and 3,400 of those prescriptions were generic (a generic dispensing rate of 56.7 percent), the third party will reimburse the pharmacy retrospectively an additional $3,000 ($0.50 per prescription × 6,000).

▓ EVALUATING THE FINANCIAL IMPACT OF THIRD-PARTY REIMBURSEMENT

This section describes several ways to examine how third-party reimbursement affects a pharmacy's financial performance. Although other factors are also important and will be discussed later in this chapter, it is essential to understand the impact of different third-party plans on a pharmacy's net profit. One important step in evaluating a third-party contract is to examine the average net profit per prescription. An average net profit comparison may be used to evaluate the effect of a change in reimbursement for a particular third-party plan or to evaluate reimbursement rates across third-party plans and private-pay prescriptions. An important part of this analysis is calculating the average cost of dispensing a prescription.

Recognizing that there are many fixed costs in pharmacies, another evaluation technique that will be discussed is differential analysis. This analysis accounts for the fact that many pharmacy expenses change little as the prescription volume increases or decreases. Finally, pro forma analysis will be discussed. This analysis factors in the different volumes of prescriptions

in different third-party plans and includes elements of both the differential analysis and the average net profit comparison.

Calculating the Cost of Dispensing a Prescription

A fundamental pharmacy management tool is calculating the average cost of dispensing a prescription. The cost of dispensing includes the *fair share* of all a pharmacy's costs related to dispensing a prescription over and above the cost of the drug product. Knowing the cost of dispensing is necessary to evaluate third-party contracts, and it is also useful in tracking pharmacy expenses. Costs can be separated into two different types of costs: fixed and variable. *Fixed costs* are costs that do not change as prescription volume changes (e.g., rent, pharmacy license, and depreciation). A variation is *semifixed costs,* which only change with large changes in prescription volume. An example of a semifixed cost would be pharmacist labor costs. Pharmacists will not be hired or fired for small changes in prescription volume, but if there are large changes in prescription volume, it may be necessary to change the number of pharmacists employed by the pharmacy or reduce pharmacist hours (e.g., full time to part time). *Variable costs* are costs that change directly as prescription volume changes (e.g., prescription vials). When differential analysis is discussed, it will be necessary to identify the average variable costs of dispensing a prescription.

Another way to classify costs is direct versus indirect. *Direct costs* are costs that are completely attributable to the prescription department (e.g., the costs of prescription vials and the prescription department computer). Pharmacist labor is considered a direct expense unless the pharmacist has managerial responsibilities in nonprescription departments. *Indirect costs* are costs that are shared between the prescription department and the rest of the store. Rent, clerical labor costs, utilities, and advertising for the pharmacy are examples of indirect expenses. Methods for allocating indirect expenses to the prescription department are discussed in the example in Table 16-2.

The overall process to calculate a *cost of dispensing* (COD) is to identify the direct and indirect costs

---

Table 16-2. Calculating the Average Cost of Dispensing per Prescription

---

Step 1: Identify costs associated with the prescription department.

Labor expenses:

Labor expenses will need to be allocated between the prescription department and the rest of the pharmacy. These expenses typically are allocated based on the percent of time spent in the prescription department. Marcie Hawkins, the pharmacy manager at Good Service Pharmacy, estimates that she spends 75 percent of her time in the prescription department. Assume that the employee pharmacist and the pharmacy technicians spend 95 percent of their time in the prescription department, so 95 percent of their wages is allocated to the cost of dispensing. The other workers spend about 50 percent of their time in the prescription department. Using these percentages and the wage information contained in the notes under the Income Statement, the total amount of labor costs allocated to the prescription department is $423,165.

Direct expenses:

Some expenses are directly related to prescription drug dispensing and should be allocated 100 percent to the prescription department. For Good Service Pharmacy, the direct expenses that are listed on the Income Statement are prescription vials and the computer. The total of these direct expenses is $17,250. *Note: Other direct expenses that may appear in a pharmacy Income Statement include delivery expenses, professional liability insurance, continuing education expenses, transaction fees, and professional license fees.*

Indirect expenses:

The rest of the expenses are indirect expenses that are not obviously linked to a particular department.

Occupancy expenses such as rent, utilities, and other facility costs often are allocated using a square-footage allocation method. Under this method, costs are allocated to the prescription department using the percentage of the store square footage occupied by the prescription department. For Good Service Pharmacy, this percentage is 25.8 percent.

The typical allocation method for other indirect expenses is percent of sales. Since the prescription department generated 75.31 percent of the total sales, 75.31 percent of each of the other expenses will be allocated to the prescription department. *Note: The percent of sales allocation method also may be used for occupancy expenses. This method usually results in a higher cost of dispensing than the square-footage allocation method because prescription departments typically generate a large percentage of sales but occupy a small percentage of the store square footage.*

The total of indirect expenses allocated to the prescription department is $237,611 ($18,384 in occupancy expenses and $219,227 in other indirect expenses). All the allocation percentages and amounts are displayed in the far right columns in Fig. 16-1.

Step 2: Sum all the prescription department costs:

Labor expenses	$423,165
Direct expenses	$17,250
Indirect expenses	$237,611
Total expenses	$678,026

Step 3: Divide the prescription expenses by the number of prescriptions dispensed.

Average cost of dispensing per prescription: $678,026/56,795 = **$11.94** associated with the prescription department, allocate the fair share of indirect costs to the dispensing process, and then divide the total prescription department expenses by the number of prescription dispensed during the same time period. It often is convenient to use one year as the time frame. To calculate the COD, you will need the most recent income (revenue and expense) statement or a pro forma income statement for the pharmacy and information on the number of prescriptions dispensed during the same time period as the statement. More information on income statements is provided in Chapter 15, and pro forma income statements are discussed later in this chapter. The calculations use the income statement and other relevant information for Good Service Pharmacy that is provided

in Table 16-3. This table also contains information about the percentage of expenses allocated to the prescription department. This information will be used to illustrate part of the process of calculating a COD, but it is not typically contained in an income statement and must be calculated separately. Table 16-2 shows the process for calculating the COD for Good Service Pharmacy. It should be noted that although the COD is calculated for the entire prescription department, the COD often varies as the percentage of prescriptions paid for by private or third-party sources changes.

It is useful to know the COD for third-party prescriptions and even the COD for a specific third-party plan, but often the necessary information for these calculations is unavailable or too time-consuming to

Table 16-3. Income Statement for Good Service Pharmacy, 2007

	2007	Sales (%)	Prescription Dept. Allocation for COD	Allocation for COD (%)
Sales				
Prescription sales	3,975,650	75.31		
Other sales	1,303,475	24.69		
Total sales	5,279,125	100.00		
Cost of goods sold	4,006,856	75.90		
Gross margin	1,272,269	24.10		
Expenses				
Labor	586,286	11.11	423,165	
Rent	52,059	0.99	13,431	25.80
Utilities/other facility costs	19,196	0.36	4,953	25.80
Prescription vials/labels	9,750	0.18	9,750	100
Computer	7,500	0.14	7,500	100
Advertising	16,128	0.31	12,146	75.31
All other expenses	274,971	5.21	207,081	75.31
Total expenses	965,890	18.30		
Net profit (before taxes)	306,379	5.80		

Notes:
1. Number of prescriptions dispensed in 2007 = 56,795.
2. Prescription COGS = 76.88 percent of the total COGS.
3. Labor costs (wages plus benefits): Pharmacy manager = $125,583 (75 percent in prescription department); employee pharmacist = $115,279 (95 percent in prescription department); pharmacy technicians = $103,890 (95 percent in prescription department); and other staff = $241,534 (50 percent in prescription department).
4. The pharmacy department occupies 25.80 percent of the store square footage.

obtain. In this example, the overall average COD for Good Service Pharmacy of $11.94 per prescription is used.

Average Net Profit Comparison

The basic formula for calculating an *average net profit comparison* is included in Table 16-4. The average cost of goods sold per prescription is subtracted from the average price (for private-pay prescriptions) or average reimbursement rate to give the average gross margin. Gross margin may also be referred to as *gross profit*. The average cost of dispensing is subtracted from the gross margin to yield the average net profit per prescription. The average net profit can be calculated for all prescriptions dispensed at the pharmacy, for selected third-party plans, or for a particular third-party plan before and after a change in reimbursement. The same formula is used on an aggregate basis to conduct a pro forma analysis. Table 16-4 shows an average net profit comparison for the current and new Better Health reimbursement rates from the scenario. In this example, assume that the COD will not change and that the average COD for Better Health prescriptions is the same as for all other prescriptions. Also assume that the average cost of goods sold (COGS) will not change. When conducting an average net profit comparison across different third-party plans, the most accurate approach would be to calculate the average COGS separately for each plan because each plan may have a very different prescription drug mix. In reality, it often is assumed that the average COGS is the same to simplify the analysis. When conducting an average net profit comparison, the need for accurate COGS data must be balanced with practical constraints.

Note: In practice, it may be difficult to determine the average COGS. The information on the COGS that is provided in the computer records often is not an actual reflection of the true COGS. One way to calculate the average COGS is to examine invoices that the pharmacy receives from the wholesaler. However, the invoice price also may be somewhat inaccurate because the pharmacy may receive an extra price discount or rebate from the wholesaler at the end of the year or during some other time period if the pharmacy reaches target purchase levels.

The net profit comparison of the current and new Better Health reimbursement rates reveals that while Good Service Pharmacy is making a slim profit under the current rate, it would lose $4.92 on an average Better Health prescription if it accepted the new contract. Although this result would seem to make the decision about accepting the contract clear, this analysis is only one of several relevant financial analyses, and other factors need to be considered. It may also be useful to conduct an average net profit comparison across other third-party plans and private-pay prescriptions at Good Service Pharmacy to see how Better Health compares.

Differential Analysis

Another analysis to consider is a *differential analysis*. The net profit comparison makes it appear as if accepting the new Better Health contract would be a very bad idea because the pharmacy would lose an average of $4.92 per prescription. However, this analysis does not account for the fact that some pharmacy expenses are fixed and will not change if there is a change in prescription volume. Prescription departments almost always have a large percentage of fixed expenses, and this tendency results in economies of scale[1] because the average fixed cost per prescription decreases as the number of prescriptions increases. One example of this is pharmacist labor costs. Generally, having a prescription department requires at least one full-time pharmacist, and the average cost of dispensing will be much different if this pharmacist dispenses 20 prescriptions per day or 100 prescriptions per day.

A differential analysis compares the differential (marginal) revenue with the differential (marginal) cost of dispensing a prescription for a selected third-party plan. The differential revenue minus the differential cost is called the *contribution margin*. The differential revenue is the average gross margin, and the differential cost is the variable cost per prescription. The decision rule is to accept all third-party plans if they generate a contribution margin greater than zero. This analysis is particularly useful when deciding whether

---

[1] Economics of scale occur when the average cost per unit decreases as the number of units produced increases.

Table 16-4. Conducting an Average Net Profit Comparison

Step 1: Calculate the current average reimbursement rate.

If the total reimbursement for the Better Health prescriptions and the number of Better Health prescriptions is known then divide the total reimbursement by the number of prescriptions to obtain the average reimbursement. If either of those pieces of information is unknown then use the reimbursement rate formula to obtain an estimate of the average reimbursement. To do this, the following information is needed: (1) the average AWP for prescriptions sold in the pharmacy or (2) the average COGS and the discount from AWP that the pharmacy receives from their drug wholesaler. For this example, assume that Good Service Pharmacy purchases drugs from their wholesaler at AWP – 28% and their average prescription COGS is $54.24. Use an algebraic maneuver to calculate the average AWP from the average COGS and the purchase formula:

$$AWP - 28(AWP) = \$54.24$$
$$.72AWP = \$54.24$$
$$AWP = \$75.33$$

Now use this average AWP to determine the average reimbursement under the current reimbursement formula.

Current B.H. Formula: AWP – 15% + $2.50
average reimbursement = $75.33 – 0.15($75.33) + $2.50 = $66.53

Step 2: Calculate the new average reimbursement rate

The new average reimbursement rate is also calculated using the average AWP and the reimbursement formula.

New B.H. Formula: AWP – 20% + $1.00
average reimbursement = $75.33 – 0.20($75.33) + $2.50 = $61.26

Step 3: Calculate the Average Net Profit

Subtract the average COGS per prescription from the average reimbursement to obtain the average gross margin. Then subtract the average COD that was calculated earlier from the gross margin to obtain the net profit.

Results of a Average Net Profit Comparison

	Formula	Current B.H. Rate ($)	New B.H. Rate ($)
	Price/Reimbursement	66.53	61.26
–	Cost of Goods Sold (COGS)	54.24	54.24
=	Gross margin	12.29	7.02
–	Cost of Dispensing (COD)	11.94	11.94
=	Net Profit	0.35	–4.92

to accept a contract that would increase the prescription volume, but it also may be used to evaluate continuing with an existing plan if it is framed in terms of losing existing volume. Table 16-5 shows an example of a differential analysis for the new Better Health contract.

The contribution margin under the new Better Health contract is $5.11, suggesting that it should be accepted. The pharmacy would have some excess capacity if it did not accept the new contract, unless it could make up the prescription volume elsewhere. The differential analysis result is contrary to the result of the average net profit analysis, but the pro forma analysis will help to reconcile these opposing results.

Pro Forma Analysis

The decision about accepting a third-party contract clearly will be affected by whether 5 or 50 percent

---

Table 16-5. Conducting a Differential Analysis

Step 1: Calculate the differential revenue (average gross margin).
The marginal revenue is the average gross margin per prescription. Recall from Table 16-4 that the average gross margin under the new Better Health contract is $7.02 per prescription.

Step 2: Calculate the differential cost (average variable cost).
The differential cost is the average variable cost, and to calculate this cost, it is necessary to divide the average COD into the fixed and variable components. The most obvious variable expenses is prescription vials and labels. If the total prescription vial and label cost is divided by the number of prescriptions, the cost for the vial and label is $0.17 for each prescription. The other direct cost was the computer, but that is a fixed expense. It is assumed that the indirect expenses do not vary directly with prescription volume; for example, the rent and advertising costs will not change just because the prescription volume changes.

Determining whether the labor expenses are fixed or variable is somewhat challenging and may be different for different scenarios; that is, a 5 percent change in prescription volume will have different effects than a 50 percent change in prescription volume. For this analysis, the effect of a 20 percent decrease in prescription volume will be considered because about 20 percent of the prescriptions are from Better Health Insurance, and it is assumed that the pharmacy would lose all those prescriptions if the contract is declined. The pharmacy currently has two pharmacists, the pharmacy manager and the staff pharmacist, and pharmacy manager believes that the pharmacy needs both of them because of the number of hours the pharmacy is open. As a result, pharmacist labor will be treated as a fixed expense. The pharmacy manager believes that the pharmacy technician hours could be reduced if the prescription volume decreased, so technician labor is treated as a variable expense. Assume that the pharmacy technician labor expenses will be reduced by 20 percent if the prescription volume is reduced by 20 percent (a 1:1 ratio), so the average variable technician cost is the total prescription department technician expense divided by the number of prescriptions ($98,696/56,795). *Note: Recall that 95 percent of the technician time is allocated to the prescription department.* This equals $1.74 per prescription. There are no other variable costs other than the prescription vials and the technician labor, so the total variable cost per prescription is $1.91 ($0.17 + $1.74).

Step 3: Calculate the contribution margin.
The contribution margin is the differential revenue minus the differential cost:

$$DR - DC = \$7.02 - \$1.91 = \$5.11$$

The contribution margin is positive, suggesting that the contract should be accepted.

of the pharmacy's prescriptions are dispensed under that third-party plan. The *pro forma analysis* incorporates this important factor. A pro forma analysis is a projection of what the income statement for the pharmacy would look like both if the contract is accepted and if it is rejected. In the case of Good Service Pharmacy, if it accepts the new contract, it will maintain prescription volume and therefore have similar costs. However, it will have lower prescription revenue owing to the decreased Better Health reimbursement rate. If it declines the contract, it will have lower prescription volume, resulting in less revenue but also in lower costs. The pro forma analysis provides a comparison of the total net profit under both scenarios.

To conduct a pro forma analysis, it is necessary to construct two income statements using information from the current income statement and knowledge about the pharmacy and the third-party contract being evaluated. Information from the average net profit comparison and the differential analysis also will be needed. An example of a pro forma analysis for Good Service Pharmacy is presented in Table 16-6. The

---

Table 16-6. Conducting a Pro Forma Analysis

Step 1: Constructing the "Accept Better Health Contract" projected income statement.
The only information in the income statement that will change if the pharmacy accepts the new Better Health contract is the prescription sales. Recall that the pharmacy dispensed 56,795 prescriptions last year and that 11,359 (20 percent) of those prescriptions were Better Health. To determine the decrease in prescription sales, multiply the number of Better Health prescriptions by the average decrease in reimbursement per prescription. The average decrease in reimbursement may be obtained from the average net profit comparison in Table 16-4 ($66.53 – $61.26 = $5.27). The total decrease in prescription sales is $59,862 (11,359 × $5.27). Subtracting this amount from the current prescription sales gives the projected prescription sales of $3,915,788. The rest of the income statement can be constructed using the other information in the current income statement.
Note: It was assumed that the total prescription volume, the average COGS, and the average COD did not change. While these assumptions may be inaccurate, it is still possible to obtain an accurate comparison by using comparable assumptions for both scenarios.

Step 2: Constructing the "Decline Better Health Contract" projected income statement.
This step is somewhat more complex because several pieces of information will change. The prescription sales, COGS, and operating expenses all will decrease. To calculate the decrease in prescription sales, multiply the current Better Health average reimbursement by the number of Better Health prescriptions ($66.53 × 11,359 = $755,714) and subtract this amount from the current prescription sales to get the new prescription sales of $3,219,936.
To calculate the new COGS, multiply the average COGS by the number of Better Health prescriptions ($54.24 × 11,359 = $616,112) and subtract this amount from the current COGS ($4,006,856 – $616,112 = $3,390,744).
To calculate the new operating expenses, remember that some of the expenses are fixed. Recall from the differential analysis that the prescription vials/labels and technician labor are the variable expenses. The prescription vial/label expense will decrease by the average cost per prescription multiplied by the number of Better Health prescriptions ($0.17 × 11,359 = $1,931). The labor costs will decrease by the average technician cost per prescription (already calculated in the differential analysis) multiplied by the number of Better Health prescriptions ($1.74 × 11,359 = $19,765).
The rest of the income statement can be constructed using the other information in the current income statement.

(Continued)

Table 16-6. Conducting a Pro Forma Analysis *(Continued)*

Step 3: Compare Net Profit for the Two Projected Income Statements

The net profit under the "accept" scenario is $246,517 and the net profit under the "decline" scenario is $188,473, so the pharmacy would make $58,044 more profit if they accept the contract.

Step 4: Sensitivity analysis.

Sensitivity analysis is a very important step in doing a pro forma analysis, and it involves changing one or more of the assumptions and seeing how that change affects the results. One assumption was that the pharmacist labor costs are fixed, so an example of a sensitivity analysis would be to change this assumption. The manager estimates that if she reduced the employee pharmacist from full time to half time with limited benefits under the "Decline Better Health Scenario," the labor costs would decrease by approximately $60,000. This would increase the net profit under this scenario to $248,473, which is slightly more than the "Accept Better Health Scenario." The correct conclusion depends on whether the manager is willing to make the decision to reduce the pharmacist's hours.

Note: Other sensitivity analyses also are possible. For example, the amount of other sales and COGS could be decreased under the "Decline Better Health Scenario" to account for lower OTC sales resulting from less store traffic.

Results from the Pro Forma Analysis for Good Service Pharmacy

Sales	Original ($)	Accept Better Health ($)	Decline Better Health ($)
Prescription sales	3,975,650	3,915,788	3,219,936
Other sales	1,303,475	1,303,475	1,303,475
Total sales	5,279,125	5,219,263	4,523,411
Cost of goods sold	4,006,856	4,006,856	3,390,744
Gross margin	1,272,269	1,212,407	1,132,667
Expenses			
Labor	586,286	586,286	566,521
Rent	52,059	52,059	52,059
Utilities	19,196	19,196	19,196
Prescription vials/labels	9,750	9,750	7,819
Computer	7,500	7,500	7,500
Advertising	16,128	16,128	16,128
All other expenses	274,971	274,971	274,971
Total expenses	965,890	965,890	944,194
Net profit (before taxes)	306,379	246,517	188,473

results show that although both scenarios result in less net profit than the current situation, declining the new contract would result in $58,044 less net profit than accepting the contract. However, under the sensitivity analysis, if the manager were willing to reduce the employee pharmacist's hours to part time, declining the contract would be a slightly better scenario.

It is important to note that the pro forma analysis did not incorporate different reimbursement rates for brand-name and generic drugs. If accurate information on percent of generic drugs dispensed under a particular third-party plan is available and it is possible to calculate the different reimbursement rates and COGS for generic and brand-name drugs, it would be useful to incorporate this information into the pro forma analysis. At a minimum, if the third party used MAC reimbursement for generic drugs, pharmacy managers should consider the source of the MAC rates and their relative generosity level.

OTHER CONSIDERATIONS IN EVALUATING A THIRD-PARTY CONTRACT

Understanding the financial impact of a third-party contract clearly is important when making a decision about whether to accept or decline a third-party contract, but other factors also have a role in the decision. One factor that needs to be considered is the effect of the decision on pharmacy customers. If the decision is made to reject the contract, customers who have that third party may be forced to go elsewhere to obtain their prescriptions. This may mean angering, distressing, or inconveniencing some pharmacy customers. Many customers may not understand the pharmacy's decision and subsequently direct their anger toward the pharmacy staff. Pharmacists employed by the pharmacy also may be distressed by losing customers with whom they have established relationships.

Pharmacy image is another concern. Some pharmacies want to avoid the reputation of being a pharmacy that "does not accept many insurance plans," and this image may occur if a large third-party contract is declined. Conversely, a pharmacy may want to have an image as a high-quality service pharmacy, and accepting a contract with a low reimbursement rate may jeopardize the pharmacy's ability to provide good service. If the low reimbursement rate means that pharmacists have to dispense more prescriptions, therefore having less time for their patients, then the quality of patient care at the pharmacy may be affected.

Pharmacies also need to consider the impact of the decision on any remaining private-pay customers. If the pharmacy accepts a lower reimbursement rate contract,

it may attempt to make up the lost revenue from other sources. One source of revenue is to raise the private-pay prices, sometimes referred to as *cost shifting*. The problem with this approach is that it may result in the pharmacy being less competitive with other pharmacies, and perhaps more important, it places the burden of high prescription prices on those who may be least able to afford them. Having a good understanding of the pharmacy's competitors and customer base is necessary to determine the importance of this factor.

Another critical factor to consider is the signal that the pharmacy's decision sends to other third parties. Accepting a low reimbursement rate from one third-party may encourage other third parties to lower their rates to comparable levels. As long as pharmacies continue to accept declining rates, the third parties are likely to continue offering progressively lower rates. Conversely, declining a low reimbursement rate contract may send a signal that the pharmacy is not willing to accept poor reimbursement rates.

One last factor to consider is the effect of the decision on other sources of revenue. In the pro forma analysis it was assumed that other sales would not be affected. In reality, if prescription volume decreased by 20 percent, it is likely that other sales would decrease as well. If there is less store traffic, there likely will be fewer over-the-counter (OTC) product sales and fewer sales of other products in the pharmacy. This loss of other sales may be more important for a store where other sales are a large percentage of total sales. OTC or other sales also sometimes are used as a justification to accept a third-party contract with a low reimbursement rate. The argument is that "even though we lose money on each prescription, we will make it up with OTC sales." While prescription customers may purchase some OTC or other products, managers need to be careful with this argument because only the profit on the OTCs will help to compensate for the prescription losses. In one study, researchers found that the average OTC purchase per prescription was $1.24, but pharmacies would have needed an average OTC purchase of $11.27 per third-party prescription to compensate for accepting lower third-party reimbursement (Huey, Jackson, and Pirl, 1995).

Third-Party Contract Terminology

It is important to understand the terminology commonly used in third-party contracts. For a more thorough discussion of this issue, see Fridy, DeHart, and Monk-Tutor (2002). Basic elements of a third-party contract include provider rights and responsibilities, transmission of claims process, requirements for pharmacy participation in the third-party network, and third-party rights and responsibilities. Some common provider rights and responsibilities relate to record keeping, collecting patient copayments, complying with third-party formularies, and maintaining professional standards. The section on requirements for pharmacy participation usually is where the reimbursement rate and the timing of reimbursement are described. It also will specify the procedure for changes in the contract. Most changes in the contract occur at the request of the third party. Pharmacies certainly can request changes in a contract but often are not successful in getting the third party to accept the changes (Fridy, DeHart, and Monk-Tutor, 2002). Third-party rights and responsibilities may include the right to inspect/audit pharmacy records and the provision of help-desk support. There also may be language about the confidentiality of information and plan sponsor trademarks.

One thing to consider in a third-party contract is the length of time before the pharmacy will be reimbursed by the third party. If the third party's reimbursement cycle is longer than the pharmacy's payment cycle with its vendors, this may create a cash-flow problem for the pharmacy (see Chapter 15). The length of time before the pharmacy receives payment also will be influenced by the percentage of claims rejected or challenged by the third party. Although electronic "real time" transmission of claims makes it possible to determine at the time of dispensing whether the prescription claim will be accepted, some rejected claims still will be identified during the claim reconciliation process. Having to resubmit rejected claims to the third party or having to try to obtain payment from the patient delays payment for the prescription. One study reported that the median payment time for Medicare prescription drug plan claims was 29 days, but almost 41 percent of the December 2006 claims were not paid within 30 days (Shepherd, Richards and Winegar, 2007).

A requirement of most third-party contracts with pharmacies is that the pharmacy *accept assignment.* This clause means that the pharmacy agrees to charge the patient no more than the amount specified by the contract. In other words, a pharmacy that has accepted assignment cannot charge a third-party patient more to make up for a decrease in the third-party reimbursement rate. It is important to be careful that the assignment is confined to payment for prescription dispensing. The pharmacy manager should clarify that accepting assignment does not preclude the pharmacy from charging third-party patients for additional professional services.

Two clauses seen occasionally in pharmacy contracts are the *most favored nation clause* and the *all-products clause.* The most favored nation clause requires pharmacies to extend their lowest price or reimbursement rate to that third party. It is customary for third parties to require that the pharmacy charge the third party its U&C price if it is lower than the third party's reimbursement formula price. However, having to give the third party the lowest reimbursement rate of all the other third-party rates is not customary. The all-products clause requires pharmacies to participate in all the third party's plans if it wants to participate in one plan. A pharmacy may want to choose only some of a third party's plans depending on the reimbursement rate and number of customers affected. Some states prohibit all-products clauses. These clauses became especially problematic with the advent of discount cards and more recently with the implementation of Medicare Part D. *Discount cards* are given or sold to people who do not have insurance coverage for prescription drugs. People who have a discount card pay a price that is determined by a reimbursement formula rather than the U&C pharmacy price. As noted earlier, the reimbursement price usually is less than the pharmacy's U&C price, so pharmacies receive less revenue. Some of the discount cards are administered by PBMs and other third parties, and pharmacies may prefer not to accept a third party's discount card even if they accept patients with insurance from that third party. Pharmacies generally do not like discount cards because they lower revenue and further decrease the pharmacy's pricing flexibility.

Responding to Reductions in Third-Party Reimbursement

As was shown in the pro forma analysis, Good Service Pharmacy's net profit will decrease regardless of whether it accepts or rejects the new Better Health contract. Decreasing third-party reimbursement is a common occurrence, and pharmacies need to develop strategies to maintain their profit levels as reimbursement rates decrease. To accomplish this goal, pharmacy managers need to consider developing alternative sources of revenue or decreasing their expenses.

One source of revenue is to increase prescription volume by attracting new third-party or private-pay customers. As discussed earlier in this chapter, pharmacies tend to have a high percentage of fixed costs, so there usually are economies of scale to be achieved by dispensing more prescriptions. This strategy seems to have been used widely by pharmacies, and although it provides a short-term solution, it may not be a viable long-term strategy because the new private-pay patients may become third-party patients in the future, and the other third-party prescription reimbursement rates also likely will decline over time.

Another strategy for pharmacies to consider is diversifying their sources of revenue. A pharmacy that obtains most of its revenue from prescription drugs is more vulnerable to decreasing reimbursement rates than a pharmacy with other significant sources of revenue. One possible source of revenue is payment for pharmacist cognitive services, either from patients or from third parties. Medication therapy management (MTM) services under Medicare Part D are one opportunity in this area (see Chapters 17 and 24 through 27). It should be noted that obtaining third-party payment for pharmacist services likely will result in many of the same problems as third-party payment for prescriptions (Ganther, 2002). As long as the third-party contract does not prevent pharmacists from charging patients directly for their services, obtaining payment for pharmacist services from patients is possible for both third-party and private-pay patients. Another source of revenue is sales of items such as OTC products, durable medical equipment, and other health- or non-health-related products. Pharmacies that have the space for additional products may want to consider developing this source of revenue, but it is important to stay informed about ongoing reimbursement changes for these products, particularly in the Medicare program.

Another strategy to preserve net profit when reimbursement rates are decreased is to decrease expenses. The largest prescription department expense is labor, so labor costs are important to evaluate. The most expensive labor cost in most pharmacies is pharmacist labor, so pharmacies need to evaluate carefully how pharmacists are spending their time. Having pharmacists spend their time doing tasks that do not require a pharmacist's expertise is an inefficient use of resources. Pharmacy managers should consider using other pharmacy personnel such as pharmacy technicians and clerks to do some of the tasks associated with the dispensing of prescriptions, for example, counting tablets and reconciling third-party claims. Other pharmacy personnel costs and nonlabor costs of the pharmacy department should also be evaluated.

■ CONCLUSION AND FUTURE THIRD-PARTY REIMBURSEMENT ISSUES

What now should be apparent is that the decision to accept or reject a third-party contract often is very difficult. Even after the pharmacy manager answered the questions listed in the scenario, she still has to use her judgment about accepting the new Better Health contract with its low reimbursement rate (Table 16-7). It is important to understand and use the tools that were described in this chapter, but they do not necessarily yield an easy answer. Regardless of the manager's decision, the pharmacy faces lower net profit unless it finds other sources of revenue or decreases its expenses.

A third-party payer issue that will continue to be important is declining reimbursement rates. Private third-party reimbursement rates are likely to continue to decrease. Medicare prescription drugs plans now are

Table 16-7. Revisiting the Scenario

In the scenario described at the beginning of the chapter, the pharmacy manager at Good Service Pharmacy (Marcie Hawkins) was faced with the decision to accept or reject a new contract from Better Health Insurance. The reimbursement rates in the new contract were significantly lower than the current rates, and 20 percent of the pharmacy's prescriptions would be affected.

1. How much would the change in reimbursement affect the net profit on an average Better Health Prescription? Would they be losing money on each Better Health prescription they dispense?

The average net profit comparison showed that the average decrease in net profit from the change in reimbursement would be $5. 27. Under the new reimbursement rate, the pharmacy would lose an average of $4.92 on each Better Health Prescription it dispenses.

2. Would Good Service Pharmacy be better off financially by accepting or declining the contract? How do you determine whether it is worse to accept a very low reimbursement rate or lose about 20 percent of your prescription volume?

The results from both the differential analysis and the pro forma analysis show that Good Service Pharmacy would be better off financially by accepting the contract. Although the level of net profit in either case would be less than the current level of net profit, the pro forma analysis shows that net profit if the pharmacy accepts the contract would be $58,044 more than the net profit if it declines the contract. In this case, losing 20 percent of the pharmacy's prescription volume is worse than accepting a low reimbursement rate. The reason for this result is the high percentage of fixed costs in the prescription department. If the pharmacy was willing to make changes to reduce its fixed costs (e.g., reduce pharmacist hours), then the pharmacy might be better off declining the contract.

3. What other factors need to be considered? Could the contract be renegotiated? What effect would signing or declining the contract have on its customers?

The pharmacy manager knows that if she accepts the contract, the pharmacy risks sending a signal to other third parties that it will accept low reimbursement rates. The pharmacy may also have to raise its cash prices or decrease its level of service to decrease costs, but this may be necessary in either scenario. If she declines the contract, the pharmacy will lose long-term customers and may get a reputation for being a pharmacy that does not accept insurance plans. It may also have to reduce a pharmacist's hours. It is unlikely that the contract could be renegotiated, although Marcie could decline the contract and see how Better Health Insurance responds.

4. Good Service Pharmacy will lose revenue regardless of whether the new Better Health contract is accepted or rejected. Is there any way for Good Service Pharmacy to make up the lost revenue? Or decrease its expenses?

The pharmacy could raise cash prices to make up for the lost revenue, or it could try to attract new customers to generate new prescription volume. It also could try to generate revenue from pharmacist services or selling more products (e.g., OTC products or durable medical equipment). Its largest expenses are labor costs, so the best way to decrease its cost of dispensing would be to decrease its staffing levels.

In the end, Marcie decides to accept the new Better Health Insurance contract. The financial impact of losing 20 percent of the pharmacy's business was substantial, and she was not willing to lose Mrs. Anderson and other Better Health customers. However, she is very worried about what other third parties will do in the future and how she can make up the lost revenue. She decides that developing other sources of revenue is a better option for the pharmacy's future than reducing the pharmacy staff, so she decides to try to implement and obtain payment for some pharmacist services. This includes participating in any available Medicare Part D medication therapy management services. She also hopes to expand the pharmacy's sales of durable medical equipment.

major players in the third-party prescription drug market, and there is concern about their low reimbursement rates. There are some opportunities to obtain reimbursement for MTM services from Medicare drug plans, but these reimbursement levels also need to be evaluated by managers.

Decreasing Medicaid reimbursement rates also are an issue. Whenever states are faced with budget shortfalls or rapidly rising prescription drug costs in the Medicaid program, there is renewed pressure to decrease pharmacy reimbursement rates. The change to AMP-based reimbursement for generic prescription drugs dispensed through Medicaid is an important trend that needs to be monitored carefully. Some state Medicaid programs may increase generic drug dispensing fees or make other changes to compensate pharmacies for the lost revenue from the new AMP-based reimbursement, but they are not required to do so. Other third parties also may use the new federal AMP-based MAC list for their generic drug reimbursement, potentially broadening the impact of this change. It is also possible that third parties will start to use AMP as the basis for brand-name drug reimbursement.

It is crucial that pharmacy managers understand the impact of third-party payers on pharmacies as well as understand and use the decision-analysis tools described in this chapter to evaluate carefully third-party contracts. It also is important that pharmacy managers and owners manage expenses carefully and think creatively about developing new sources of revenue. Third-party payment for prescriptions will continue to be an important issue in pharmacy in the future, and pharmacy managers need to be aware continually of changing reimbursement levels and other third-party issues.

REFERENCES

Academy of Managed Care Pharmacy (AMCP) Task Force on Drug Payment Methodologies. 2007. *AMCP Guide to Pharmaceutical Payment Methods,* Version 1.0. Alexandria, VA: AMCP, October, 2007.

Brooks JM, Doucette WR, Sorofman BA. 1999. Factors affecting bargaining outcomes between pharmacies and insurers. *Health Serv Res* 34:439.

Caroll NV. 1991. Costs of dispensing private-pay and third-party prescriptions in independent pharmacies. *J Res Pharm Econ* 3:3.

Fridy K, DeHart RM, Monk-Tutor MR. 2002. Negotiating with third-party payers: One community pharmacy's experience. *J Am Pharm Assoc* 42:780.

Ganther JM. 2002. Third-party reimbursement for pharmacist services: Why has it been so difficult to obtain and is it really the answer for pharmacy? *J Am Pharm Assoc* 42:875.

Huey C, Jackson RA, Pirl MA. 1995. Analysis of the impact of third-party prescription programs on community pharmacy. *J Res Pharm Econ* 7:57.

National Association of Chain Drug Stores (NACDS). 1999. *Pharmacy Activity Cost and Productivity Study.* Alexandria, VA: NACDS, November, 1990.

National Association of Chain Drug Stores (NACDS). 2007. *NCPA-Pfizer Digest.* Alexandria, VA: NACDS, October.

Office of the Inspector General (OIG). 2001. Medicaid pharmacy: Actual acquisition cost of brand name prescription drug products. Report A-06-00-00023. Washington, DC: OIG, August, 2001.

Office of the Inspector General (OIG). 2002. Medicaid pharmacy: Actual acquisition cost of brand name prescription drug products. Report A-06-01-00053. Washington, DC: OIG, March, 2002.

Schafermeyer KW, Schondelmeyer SW, Thomas J, et al. 1992. Analysis of the cost of dispensing third party prescriptions in independent pharmacies. *J Res Pharm Econ* 4:3.

Schneider A, Elam L. 2002. Medicaid: Purchasing prescription drugs. Kaiser Family Foundation Report. Menlo Park, CA: Kaiser Family Foundation, January, 2002.

Shepherd MD, Richards KM, Winegar AL. 2007. Prescription drug payment times by Medicare Part D plans: Results of a national study. *J Am Pharm Assoc* 47(6): e20.

Thornton. 2007. Cost of dispensing study. Grant Thornton report commissioned by Coalition for Community Pharmacy Action. Washington, DC: Coalition for Community Pharmacy Action, January, 2007.

U.S. Department of Health and Human Services (US-DHHS). 2000. Report to the President: Prescription Drug Coverage, Spending, Utilization, and Prices. Washington, DC: Office of the Assistant Secretary for Planning and Evaluation, US Department of Health and Human Services.

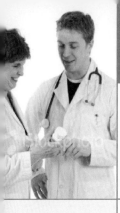

17

MEDICARE PART D

Karen B. Farris

About the Author: Dr. Farris is Associate Professor of Pharmaceutical Socioeconomics at the University of Iowa College of Pharmacy. She received a B.S. in pharmacy from the University of Tennessee, Memphis, and a Ph.D. from the University of Michigan. She serves as Vice-Chair of Post-Graduate Education in the Division of Clinical & Administrative Pharmacy and is Chair of the College's Assessment Committee. She has been a teacher and researcher in pharmacy since 1993 and taught at the University of Alberta Faculty of Pharmacy in Edmonton, Alberta, Canada, from 1993 to 2000 before returning to the United States and the University of Iowa. Her research uses social theories to examine the roles of community pharmacists, how pharmacists can influence medication use, and how older adults manage their medications. Dr. Farris has published over 70 peer-reviewed articles, professional articles, letters, and book chapters and has worked with 25 graduate students and 10 student pharmacists completing research under her direction. Her teaching for professional students focuses on the social/behavioral context of the medication use process, with particular emphasis on patient and pharmacist influences. Her graduate teaching includes health behavior models and research methods. She received the American Association of Colleges of Pharmacy Lyman Award for best published paper in the *American Journal of Pharmaceutical Education* in 2005 and was name Fellow of the American Pharmacists Association in 2006.

▮ LEARNING OBJECTIVES

After completing this chapter, students should be able to

1. Explain the variety of benefit designs in the Medicare Part D program.
2. Understand enrollment issues for Medicare beneficiaries, low-income Medicare beneficiaries, and dual-eligible beneficiaries.
3. Identify medication therapy management (MTM) opportunities available via Medicare Part D.

4. Consider management issues brought about by Medicare Part D, including stakeholder relationships and financial viability.
5. Understand new quality initiatives driven by the Centers for Medicaid and Medicare Services (CMS) and their possible impact on pharmacy operations and management.
6. Identify sources of information about Medicare Part D programs.

■ SCENARIO

Sam Bell has been the pharmacist-owner of Bell's Pharmacy, an independent pharmacy in a rural Tennessee town, for almost 45 years. Over time, he has seen his business change significantly. When he first owned the pharmacy, there was a small prescription department. Much of the pharmacy was dedicated to over-the-counter (OTC) products and gift merchandise. During the 1990s, Sam reduced the focus on gifts and placed more emphasis on dispensing prescription medications. Over the past 5 years, he has renovated the pharmacy so that over 50 percent of his floor space is devoted to dispensing and patient counseling. His pharmacy is staffed with one or two pharmacists and two or three pharmacy technicians Monday through Saturday. The pharmacy's prescription volume has grown over the past decade from 200 prescriptions per day to approximately 300 per day. He has good relationships with the physicians in town, but he does not offer value-added services such as disease-state monitoring, screenings, or vaccinations. His patients admire him and continue to support his pharmacy. In 2006, when Medicare Part D was introduced, he was concerned about the impact that additional third-party prescriptions would have on his cash flow. He determined that he would avoid accepting contracts requiring that he dispense 90-day supplies of medications because he thought this would reduce his profitability. While he receives electronic payments from most third parties, he has experienced some payment delays. He also has to manage a greater number of third-party plans now than he did in the past, increasing the administrative burden on his pharmacists and staff. While his pharmacy has remained financially viable since Medicare Part D was implemented, he has experienced lower profit margins. At the same time, his patients and the community have expressed their gratitude for his assistance during Medicare enrollment periods and for helping them better understand the issues related to the many Medicare Part D prescription drug plans.

■ CHAPTER QUESTIONS

1. Are patients at Bell's Pharmacy likely to benefit from Medicare Part D?
2. Why is Medicare Part D threatening to Bell's Pharmacy?
3. What positive things have happened to Sam Bell since Medicare Part D was implemented?
4. What management strategies can Sam Bell use to maintain the financial viability of his pharmacy?
5. What alternative revenue streams are available for Sam Bell to consider?

■ INTRODUCTION

An entire book could be written about Medicare Part D and all its intricacies. The purpose of this chapter is to consider the management issues and concerns as they relate to Medicare Part D because the preceding chapter covered the primary components and descriptions of third-party coverage. Medicare Part D, in reality, simply provides an opportunity for even more people (especially older adults) to access third-party coverage for prescription drugs. However, Medicare Part D also has provided pharmacies with new challenges (e.g., effectively eliminating the base of cash-paying customers) and opportunities (e.g., ability to bill for professional services in some instances). This chapter will begin with a review of Medicare Part D's organization and enrollment procedures. New programs arising from Part D, such as medication therapy management (MTM), will be discussed. Finally, management considerations for considering contracts and reimbursement, operations, customer relations, and development of value-added services are reviewed. Throughout this chapter, evidence from studies is presented detailing the impact of Medicare Part D on pharmacies, patients, and the health system.

■ MEDICARE PART D PROGRAMS

Medicare was established in 1965 by President Lyndon Johnson, 20 years after President Truman asked for a national health insurance plan. Medicare originally included coverage for medications provided in hospitals and doctor's offices, but not for outpatient medications that are typically dispensed in community pharmacies. At that time, there was not a large outcry to include outpatient prescription drug coverage among policymakers, health professionals, or patients because hospital care was the least predictable expense (Morgan, 2004; Oliver, Lee, and Lipton, 2004). However, in 1967, the Task Force on Prescription Drugs was established to study the impact of including prescription medicines in Medicare. Its final report in 1969 concluded that older adults would benefit from a prescription medicine insurance program in Medicare and that it would be economically feasible. Yet the recommendations in that report were not adopted at that time because the Nixon administration never acted on the recommendation that an out-of-hospital drug insurance program under Medicare should be implemented, stating instead that "we have done as much as we need to do." Instead, Congress extended eligibility for Medicare to individuals with disabilities and with end-stage renal disease in 1972 (Oliver, Lee, and Lipton, 2004).

The Medicare Catastrophic Coverage Act of 1988 was passed and included coverage for outpatient prescription medicines under Medicare Part B. Coverage was to go into effect in 1991. Owing to public campaigns led by the National Committee to Preserve Social Security and Medicare, along with a 40-group coalition of unions and grass roots organizations, many older adults became convinced that the cost of the program would outweigh the benefits because enrollment was mandatory and higher-income older adults would pay for the brunt of the program. The resulting political pressure from older adults resulted in the act being repealed by Congress in 1989 before coverage ever took place.

In 1993–1994, the Health Security Act also added outpatient prescription drugs as part of Part B, but President Clinton could not get health reform passed. It was not until the passage of the landmark Medicare Prescription Drug, Improvement and Modernization Act of 2003 (MMA) that a voluntary prescription drug benefit was added to the Medicare program (Oliver, Lee, and Lipton, 2004). The MMA also made other changes in Medicare, including improving payments to rural hospitals, renaming and expanding the managed-care plans under Medicare (*Medicare Advantage*), allowing health savings accounts for individuals with high-deductible health insurance plans, and implementing higher Part B premiums for high-income beneficiaries.

Medicare Part D is the government-sponsored prescription drug insurance program initiated in 2006. The Centers for Medicare and Medicaid Services (CMS) is the federal agency responsible for administering Medicare, Medicaid, the state children's health insurance programs (SCHIPs), and several other health-related programs. To learn more about CMS and their programs, please visit http://new.cms.hhs.gov/home/aboutcms.asp. While some CMS programs are administered primarily by the federal government (e.g., Medicare Parts A and B) and others are administered in cooperation with state governments (e.g., Medicaid and SCHIPs), the MMA required that CMS use privately owned third-party drug plans (see Chapter 16) to develop and administer Medicare Part D. In the time between passage of the MMA in 2003 and implementation of Medicare Part D in 2006, most privately owned third-party drug plans developed numerous prescrip-

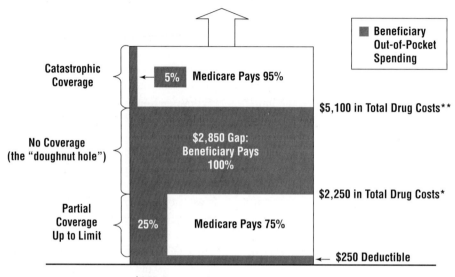

Standard Medicare Prescription Drug Benefit, 2006

Beneficiary Out-of-Pocket Spending

Catastrophic Coverage ← 5% **Medicare Pays 95%**

$5,100 in Total Drug Costs**

No Coverage (the "doughnut hole") $2,850 Gap: Beneficiary Pays 100%

$2,250 in Total Drug Costs*

Partial Coverage Up to Limit 25% **Medicare Pays 75%**

← **$250 Deductible**

$386 Average Annual Premium***

Note *Equivalent to $750 in out-of-pocket spending. **Equivalent to $3,600 in out-of-pocket spending ***Annual amount based on $32.20 national average monthly beneficiary premium (CMS, August 2006). SOURCE: Kaiser Family foundation illustration of standard Medicare drug benefit decribed in the Medicare Modernization Act of 2003.

Figure 17-1. Standard medicare prescription drug benefit for 2006. (From the Medicare Prescription Drug Benefit - An Updated Fact Sheet (#7044-04), The Henry J. Kaiser Family Foundation, June 2006.) Source: http://www.kff.org/medicare/medicarebenefitataglance.cfm, accessed on June 19, 2008.

tion drugs plans (PDPs), thus giving Medicare beneficiaries who voluntarily enroll many choices among drug plans that fit their needs. Beneficiaries also may elect to purchase Medicare Advantage (MA-PD) plans, which provide all Medicare-covered services including drugs.

The MMA defined a standard drug insurance benefit. This standard benefit represents the minimum level of service that any PDP must provide. The standard benefit has the characteristics described below and in Fig. 17-1. Note how the benefit has changed in just two short years because the numbers for 2008 are also included below (Kaiser Family Foundation, 2006a, 2006b).

- Beneficiaries pay an annual premium. The average premium was $386 in 2006 and $304 in 2008.

- Beneficiaries pay 100 percent of drug costs until covered drugs costs reach an initial deductible. The deductible was $250 in 2006 and $275 in 2008.
- After the initial deductible is met, plans pay 75 percent and beneficiaries pay 25 percent of covered drug costs until beneficiaries' costs meet the initial coverage limit. The initial coverage limit was $2,250 in 2006 and $2,510 in 2008.
- Beneficiaries then pay 100 percent of drug costs above the initial coverage limit until the catastrophic or total drug cost threshold is met. The total drug cost threshold was $5,100 in 2006 and $5,726 in 2008. This lack of coverage between the initial coverage limit and the total drug cost threshold is commonly called the *donut hole* or *coverage gap*.
- After the total drug cost threshold is met, beneficiaries pay the greater of 5 percent coinsurance or

copayments of $2.25 per generic drug and $5.60 per brand-name drug and plans pay the remainder of drug costs. When Part D began in 2006, the copayments were $2.15 per generic drug and $5.35 per brand-name drug.

In practice, most prescription drug benefit plans available to Part D enrollees are not exactly like the standard benefit just described. Rather, plans may provide *actuarially equivalent* standard coverage, meaning that two or more plans have payment streams with the same present value based on appropriate actuarial assumptions. In layperson's terms, this means that any plan not exactly like the standard plan must use a two-prong test to show that it has a "value of which is at least equal to the value of the coverage the same beneficiaries would receive under the defined standard prescription drug coverage." The first test is the *gross value test,* "where the expected amount of paid claims for Medicare beneficiaries under the sponsor's alternative basic plan must be at least equal to the expected amount of paid claims for the same beneficiaries under the defined standard prescription drug coverage, including catastrophic coverage available when an individual's out-of-pocket expenses exceed a specified threshold." The second test is the *net value test,* in which "the net value of the sponsor's alternative basic plan must be at least equal to the net value of the defined standard prescription drug coverage," where net value of a plan is calculated by subtracting the retiree premium from the gross value of the plan (CMS, 2005).

To complicate matters a bit more, plans may also offer basic alternative coverage or enhanced alternative coverage. *Basic alternative coverage* is alternative prescription drug coverage that is actuarially equivalent to defined standard prescription drug coverage, whereas *enhanced plans* are prescription drug plans whose value exceeds the defined standard coverage. Importantly, when plans are alternative, then the Part D sponsors must use the defined standard coverage (and not the actuarially equivalent standard coverage) as a point of comparison (Kaiser Family Foundtion, 2007b).

Because plans do not have to look like the standard benefit, they vary in their monthly premiums, initial deductibles, copays or coinsurance, coverage gap, catastrophic threshold, and formulary design. In actuality, there has been a great deal of variability in the PDPs available to beneficiaries. In 2006, 17 percent of plans provided the standard benefit, 52 percent were actuarially equivalent, and 30 percent had an enhanced benefit (Cubanski and Neuman, 2006). According to the Kaiser Family Foundation, there were 1,429 standalone PDPs available nationwide in in 2006. The majority of PDPs had monthly premiums of between $20 and $50. The majority of PDPs nationwide (60 percent) have no deductible. Among the 10 PDPs with the highest enrollment in 2006, representing 66 percent of all enrollees in PDPs, most used tier coverage. However, most plans (71 percent of PDPs) did not provide any gap coverage. Among PDPs, the number offering an enhanced benefit was 42 percent in 2006. For these enhanced benefits, 89 percent of all enrollees had no gap coverage, whereas 8 percent had generic-only medications for gap coverage and 4 percent had brand-name and generic coverage in the gap (Hoadley et al., 2006).

In 2007, there were 1,875 standalone PDPs available nationwide. Many plans had premium increases from 2006, and more plans offered gap coverage to provide prescription drug coverage in the donut hole. In 2007, "the average unweighted monthly premiums for PDPs without gap coverage was $30.17, $51.11 for plans with gap coverage for generics, and $93.46 for plans with gap coverage including brand-name drugs." Among PDPs, the number offering an enhanced benefit increased to 47 percent in 2007 (Hoadley et al., 2006).

Specific comparisons may help to explain the variety of options available to enrollees. In 2007, there were three American Association of Retired Persons (AARP)-associated plans: Medicare Rx had an average monthly premium of $27.83, Medicare Rx Saver had a premium of $17.83, and Medicare Rx Enhanced had a premium of $46.30 (Hoadley et al., 2006). Humana also had three plans with premiums of $15.17, $22.03, or $80.43 for standard, enhanced, and complete coverage, respectively. As well as variation in premiums, there also was variation in other benefit cost-sharing characteristics, such as copays and tiered medications.

For example, in Maryland, enrollees in AARP Medicare Rx had a $6.00 copay on tier 1 medications, $28.00 on tier 2 medications, $69.10 on tier 3 medications, and a 33 percent copay on specialty-tier medications. The fact that all plans do not look alike provides a competitive environment where enrollees are required to weigh aspects of plans such as premiums, copays, coverage gap, and formulary considerations to determine which plan best suits their needs. In addition, some plans are available within specific Medicare regions, and some plans are available at a national level. While the specific plan characteristics and availability may change from year to year, these data show that actuarially equivalent plans are the norm. Again, this feature of Medicare Part D allows plan sponsors to differentiate their benefit plans and then market them to specific components of the older adult market (e.g., higher-income older adults may be targeted to receive information about enhanced-benefit plans). In summary, most beneficiaries can choose from among at least 50 stand-alone PDPs and multiple MA-PD plans (Hoadley et al., 2006).

Recall that enhanced plans are those whose value exceeds the defined standard coverage. Typically, these plans may offer lower deductibles, reduced coinsurance or copayments, and/or reductions in cost sharing in the donut hole, also known as *providing gap coverage.* For example, there were 12 PDPs in 2007 with premiums exceeding $100 per month, and all these PDPs were among the 27 PDPs that offered full coverage of on-formulary drugs in the coverage gap (Hoadley et al., 2006).

For low-income individuals, Medicare Part D appears to have been especially helpful. Individuals may receive low-income subsidies (LISs) to enroll into a prescription drug plan. As of 2007, individuals who exceed Medicaid eligibility but have incomes below 135 percent of poverty and resources below $6,120 per individual or $9,190 per couple pay no monthly premiums, no deductible, and copayments of $2.15 for generics and $5.35 for brand-name drugs. There is no coverage gap, and they do not need to make copayments after they have reached $3,850 out-of-pocket drug expenditures. Individuals with incomes below 150 percent of poverty and resources below $10,210 per individual

also are eligible to participate with lower premiums and deductibles than the standard benefit (Kaiser Family Foundation, 2007a). While these specific numbers may change in the future, they illustrate the benefit characteristics and cost-sharing opportunities for individuals meeting specific income requirements. While low-income subsidies are available, it has been a challenge to increase awareness of the subsidies among those who are eligible. Up to 48 percent of individuals with incomes at or below 150 percent of poverty who were not receiving the low-income subsidy were not aware that they could obtain a subsidy (Neuman et al., 2007).

Medicare-eligible individuals may enroll in prescription drug plans when they first become eligible for Medicare (±3 months of turning age 65 years). Individuals with disabilities may enroll ± 3 months after the twenty-fifth month of cash disability payments. To decrease the impact of adverse selection (i.e., a higher tendency to enroll among beneficiaries who are older and use more drugs combined with a lower tendency to enroll among those who are younger and use fewer drugs), individuals who do not enroll in a Part D drug plan when they first become eligible are penalized if they attempt to enroll at a later date. These penalties are typically a 1 percent increase in the monthly premium for each month they delay enrollment. Low-income beneficiaries, including those designated as having dual eligibility for Medicare and Medicaid, may be enrolled automatically by CMS or its Part D partners in a plan with a no premium and can later switch to another plan of their own choice. Medicare-eligible individuals also can opt to keep any current prescription drug coverage that they currently have offered through their employer, Veterans Administration, or other health plan.

At the end of February 2006, the U.S. Department of Health and Human Services indicated that just over 43 million Medicare-eligible individuals had access to prescription drug coverage under Part D (Kaiser Family Foundation, 2006c). In early 2007, coverage from Part D was provided to 23.9 million individuals (Fig. 17-2), with 15.2 million (35 percent of Medicare-eligible beneficiaries) retaining their employee/union, VA, or other coverage. An estimated 4 million beneficiaries had no prescription drug coverage (Table 17-1) (Kaiser Family Foundation, 2006c).

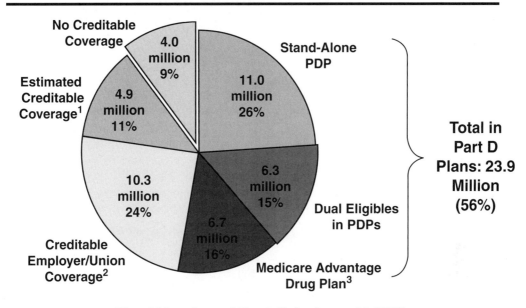

HHS Estimates of Prescription Drug Coverage Sources Among Medicare Beneficiaries, as of January 2007

No Creditable Coverage — 4.0 million 9%

Estimated Creditable Coverage[1] — 4.9 million 11%

Stand-Alone PDP — 11.0 million 26%

Dual Eligibles in PDPs — 6.3 million 15%

Medicare Advantage Drug Plan[3] — 6.7 million 16%

Creditable Employer/Union Coverage[2] — 10.3 million 24%

Total in Part D Plans: 23.9 Million (56%)

Total Number of Beneficiaries = 43 Milliom

SOURCE: HHS, January 30, 2007. Data as of January 16, 2007.

Figure 17-2. Extent of prescription drug insurance coverage among medicare beneficiaries. (The Medicare Prescription Drug Benefit - An Updated Fact Sheet (#7044-07), The Henry J. Kaiser Family Foundation, October 2007.) Source: http://www.kff.org/medicare/medicarebenefitataglance.cfm, accessed on June 19, 2008.

Early evidence suggests that Medicare Part D is working well for beneficiaries. For example, access to medications appears to be adequate. While there are many plans, and each plan may have different formularies, an analysis comparing plans available in California and Hawaii showed that among eight treatment categories that are used most commonly by older adults in the National Ambulatory Medical Care Survey, seven of the eight classes had one "widely covered" medication. A widely covered medication was one with a co-payment of $35 or less. Coverage for the studied drugs ranged from 7 to 100 percent of the formularies and averaged 69 percent across all drugs. The percentage of formularies covering each drug (averaged across all drugs in the class) was highest for thiazide diuretics (90

percent), followed by beta blockers (85 percent), selective serotonin reuptake inhibitors (69 percent), calcium channel blockers (66 percent), angiotensin-converting enzyme (ACE) inhibitors (66 percent), statins (49 percent), and angiotensin receptor blocker (ARB) (39 percent).

In terms of costs, it also seems that Medicare Part D has helped beneficiaries (Tseng et al., 2007). The prescription drug costs for 472 patients with atrial fibrillation were compared for one AARP plan, the Part D standard benefit plan, and no prescription drug coverage. Total prescription drug costs were lowest under the AARP plan. The primary concern raised by some beneficiaries relates to the coverage gap. Another study found that while 27 to 46 percent of patients entered

Table 17-1. Distribution of Seniors by Primary Source of Drug Coverage, 2006

	Part D	Employer	VA	Other	None
Raw N	8,777	4,236	452	1,170	1,437
Total	50.2%.	30.8%	3.1%	7.5%	8.5%
Age (years)					
65–74[a]	50.4	33.6	2.5	6.3	7.2
75–34	49.8	29.5**	3.9**	8**	8.9**
85+	50.6	22.4**	3.1	10.9**	12.9**
Sex					
Male[a]	44.9	34.5	6.8	5.8	7.9
Female	53.9**	28.2**	0.5**	8.6**	8.8
Urban/rural location					
Urban[a]	50.1	32.0	2.7	7.3	7.9
Rural	50.6	27.1**	4.2**	7.8	10.3**
Race/ethnicity					
White[a]	48.4	32.5	3.4	7.8	3.0
African American	61.7**	21.4**	1.4**	3.9**	11.6**
Nonwhite Hispanic	66.1**	16.8**	1.2**	5.8	10.1
Asian	54.3	26.6	0.7**	5.1	13.3
Other	47.7	28.4	0.5**	12.5	11.0
Education					
Less than high school	63.1**	15.5**	2.9	6.6	11.8**
High school graduate	48.9**	31.1**	3.4	8.3	8.2**
Some college or more[a]	44.6	39.0	2.9	7.1	6.4
Poverty level					
≤100%	74.1**	4.7**	1.9**	5.6**	13.7**
101–150%	63**	13.4**	2.9	9.8**	10.9**
151–200%	54**	25.4**	5.4**	7.5	7.6
>200%[a]	39.7	43.5	3.0	7.1	6.6
Chronic conditions					
None[a]	40.5	26.7	1.8	7.9	23.1
1 or 2	50**	33.2**	2.8**	7.1	6.9**
3 or more	54**	29.6**	3.9**	7.7	4.8**
Number or prescriptions					
None[a]	41.6	26.5	2.0	7.8	22.2
1 or 2	49.6**	30.7**	2.0	7.7	10**
3 or 4	52.6**	30.1**	3.0	8.3	6**
5 or 6	50.1**	33**	3.9**	7.1	5.9**
7 or more	53.2**	32.4**	4.1**	6.5	3.9**
Drug coverage, 2005					
None[a]	60.7	7.4	4.6	7.1	20.2
Any	45.5**	43.6**	2.4**	7.4	1.1**

Source: Neuman et al., 2007, p. w633.

Notes: Weighted percentages: nonweighted Ns. Characteristics in rows add to 100 percent. "Other coverage" includes respondents who said that they have drug coverage and said yes to having other programs or insurance that pay to their prescription medicines; it includes respondents who confirmed that they had drug coverage but did not indicate the source. VA is Department of Veterans Affairs.

[a]Reference group.

**p <0.05.

the coverage gap in the AARP plans, only 3 to 11 percent exited the coverage gap to receive catastrophic coverage (Evans-Molina et al., 2007). While access to needed medications appears to have improved with Medicare Part D, it has been estimated that 20 percent of individuals taking at least one prescription drug still report that they did not fill or delayed filling a prescription owing to cost (Neuman et al., 2007).

From the perspective of pharmacies, Medicare Part D has created a number of concerns. No nationwide survey of pharmacists has been conducted since June 2006; thus it is difficult to understand the full impact of Medicare Part D on pharmacies. Pharmacists reported that their cash-paying customer base was greatly diminished. Pharmacists mentioned that the administrative burden of managing so many insurance plans had increased. Pharmacies found it particularly burdensome to manage individuals with dual eligibility in Medicare and Medicaid. All Medicaid patients were switched to Medicare plans, often by CMS, and the eligibility and payment delays were significant (often 5 or more weeks)(Kaiser Family Foundation, 2006a; General Accounting Office, 2007).

Anecdotally, there have been reports of pharmacy closings, late payments, increased administrative burden, and loss of patients. One survey of 22 rural pharmacy owners recently summarized their experiences. Among these pharmacy owners, four had accepted all PDP contracts, but others were more selective in which contracts they signed. The pharmacy owners expressed concern about the low reimbursements by some plans and that signing such contracts would risk financial viability. For example, the best reimbursement rate reported by these pharmacy owners was average wholesale price (AWP) less 10 percent to a low of AWP less 30 percent. Dispensing fees ranged from $1.00 to $4.00 with a median of $1.75 (Radford et al., 2007).

In summary, MMA and Medicare Part D represent the single greatest policy change to affect pharmacy in the past 20 years, since the Omnibus Budget Reconciliation Act of 1990 and its counseling requirements. Medicare Part D has resulted in a majority of patients receiving prescription drugs now having prescription drug insurance to pay for their drugs. This has improved access for older adults, particularly low-income individuals. However, its impact on pharmacy and pharmacy access (not pharmaceutical access) owing to financial viability remains unclear. Pharmacies where prescriptions drugs are the primary source of revenue, such as rural independent pharmacies, may be particularly vulnerable to this significant health policy change.

MEDICATION THERAPY MANAGEMENT

One aspect of MMA and Medicare Part D that is positive for enrollees and pharmacy is the introduction of medication therapy management (MTM). MTM is a quality improvement activity required by CMS of the contracting plan sponsors that provide the Part D prescription drug insurance for individuals who are considered "high users" of Medicare services (i.e., beneficiaries with multiple chronic conditions, using multiple chronic medications, and with drug costs exceeding $4,000 in 2006). Generally, the goals of MTM are to enhance understanding of medications, improve medication adherence, and reduce adverse drug events. For example, pharmacists are being reimbursed for comprehensive medication reviews so that they can identify ways that medication therapy can be improved. Pharmacists also may be prompted by MTM plans and reimbursed for specific interventions such as discontinuing use of high-risk medications and identifying and improving medication adherence (Mirixa Clinical Solutions, 2007; Outcomes MTM System, 2007; Outcomes Medicare Plans, 2007).

From pharmacy's perspective, MTM is a set of services provided by pharmacists to improve outcomes from medications (Table 17-2). A positive aspect of the MMA is that pharmacists were named as one provider of MTM, and this has provided pharmacists with a long-sought opportunity to bill some insurance plans for their clinical services. At the same time, the plan sponsors, not Medicare, were given full control over what MTM services actually entail, who can provide the services, and how they will be reimbursed. What remains problematic for pharmacists is that the

Table 17-2. Medication Therapy Management Services Definition and Program Criteria

Medication Therapy Management is a distinct service or group of services that optimize therapeutic outcomes for individual patients. Medication Therapy Management Services are independent of, but can occur in conjunction with, the provision of a medication product.

Medication Therapy Management encompasses a broad range of professional activities and responsibilities within the licensed pharmacist's, or other qualified health care provider's, scope of practice. These services include but are not limited to the following, according to the individual needs of the patient:

a. Performing or obtaining necessary assessments of the patient's health status;

b. Formulating a medication treatment plan;

c. Selecting, initiating, modifying, or administering medication therapy;

d. Monitoring and evaluating the patient's response to therapy, including safety and effectiveness;

e. Performing a comprehensive medication review to identify, resolve, and prevent medication-related problems, including adverse drug events;

f. Documenting the care delivered and communicating essential information to the patient's other primary care providers;

g. Providing verbal education and training designed to enhance patient understanding and appropriate use of his/her medications;

h. Providing information, support services and resources designed to enhance patient adherence with his/her therapeutic regimens;

i. Coordinating and integrating medication therapy management services within the broader health care-management services being provided to the patient.

A program that provides coverage for Medication Therapy Management Services shall include:

a. Patient-specific and individualized services or sets of services provided directly by a pharmacist to the patient*. These services are distinct from formulary development and use, generalized patient education and information activities, and other population-focused quality assurance measures for medication use.

b. Face-to-face interaction between the patient* and the pharmacist as the preferred method of delivery. When patient-specific barriers to face-to-face communication exist, patients shall have equal access to appropriate alternative delivery methods. Medication Therapy Management programs shall include structures supporting the establishment and maintenance of the patient*-pharmacist relationship.

c. Opportunities for pharmacists and other qualified health care providers to identify patients who should receive medication therapy management services.

d. Payment for Medication Therapy Management Services consistent with contemporary provider payment rates that are based on the time, clinical intensity, and resources required to provide services (e.g., Medicare Part A and/or Part B for CPT & RBRVS).

e. Processes to improve continuity of care, outcomes, and outcome measures.

---

*In some situations, Medication Therapy Management Services may be provided to the caregiver or other persons involved in the care of the patient.

Approved on July 27, 2004 by the Academy of Managed Care Pharmacy, the American Association of Colleges of Pharmacy, the American College of Apothecaries, the American College of Clinical Pharmacy, the American Society of Consultant Pharmacists, the American Pharmacists Association, the American Society of Health-System Pharmacists, the National Association of Boards of Pharmacy**, the National Association of Chain Drug Stores, the National Community Pharmacists Association and the National Council of State Pharmacy Association Executives.

**Organization policy does not allow NABP to take a position on payment issues.

Source: www.pharmacist.com/AM/Template.cfm?Section=Home&TEMPLATE=/CM/ContentDisplay.cfm& CONTENTID=4577; accessed on November 21, 2007.

legislation prevents MTM from being a billable service to the beneficiary with coverage through Medicare reimbursement. Instead, pharmacists are paid for MTM from administrative fees given to the plan sponsors from CMS or via revenue from premiums.

MTM services in Medicare Part D have been slower to be developed by the PDPs than the prescription drug benefits, but the momentum for MTM grew in 2007. This was not unexpected because plans wanted to get their prescription drug benefits functional by January 2006, with quality assurance activities such as MTM to follow. Two studies of the implementation of MTM by PDPs were conducted late in 2006. Among 70 health insurance plans representing coverage for 12.1 million enrollees, 90 percent had MTM programs with eligibility based on the number of chronic conditions (median was three), and 95 percent had eligibility based on the number of medications (median was six). In terms of the services delivered by their 21 distinct types of MTM programs, patient education (75 percent of programs), patient adherence (70 percent), and medication review (60 percent) were most common. Almost all programs used in-house call centers and mailed materials. Only four programs used community pharmacists to provide face-to-face consultations with eligible beneficiaries (Touchette et al., 2006). Results from the second study found similar results, with most programs using managed-care pharmacists and nurses to provide MTM (Boyd, Boyd, and Zillich, 2006). There were few opportunities for pharmacists in settings such as community pharmacies or clinics to provide MTM services for their beneficiaries. Since these studies, successful MTM program have been implemented, and research to quantify their impact will be forthcoming over the next few years (Mirixa Clinical Solutions, 2007; Outcomes MTM System, 2007; Outcomes Medicare Plans, 2007).

To date, there are few data available about the beneficiaries who are eligible for MTM and the outcomes related to MTM programs. Daniel and Malone (2007) examined 2002–2003 Medicare Expenditure Panel Survey (MEPS) data to characterize beneficiaries eligible for MTM. According to their analysis, 9.2

percent of Medicare beneficiaries would be eligible for MTM services based on the cost criterion of $4,000 adjusted dollars. Eligible individuals had an average of 5.2 medical conditions and 10.8 unique medications (82.2 prescriptions in 1 year) compared with 2.9 medical conditions and 4.6 unique medications among ineligible individuals. Factors predictive of MTM eligibility included age; having assistance with activities of daily living; having limitations in walking, lifting, bending, or housework; and having three or more chronic conditions. Thus individuals eligible for MTM are those high-risk individuals who are likely to benefit from pharmacists' care.

One positive advancement for pharmacy is that Current Procedural Terminology (CPT) codes have been developed specifically for MTM services provided by pharmacists. These codes are a standard used within health care to bill for goods and services. Separate codes have been developed for an initial encounter of 15 minutes of MTM service for a new patient (99605), initial encounter of 15 minutes of MTM service for an established patient (99606), and additional 15-minute increments (99607). While there has yet to be widespread use of these CPT codes by pharmacists, it is anticipated that their use will increase as plans implement MTM services involving pharmacists (American Society of Health-System Pharmacists, 2007).

As of 2008, pharmacies and pharmacists need to use a National Provider Identifier (NPI). This number will be used by all covered providers and health plans in transactions related to administration and financial transactions under the Health Insurance Portability and Accountability Act (HIPAA). Specifically, pharmacists will need to use their NPIs when billing PDPs for MTM services. The NPI is a numeric 10-digit unique identifier for providers (CMS, 2007b). It is available to any health care professional simply by completing an online form available at https://nppes.cms.hhs.gov/NPPES/Welcome.do.

Medicare Part D has increased prescription drug access for millions of older adults. The private administration of the program has resulted in many choices among plans, which has an impact on both patients and pharmacies. MTM developed in 2007, and it has

Table 17-3. Advantages and Disadvantages of Medicare Part D	
Advantages	**Disadvantages**
Increased dispensed prescriptions	Reduced reimbursement per prescription
Increased access to needed medications for Medicare-eligible individuals	Largest cash-paying client base eliminated
Medication therapy management available for high users of medications	Reimbursement can be slow
Tricare access standard ensures access to pharmacy	Assignment of dual eligibles to Part D plans resulted in eligibility delays
Subsidies available for low-income enrollees	Too many plans resulted in patient confusion
Significant variability in available plans	Patients choose plans not available in your pharmacy
CMS has access to prescription utilization data for all older adults for future research	Donut hole/gap coverage is confusing and unlike other insurance
Catastrophic coverage is available	

advantages and disadvantages in its current structure and operations (Table 17-3). The long-term impact of MTM services on patients, pharmacists, pharmacies, and Part D programs remains unclear. In the next section we discuss some of the primary management concerns that have arisen with Part D.

▣ MANAGEMENT

In Chapter 2 the management process was displayed as a cube describing the level, activities, and resources that all pharmacists manage (see Fig. 2-1). Three key resources that pharmacists must manage to effectively integrate Part D into their practices are people, money, and information. Pharmacists must also effectively plan, organize, take action, and evaluate their activities to monitor the impact of Part D on their practices. Finally, pharmacy organizations, managers, and pharmacists need to consider how to lead the development and implementation of MTM services and other quality assurance activities so that Part D plan sponsors will look to pharmacy for assistance in ensuring high-quality drug therapy and patient outcomes for their Medicare beneficiaries.

In considering the key relationships pharmacists must enter to effectively participate in Part D, CMS, plan sponsors (including PDPs and MA-PDs), and pa-

tients come instantly to mind. Since CMS is a government agency charged with oversight of Medicare Part D, pharmacists must develop relationships with CMS to better understand the intricacies of the program. CMS has taken steps to increase its knowledge of the pharmacy community by hiring pharmacists to work in national and regional offices and liaise with pharmacists and pharmacy organizations. CMS also communicates with pharmacists regularly via e-mail and pharmacy-oriented Web pages (www.cms.hhs.gov/Pharmacy/). Community pharmacists have increased their interactions with CMS, which historically had been limited to questions regarding coverage of specific products such as medical equipment or diabetic supplies. Now pharmacists interact daily with Medicare-related systems to determine beneficiary eligibility and copayments for medications.

An important caveat that may not have been fully recognized is that CMS may view plan sponsors (PDPs) as their primary "customer" for Part D rather than pharmacies or pharmacists. This view arises because the plan sponsors are the contractors with CMS for delivering Part D, not pharmacies or pharmacists. Therefore, it is equally if not more important for pharmacists to develop relationships with plan sponsors to better understand the intricacies of participation in their various plans.

Plan sponsors are usually insurance companies and pharmaceutical benefit managers. The sponsors providing the plans with highest Medicare Part D enrollments in 2006 included United Healthcare, Humana, Wellcare, Wellpoint, Member Health, Caremark, and Pennsylvania Life Insurance Company (Hoadley et al., 2006). Pharmacies are required to sign contacts with plan sponsors to provide medications and other services for patients covered under their plans. Thus pharmacies are required to evaluate the financial viability of each contract to ensure that profits can be generated. This requires pharmacists to understand their cost to dispense and to consider the reimbursement under each contract. Conducting differential analysis to compare different net profits under current and new reimbursements rates benefits pharmacies so that they understand how reimbursement rates affect net profit. In addition, pro forma analysis may be conducted to better anticipate the implications of choosing to participate or not participate in any particular plan. These analyses are described in Chapter 16.

Similar to participation in other private third-party drug plans, individual pharmacies have relatively little leverage in negotiating with plan sponsors on reimbursement rates. The only exception to this is the Tricare standard, used to ensure access to pharmacies by beneficiaries. It states that at least 70 percent of beneficiaries, on average, must live within 15 miles of a retail pharmacy. Some pharmacies have been able to negotiate higher reimbursement rates because of this standard (Radford et al., 2007). Data that may define high-quality care in pharmacy, such as dispensing error rates, percentage of patients counseled, or percentage of patients receiving follow-up on new prescriptions, generally have yet to be considered in setting reimbursement rates with plan sponsors.

Making decisions about which PDP contracts to accept can take a great deal of time. In 2007, there were 1,875 different PDPs, and there were 23 plans that were national, near national, or covered in 10 + Medicare regions (Hoadley et al., 2006). While large chain pharmacy organizations typically have administrative staff who are responsible for evaluating participation in various drug plans, smaller chain and independently owned pharmacies often do not have the resources to give all the plans they are presented with such a thorough review. This can lead to accepting plans that have an adverse financial impact on their pharmacies, as well as not accepting plans that may in fact improve their financial standing.

Small chain and independently owned pharmacies may gain leverage in their negotiations with drug plans if they were allowed to join together and bargain as a group, often referred to as *collective bargaining*. However, federal and state antitrust laws typically prevent competitors from acting together on contracts such as those with the sponsors of Medicare Part D drug plans. The National Community Pharmacists Association, a trade association representing the interest of independently owned pharmacies and pharmacists, continues to advocate for such opportunities.

In their effort to interact more effectively with prescription drug plans, small chains and independent pharmacies often choose to use third-party networks such as AccessHealth (www.mckesson.com/en_us/ McKesson.com/Forpercent2BPharmacies/Independent percent2BRetail/Managedpercent2BCare/AccessHeal th.html) through McKesson or Leader Pharmacies through Cardinal Health (www.cardinal.com/us/en/ pharmacies/offerings/leader/index.asp) to assist them with third-party contracts, group purchasing pricing, business development opportunities, and advocacy. For example, money management tools offered by AccessHealth include consolidated reimbursement for PDPs, electronic funds transfer, online claim reports, reconciliation assistance with problematic claims, and online purchasing tools to facilitate real-time order and inventory status.

The information technology demands of Part D remain unclear as they relate to electronic prescribing and its impact on pharmacy. Currently, pharmacies interact with PDPs electronically to determine eligibility and adjudicate claims. The MMA directed the Secretary of Health and Human Services to establish federal standards for e-prescribing. Five pilot studies conducted in 2005–2006 tested six standards, showing that three standards are ready for implementation. Standards related to prior authorization, structured

Table 17-4. Web-Based Medicare Part D Resources

For pharmacists:
www.medicare.gov/pdphome.asp
www.cms.hhs.gov/center/pharmacist.asp
www.cms.hhs.gov/PrescriptionDrugCovGenIn/
www.cms.hhs.gov/MLNProducts/23_DrugCoverage.asp#TopOfPage
www.medicare.gov/MPDPF/Public/Include/DataSection/Questions/SearchOptions.asp
www.medicare.gov/MPDPF/Public/Include/DataSection/Questions/EnrollDirectly.asp
www.pqaalliance.org
www.qualitymeasures.ahrq.gov/
www.ahrq.gov/qual/
http://healthit.ahrq.gov/portal/server.pt?open=512&objID=650&parentname=CommunityPage&parentid=
    19&mode=2&in_hi_userid=3882&cached=true

To review reports about medication use trends including Medicare Part D:
http://kff.org/rxdrugs/index.cfm

To review and join mailing lists from CMS about a variety of topics:
www.cms.hhs.gov/apps/mailinglists/

To download Part D formularies:
www.epocrates.com/resources/medicare-partd/

For patients:
www.mymedicarematters.org/
www.shiip.state.ia.us/ (every state has a SHIIP office)
www.medicare.gov/pdphome.asp.
www.medicare.gov/MPDPF/Public/Include/DataSection/Questions/MPDPFIntro.asp.
www.healthfinder.gov/
www.talkingquality.gov/

SIG (prescription instructions), and RxNorm (standard name, dose, and form availability) were not considered ready for implementation because of numerous approaches used in these three areas across health information technology. Electronic prescribing is not required under MMA, but plans are to have it available should providers choose to use it. As standards are developed, the adoption of e-prescribing is expected to improve patient safety by reducing prescribing and dispensing errors (Agency for Healthcare Research & Quality, 2007).

Pharmacists and pharmacy organizations must continually monitor Part D changes and assess the pos-

sible impact on practice. Information resources about Part D for pharmacists and patients are widely available (Table 17-4).

■ EPILOGUE: WHAT HAVE WE LEARNED SO FAR?

Medicare Part D is in its relatively early stages of implementation. There is still much to be learned about the impact of the program on patients, pharmacists, and pharmacies and the general health care system. Fortunately, a number of program evaluations have already taken place. The results of these studies will help policymakers, pharmacists, and patients further refine their programs and make more informed choices.

In November 2006, the Kaiser Family Foundation interviewed a nationally representative sample of older adults about Medicare Part D. At the time of their initial enrollment (November 2005–January 2006), only 30 percent of respondents had a favorable opinion about the Medicare Part D benefit, and 47 percent had an unfavorable opinion. By the following November, 42 percent had a favorable opinion, and only 34 percent were unfavorable. The majority agreed or somewhat agreed (68 percent) that Part D helped them save money on prescriptions, and 56 percent agreed or somewhat agreed that the program "helps people like me." However, the majority (78 percent) also agreed or somewhat agreed that the program is too complicated, and 60 percent of all respondents would prefer to actually have fewer drug plans from which to choose (Kaiser Family Foundation, 2006b).

Simplifying Part D for patients is where pharmacists have been helpful and can continue to build goodwill among their patients. In a Kaiser Family Foundation national survey of pharmacists conducted in the spring of 2006, pharmacists were positive about Part D's impact on cost and access to medications for their patients, especially for individuals with low incomes (Kaiser Family Foundation, 2006d). Pharmacists also reported that they themselves had been a good resource in terms of information about Part D and navigation of the system to obtain medications for their patients. Almost all pharmacies indicated that they talked with patients about enrolling in Medicare Part D and answered their patients' questions about the program. However, pharmacists also indicated frustration with administering the plans under Medicare Part D. Over half of respondents (53 percent) felt that the administrative burden of filling prescriptions under Part D plans exceeded that of traditional prescription drug insurance plans. Over 40 percent of pharmacists indicated that reimbursement under Part D plans was lower than other plans, and 29 percent reported waiting longer for reimbursement. Pharmacists in chain and independently owned pharmacies had differing views on Part D. For example, 78 percent of independent pharmacies felt that reimbursement was lower for Part D drug plans, whereas only 29 percent of chain pharmacists reported lower reimbursement. More than one-quarter (27 percent) of respondents from independently owned pharmacies stated that their pharmacies had to take out loans because of cash-flow problems resulting from reimbursement delays versus 1 percent of chain pharmacists who reported similar problems. In terms of overall financial perspectives, 44 percent of independent and 7 percent of chain pharmacists reported that Part D placed "a lot" of burden on their pharmacy (Kaiser Family Foundation, 2006d).

Pharmacists must weigh financial issues and customer-service issues. In terms of financial issues, pharmacies must determine whether the reimbursement is sufficient to participate in the plan. For customer service, pharmacies must determine if the plans they participate in are those aligned with the ones customers will select. MTM may provide opportunities for pharmacists to generate additional streams of revenue. MTM for the plan sponsors is a quality assurance activity and not a service wherein they receive additional payment from CMS for its provision.

One final issue that may become important in the coming years is that CMS was instrumental in helping to establish the Pharmacy Quality Alliance (pqaalliance.org). This multistakeholder organization is charged with measuring, collecting, and reporting performance at the pharmacy and pharmacist levels. For example, pharmacists and/or pharmacies may be compared regarding the percent of Medicare-eligible patients receiving a high-risk medication that is contained on an approved list or the percent of patients having 60 to 80 percent of the daily supply of medication over a 6-month period. In 2007, the Pharmacy Quality Alliance began testing measures that are likely to be used to evaluate the quality of pharmacies, pharmacists, and pharmacist services. This initiative is consistent with the Hospital Quality Alliance and Ambulatory Care Quality Alliance, wherein credible and user-friendly information about the quality of care is or will be available for comparison by the public (www.hospitalcompare.hhs.gov). We remain a few years off from comparing pharmacies based on quality

Table 17-5. Answers to Scenario Questions

In the scenario, Sam Bell is faced with declining profits and loyal patients. He has a good business in rural Tennessee but new avenues of revenue may be necessary.

1. Are patients in Bell's Pharmacy likely to benefit from Medicare Part D?

   People receiving Medicaid and individuals receiving the lower-income subsidy will benefit from Medicare Part D plans because their enrollment is subsidized fully or to some extent. Individuals receiving the low-income subsidy are those least likely to have other insurance and have difficulty paying case prices for prescription drugs.

2. Why is Medicare Part D threatening to Bell's Pharmacy?

   Medicare Part D is threatening to the financial viability of Bell's Pharmacy because of (1) lower reimbursement, (2) slower reimbursements, and (3) increased administrative time for prescriptions.

3. What positive things have happened to Sam Bell since Medicare Part D was implemented?

   Sam Bell has always been a respected businessman in his community. Since Medicare Part D has been implemented, Sam dispenses more prescriptions, and he does not think that his paitent base has been affected to a great extent. Sam spent considerable time with patients helping them sort out plans during the enrollment period. This extra effort has won the hearts of his patients.

4. What management strategies can Sam Bell use to maintain the viability of his pharmacy?

   Avoiding contracts with 90-days supply of medications is one strategy to help avoid losing profit per prescription.

   Sam Bell also would benefit by conducting a differential analysis as well as a pro forma analysis to fully realize the impact of Medicare Part D on his net profit. Examining the income-expense statements certainly suggests that Medicare Part D has decreased profits, but these analyses would provide useful information for Sam each year as he faces new contracts.

   He already is a member of a buying group, and he uses electronic funds transfer to facilitate timely deposits from plans.

   He recently stopped his internal charge accounts. He gave his clients/patients a 3-month notice about this change, and almost all clients were positive about the change. In a few limited cases, he worked out alternative payment arrangements to assist some long-term, limited-income individuals. This business decision has contributed to reduced administrative burden in the pharmacy and improved cash flow as well.

5. What alternative revenue streams are available for Sam Bell to consider?

   Sam is not currently an MTM provider. He should calculate the expenses required to provide these services balanced against the revenues they would generate to determine whether to proceed with these activities. It is likely that he has numerous enrollees in plans offering MTM, and he may benefit financially as well as professionally by providing MTM to his patients.

   There are local employers in his rural community that may benefit from health screenings. Sam could approach these employers with cardiovascular risk screening, for example, and even develop a set of services related to cardiovascular risk reduction set.

   Additional revenue could be generated via administration of vaccines. In some states, pharmacists can administer vaccines, charging for the product as well as administration.

   Sam could determine if his state allows collaborative practice agreements. If so, he could develop a clinical service such as warfarin management, diabetes management, or hypertension management and bill these services using 1,500 billing codes.

of care provided in the pharmacy, but pharmacists need to monitor this initiative and take an active part is helping shape its future.

REVISITING THE SCENARIO

Sam Bell has been able to increase prescription volume and is selective about the plans that he accepts. He uses a third-party network for some aspects of his business management. A financial analysis to determine which plans to accept would be beneficial rather than simply using 90-day supply as the key criterion (Table 17-5).

CONCLUSION

Medicare Part D is a voluntary prescription drug insurance plan administered by numerous health plans and offered to all Medicare enrollees. It has increased access to prescription medications for many Americans, particularly low-income Medicare beneficiaries. While there is a standard Part D benefit, there are many plans to choose from because plans can be actuarially equivalent. Pharmacists assist older adults in managing the intricacies of numerous Part D plans, especially during yearly enrollment. One component of Part D plans that presents a great opportunity for pharmacists is MTM. Pharmacists must continually monitor the impact of Part D, such as determining which plans to participate in and whether and with whom to provide MTM. Finally, pharmacists must stay well informed about upcoming Part D plan changes and associated changes in practice such as NPI, e-prescribing, and pharmacy quality assurance.

QUESTIONS FOR FURTHER DISCUSSION

1. How and why has the standard benefit changed since 2006?
2. What trends are notable in benefit design of prescription drug plans since the first year of Part D?
3. What legislation has been considered to "fix" Medicare Part D, especially from a pharmacist's viewpoint?
4. What quality measures have been proposed and tested to compare prescription drug plans and pharmacies?

REFERENCES

Agency for Healthcare Research & Quality. 2007. National Resource Center for Health Information Technology. Electronic Prescribing. http://healthit.ahrq.gov/portal/server.pt?open=514&objID=5554&mode=2&holderDisplayURL=http://prodportallb.ahrq.gov:7087/publishedcontent/publish/communities/k_o/knowledge_library/key_topics/health_briefing_03282006124741/electronic_prescribing.html; accessed on November 21, 2007.

American Society of Health-System Pharmacists. 2007. Pharmacists' CPT codes become permanent. Available at www.ashp.org/s_ashp/article_news.asp?CID=167&DID=2024&id=23065; accessed on November 21, 2007.

Boyd ST, Boyd LC, Zillich AJ. 2006. Medication therapy management survey of the prescription drug plans. *J Am Pharm Assoc* 46:692.

CMS. 2007a. Guidance on the Actuarial Equivalence Standard for the Retiree Drug Subsidy; available at www.cms.hhs.gov/EmployerRetireeDrugSubsid/Downloads/ActrlEqvlncStdforRDS.pdf, accessed on November 7, 2007.

CMS. 2007b. National Provider Identifier Standard; available at www.cms.hhs.gov/NationalProvIdentStand/; accessed on November 21, 2007.

CMS. 2007c. *Prescription Drug Benefit Manual,* Chapter 5: Benefits and Beneficiary Protections. Available at www.cms.hhs.gov/PrescriptionDrugCovContra/Downloads/PDMChap5BeneProtections˙03.09.07.pdf; accessed on November 7, 2007.

Cubanski J, Neuman P. 2007. Status report on Medicare Part D enrollment in 2006: Analysis of plan-specific market share and coverage. *Health Affairs* 26:w1 (published online November 21, 2006; 10.1377/hlthaff.26.1.w1).

Daniel GW, Malone DC. 2007. Characteristics of older adults who meet the annual prescription drug expenditure threshold for Medicare medication therapy management programs. *J Manag Care Pharm* 13:142.

Evans-Molina C, Rean S, Henault LE, et al. 2007. The new Medicare part D prescription drug benefit: An estimation of its effect on prescription drug costs in a Medicare population with atrial fibrillation. *J Am Geriatr Soc* 55:1038.

General Accounting Office. 2007. Challenges in enrolling new dual-eligible beneficiaries; available at www.gao.gov/cgi-bin/getrpt?GAO-07–272; accessed on November 8, 2007.

Hoadley J, Hargrave E, Merrell K, et al. 2006. Benefit Design and Formularies of Medicare Drug Plans: A Comparison of 2006 and 2007 Offerings, a First Look; available at www.kff.org, report no. 7589; accessed on November 7, 2007.

Kaiser Family Foundation. 2006a. Standard Medicare Drug Benefit; available at www.kff.org/medicare/medicarebenefitataglance.cfm; accessed on November 14, 2007.

Kaiser Family Foundation. 2006b. Chartpack: Seniors and the Medicare Prescription Drug Benefit, December; available at www.kff.org/kaiserpolls/7604.cfm; accessed on November 7, 2007.

Kaiser Family Foundation. 2006c. Tracking Prescription Drug Coverage under Medicare: Five Ways to Look at the New Enrollment Numbers, February; available at http://kff.org/medicare/7466.cfm; accessed on November 8, 2007.

Kaiser Family Foundation. 2006d. National Survey of Pharmacists, November; available at www.kff.org/kaiserpolls/upload/7585.pdf, accessed on November 7, 2007.

Kaiser Family Foundation. 2007a. Prescription Drug Sources Among Medicare Beneficiaries; available at www.kff.org/medicare/med043007oth.cfm; accessed on November 21, 2007.

Kaiser Family Foundation. 2007b. Additional Help with Prescription Drug Costs for Low-Income People on Medicare (For 2007 Benefits and Cost-Sharing). Available at www.kff.org/medicare/med062804oth.cfm; accessed on November 7, 2007.

Kaiser Family Foundation. 2007c. Medicare Prescription Drug Benefit: An Updated Fact Sheet, October; available at www.kff.org/medicare/upload/7044_07.pdf; accessed on November 7, 2007.

Mirixa Clinical Solutions. 2007. Available at www.mirixa.com/media/8760/mirixa percent20clinical percent202.pdf; accessed on November 21, 2007.

Morgan PC, for the Congressional Research Service at the Library of Congress. 2004. Health Care Spending: Past Trends and Projections, Order Code RL31094; available at http://kuhl.house.gov/UploadedFiles/healthspending.pdf; accessed on November 14, 2007.

Neuman P, Strollo MK, Guterman S, et al. 2007. Medicare prescription drug benefit progress report: Findings from a 2006 national survey of seniors. *Health Affairs* 26:w630; published online August 21, 2007; available at 10.1377/hlthaff.26.5.w630.

Oliver TR, Lee PR, Lipton HL. 2004. A political history of Medicare and prescription drug coverage. *Milbank Q* 82:283.

Outcomes MTM System. 2007. Available at www.getoutcomes.com/aspx/Welcome/outcomesmtmsystem.aspx; accessed on November 21, 2007.

Outcomes Medicare Plans. 2007. Available at www.getoutcomes.com/aspx/Sponsors/medicareplans.aspx; accessed on November 21, 2007.

Radford A, Slifkin R, Fraser R, et al. 2007. The experience of rural independent pharmacist with Medicare Part D: Reports from the field. *J Rural Health* 23:286.

Touchette DR, Burns AL, Bough MA, Blackburn JC. 2006. Survey of medication therapy management programs under Medicare Part D. *J Am Pharm Assoc* 46:683.

Tseng CW, Mangione CM, Brook RH, et al. 2007. Indentifying widely covered drugs and drug coverage variation among Medicare Part D formularies. *JAMA* 297:2596.

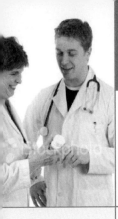

18

BUDGETING

David A. Gettman

A **bout the Author:** Dr. Gettman is an Associate Professor in the Department of Pharmaceutical, Administrative, and Social Sciences at the University of Appalachia College of Pharmacy. He received a B.S. in pharmacy from the University of Montana, an MBA from the College of William and Mary, and a Ph.D. in pharmacy health care administration from the University of Florida. He has practiced pharmacy in numerous settings, including community, hospital, nursing home, hospice, and both the U.S. Navy and U.S. Air Force. In addition to pharmacy management, Dr. Gettman has taught pharmacy law, health care ethics, health care delivery, pharmacoepidemiology, pharmacoeconomics, biostatistics, and research design. The author of numerous publications, he has also made over 100 different presentations to various professional health care groups at the state, national, and international levels.

▩ LEARNING OBJECTIVES

After completing this chapter, students should be able to

1. List and explain five purposes of budgeting systems.
2. Describe the similarities and differences in the operational budgets prepared by pharmaceutical manufacturers, health system pharmacies offering value-added services, community pharmacies selling merchandise, and nonprofit pharmacy organizations.
3. Explain the concept of activity-based budgeting and the benefits it brings to the budgeting process.
4. Describe each of the budget schedules that make up a master budget.
5. Discuss the role of assumptions and predictions in budgeting.
6. Describe a typical pharmacy organization's process of budget administration.
7. Understand the importance of budgeting product life-cycle costs.
8. Discuss the behavioral implications of budgetary slack and participative budgeting.

SCENARIO

Mary Quint, Pharm.D., has just taken a position managing the production and distribution of total parenteral nutrition (TPN) for a business unit called Home TPN Care. Home TPN Care is part of a local university's health system that includes a large teaching hospital, several clinics, and numerous ancillary services. Procurement, receiving, insurance verification, claims processing, and cash application operation activities are all completed within Home TPN Care located 5 miles away from its main hospital. Home TPN Care consistently generates a positive net margin that contributes to the health system's margin targets and support of non-revenue-generating activities. Clinical, patient care, quality, and process improvement programs are integrated into the health system's strategic plan.

Home TPN Care is a licensed pharmacy and home infusion provider responsible for providing a wide range of products and services to safely and effectively facilitate care to patients in the convenience and comfort of their homes. Since 2001, Home TPN Care has been providing infusion medications, nutritional therapy, specialty drugs, high-tech infusion nursing, and care management services throughout the region. An interdisciplinary team consisting of pharmacists, nurses, and dietitians, along with technical, administrative, and support staff, provides pharmacy manufacturing (i.e., compounding), equipment management, dispensing, delivery, and care management services to ensure that patient home regimens are safe and effective throughout the course of therapy. The staff has direct access to up-to-date and complete medical and patient drug information that facilitates effective and efficient collaboration with physicians and other caregivers within the organization. To ensure a smooth transition to home care, Home TPN Care has a training and education team. This team consists of nurses and dietitians who work with patients and the referring health care team to ensure that home care needs are identified prior to hospital discharge and infusion nurses who provide care for patients in their homes.

Although Home TPN Care resides within the home care service division in the health system's organizational structure, an administrative relationship exists between Home TPN Care and the health system's department of pharmacy services. Thus many administrative, pharmacy practice, and educational activities are collaborative and integrated. There is Home TPN Care representation on several department of pharmacy committees. Additionally, most of Home TPN Care's professionals hold academic appointments within the university, reflecting a commitment to teaching, experiential training, and research.

Dr. Quint has been advised that among her many new job responsibilities, she will need to develop a master budget, or profit plan, for Home TPN Care. It was obvious to her that she would need to review the materials she studied in her pharmacy management course about budgeting before she could tackle this important challenge.

CHAPTER QUESTIONS

1. How does a budget facilitate communication and coordination in a pharmacy organization?
2. What is a master budget, and what are the parts of a master budget?
3. What is meant by the term *operational budgets*?
4. How does activity-based budgeting differ from more traditional budgeting methods?
5. How does e-budgeting make use of the Internet?
6. What is the purpose of a budget manual?
7. What is zero-base budgeting?
8. What is budgetary slack, and what problem(s) can it cause?

INTRODUCTION

Developing a budget is a critical step in planning any economic activity. This is true for pharmacy businesses, for individual pharmacists, and for governmental agencies that regulate both pharmacy businesses and individual pharmacists. As individuals, we all must budget our money to meet day-to-day expenses and plan for major capital expenditures, such as buying a car. Similarly, pharmacy businesses of all types and governmental agencies must make financial plans to carry out routine operations, to plan for major expenditures, and to help in making financial decisions.

PURPOSES OF BUDGETING SYSTEMS

A *budget* is a detailed plan, expressed in quantitative terms, that specifies how resources will be acquired and used during a specified period of time. The procedures used to develop a budget constitute a *budgeting system*. Budgeting systems have five primary purposes.

Planning

The most obvious purpose of a budget is to quantify a plan of action. The budgeting process forces people who make up an organization to anticipate or react to changes in the environment. For example, the U.S. Food and Drug Administration's (FDA) approval of capecitabine, an oral form of fluorouracil, in 1998 and imatinib mesylate, an oral agent use in the treatment of chronic myeloid leukemia, in 2001 signaled a new period in budget planning for pharmacy benefits. This was of particular concern for small, self-insured employers, for whom a drug with a cost of $25,000 per year of therapy for one patient could increase total pharmacy benefit costs by 10 percent or more (Curtiss, 2006).

Facilitating Communication and Coordination

For any organization to be effective, each manager throughout the organization must be aware of plans made by other managers. The budgeting process pulls together the plans of each manager in an organization. For example, pharmaceutical companies who market products with "blockbuster" potential are often developed by groups of researchers and project managers around the world. These managers require coordinated financial information at the local, national,

and global levels (Cowlrick, Dumon, and Bauleser, 2002).

Allocating Resources

Any organization's resources are limited, including pharmacies and pharmacy departments. Budgets provide one means of allocating resources among competing uses. Hospitals, for example, must make difficult decisions about allocating their revenue among services (e.g., pharmacy, laboratory, and nursing), maintenance of property and equipment (e.g., beds, laminar flow hoods, and vehicles), and other community services (e.g., child care services and programs to prevent alcohol and drug abuse). In particular, allocating resources to pharmacy initiatives to improve patient safety as a result of drug-related deaths has had to compete with other areas where dollars are also needed to improve patient care (Tierney, 2004).

Controlling Profit and Operations

A budget is a plan, and plans are subject to change. A budget serves as a useful benchmark with which actual results can be compared. For example, a pharmacy business can compare its actual sales of prescriptions for a year against its budgeted sales. Such comparisons can help managers evaluate the pharmacy's effectiveness in selling prescriptions. Nevertheless, pharmacy managers must be prepared for a financial crisis. Taking the initiative to acquire appropriate data, to translate those data into relevant information, and to seek benchmarks for comparison is important. Once the crisis has passed, attention must be given to updating and maintaining databases, supporting the staff, and improving morale. Scenario planning can help to identify measures that might be taken if another crisis should develop (Demers, 2001).

Evaluating Performance and Providing Incentives

Comparing actual results with budgeted results also helps pharmacy managers evaluate the performance of individuals, departments, or entire corporations. Since budgets are used to evaluate performance, they can also be used to provide incentives for people to perform well. Many health care organizations are beginning to implement pay-for-performance (P4P) programs that will tie monetary incentives for pharmacy personnel to hospital quality scores (Gregg, Moscovice, and Remus, 2006).

TYPES OF BUDGETS

Different types of budgets serve different purposes. A *master budget,* or *profit plan,* is a comprehensive set of budgets covering all phases of a pharmacy organization's operations for a specified period of time.

Budgeted financial statements, often called *pro forma financial statements,* show how the pharmacy organization's financial statements will appear at a specified time if operations proceed according to plan. Budgeted financial statements include a budgeted income statement, a budgeted balance sheet, and a budgeted statement of cash flows.

A *capital budget* is a plan for the acquisition of capital assets, such as buildings and equipment. A *financial budget* is a plan that shows how the pharmacy business will acquire its financial resources, such as through the issuance of stock or incurrence of debt.

Budgets are developed for specific time periods. *Short-range budgets* cover a year, a quarter, or a month, whereas *long-range budgets* cover periods longer than a year. *Rolling budgets* are continually updated by periodically adding a new incremental time period, such as a quarter, and dropping the period just completed. Rolling budgets are also called *revolving budgets* or *continuous budgets.*

THE MASTER BUDGET: A PLANNING TOOL

The *master budget,* the principal output of a budgeting system, is a comprehensive profit plan that ties together all phases of a pharmacy's operations. The master budget consists of many separate budgets, or schedules, that are interdependent. Figure 18-1 portrays these interrelationships in a flowchart.

Sales of Services or Goods

The starting point for any master budget is a *sales revenue budget.* For many pharmacy departments, this

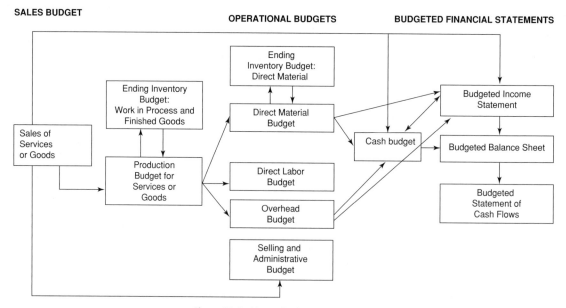

Figure 18-1. Master budget components.

budget begins with a sales forecast for prescription drug spending. A pharmacy manager would need to keep abreast of how changes in government expenditures (e.g., Medicare prescription drug coverage) might change the distribution of drug spending among payers and affect aggregate spending (Poisal et al., 2007).

Sales Forecasting

All pharmacies have two things in common when it comes to forecasting sales of services or goods. Sales forecasting is a critical step in the budgeting process, and it is very difficult to do accurately.

Various procedures are used in sales forecasting, and the final forecast usually combines information from many different sources. Many pharmacy corporations have a market research staff whose job is to coordinate the corporation's sales forecasting efforts. Typically, everyone from key executives to the firm's sales personnel will be asked to contribute sales projections.

Major factors considered when forecasting sales include the following:

1. Past sales levels and trends
    a. For the firm developing the forecast (e.g., Walgreen's)
    b. For the entire industry (e.g., the chain drug store industry)
2. General economic trends (Is the economy growing? How fast? Is a recession or economic slowdown expected?)
3. Economic trends in the pharmaceutical industry (In the drug store industry, for example, are customers getting older, thereby implying increased demand for prescriptions?)
4. Other factors expected to affect sales in the industry (Is an unusually cold winter expected, which would result in increased demand for cold remedies in chain drug stores located in northern climates?)
5. Political and legal events (For example, are there any significant over-the-counter switches by the FDA that would affect the demand for prescriptions?)
6. The intended pricing policy of the pharmacy
7. Planned advertising and product promotion
8. Expected actions of competitors
9. New services contemplated by the pharmacy or other pharmacies (For example, drug stores are continuing to develop value-added services, which may increase the demand for certain categories of prescriptions.)
10. Market research studies

The starting point in the sales forecasting process is generally the sales level of the prior year. Then the market research staff considers the information discussed earlier, along with input from key executives and sales personnel. In many pharmacy organizations, elaborate econometric models are built to incorporate all the available information systematically. Statistical methods, such as regression analysis and probability distributions for sales, are often used. A great deal of effort goes into the sales forecast because it is such a critical step in the budgeting process. A slightly inaccurate sales forecast, coming at the very beginning of the budgeting process, likely will disrupt all the other schedules comprising the master budget.

Operational Budgets

Based on the sales budget, a pharmacy organization develops a set of operational budgets that specify how its operations will be carried out to meet the demand for its goods or services. The budgets constituting this operational portion of the master budget are illustrated in Fig. 18-1.

Pharmacy Organizations with Manufacturing

A pharmacy organization that conducts manufacturing operations develops a *production budget,* which shows the number of product units to be manufactured. Coupled with the production budget are ending *inventory budgets* for raw material, work in process, and finished goods. For example, home infusion pharmacies plan to have some inventory on hand at all times to meet peak demand while keeping production at a stable level. From the production budget, this pharmacy develops budgets for the direct materials, direct labor, and overhead that will be required in the production process. A budget for selling and administrative expenses is also prepared.

Pharmacy Organizations with Merchandising

The operational portion of the master budget is similar in a pharmacy organization with merchandising, but instead of a production budget for goods, a merchandiser develops a budget for merchandise purchases. For example, a chain drug store pharmacy will not have a budget for direct material because it does not engage in production. However, the chain drug pharmacy will develop budgets for labor (or personnel), overhead, and selling and administrative expenses.

Pharmacy Organizations with Value-Added Services

Based on the sales budget for its services, a service-oriented pharmacy organization develops a set of budgets that show how the demand for those services will be met. Pharmacy departments in hospitals are focusing their efforts on improving the efficiency of product-related functions mainly through automation and redeploying staff to value-added clinical functions. Services added under these transformations include intravenous-to-oral conversion, dosage adjustments for patients with renal impairment, medication therapy management (MTM) services, and participation in rounds in all areas of the hospital. The introduction of clinical pharmacy services as part of hospital-wide reengineering programs has been associated with positive benefit-cost ratios and a substantial net cost savings (Schumock, Michaud, and Guenette, 1999).

Cash Budget

This budget shows expected cash receipts as a result of selling goods or services and planned cash disbursements to pay the bills incurred by the pharmacy. Pharmacies prepare cash budgets to allow them to anticipate changes in cash flows over a period of time.

Summary of Operational Budgets

Operational budgets differ because they are adapted to the operations of individual pharmacies in various industries. However, operational budgets are also similar in important ways. In each pharmacy, they encompass a detailed plan for using the basic factors of production—material, labor, and overhead—to produce a product and/or provide a service.

Budgeted Financial Statements

The final portion of the master budget, depicted in Fig. 18-1, includes a budgeted income statement, a budgeted balance sheet, and a budgeted statement of cash flows. These budgeted financial statements show the overall financial results of the pharmacy organization's planned operations for the budget period.

Nonprofit Organizations

The master budget for a nonprofit organization includes many of the components shown in Fig. 18-1. However, there are some important differences. Many nonprofit organizations provide services free of charge. Hence there is no sales budget as shown in Fig. 18-1. However, such organizations do begin their budgeting process with a budget that shows the level of services to be provided. For example, the budget for a free clinic would show the planned levels of various public services, such as the hours of operation for the outpatient pharmacy. Nonprofit organizations also prepare budgets showing their anticipated funding. A free clinic budgets for revenue from both public (e.g., support from government agencies) and private sources (e.g., donations).

■ ACTIVITY-BASED BUDGETING

The process of constructing a master budget can be significantly enhanced if the concepts of *activity-based costing* (ABC) are applied. ABC uses a two-stage cost-assignment process. In stage 1, overhead costs are assigned to cost pools that represent the most significant activities. The activities identified vary across pharmacy organizations, but examples include such activities as purchasing, materials handling, prescription processing, scheduling, inspection, quality control, purchasing, and inventory control.

After assigning costs to the activity cost pools in stage 1, cost drivers are identified that are appropriate for each cost pool. Then, in stage 2, the overhead costs are allocated from each activity cost pool to cost objects (e.g., prescriptions, value-added services, and patients)

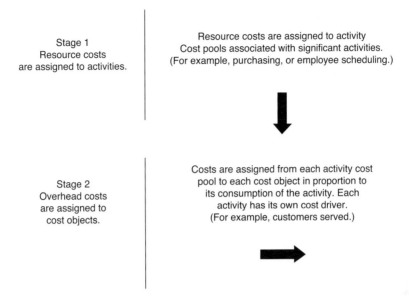

Figure 18-2. Activities-based costing system.

in proportion to the amount of activity consumed. Figure 18-2 portrays the two-stage allocation process used in ABC systems.

Applying ABC concepts to the budgeting process yields *activity-based budgeting* (ABB). Under ABB, the first step is to specify the products or services to be produced and the customers to be served. Then the activities that are necessary to produce these products and services are determined. Finally, the resources necessary to perform the specified activities are quantified. Conceptually, ABB takes the ABC model and reverses the flow of the analysis, as depicted in Fig. 18-3. As portrayed in the figure, ABC assigns resource costs to activities, and then it assigns activity costs to products

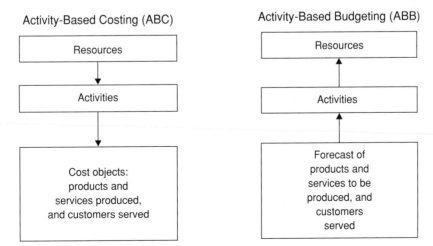

Figure 18-3. Activities-based costing versus activity-based budgeting.

and services produced and customers served. ABB, on the other hand, begins by forecasting the demand for products and services as well as the customers to be served. These forecasts then are used to plan the activities for the budget period and budget the resources necessary to carry out the activities.

USING ACTIVITY-BASED BUDGETING TO PREPARE THE MASTER BUDGET

The process of constructing a master budget requires the pharmacy manager to use 13 different schedules that are displayed in Table 18-1.

Financial Planning Models

Pharmacy managers must make assumptions and predictions in preparing budgets because pharmacies, like any other business or organization, operate in a world of uncertainty. One way of coping with that uncertainty is to supplement the budgeting process with a financial planning model. A *financial planning model* is a set of mathematical relationships that expresses the interactions among the various operational, financial, and environmental events that determine the overall results of an organization's activities. A financial planning model is a mathematical expression of all the relationships expressed in the flowchart in Fig. 18-1.

In a fully developed financial planning model, all the key estimates and assumptions are expressed as general mathematical relationships. Then software programs (e.g., Microsoft Excel) are used to determine the impact of different combinations of these unknown variables. "What if" questions can be answered about such unknown variables as inflation, interest rates, the value of the dollar, demand, competitors' actions, union demands in forthcoming wage negotiations, and a host of other factors.

BUDGET ADMINISTRATION

In small organizations, the procedures used to gather information and construct a master budget are usu-ally informal. In contrast, larger organizations use a formal process to collect data and prepare the master budget. Such organizations usually designate a budget director or chief budget officer. This is often the organization's controller (or comptroller in government organizations). The budget director specifies the process by which budget data will be gathered, collects the information, and prepares the master budget. To communicate budget procedures and deadlines to employees throughout the organization, the budget director often develops and disseminates a budget manual. The budget manual states who is responsible for providing various types of information, when the information is required, and what form the information is to take. For example, the budget manual for a pharmacy retail chain might specify that each regional director is to send an estimate of the following year's sales, by product line, to the budget director by September 1. The budget manual also states who should receive each schedule when the master budget is complete.

A budget committee, consisting of key senior executives, often is appointed to advise the budget director during preparation of the budget. The authority to give final approval to the master budget usually belongs to the board of directors or a board of trustees in many nonprofit organizations. Usually the board has a subcommittee whose task is to examine the proposed budget carefully and recommend approval or any changes deemed necessary. By exercising its authority to make changes in the budget and grant final approval, the board of directors or trustees can wield considerable influence on the overall direction the organization takes.

e-Budgeting

As more pharmacy organizations operate globally, the Internet is playing an important role in the budgeting process. e-Budgeting is an increasingly popular Internet-based budgeting tool that can help to streamline and speed up an organization's budgeting process. The e in e-budgeting stands for both electronic and enterprise-wide. Employees throughout an organization and at all levels can submit and retrieve budget

Table 18-1. Thirteen Scjedules Used to Construct a Master Budget

Schedule	Description
Sales budget	Displays the projected sales in units for each quarter and then multiplies the unit sales by the sales price to determine sales revenue
Production budget	Shows the number of units of services or goods that are to be produced during a budget period
Direct-material budget	Shows the number of produced units and the cost of material to be purchased and used during a budget period
Direct-labor budget	Shows the number of hours and the cost of the direct labor to be used during the budget period
Manufacturing-overhead budget	Shows the cost of overhead expected to be incurred in the production process during the budget period
Selling, general, and administrative (SG&A) expense budget	Lists the expenses of administering the firm and selling its units (e.g., prescriptions)
Cash receipts budget	Details the expected cash collections during a budget period
Cash disbursements budget	Details the expected cash payments during a budget period
Cash budget	Details the expected cash receipts and disbursements during a budget period
Budgeted schedule of cost of goods manufactured and sold	Details the direct material, direct-labor, and manufacturing-overhead costs to be incurred, and shows the cost of the goods to be sold during the budget period
Budgeted income statement	Shows the expected revenue and expenses for the budget period, assuming that planned operations are carried out
Budgeted statement of cash flows	Provides information about the expected sources and uses of cash for operating activities, investing activities, and financing activities during a particular period of time
Budgeted balance sheet	Shows the expected end-of-period balances for the company's assets, liabilities, and owner's equity, assuming that planned operations are carried out

information electronically via the Internet. Budgeting software is used and made available on the Web so that budget information submitted electronically from any location is in a consistent organization-wide format. Managers in pharmacy organizations using e-budgeting have found that it greatly streamlines the entire budgeting process. In the past, these organizations have compiled their master budgets on hundreds of spreadsheets, which had to be collected and integrated by the corporate controller's office. One result

of this cumbersome approach was that a disproportionate amount of time was spent compiling and verifying data from multiple sources. Under e-budgeting, both the submission of budget information and its compilation are accomplished electronically by the Web-based budgeting software. Thus e-budgeting is just one more area where the Internet has transformed how the workplace operates in the era of e-business. Examples of this type of software include OutlookSoft, Cognos, and WebFOCUS.

ZERO-BASE BUDGETING

Zero-base budgeting is used in a wide variety of organizations. Under zero-base budgeting, the budget for virtually every activity in the organization is initially set to zero. To receive funding during the budgeting process, each activity must be justified in terms of its continued usefulness. The zero-base-budgeting approach forces management to rethink each phase of an organization's operations before allocating resources.

Some organizations use a *base-budgeting* approach without going to the extreme of zero-base budgeting. Under this approach, the initial budget for each of the organization's departments is set in accordance with a base package, which includes the resources required for the subunit to exist at an absolute minimal level. Below this level of funding, the subunit would not be a viable entity. Any increases above the base package would result from a decision to fund an incremental package, which describes the resources needed to add various activities to the base package. The decision to approve such an incremental budget package would have to be justified on the basis of the costs and benefits of the activities included. Base budgeting has been effective in many organizations because it forces managers to take an evaluative, questioning attitude toward each of the organization's programs.

INTERNATIONAL ASPECTS OF BUDGETING

As the economies and cultures of countries throughout the world become intertwined, more companies are becoming multinational in their operations. Firms with international operations face a variety of additional challenges in preparing their budgets. First, a multinational firm's budget must reflect the translation of foreign currencies into a single currency (i.e., U.S. dollars). Since almost all the world's currencies fluctuate in their values relative to each other, this makes budgeting for those translations difficult. Second, it is difficult to prepare budgets when inflation is high or unpredictable. While the United States has experienced several periods of price inflation in the range of

10 percent increases per year, some foreign countries have experienced hyperinflation, sometimes with annual inflation rates well over 100 percent. Predicting such high inflation rates is difficult and further complicates a multinational's budgeting process. Finally, the economies of all countries fluctuate in terms of consumer demand, availability of skilled labor, laws affecting commerce, and other factors. Companies with offshore operations face the task of anticipating such changing conditions in the budgeting processes.

BUDGETING PRODUCT LIFE-CYCLE COSTS

A relatively recent focus of the budgeting process is to plan for all the costs that will be incurred during the introduction of a new product into the marketplace before a commitment is made to the product. The introduction of a new product may involve unanticipated costs during the following five phases:

- Product planning and concept design
- Preliminary design
- Detailed design and testing
- Production
- Distribution and customer service

For example, for a pharmaceutical manufacturer to justify a new drug's introduction, the sales revenues it will generate must be sufficient to cover all these costs. Thus, planning these costs is a crucial step in making a decision about the introduction of a new drug. Management must be fairly certain before a commitment is made to the drug that these costs will be covered.

BEHAVIORAL IMPACT OF BUDGETS

There is no other area where the behavioral implications are more important than in budgeting. A budget affects virtually everyone in an organization—those who prepare the budget, those who use the budget to facilitate decision making, and those who are evaluated using the budget. The human reactions to the budgeting process can have considerable influence on an organization's overall effectiveness.

A great deal of study has been devoted to the behavioral effects of budgets. Two key issues that a pharmacy manager should clearly understand are budgetary slack and participative budgeting.

Budgetary Slack: Padding the Budget

The information on which a budget is based comes largely from people throughout an organization. For example, the sales forecast for a retail pharmacy chain relies on market research and analysis by market research staff but also incorporates the projections of sales personnel. If a territorial sales manager's performance is evaluated on the basis of whether the sales budget for the territory is exceeded, what is the incentive for the sales manager in projecting sales? The incentive is to give a conservative, or cautiously low, sales estimate. The sales manager's performance will look much better in the eyes of top management when a conservative estimate is exceeded than when an ambitious estimate is not met. At least that is the perception of many sales managers, and in the behavioral area, perceptions are what count most.

When a manager provides an inpatient pharmacy departmental cost projection for budgetary purposes, there is an incentive to overestimate costs. When the actual cost incurred in the department proves to be less than the inflated cost projection, the supervisor appears to have managed in a cost-effective way.

These illustrations are examples of padding the budget. *Budget padding* means underestimating revenue or overestimating costs. The difference between the revenue or cost projection that a person provides and a realistic estimate of the revenue or cost is called *budgetary slack*. For example, if a pharmacy manager believes the annual utilities cost will be $18,000 but gives a budgetary projection of $20,000, the manager has built $2,000 of slack into the budget.

Why do people pad budgets with budgetary slack? There are three primary reasons. First, people often perceive that their performance will look better in their superiors' eyes if they can "beat the budget." Second, budgetary slack often is used to cope with uncertainty.

A pharmacy manager may feel confident in his or her cost projections. However, the pharmacy manager also may feel that some unforeseen event during the budgetary period could result in unanticipated costs. For example, an unexpected laminar flow hood breakdown could occur. One way of planning ahead for unforeseen events such as a laminar flow breakdown is to pad the budget. If nothing goes wrong, the pharmacy manager can beat the cost budget. If some negative event does occur, the pharmacy manager can use the budgetary slack to absorb the impact of the event and still meet the cost budget.

The third reason why cost budgets are padded is that budgetary cost projections are often cut by others in the resource-allocation process. Thus the process of preparing budgets can result in a vicious cycle. Budgetary projections are padded because they will likely be cut, and they are cut because they are likely to have been padded.

How does an organization solve the problem of budgetary slack? First, it can avoid relying on the budget as a negative evaluation tool. If a pharmacy manager is harassed by a higher-level manager every time a budgetary cost projection is exceeded, the likely behavioral response will be to pad the budget. In contrast, if the pharmacy manager is allowed some managerial discretion to exceed the budget when necessary, there will be fewer tendencies toward budgetary padding. Second, pharmacy managers can be given incentives not only to achieve budgetary projections but also to provide *accurate* projections. This can be accomplished by asking pharmacy managers to justify all or some of their projections and by rewarding pharmacy managers who consistently provide *accurate* estimates (as opposed to rewarding managers who perform under their cost projections and punishing managers who exceed their cost projections).

Participative Budgeting

Most people will perform better and make greater attempts to achieve a goal if they have been consulted in setting the goal. The idea of participative budgeting is to involve employees throughout an organization in the budgetary process. Such participation can give employees the feeling that "this is our budget" rather than the all-too-common feeling that "this is the budget you imposed on us."

While participative budgeting can be very effective, it can also have shortcomings. Too much participation and discussion can lead to vacillation and delay. Also, when those involved in the budgeting process disagree in significant and irreconcilable ways, the process of participation can accentuate those differences. Finally, the problem of budget padding can be severe unless incentives for accurate projections are provided.

REVISITING THE SCENARIO

Mary Quint, Pharm.D., knows that a budget is often used as the basis for evaluating a pharmacy manager's performance. Actual results are compared with budgeted performance levels, and those who outperform the budget often are rewarded with promotions or salary increases. In many cases, bonuses are tied explicitly to performance relative to a budget.

Serious ethical issues can arise in situations where a budget is the basis for rewarding managers. For example, suppose Home TPN Care's top-management personnel will split a bonus equal to 10 percent of the amount by which the actual business unit profit exceeds the budget. This may create an incentive for the pharmacy manager supplying data to pad the profit budget. Such padding would make the budget easier to achieve, thus increasing the chance of a bonus.

Alternatively, there may be an incentive to manipulate the business unit's actual results to maximize management's bonus. For example, year-end sales could be shifted between years to increase reported revenue in a particular year. Budget personnel could have such incentives for either of two reasons: (1) They might share in the bonus, or (2) they might feel pressure from the managers who would share in the bonus.

Dr. Quint has put herself in the position of Home TPN Care's controller. Her bonus, and that of her boss, the health system's vice president, will be determined in part by Home TPN Care's income in comparison with the budget. She can see from budgets submitted in the past that the organization's management usually has cut the unit's budgeted expenses, thereby increasing the business unit's budgeted profit. This, of course, makes it more difficult for her business unit to achieve the budgeted profit. Moreover, it makes it less likely that she and her business unit colleagues will earn a bonus. Now her boss is pressuring her to pad the expense budget because "the budgeted expenses will just be cut anyway at the organizational level." Is padding the budget ethical under these circumstances?

CONCLUSION

The budget is a key tool for planning, control, and decision making in virtually every organization. Budgeting systems are used to force planning, to facilitate communication and coordination, to allocate resources, to control profit and operations, and to evaluate performance and provide incentives. Various types of budgets are used to accomplish these objectives.

Since budgets affect almost everyone in an organization, they can have significant behavioral implications and can raise difficult ethical issues. One common problem in budgeting is the tendency of people to pad budgets. The resulting budgetary slack makes the budget less useful because the padded budget does not present an accurate picture of expected revenue and expenses.

QUESTIONS FOR FURTHER DISCUSSION

1. Use an example to explain how a budget could be used to allocate resources in a hospital pharmacy.
2. Give an example of how general economic trends would affect sales forecasting in the pharmaceutical industry.
3. Give three examples of how an independent community pharmacy could use a budget for planning purposes.
4. Discuss the importance of predictions and assumptions in the budgeting process.
5. How can the pharmacy department of a large urban hospital help to reduce the problems caused by budgetary slack?

6. Why is participative budgeting often an effective pharmacy management tool?

7. List the steps you would go through in developing a budget to meet your independent community pharmacy expenses.

REFERENCES

Cowlrick I, Dumon J, Bauleser M. 2002. Managing medical information effectively facilitates the quality and time to delivering the final product. *Drug Info J* 36:825.

Curtiss FR. 2006. Pharmacy benefit spending on oral chemotherapy drugs. *J Manag Care Pharm* 12:570.

Demers RF. 2001. Operational and financial principles of "managing up" *Am J Health-Syst Pharm* 58:S7.

Gregg W, Moscovice I, Remus D. 2006. The Implementation of Pay-for-Performance in Rural Hospitals: Lessons from the Hospital Quality Incentive Demonstration Project. Available at www.uppermidwestrhrc.org/pdf/pay_for_performance.pdf.

Poisal JA, Truffer C, Smith S, et al. 2007. Health spending projections through 2016: Modest changes obscure Part D's impact. *Health Affairs* 26:w242 (published online February 21, 2007;10.1377/ hlthaff.26.2.w242).

Schumock GT, Michaud J, Guenette AJ. 1999. Reengineering: An opportunity to advance clinical practice in a community hospital. *Am J Health-Syst Pharm* 56: 1945.

Tierney M. 2004. Lessons from patient deaths: An Ontario pharmacist responds to Calgary's patient safety review. *Can Pharm J* 137:8;9.

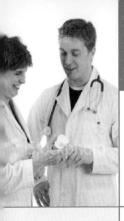

19

PERSONAL FINANCE

David A. Latif

About the Author: Dr. Latif is Professor of Pharmacy Administration and Chair of the Department of Pharmaceutical and Administrative Sciences at the University of Charleston School of Pharmacy. He earned an MBA from Augusta State University and a Ph.D. in social and behavioral pharmacy from Auburn University. His current research interests include examining the relationship between pharmacists' moral reasoning, work climates, and performance measures. Additional research and teaching interests include financial management, education, leadership, and the relationship between emotional intelligence and organizational effectiveness. Dr. Latif has published over 60 articles in pharmacy and business journals relating to his research interests.

▪ LEARNING OBJECTIVES

After completing this chapter, students should be able to

1. Describe why pharmacy students and pharmacists should be knowledgeable about their personal finance situation.
2. Identify and describe each component of the financial planning process.
3. Identify and describe the components of personal financial statements and budgeting.
4. Identify sources of credit and the costs of credit alternatives.
5. Describe factors that influence the amount of money needed for retirement. Compare and contrast methods of saving money for retirement.
6. Describe and discern among alternative asset classes.
7. Describe and explain asset allocation and its importance in reaching one's financial goals.
8. Compare index mutual fund investing with managed mutual fund investing.
9. List and explain the seven principles of effective personal finance.

■ SCENARIO

Daniel Keene has just graduated from a private pharmacy school with a doctor of pharmacy degree. He has several job offers from various pharmacies, all at salaries in the $100,000 per year range. He is told that with the sign-on bonus and overtime, he potentially can be making close to $120,000 per year. Daniel can hardly contain his excitement. He thinks to himself, "This degree was really worth getting." He begins to dream about what his life will be like from this point forward. His income was below the poverty line during the past 4 years. Now he will be in the top fifth of all income earners in the United States. Daniel begins thinking of all the sacrifices he has made to go to pharmacy school. For example, he drives a beat-up 1993 Honda Civic. Now he can afford a much nicer car. Daniel wonders, "Maybe I should buy a Lexus." Likewise, Daniel lives in a $400-per-month one-bedroom apartment. He contemplates buying a house. But how much of a house should he buy, and where can he get the most value? What type of mortgage should he get? Is it better to just rent for a few years to see if he likes his job? How much down payment should he put down if he decides to buy a house? Many additional thoughts are running through Daniel's head. They include

- "What should I do with my money? Should I save for the future or pay off my debts? If I choose to save, how much money should I put into stocks? How much should I put into bonds and cash? With the stunning declines in the stock market during the early 2000s, should I even own stocks? What is risk tolerance?"
- "Should I begin retirement planning immediately, or should I wait a few years?"
- "If I do decide to begin contributing to retirement plans, how much of my salary should I contribute and to what plan(s) [e.g., 401(k)/403(b), Roth IRA, traditional IRA, or regular savings account]?"
- "Should I use my credit card to buy things?"

Daniel thinks to himself, "I did not realize I would be faced with making so many decisions." Then a disturbing thought went through his head, "What about my $130,000 in student loans! How should I pay them back? Is any part of these loans tax deductible?"

After much reflection, Daniel realizes that he must get educated in personal finance. He wishes that he had been offered a course on it in pharmacy school. He decides to buy a good personal finance book to find the answers to his many questions.

■ CHAPTER QUESTIONS

1. Assume that a fourth-year pharmacy student has two job offers on graduation. One is to work as a staff pharmacist at a chain pharmacy for $100,000 per year. The other is a 1-year residency in a hospital for $40,000. Without considering the impact of taxes and qualitative factors, what is the 1-year financial opportunity cost of taking the residency over the chain offer?
2. Time value of money:
   a. What is the future value of $450 six years from now at a 7 percent annual interest rate?
   b. Assume that you contribute $5,000 per year to a Roth IRA for 20 years. What is the value of the IRA at the end of 20 years assuming a 10 percent annual interest rate?
   c. What is the amount a person would have to deposit today (present value) at a 6 percent interest rate to have $1,000 five years from now?
   d. Assume that your $150,000 student loan interest rate is 6 percent. To pay it off over 10 years, what will be your annual payment?
3. John Hardesty obtained a $200,000 thirty-year mortgage on his house at 7 percent interest. Not including property taxes and other costs, his monthly payment is $1,331. How much interest will John have paid at the end of 30 years?
4. What would a personal net worth statement help a recent pharmacy graduate assess?
5. Estimate your retirement needs based on the guidelines presented in this chapter.

INTRODUCTION

A National Bureau of Economic Research study reported that instruction in personal financial management prior to entering the workforce has the long-term effect of increasing a person's late savings and wealth (Garman and Bagwell, 1998). Specifically, the research reveals that 15 to 20 years after high school, wealth is greater by 1 year of earnings for those who received personal finance instruction compared with those who did not. To illustrate, if a 35-year-old who had a personal finance education earns $100,000 per year and has a net worth of $300,000, a similar person (i.e., same age and same yearly earnings) who did not have a personal finance education would have a net worth of only $200,000.

Doctor of pharmacy graduates face two immediate impediments to prudent financial planning on graduation. The first impediment is dealing with their student loans. Pharmacy education is an expensive undertaking. It is not unusual for a new pharmacy graduate to have over $100,000 of student loan debt after 6 or more years of college.

The second impediment to prudent financial planning is a prevailing perception that the sacrifice of 4 years of pharmacy school and of being "poor" must be rewarded immediately with significant material purchases. For example, many students may feel the need to purchase an expensive new car or as much house as they can get a loan for. A guiding principle that should be remembered is the simple economic law of unlimited wants and limited resources. By purchasing a lower-priced car and house, one will have more money (limited resource) for other important things.

Employee pharmacists must make many decisions regarding financial management. Among the most important is the specific types and extent of benefits provided by the employer. Benefits often amount to an additional 30 percent of an employee's salary and include such things as health, life, and disability insurance and retirement planning issues such as 401(k) contributions and defined pension benefits.

Pharmacy owners may face greater concerns relating to personal financial management than employee pharmacists. Decisions relating to adequate insurance coverage for property and liability losses, adequate and affordable health and disability insurance, and retirement planning issues require a considerable amount of financial knowledge. Although pharmacy employees probably have a retirement plan available (with employer contributions), pharmacy owners must establish a retirement plan, such as a Keogh plan, for the business.

The changing face of retirement has made financial planning knowledge more important than ever for pharmacists. Life expectancies have increased significantly over the past 100 years (American Counsel for Life Insurance, 2006). For example, an American born in 1900 could expect to live 47.6 years, whereas one born in 2002 can expect to live to 77.3 (averages of male and female). These expectations are median averages. In other words, a person born in 2002 has a life expectancy of 77.3 years. This means that half of those born in 2002 are expected to live longer than 77.3 years and half are expected to live less than 77.3 years. Many Americans can expect to live at least a quarter of their lives in retirement. To retire comfortably for this amount of time, people should apply the principles of effective personal financial management throughout their lives.

BENEFITS AND COSTS OF PERSONAL FINANCE EDUCATION

Financial matters affect not only one's personal and family life but also one's workplace behavior. Brown (1979) reported that workers who experience financial problems negatively affect their employers. This is true regardless of occupation or level of income. Brown observed that the poor financial behaviors of employees often result in one or more counterproductive work behaviors (e.g., absenteeism or productivity loss from lack of focus).

Table 19-1.	Costs of Poor Employee Financial Behaviors on Employers

1. Absenteeism
2. Tardiness
3. Fighting with coworkers and supervisors
4. Sabotage the work of coworkers
5. Job stress
6. Reduced employee productivity
7. Lower employee morale
8. Loss of customers who seek better service
9. Loss of revenue from sales not made
10. Disability and worker compensation claims
11. Substance abuse
12. Increased use of health care resources
13. Thefts from employers
14. Lack of focus on strategic goals of employer
15. Use of employer time to deal with poor financial behaviors of employees

Source: Adapted with permission from Garman, Leech, and Grable, 1996.

Table 19-2.	Behaviors Associated with Poor Personal Financial Management

1. Regularly spending too much money
2. Regularly overusing credit
3. Regularly reaching the maximum limit on a credit card
4. Regularly running out of money
5. Typically having a low or nonexistent emergency fund savings account
6. Regularly being unable to pay due bills (e.g., utilities, rent, child care, credit cards)
7. Habitually receiving "overdue notices" from creditors
8. Typically having liabilities in excess of assets
9. Regularly losing money to rip-offs and frauds
10. Regularly losing money by gambling or buying lottery tickets and/or gambling in an attempt to fix one's financial situation

Source: Adapted with permission from Garman, Leech, and Grable, 1996.

Job productivity suffers because of the impact poor personal financial behaviors have on family life (Garman, Leech, and Grable, 1996). For example, poor personal financial decisions may lead to loss of transportation, loss of the ability to obtain credit and adequate housing, arguments with relatives, emotional stress, spouse/child abuse, and divorce. These decisions manifest in dysfunctional work behaviors such as absenteeism, tardiness, and reduced job productivity. Table 19-1 summarizes the potential costs associated with poor employee financial behaviors.

A major cause of financial problems is the financial illiteracy of individuals (Garman, Leech, and Grable, 1996). *Financial illiteracy* refers to an inadequate knowledge of personal finance facts and concepts for successful personal financial management. According to Garman, Leech, and Grable (1996), financial illiteracy is widespread among Americans owing to a lack of knowledge in personal finance, the complexities of financial life, a feeling of being overburdened with

numerous choices in financial decision making, and a lack of time to learn financial planning concepts. Table 19-2 lists examples of personal financial mistakes and careless behaviors.

This chapter describes a six-step process that has been proven to be useful in beginning to manage one's personal finances. Personal financial statements, the use of credit, investment strategies, and retirement planning also are discussed. The chapter concludes with seven principles of effective personal finance.

■ THE FINANCIAL PLANNING PROCESS

It would be very difficult for a homebuilder to build a house without blueprints. It would be equally difficult for one to take a cross-country automobile trip without a map. Likewise, it is difficult for people to reach financial goals without planning. *Personal financial planning* is the process of managing one's money to achieve economic satisfaction (Kapoor, Dlabay, and Hughes, 2004). The primary purpose of this process is to allow one to control one's financial situation by identifying and developing a plan to meet specific needs and goals. According to Kapoor, Dlabay, and Hughes (2004), the financial planning process includes six steps.

Step 1: Determine Your Financial Situation

The first step requires that one assess one's current situation regarding income, savings, living expenses, and debts. This step requires that one prepare a list of current asset and debt balances, along with present expenditures. Personal finance statements (discussed later in this chapter) can be a useful tool for this step.

Step 1 Example
Daniel Keene will graduate from pharmacy school within the next 2 months. During school, Daniel has worked part time as a pharmacy technician. He has a savings fund of $2,000 and over $130,000 in student loans. What additional information should Daniel have available when planning his personal finances?

Step 2: Develop Financial Goals

The purpose of this step is to differentiate a person's needs from his or her wants. This analysis involves identifying how one feels about money. Are feelings based on objective information? Are priorities based on social pressures, needs, or desires? It is important to understand that while wants are unlimited, resources are limited. People should set their financial priorities around satisfying needs (e.g., food, clothing, shelter, and transportation) before considering to what extent their wants can be satisfied.

Step 2 Example
Daniel Keene has several goals, including paying off his student loans, doing a residency, and buying a house. What other goals might be appropriate for Daniel?

Step 3: Identify Alternative Courses of Action

Many factors influence potential alternative courses of action. Considering all possible alternatives helps people to make more effective financial decisions. The most common categories include

- *Continuing along the same course of action.* For example, one might decide that saving 5 percent of one's gross income is adequate for one's financial goals.
- *Expanding the current situation.* Alternatively, one might decide that 10 percent of one's salary is a more appropriate amount to save to meet important goals.
- *Changing the current situation.* One might decide that aggressive stock investments are too risky given the stock market environment. Therefore, a more conservative investment approach is warranted.
- *Taking a new course of action.* Some people may decide that instead of investing their monthly savings, they will divert it toward paying off debts such as student loans.

Step 3 Example
Daniel Keene has numerous alternative courses of action available to him. He can postpone a residency to earn "quick" money by working for a community pharmacy on graduation. This money could be used to help pay off his loans and/or to put a down payment on a house. What additional alternatives might Daniel consider?

Step 4: Evaluate Alternatives

People need to evaluate from among their possible courses of action. Life situation, personal values, current economic conditions, and many other factors can be taken into consideration. For example, if interest rates are low, would it be better to buy a house in the near future rather than take a chance on rates increasing in 2 years? Every decision you make has a consequence, or opportunity cost. For instance, the opportunity cost of going to pharmacy school is not only the tuition cost of going to school but also the amount of money you could have earned in the mean time had you not gone to school. Similarly, investing 10 percent of your salary in the stock market may require that you go on a less expensive vacation (opportunity cost) than if you did not save the 10 percent.

Uncertainty or risk is part of every financial decision. Even seemingly safe, conservative financial decisions entail risk. For example, investing 10 percent of your salary in a savings account in the hope of being able to one day retire based on its performance may be risky because, historically, savings account returns have been among the lowest returns of any asset class (especially when one considers the effects of inflation).

Step 4 Example

Daniel Keene must consider his income needs as he evaluates his alternative courses of action. Should he go straight to the residency? Or should he work a year in a community pharmacy first? What risks and tradeoffs should Daniel consider?

Step 5: Create and Implement a Financial Action Plan

This is the step where one develops an action plan. At this stage, goals already have been decided on, and a decision must be made on how to achieve them. For example, if Daniel wishes to pay his student loans off more quickly, he must decrease his spending in certain categories (e.g., eating out). Alternatively, he can increase his salary by working overtime or by moonlighting at another pharmacy. Once one of his goals is achieved, Daniel should focus on the next one in priority.

Step 5 Example

Daniel Keene has decided to work full time for 2 years to pay down his student loans and to purchase a home. What are the benefits and costs of this course of action?

Step 6: Reevaluate and Revise Your Plan

Personal financial planning is a dynamic process. As such, it is imperative that you review your plan regularly. Many financial planners recommend a complete review at least once a year. Changing personal, social, and economic conditions may require a more frequent review.

Step 6 Example

Over the next 12 months, Daniel Keene should review and reassess his educational, financial, and personal situation. What circumstances might affect his need to take a different course of action?

■ PERSONAL FINANCIAL STATEMENTS

As described in step 1 above, you must know where you are presently before you can go somewhere else. Personal financial statements tell you where you are in your financial journey. Among the most pertinent financial statements are personal balance sheets, cashflow statements, and the development of a monthly budget.

Personal Balance Sheet

A logical starting point for an individual or family is to determine the present financial statement. In essence, this entails determining what is owned, what is owed, and what is left over.

What is owned (assets) − what is owed (liabilities) = net worth

It is not uncommon for pharmacy students to have a negative net worth. For example, if all of Daniel Keene's possessions are worth $10,000 and he owes $130,000 in student loans, then his net worth is −$120,000.

Table 19-3 provides an example of determining one's net worth. Assets are cash and other tangible property with monetary value. In this example, assets are divided into current assets and long-term assets. Liquid assets are current assets that are easily converted to cash. For example, a checking account is a liquid asset. Long-term assets include such items as real estate, personal possessions, and investment assets. Real estate may include the value of one's house and/or any rental property that one might own. Personal possessions might include such items as the market value of a person's car, furniture, jewelry, and computer. Investment assets include such items as the market value of mutual funds and retirement accounts.

Liabilities are often categorized as current and long term. Current liabilities include debts that must be paid within a year. These might include the following: credit-card balances, balance due on your automobile loan, tax payments, and insurance premiums. Long-term liabilities include such items as mortgage and student loans.

Table 19-3. Net Worth Example

Assets

Current assets	
Cash	
Savings account	
Checking account	
Certificate of deposits	
Other current assets	$3,000
Total current assets	$3,000
Long-term assets	
Homes	
Furnishings	
Automobile	$8,000
Electronic equipment	$2,200
Appliances	$1,200
Other property	
Total property	$11,400
Investments	
Stocks and bonds	$2,575
Retirement plan assets	
Other investments	
Total investments	$2,575
Total assets	$16,975
Liabilities	
Current liabilities	
Credit-card debt	$1,250
Short-term installment loan	$450
Short-term personal loan	$750
Other current liabilities	
Total current liabilities	$2,450
Long-term liabilities	
Mortgage	
Student loan	$110,000
Other long-term liabilities	
Total long-term liabilities	$110,000
Total liabilities	$112,450
Net worth	
Total assets – total liabilities	($95,475)

Cash-Flow Statement

This statement answers the question, "Where did all my money go?" Many events continually affect your cash flow. For example, paying living expenses and receiving a paycheck affect cash flow. *Cash flow* is simply the inflow and outflow of cash during a period of time (e.g., 1 month). Table 19-4 provides an example of a cash-flow statement. Cash inflows include income from salary and interest and investment earnings. Cash outflows can be divided into two categories: fixed expenses and variable expenses. *Fixed expenses* are stable expenses that do not vary frequently and include rent or mortgage payments, loan payments, cable television payments, and insurance premiums. *Variable expenses* include items that one might have control over, such as food purchases, entertainment, and clothing purchases.

Budget

A *budget* (see Chapter 18) is a spending plan that may help you live within your means, spend money wisely, and develop critical financial management habits (Fullen and Fitzgerald, 1991; Kapoor, Dlabay, and Hughes, 2004). A budget is useful because it is a tool you can use to make adjustments to your monthly cash flow and spending habits. Using the information from the cash-flow statement, you can project any adjustments to your cash outflows. This is particularly true of the variable expense section on the cash-flow statement. For example, if Daniel Keene finds that he spent $200 eating out last month (which he feels is too much), he might budget $100 for next month. The budget is an anticipated blueprint of future expenditures. As another example, the Bakers are a family of four who have carefully examined their expenditures for the past 3 months. They were surprised to find that they were spending $1,500 per month on clothing, groceries, and eating out. Armed with this information, they decided to budget 20 percent less ($300 per month) on these categories than they spent on them during the prior 3 months. Assuming that the Bakers stick to their budget, they will have $3,600 more at the end of 1 year than before they began the budget process

(assuming that all other expenditures and earnings remain the same).

▮ CONSUMER CREDIT

"Charge it!" "Put it on my account!" "Add it to my student loan!" As these statements indicate, buying on credit is a way of life in the United States. Simply stated, *credit* is an arrangement to receive cash, goods, or services now and pay for them in the future (Rejda and McNamara, 1998). Consumer credit is differentiated from other types of credit (i.e., business credit) in that it is credit for personal and family needs (except a home mortgage). According the 2004 Survey of Consumer Finance, the median value of credit-card balances and installment loans for a typical family in 2004 was $13,700 (Bucks et al., 2006). Installment loans describe consumer loans that require fixed payments and a fixed term (e.g., an automobile loan).

There are advantages and disadvantages to credit. One advantage is that it allows people to use goods and services now rather than later. For example, it may take many years to save the $125,000 (or more) it can cost to attend pharmacy school. If loans were not available, many students would never be able to attend pharmacy school. By getting low-interest (and for many, tax-deductible) loans, students are able to go to school now rather than later. It lets them begin earning pharmacist salaries within 4 years of beginning pharmacy school (as opposed to saving for many years prior to going to pharmacy school). With the salaries pharmacists earn, most lenders feel that there is a reasonably low risk that these students will not be able to pay back their loans after they graduate and enter the workforce.

Using credit cards is another common example of consumer credit. Credit cards allow people to make purchases even when they may not have enough cash on hand to pay for them. Many people feel more comfortable making purchases on credit cards instead of carrying large amounts of cash. In addition, they are a convenient way to consolidate individual purchases into one single monthly payment. Many large corporations

Table 19-4. Cash-Flow Statement Example

Income (cash inflows) (monthly)		
Salary (gross)		$6,550
Less deductions		
Federal income tax	$525	
State income tax	$130	
Social Security	$502	
Total deductions	$1,157	$5,393
Interest earned on savings		$95
Earnings from investments		
Total income		$5,488
Cash outflows		
Fixed expenses		
Rent		$1,500
Loan payment		$1,000
Cable television		$50
Monthly train ticket		$75
Insurance		$150
Other fixed outflows		
Total fixed outflows		$2,775
Variable expenses		
Food at home		$325
Food away from home		$250
Clothing		$200
Telephone		$125
Electricity		$60
Personal care (e.g., cosmetics and dry cleaning)		$60
Medical expenses		$55
Entertainment		$300
Gifts		$50
Donations		$50
Total variable outflows		$1,475
Total outflows		$4,250
Cash surplus (or deficit)		$1,238
Allocation of surplus		
Savings		$1,238

issue their own credit cards to the public. They provide incentives in the form of rebates to users of their cards. Likewise, using a credit card for such things as airplane travel and car rentals often includes, at no additional cost, added benefits such as accident insurance.

Credit also has disadvantages if it is not used prudently. For instance, if you do not pay your credit-card balances in full each month, prohibitive interest expenses can be incurred. Interest rates are often 15 to 20 percent on credit cards, so if you only pay the minimum amount due each month, you will be paying the debt for decades. One of the biggest disadvantages of credit in general and credit cards in particular is the temptation to overspend. Overspending can lead to serious long-term financial problems and poor family relationships and may reduce the likelihood of reaching your financial goals. Therefore, it is imperative that pharmacists continually question their potential purchases from a cost-benefit standpoint. For example, most people in the 25 percent federal tax bracket and 6 percent state tax bracket must earn $1,630 for every $1,000 they spend on their lifestyle (this figure includes employee Social Security and Medicare taxes).

ASSET CLASSES AND ASSET ALLOCATION

The following are facts about investments:

- Since 1940, there have been only 2 years without inflation.
- To earn long-term returns, you have to accept short-term risk.
- The only prices that count are the prices at which you buy and sell; *everything else is a distraction.*
- You should only invest in equities if you will not need the money in the near future.
- Past performance is a poor indicator of future results.

The broad equity market, as measured by the Standard & Poor's 500 Index (S&P 500), experienced a historical high in March of 2000. By February of 2003, it had declined approximately 45 percent. However, even before these significant declines, the typical investor did significantly worse than the average return in the asset classes of stocks and bonds. According to Dalbar, Inc., an investment research firm, the S&P 500 returned an average of 11.81 percent annually between January 1987 and December 2006 (Dalbar, 2007). However, the typical investor in stock market mutual funds gained only 6.19 percent per year. The major reason for this underperformance is that investors typically buy high and sell low. In other words, they wait too long to get into an asset class (i.e., until after it has gone up substantially) and sell after it has declined (i.e., right before it is set to increase in value). How can investors increase the probability of approximating the market return? Three key concepts that will increase investors' chances are identifying tolerance for risk, asset diversification, and index investing.

Risk and Risk Tolerance

If your investments declined 30 percent in a year, would you sell them and commit your remaining assets to a guaranteed savings account? Your answers to questions such as this one determine the percentage of your investment funds that should be committed to the three major asset classes of stocks, bonds, and cash (i.e., stable money market funds or bank savings accounts). The following is a law of finance: "To receive higher returns, one must take greater risks." There are two basic sources of risk: (1) changing economic conditions and (2) changing conditions of the security issuer. Changing economic conditions include inflation risks, business cycle risks, and interest rate risks.

Inflation risk occurs when inflation increases, but the return on one's investment does not keep pace with it. An example might be your savings account paying 1 percent interest when inflation is 3 percent. *Business-cycle risk* refers to the fact that your investments may mirror the fluctuations in the business cycle. For example, stocks typically decline when the economy first enters a recession because the earnings of companies normally decline during recessions. *Interest-rate risk* may occur when interest rates rise, but you have locked into a lower rate on a long-term bond. For example, if you purchase a 4 percent bond for 10 years, you face the real possibility that if interest rates rise, the value of the bond will decline.

A second source of risk is the changing condition of the issuer. These risks include *management risk* (e.g., the company in which you invest has poor managers), *business risks* (e.g., the risks associated with the company's products), and *financial risks* (e.g., the company may borrow too much money and have to declare bankruptcy). Therefore, you cannot expect to receive a greater return for a nondiversified company-specific high-risk investment (e.g., committing all your investment capital to one or two stocks). This is so because the market may do quite well, but one or two companies (the one's you picked) may go bankrupt owing to management, business, and/or financial risk specific to a few companies.

In general, the greater the variability of an investment, the greater is its risk. However, the longer the risky investment is held, the greater are the chances of earning a higher return as opposed to a "safe" investment (i.e., savings account). For example, between 1926 and 2005, the worse 1-year performance of the U.S. stock market was –43.3 percent, and the best performance was 54.2 percent (Ibbotson, 2006). Extending the return performance to 20 years reveals that the worse 20-year performance of stocks was an annualized return of 3.1 percent, whereas the best 20-year annualized return was 17.8 percent. Therefore, it is imperative that you examine your tolerance for risk and, based on that tolerance, construct a diversified portfolio of investments that not only meet your financial goals but are also consistent with your tolerance for risk.

Asset Allocation

As discussed previously, if you cannot tolerate your investment portfolio declining by 30% percent in one year, you do not want to have an all-stock portfolio (because the largest historical one year decline was 43.3%). But how should you allocate your resources? Suppose that you can tolerate a 20% decline or a 10% decline? Based on historical returns and using large stocks and long-term bonds as major asset classes to design a portfolio, you should not have more than 40% stocks in your portfolio if you cannot tolerate a greater than 20%

loss (Ibbotson, 2006). If you cannot tolerate a greater than 10% loss to your portfolio you should not have more than 20% in stocks. By designing a portfolio based on your risk tolerance, you significantly increase the probability that you will stick with it when the going gets tough. Therefore, you will be more likely to attain the market returns rather than typical investor returns.

Index Investing

Investing in an index mutual fund is an attempt to match, after expenses, the performance of a group of stocks. For example, the S&P 500 is a broad measure of the U.S. stock market performance. Investing in an index mutual fund following the S&P 500 will result in slightly lower returns than the index (owing to fund expenses). Historically, expense ratios are much lower for investments in index funds than for investments in managed stock mutual funds (those in which "experts" invest only in stocks that they believe will exceed the overall average market return). Although managed mutual funds have the goal of beating the index on which they are judged, they rarely do (owing, in part, to increased expenses). For example, during the 25-year period between December 31, 1980, and December 31, 2005, the average managed equity mutual fund earned 10 percent per year, whereas an S&P 500 index mutual fund earned 12.3 percent per year (Bogle, 2006). Stated another way, $10,000 grew to $108,347 in the average equity mutual fund but grew to $181,758 in a S&P 500 index fund over the same period of time.

Time Value of Money

Having a dollar today is worth more than receiving a dollar some time in the future. Conversely, paying a dollar at a later date is more desirable than paying it now. These statements make sense because any sum of money today can be invested to earn interest and thereby grow to a larger amount. For example, without considering taxes and commissions, you can use a business calculator to determine how much $10,000 will grow to in 10 years assuming an annual 8 percent interest rate. The answer, $21,589, is derived in the following manner: $10,000 \times 1.08^{10} = \$21,589$ (1.08 to the tenth power is simply the interest rate factor over the next 10 years). Using Table 19-5, we can determine what $10,000 invested in stocks from 1926 to 2005 would have grown to (disregarding taxes and commissions): $10,000 × 1.104^{80} = $27,385,828. Stocks averaged 10.4 percent per year during the past 80 years, which would have increased an initial $10,000 investment to over $27 million.

To put the concept of time value of money in perspective, consider the tale of the two investors investing in an IRA (maximum contribution for 2008 for those aged 49 and under is $5,000). As depicted in Table 19-5 (assumes a tax-deferred return of 9 percent per year), Investor A contributed $5,000 per year from age 22 through age 30 and then terminated contributions (total of $45,000 invested). Investor B began her $5,000 contributions at age 31 but continued until retiring at age 65 (total of $175,000 invested). Despite contributing $130,000 less, Investor A had $1,347,359 at age 65, whereas Investor B had only $1,086,982. Because of the time value of money, the earlier one begins investing, the more one can accumulate (and the less one needs to save).

▨ RETIREMENT PLANNING

Significant changes have taken place in company retirement plans during the last few decades. Traditionally, employers provided employees with *defined-benefit plans,* which used a formula based on years of service to determine benefits. For example, an individual working for a company for 20 years may receive 50 percent of his or her final year's salary in a pension. During the past 30 years, more and more employers have transferred the responsibility of retirement planning and future benefits to the employee through *defined-contribution plans.* Defined-contribution plans give employees control over and responsibility for their pensions through vehicles such as 401(k) plans (for for-profit companies) and 403(b) plans (for not-for-profit organizations). Thus, if employees do not participate in their company retirement plans and invest wisely in them, there is a possibility that they will not have a comfortable retirement.

A question many employees have is, "How much money do I need to retire and maintain my preretirement lifestyle?" According to a growing field of research on investment withdrawals, in order to have a 100 percent inflation-adjusted probability of not running out of money over a 30-year period (based on the historical performance of stocks, bonds, cash, and inflation), retirees should not withdraw more than 4 to 5 percent of their investment portfolios on an annual basis (Cooley, Hubbard, and Waltz, 1998). A typical couple needs to plan for a minimum of 20 years of income at retirement (Burns, 1997). In essence, if you have 20 years of income in investments or some other vehicle, you will be secure. Where do you get those years of income?

You do not need to have 20 years' worth of income, only the equivalent. Social Security will replace a portion of your income. If the figure is 25 percent, as it is for those earning the wage-base maximum, this means that it is the rough equivalent of 5 years of income (25 percent × 20 = 5).

Home ownership can provide "income years" through a trade-down. For example, moving from a $400,000 house to a $200,000 house in retirement will allow you to have $200,000 of new investment money (which can support your entire shelter bill, including utilities, property insurance, and upkeep). The trade-down option is the single largest lever people have on their retirement security. It can replace 2 to 4 years of income.

Personal savings, pension plans, and retirement savings from such vehicles as 401(k) or 403(b) plans will replace the remaining "years of income." It does not require financial acumen or brilliance to have financial stability. Anyone can achieve financial security by being a regular saver and a homeowner and having stable employment.

According to Burns (1997), the blueprint for financial security can be narrowed down to seven key principles:

1. Spend less than you earn (e.g., save 10 percent of all wages).
2. Pay yourself first (e.g., have 10 percent taken from your paycheck each period, and invest it).

Table 19-5. The Impact of Time Value of Money at 9 percent Interest

Age (Years)	Contributions Made Early ($)	Age (Years)	Contributions Made Later ($)
22	5,000	22	
23	5,000	23	
24	5,000	24	
25	5,000	25	
26	5,000	26	
27	5,000	27	
28	5,000	28	
29	5,000	29	
30	5,000	30	
31		31	5,000
32		32	5,000
33		33	5,000
34		34	5,000
35		35	5,000
36		36	5,000
37		37	5,000
38		38	5,000
39		39	5,000
40		40	5,000
41		41	5,000
42		42	5,000
43		43	5,000
44		44	5,000
45		45	5,000
46		46	5,000
47		47	5,000
48		48	5,000
49		49	5,000
50		50	5,000
51		51	5,000
52		52	5,000
53		53	5,000
54		54	5,000
55		55	5,000
56		56	5,000
57		57	5,000
58		58	5,000
59		59	5,000

(Continued)

Table 19-5. The Impact of Time Value of Money at 9 percent Interest *(Continued)*

Age (Years)	Contributions Made Early ($)	Age (Years)	Contributions Made Later ($)
60		60	5,000
61		61	5,000
62		62	5,000
63		63	5,000
64		64	5,000
65		65	5,000
Amount available at 65	1,347,359		1,086,982

3. Take advantage of free money [always take advantage of employer matching on 401(k) or 403(b) plans].
4. Keep investment expenses low (the more you pay in investment expenses, the less you will have ultimately).
5. Owe as little as possible (e.g., do not carry credit-card balances at high interest rates).
6. Diversify investments. Do not put all your investment eggs in one basket.
7. Trust the power of average. As noted earlier, matching the S&P 500 Index's return would have been far superior to what the typical investor actually earned.

▓ REVISITING THE SCENARIO: FINANCIAL EDUCATION

The preceding discussion of the many aspects of financial education brings us back to the scenario. Daniel Keene's situation is not unlike many recently graduated pharmacists. The sacrifices and opportunity costs in obtaining the doctor of pharmacy degree have given way to a bright future, one in which critical financial decisions must be made. As discussed earlier, many pharmacy students go from being in poverty to being in the top fifth of all income earners in the United States. Similar to patient care, there is not a one-size-fits-all financial plan. One student may have significantly different financial goals than his or her classmates. This is

why it is important that each person take the time to write down and reflect on the six-step financial planning process discussed earlier. The more knowledge you obtain on financial planning issues, the greater is the likelihood that you will reach your financial goals.

▓ CONCLUSION

Knowledge of financial planning translates into superior financial decisions concerning one's family and into a significantly higher net worth 20 years after high school graduation (Garman and Bagwell, 1998). The information in this chapter can contribute to your financial education. First, a six-step financial planning process was described. Next, specific components of personal financial statements were described and discussed, along with a discussion of credit. Then investing in various asset classes and the importance of asset allocation based on one's risk tolerance were discussed. Finally, the time value of money and retirement planning issues were discussed, along with seven principles of effective personal finance.

▓ QUESTIONS FOR FURTHER DISCUSSION

Given what you now know about personal finance, how would you help Daniel Keene answer the questions he raised in the scenario at the beginning of the chapter:

1. Once Daniel becomes a pharmacist, what should be his first financial priority: saving to purchase a home, paying off his student loan debt, or paying off his credit-card debt? What additional information would you like to have to help Daniel address this question?
2. What are the advantages and disadvantages of using credit cards to make personal purchases?
3. Assuming that Daniel will practice pharmacy for about 40 years before retiring, when would be the best time for him to start saving for his retirement?
4. Approximately how many years' worth of income should Daniel plan on saving for retirement?
5. What percentage of his annual income should Daniel plan on saving for retirement? What factors influence this decision?
6. Once Daniel starts saving for retirement, what would be the most appropriate investments for him to make—stocks, bonds, 401(k), IRA, or savings accounts? What factors should he think about before deciding where to invest his retirement savings?

REFERENCES

American Council of Life Insurance. 2006. *Life Insurance Fact Book.* Washington, DC: American Council of Life Insurance.

Bogle JC. 2006. What's Ahead for Stocks and Bonds—And How to Earn Your Fair Share. Bogle Financial Markets Research Center, www.vanguard.com/bogle_site/bogle_speeches. html; accessed on March 21, 2007.

Brown RC. 1979. Employee assistance programs in industry. In Myhre DC (ed), *Financial Counseling: Assessing the State of the Art,* p. 137. Blacksburg, VA: Financial Counseling Project Extension Division.

Bucks BK, Kennickell AB, Moore DB. 2006. Recent changes in U.S. family finances: Evidence from the 2001 and 2004 Survey of Consumer Finances. *Federal Reserve Bulletin* (March).

Burns S. 1997. The seven laws of personal finance (couch potato edition). *Dallas Morning News,* January 5.

Cooley P, Hubbard CM, Waltz DT. 1998. Retirement savings: Choosing a rate that is sustainable. *AAII J;* available at www.aaii.com/.

Dalbar, Inc. 2007. Quatitative Analysis of Investor Behavior, 2007. Available at www.dalbarinc.com/.

Fullen TL, Fitzgerald WL. 1991. Getting a leg up with financial planning. *Apothecary* April–May–June: 6.

Garman ET, Bagwell DC. 1998. The impact of high school financial curriculum requirements on adult behavior (or how to get an extra year's paycheck). *Assoc Financ Counsel Plan Educ Newsletter* 16:3.

Garman ET, Leech IE, Grable JE. 1996. The negative impact of employee poor personal financial behaviors on employers. *Assoc Financ Counsel Plan Educ Newsletter* 7:157.

Ibbotson R. 2006. *Stocks, Bonds, Bills, and Inflation (SBBI) Valuation Edition 2006 Yearbook.* New York: Wiley.

Kapoor JR, Dlabay LR, Hughes RJ. 2004. *Personal Finance,* 7th ed. New York: McGraw-Hill/Irwin.

Rejda GE, McNamara MJ. 1998. *Personal Financial Planning.* Reading, MA: Addison-Wesley.

SECTION V

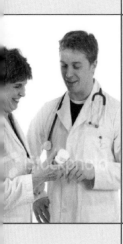

MANAGING TRADITIONAL GOODS

AND SERVICES

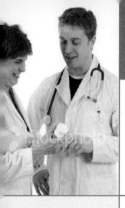

20

MARKETING THEORY

John Bentley

About the Author: Dr. Bentley is an Associate Professor in the Department of Pharmacy Administration and Research Associate Professor in the Research Institute of Pharmaceutical Sciences at the University of Mississippi School of Pharmacy. He received a B.S. in pharmacy and an MBA from Drake University and an M.S. and Ph.D. in pharmacy administration from the University of Mississippi. In addition to statistics, Dr. Bentley's teaching interests focus on the organization, delivery, financing, and outcomes of health care. His research interests include understanding the role of pharmacy practice in how medications and the medication consumption experience affect quality of life, the use of quality-of-life measures as clinical tools, and empirical investigations of ethical issues in pharmacy and research.

▪ LEARNING OBJECTIVES

After completing this chapter, students should be able to

1. Define marketing and describe its societal contributions.
2. Discuss the purpose of marketing within a business.
3. Identify orientations toward the marketplace that organizations might take when conducting marketing activities.
4. Differentiate among the concepts of needs, wants, and demands.
5. Define the concept of exchange and state its importance to marketing.
6. Describe the marketing mix and apply it to the marketing of services.
7. Describe different types of product offerings, and define the distinguishing characteristics of a service.
8. Define expectations, satisfaction, quality, value, and loyalty and describe their role in purchase behavior and the profitability of organizations.
9. Explain the concept of relationship marketing and apply it to pharmacy management.

■ SCENARIO

Jim Smyth and Sue Davidson co-own and manage the West Side Pharmacy. While looking over the books for the last year, both pharmacists begin to recognize that their pharmacy is struggling to meet its financial objectives. The two decide to ask the staff pharmacist and the technicians to help them brainstorm ideas for improving their performance. During the after-hours impromptu staff meeting, the following questions were asked: "Are there any health-related goods that we should add to the line of products we sell?" "What other services can we provide that people in our community need or want?" "What types of services can we develop given our resources?" "Should we provide the services in our pharmacy or at some other location?" "How will our services be different from the Corner Pharmacy on the other side of town?" "What should we charge for our services?" "How do we let people know that we are offering these services?" "How will we know if our patients value the goods and services we provide?" "What kinds of relationships do we need to establish with our patients to be successful?"

These are all marketing-related questions, and this chapter and the one that follows will focus on providing information to help pharmacy managers begin to address these questions. This chapter will describe and discuss some of the basic building blocks of marketing that are essential for developing and implementing a marketing plan. Chapter 21 will provide the reader with some practical tools necessary for marketing a pharmacy service.

■ CHAPTER QUESTIONS

1. What is marketing, and what is its purpose in a business setting? In a pharmacy setting?
2. What are the different philosophies that may be used to guide the marketing efforts of a company?
3. What is the difference between needs, wants, and demands?
4. What is the marketing mix?
5. What characterizes the different types of offerings that a business makes to its customers?
6. How do the concepts of expectations, satisfaction, quality, value, and loyalty relate to each other, and what is their importance to marketing?
7. What is relationship marketing, and how can it be used to enhance pharmacy practice?

■ INTRODUCTION: WHY MARKETING?

Smith (1996) has observed that marketing has received a "bad rap." Despite its contributions to society (Wilkie and Moore, 1999) and to our high standard of living (Smith, 1996), marketing has many critics. Perhaps these criticisms stem from the common perception that marketing is the "art of selling products" (Kotler and Keller, 2006). As will be discussed, this is a very myopic view of what marketing is all about. Other criticisms stem from perceptions that many marketers are unethical. While some marketers fail to act according to ethical principles, such a criticism may be levied against every endeavor, including pharmacy. The bottom line is that marketing is a function that is misunderstood by many. In the opinion of some, marketing is an often-overlooked function that is critical to the success of any organization (Smith, 2002).

Marketing is not just a function for large, multinational corporations. Indeed, the principles of marketing are just as applicable to small, independently owned pharmacies as they are to large corporations. Marketing is also critical to the profession of pharmacy. Marketing and pharmacy practice have a long history of coexisting with each other. Marketing tools have been used to help pharmacists address many issues in a variety of practice settings, such as what to charge for a prescription drug, whether to add a pharmacokinetic monitoring service or a dispensing satellite in a hospital, which over-the-counter (OTC) products to carry, and whether to use a wholesaler for all products or order directly from manufacturers.

As pharmacy continues to evolve, marketing's role grows in importance. Since articulation of the concept of pharmaceutical care (Hepler and Strand, 1990), many innovative pharmacy services have been described and implemented, ranging from comprehensive medication therapy management (MTM) services to specific disease management services, such as diabetes care, lipid management, tobacco cessation, and anticoagulation management. However, concurrent with the development and implementation of these services has been a continued growth in the literature documenting inappropriate use of medications, suggesting that a significant need still exists for services that are directed at reducing the negative consequences associated with drug therapy.

So why are these needs not being met? Concerns regarding prescriber, patient, and payer demand often are considered significant barriers to the provision of patient-centered pharmacy services (McDonough et al., 1998a). Understanding customers'* needs and using that understanding to create, deliver, and communicate value are key components of marketing. While many practitioners are interested in obtaining the necessary clinical knowledge and skills to deliver MTM services, many would argue that marketing knowledge and skills are equally important. Rovers and colleagues (1998, p. 136) succinctly summarize this point by noting that "pharmacists must build the demand and supply for pharmaceutical care services simultaneously."

As pharmacy continues its evolution from a product-focused to a service-centered practice, marketing, now more than ever, is critical to the success of the profession. The importance of understanding the nuances of marketing to the success of pharmaceutical care is recognized by Hepler and Strand (1990, p. 541), who note that "a pharmaceutical-care marketing strategy . . . would differ fundamentally from the usual strategy developed for selling drug products." In order for innovative pharmacy services to be successful in helping patients achieve optimal therapeutic outcomes, pharmacy practitioners must be able to understand the important role of marketing. This chapter will define many of the terms and concepts that are critical to understanding how to incorporate marketing effectively and efficiently into management of the pharmacy enterprise.

◼ MARKETING: DEFINITIONS AND CONCEPTS

Since the goal of this chapter is to introduce the reader to the basic building blocks of marketing, it becomes necessary to first define what *marketing* is. According to the American Marketing Association (AMA) (Keefe, 2004, p. 17), "marketing is an organizational function and a set of processes for creating, communicating and delivering value to customers and for managing customer relationships in ways that benefit the organization and its stakeholders." Included in this definition are several concepts that will be explored in subsequent sections of this chapter, namely, relationships and value. Other concepts, such as the four P's of the marketing mix (i.e., product,[†] price, place (distribution), and promotion) and the concept of exchange, are implicit in this definition. For now, it is important to recognize that this definition explicitly recognizes that marketing is about more than selling products.

Each of these preceding points suggests a broadened view of the domain of marketing, a notion that the discipline of marketing struggled with beginning in the 1960s. To many at that time, including the AMA, marketing was recognized as a set of *business* activities that existed to consummate *market* transactions between producers of goods and services and consumers (Hunt, 2002). Others proffered that marketing should be broadened (1) to include nonbusiness organizations and (2) that the societal implications of marketing activities also should be included in the domain of marketing (Hunt, 2002). After considerable

---

* While some authors appropriately argue that the terms *consumer, customer, patient,* and *client* have fundamentally different meanings, they are, for the most part, used interchangeably in this chapter (although the term *client* is not used). A discussion of the meaning and symbolism of these terms is best handled in another setting.

[†] As will be discussed later in this chapter, the concept of product in marketing can refer to any item of value offered by an organization, including tangible goods, services, and even concepts or ideas.

debate, in 1985 the AMA adopted the following definition of marketing (Keefe, 2004, p. 17): "Marketing is the process of planning and executing the conception, pricing, promotion, and distribution of ideas, goods, and services to create exchanges that satisfy individual and organizational objectives." The emphasis on *exchange* and the inclusion of *ideas* clearly demonstrate that marketing has been broadened to include non-business organizations. The 2004 AMA definition of marketing (Keefe, 2004, p. 17) takes this idea a step further and does not specifically mention what "product" is involved in the exchange but rather focuses on the creation, communication, and delivery of *value* by organizations (which very well may include nonbusiness organizations). The literature is replete with examples of how the principles of marketing have been used by charitable organizations, academic institutions, social issues groups, political candidates, and health care institutions. Hunt (2002, p. 11) remarked that "today it is noncontroversial that marketing has an important role to play in nonbusiness organizations."

While some argue that the 1985 AMA definition of marketing did not fully encompass the social role of marketing (Hunt 2002), other literature (e.g., see Hunt, 1976) and the emergence of the societal marketing concept (see next section) clearly demonstrate that a broadened view of the marketing domain includes the societal implications of marketing activities. Indeed, the 2004 definition explicitly recognizes this social role by focusing on benefits to the organization and its *stakeholders,* which include all individuals or groups affected by an organization's decisions and actions.

The preceding discussion implies that marketing includes business and social aspects. Kotler and Keller (2006) distinguished between a social definition of marketing and a managerial definition of marketing. While these managerial and social definitions shed additional light on the domain of marketing, they also serve to introduce several additional concepts that will be explored later in this chapter, namely, needs and wants. Although exchange is considered the core concept in marketing, these other concepts play a central role. Kotler and Keller's social definition reads: "Marketing is a societal process by which individuals and groups obtain what they need and want through creating, offering, and freely exchanging products and services of value with others." There is little question that marketing fulfills a social role. Several authors have suggested that marketing exists to create a higher standard of living (Smith, 2002; Kotler and Keller, 2006). While an in-depth discussion of this issue is beyond the scope of this chapter, the reader is referred to an article by Wilkie and Moore (1999) for an intriguing and insightful discussion of marketing's contribution to society.

From a managerial perspective, Kotler and Keller (2006, p. 6) defined marketing as "the art and science of choosing target markets and getting, keeping, and growing customers through creating, delivering, and communicating superior customer value." Marketing plays a demand management function within the organization, focusing partially on methods to stimulate demand but also, more important, on methods for how to control demand in order to meet the objectives of the organization. To serve a group of customers or a target market adequately, organizations must direct activities so that the right product is sold in the right quantity at the right place at the right price and at the right time. Because pharmacy is in the business of peoples' health, Smith (2002) suggests that some of these factors assume much greater importance than the stimulation of sales.

■ MARKETING SCIENCE

While there are many conceptions of what a theory is, a noted theorist in marketing suggests that the purpose of theory is to increase *scientific* understanding (Hunt, 2002). This argument, coupled with the title of this chapter, implies that at least some aspects of marketing can be fitted with the label of science. For this reason, it is worthwhile to briefly explore the question as to whether marketing is a science.

Like the broadening of the marketing debate, the debate as to whether marketing is a science has a rich history. Some authors have argued that marketing is a science, whereas others have argued that marketing is an art (e.g., see Peter and Olson, 1983; Hunt, 1976, 1983). One's view of the scope of marketing is critical to answering the question of whether or not marketing is a science. While an understanding of the nature of science is also critical, it is beyond the scope of this chapter, and the reader is referred to an excellent discussion by Hunt (2002). With respect to the scope of marketing, Hunt (1976) has proposed that all marketing content can be classified into one of eight classes or cells. One criterion that is used to define these cells is whether the marketing content is positive or normative. *Positive* marketing attempts to describe, explain, predict, and understand marketing phenomena; the focus of the analysis is descriptive—what is. *Normative* marketing attempts to prescribe what an organization, individual, or society should do; the focus is prescriptive—what ought to be done.

If one defines the scope of marketing as only normative efforts designed to assist marketing decision makers (e.g., What methods can we use to sell more product? How much should we charge for this product or service?), then marketing is not a science. However, if one considers an expanded scope of marketing to also include the positive dimensions, then marketing can be considered to be a science. As a science, what does marketing purport to do? The concept of exchange once again becomes critical because "marketing science is the behavioral science that seeks to explain exchange relationships" (Hunt, 1983). Marketing as an academic discipline has undergone significant transformation over the years (e.g., see Wilkie and Moore, 2003), and researchers in the field have become increasingly specialized. Readers interested in the science of marketing are referred to the work of McAlister, Bolton, and Rizley (2006), who have developed a compilation of scholarly articles published in marketing-related journals.

Since this chapter is more interested in the application of marketing principles to pharmacy, little more will be mentioned of the science side of marketing. The focus for the remainder of this chapter will be on the technology of marketing, or its applied side. However, it is important to remember that just as the "practice" of medicine and the "practice" of pharmacy are steeply rooted in a scientific knowledge base, so too is the "practice" of marketing. While the sheer quantity of the "product" of marketing science (i.e., the laws, principles, and theories that serve to unify, explain, and predict marketing phenomena) may be less than the quantity of the "product" of the sciences underlying medicine and pharmacy, this should not suggest that marketing is any less of a science. The scientific method is not any less appropriate to marketing than it is to other disciplines (Hunt, 2002).

■ COMPANY ORIENTATIONS TOWARD THE MARKETPLACE

For many years, marketing authors have sought to clarify the role of marketing in an organization. In essence, questions have arisen as to the type of philosophy that should guide the marketing efforts of a company. When deciding on a philosophical orientation, one needs to consider how much weight should be given to the interests of the organization, customers, and society. Kotler (2003) has described six competing concepts that organizations use as guides in the conduct of marketing activities.

The emphasis of the *production concept* is efficiency in the production and distribution of goods and services. The key assumption about consumers is that they are interested primarily in product availability and low prices. A production concept can also guide the efforts of service organizations, where the goal might be to handle as many cases as possible in a given period of time. As Kotler observes, such an orientation may lead to customer comments concerning the impersonal nature of the service delivery. A pharmacy dedicated to dispensing as many prescriptions as possible, usually without regard to medication appropriateness, and providing prescriptions at the lowest possible price relative to its competitors is practicing the production concept.

The *product concept* focuses on making good products, often as defined in the eyes of the producer, and improving them over time. The key assumptions about buyers are that they appreciate well-made products and that they can evaluate product quality. A company guided by the product concept often is focused on designing a great product (or service) and often gets little or no input from those who will benefit from its product. Kotler (2003) acknowledges that managers following this philosophical orientation might commit the "better mousetrap" fallacy. A phrase that epitomizes a product concept orientation is, "If you build it, they will come." A pharmacist who develops a smoking-cessation program that has as its sole focus the use of a technologically advanced reminder system for patients who are using nicotine-replacement therapy and believes that patients will enroll in the program and pay for the services with little other effort on his or her part is being guided by the product concept.

The *selling concept* emphasizes actions directed at stimulating consumers' interest through aggressive sales and promotion efforts. Although promotion is an important part of the marketing mix, and its use can be a critical tool in creating, delivering, and communicating value to customers, managers guided by the selling concept assume that consumers must be coaxed into buying products (or services); the focus is on hard selling, and little concern is given to customers' needs, wants, and postpurchase satisfaction. This is a common approach and is cited as a reason why the public often identifies marketing with selling and advertising (Kotler, 2003). A pharmacy that engages in an overly aggressive campaign, including the use of advertising, sales discounts, and high-pressure personal selling, is practicing the selling concept.

The *marketing concept* was proposed as a challenge to the previously discussed concepts.[‡] Rather than focus on the needs of the organization or the seller, the marketing concept suggests that the needs of the buyer are paramount. The marketing concept holds that "the key to achieving its organizational goals consists of the company being more effective than competitors in creating, delivering, and communicating superior

---

[‡] For an excellent review of the marketing concept and its implementation, referred to as *market orientation,* see Kohli and Jaworski (1990).

customer value to its chosen target markets" (Kotler, 2003, p. 19). Smith (2002, p. 9) succinctly summarizes the meaning of the marketing concept from the perspective of the pharmaceutical manufacturer: "The marketing concept states what seems obvious now but was not always practiced: It is easier to change the products and activities of the individual manufacturer to fit the market than it is to convince the entire market to use the products and services as the individual marketer prefers them."

A company guided by the marketing concept takes care to select appropriate *target markets* (i.e., distinct groups of buyers who may benefit from a given product or service mix), is focused on the needs of its customers, attempts to integrate a marketing orientation (a focus on customers' interests) into all segments of the company, and does these activities with an eye toward achieving organizational goals and objectives, notably generating profits through the creation of customer value (Kotler, 2003). The last point regarding profitability through creating customer value is not specific to for-profit firms. This precept is also important for nonprofit organizations, which instead may strive to generate funds through creating, delivering, and communicating value to their stakeholders to continue their useful work.

Increases in market diversity, changes in technology, and the need for enhanced marketing productivity have led some marketing scholars and practitioners to propose a fifth concept that moves beyond the more traditional marketing concept (Sheth, Sisodia, and Sharma, 2000). While companies guided by the marketing concept focus on segments of consumers known as *target markets,* the *customer concept* suggests that companies direct separate offers, services, and messages to individual customers (Kotler, 2003). Computers, the Internet, database software, and factory customization all have enabled such an approach to marketing. The customer concept calls for a focus on individual customer needs, sometimes leading to customization of the product or other elements of the marketing mix. The functions of the company should be integrated around customer value-added activities, and profitable growth is achieved through enhancement of customer loyalty and by focusing on the creation of lifetime value for individual customers (Kotler, 2003; Sheth, Sisodia, and Sharma, 2000).

A sixth orientation with respect to marketing thought and organizational philosophy has been proposed because of changes in our surroundings, such as deterioration of the environment, resource shortages, poverty, and neglected social services (Kotler, 2003). The previously discussed orientations give considerable weight to the interests of either the organization itself or its customers, but companies guided by these concepts still often act in ways that may not be in the best interests of society or consumers. Kotler (2003, pp. 26–27) has labeled this sixth orientation the *societal marketing concept,* which "holds that the organization's task is to determine the needs, wants, and interests of target markets and to deliver the desired satisfactions more effectively and efficiently than competitors in a way that preserves or enhances the consumer's and the society's well-being." Thus social and ethical considerations also must guide marketers' decisions; company profits, satisfaction of consumers' wants and needs, and the public interest; often conflicting end points, must be balanced.

Recognizing marketing's central role in the organization and the many forces that have shaped marketing and business practices in the past decade, Kotler and Keller (2006) proposed the *holistic marketing concept.* In essence, this philosophical orientation combines many of the features of the marketing concept, the customer concept, and the societal marketing concept. The term *holistic* communicates both the importance and complexity of marketing activities within an organization.

■ NEEDS, WANTS, AND DEMANDS

The marketing concept and the definitions of marketing discussed previously suggest that marketers must attempt to understand the needs, wants, and demands of their target markets. Briefly, a *need* is a state of felt deprivation. Needs are basic human requirements. People have physical needs (e.g., food, clothing, and shelter), social needs (e.g., the need for affection and the need to belong), and individual needs (e.g., the need for self-expression). A *want* is a desire for a specific satisfier of a need. Thus needs become wants, and these wants are shaped by culture and individual personality. A need for food can translate into wanting pizza; a need for affection may result in wanting a hug. A *demand* is a want that is backed by an ability to pay. Many people may want a vacation at a luxurious resort, but only a relative few are able and willing to purchase such a vacation.

One problem faced by health care providers is that people often do not want their goods or services. This situation is called *negative demand* (Kotler and Keller, 2006), and pharmaceutical products often are labeled as *negative goods* (Smith and Kolassa, 2001). Negative demand occurs when a major part of the market dislikes the product and may even pay a price to avoid it. There are numerous examples of negative goods besides pharmaceutical products and services, including automobile repair services, legal services, and dental work. One way to manage negative demand is to try to better understand people's true motivations for purchasing a product. For example, people purchase drill bits not because they want drill bits but because they want holes (Smith, 1996). In the same way, most people use medications not for the sake of using medications but because those medications provide benefits by alleviating, eliminating, or preventing a disease or symptoms. For example, using medications properly can allow a person to return to work or to perform activities that he or she enjoys doing.

From the health economics literature, *need* is defined as "the amount of medical care that medical experts believe a person should have to remain or become as healthy as possible, based on current medical knowledge" (Feldstein, 1999, p. 83). Economists are quick to point out that need is only one factor affecting the demand for care; demand for medical care is determined by a set of patient and provider factors, including a patient's need for care (Feldstein, 1999). Thus demand for care can be *greater than* the need; likewise, demand for care can be *less than* the need. Some might argue that certain lifestyle drugs such as Viagra are good examples of the former; MTM services are a good example of the latter.

Another important issue is the idea that a marketer's responsibility is primarily about meeting or responding to people's stated needs. Some have argued that this is too limited a view of a marketer's role (Kotler and Keller, 2006). Frequently, customers do not know what they want or need in a good or service. Think about the many goods and services available today, such as cellular telephones, 24-hour discount brokerage accounts, Internet service providers, and DVD players. Did most consumers want (or need) these things *before* they were available? For health care providers, this situation is all too common because most patients do not have the skills and knowledge that health care professionals have. Thus health care providers often recognize a patient's need that the individual patient does not recognize.

For example, assume that Mary Cooper enters a pharmacy wanting to purchase St. John's wort because her friend told her that it would help her feel better. After talking briefly with the woman, the pharmacist realizes that her symptoms are more grave than communicated initially. Given this additional information, the pharmacist refers her to a mental health care provider for further evaluation and treatment. In this case, the customer (Mary) stated a solution, not a need. The pharmacist appropriately recognized Mary's need and was able to help her by appropriately influencing her wants and demands.

The job of a marketer (and the job of a health care professional as well) is not only to understand and respond to people's *expressed* needs but also to help customers learn more about what they need and want. In essence, marketers also must understand and respond to people's *latent* needs. Narver, Slater, and MacLachlan (2004) call the former a *responsive* market orientation and the later a *proactive* market orientation. Marketers do not create needs, but they do help consumers to understand their latent needs and to translate needs into wants. An understanding of this issue is helpful in explaining pharmacy's current experiences with patient-centered services.

There is little question as to the need for patient-centered pharmacy services given the well-documented negative outcomes associated with drug therapy. McDonough and colleagues (1998a, p. 89) noted that a common misconception among pharmacists is that "patients neither want nor will be willing to pay for pharmaceutical care." While this may be true of *some* patients, this certainly is not true of *all* patients. Part of the problem lies in the fact that many patients are unaware of their needs and possible solutions (i.e., their needs are latent). McDonough (2003, p. 275) argues that "a key reason why patients do not demand pharmaceutical care is that they do not understand the concept." Patients have to see the value of the service. It is up to the profession to help translate latent needs into wants and demands.

■ THE CORE CONCEPT OF MARKETING

Central to marketing is the concept of *exchange*. Indeed, Kotler and Keller (2006) call exchange the "core concept of marketing." It is the unifying concept in marketing not only for marketing practice but also for marketing science. An *exchange* is a process of obtaining a desired product from someone by offering something in return. It is one of four ways to obtain a product, the others being self-production, coercion (or force), and begging (Kotler and Keller, 2006). Exchange is a process; when two parties reach an agreement, a transaction takes place. A *transaction* is a trade of values between two or more parties. Although the items of value often are money and a tangible good, this does not have to be the case. The items of value can be just about anything as long as they hold value for one of the parties. Thus services, ideas, experiences, events, places, material, organizations, effort, and information all can be items of value in a transaction (Kotler and Keller, 2006).

In a *transfer*, one party gives an item of value to another party while receiving nothing tangible in return. Giving to a charitable contribution is an example of a transfer. At first glance, transfers appear fundamentally different from transactions. However, in most cases, the giving party often expects something in return, such as gratitude, a change in the recipient, a positive feeling, or even a tax deduction. When observed in this light, transfers, like transactions, can be understood through the core concept of exchange. Indeed, marketers have included transfer behavior in their domain of study (e.g., see Mathur, 1996).

■ THE MARKETING MIX

Along with the concept of exchange, the 1985 AMA definition of marketing explicitly mentions several concepts that have come to be labeled as the *marketing mix.* A marketing mix is a set of tools an organization uses to pursue its objectives with respect to its target market. Although it has received criticism (e.g., Day and Montgomery, 1999) and other frameworks and classifications have been proposed (e.g., Van Waterschoot and Van den Bulte, 1992), McCarthy's (1960) schema has stood the test of time. He proposed that the tools of the marketing mix be classified into four broad groups: product, price, place, and promotion. These concepts have come to be called the *four P's of marketing.* While customer responses may be influenced by many variables outside the direct control of a company, the four P's represent variables within a company's control that can influence customer responses.

Depending on whom one reads, other P's have been added to the marketing mix. Perhaps most notably, positioning often is included as a fifth P. The following section provides a brief introduction to the variables in the marketing mix. Chapter 21 will provide more details concerning marketing-mix decisions.

Product

Product refers to an organization's offering. It is not limited to tangible goods but, as described earlier, can be any item of value or combination thereof. Thus, to marketers, the term *product* has a very broad meaning. In the delivery of pharmaceutical care, the product most often provided is a service. The next section will explore some fundamental differences between phys-

ical goods and services and will explore briefly some special considerations needed for the marketing of services.

Problems can emerge when organizations narrowly define their product (or business). Theodore Levitt (1960) labeled this *marketing myopia.* Marketing myopia is often a result of the application of the product concept as a philosophical guide to marketing activities. This is common when a firm defines its business by a product rather than in terms of what customer needs are filled by its activities. Common examples include the railroad and movie industries. These industries nearly disappeared because they assumed that they were in the railroad and movie businesses, respectively, rather than the transportation and entertainment businesses. As other businesses emerged (e.g., the airline and automobile industries and the television and theme park industries), those in the railroad and movie businesses faced a fight for the consumer's dollar against competition generated by unanticipated sources. Pharmacists and pharmacies also need to determine why people use their products and services. To simply say that they are in the business of dispensing medications prescribed by physicians is too myopic.

Another problem related to marketing myopia occurs when a single product becomes an organization's reason for being. The product of an organization is an offering that presents the consumer with a set of benefits that can be used to satisfy needs. Many different products (often seemingly disparate products) may be capable of meeting customer needs. If a company becomes too wrapped up in its product, it may miss the opportunity to fulfill the needs of the market. Pharmacist-delivered MTM services are a type of product that has the potential to fall victim to such a problem. Although MTM services are valuable for patients, for the profession, and for society, this does not imply that such services should be and will be a success. Just because pharmacists have the requisite clinical knowledge and skills to provide these services is not enough. Pharmacists must understand that these services represent an offering with a set of benefits that helps to meet the needs of customers and society. Pharmacists (and the profession) must be able to create, deliver, and communicate the value of what they do. Keep in mind that others (e.g., physicians, nurses, and information from the Internet) can also provide the benefits that pharmacists are purporting with MTM services. What seems like a relatively simplistic point is the key to widespread acceptance of pharmacist-delivered MTM services.

Price

A producer should set a price after considering several variables, including the cost function (i.e., the cost of producing, distributing, and selling the product, including a reasonable return for effort and risk), competitors' prices, and the demand for the product (including the target market's perception of the benefits)(Kotler and Keller, 2006). To a consumer, *price* is what is given up or sacrificed to obtain a product (Zeithaml, 1988). Some researchers have distinguished between an *objective* price (the actual price of a product) and a *perceived* price (what is encoded by the consumer, e.g., "expensive" or "cheap") (Zeithaml, 1988). It is also important to recognize that from the perspective of the consumer, the monetary price charged by a producer is not the only cost associated with buying a product (Lovelock and Wright, 2002; Zeithaml, 1988). Nonmonetary outlays include the costs associated with the time, effort, and discomfort that are related to the processes of searching for, purchasing, and using the product. For example, if a consumer has to travel a long distance to purchase a product, a sacrifice has been made that adds to what the consumer has given up to acquire that product.

While pricing decisions about drug products and other merchandise can be difficult for pharmacists, the pricing of patient care service raises additional considerations. Perhaps the most significant issue that needs to be addressed by the profession and its practitioners is the reluctance of pharmacists to request compensation for the services they provide (McDonough and Sobotka, 2003). Some pharmacists feel that they must give their services away initially to develop demand for them in the future. However, consumers generally are reluctant to start paying for something that they have been able to obtain for free in the past. Most consumers are willing to pay lawyers for legal advice and auto mechanics for service primarily because (1) they have expertise that most consumers do not have and (2) they have a tradition of charging for their services exclusive of charging for the goods they also might sell. While pharmacists have expertise in drug therapy not held by most consumers, they have had a difficult time obtaining payment for their professional services. This is likely because pharmacists, unlike lawyers, auto mechanics, and many other service professionals, do not have a history of charging for their services separate from their goods. When consumers obtain a prescription drug from a pharmacy, they are provided one price that has not been broken down into a "good" and a "service" component. This causes consumers to assume that either (1) there are no services that accompany prescription drug products, or (2) the services that come with these products are included with the price of the drug.

Place

Place, or *distribution,* refers to any activity designed to create utility by having the product available when and where targeted customers want to buy it. Many companies are considered successful because of their ability to deliver value in the distribution of products and services. Indeed, companies such as FedEx have made significant contributions to the success of many other companies that rely on prompt, efficient, and affordable delivery of goods (Siecker, 2002). In today's world of overnight delivery, telecommunications, and the Internet, speed and convenience are important elements in determining the distribution strategies of many firms (Lovelock and Wright, 2002). For a pharmacy, *place* may refer to providing a private area for counseling and providing other professional services (McDonough, Sobotka, and Doucette, 2003) or evaluating whether providing services at the work site for an employer group is feasible.

Promotion

Promotion activities seek to inform, remind, and persuade the target market about an organization and its offerings. Promotion activities also encourage members of the target market to take action at specific times. While advertising may be an important promotional tool, other tools in the promotion mix include sales promotion, public relations (including publicity), direct marketing, and personal selling.

Many pharmacies have used these tools successfully to spread the word about new and existing goods and services. Newspaper, radio, and television advertisements are used commonly by pharmacies. Pharmacies also employ promotional tools such as telephone book listing, coupons, newsletters, brochures, prescriber and patient mailings, health screenings, and presentations to civic groups. Some pharmacies have worked with the media to inform the public about their participation in public health events such as the Great American Smokeout or Talk About Prescriptions month.

With respect to MTM services, promotion plays an essential role in the translation of needs into wants and demands. Depending on the individual situation, all elements of the promotion mix may have a role in communicating the value of a pharmaceutical service, and pharmacists should evaluate all of them for implementation and use. McDonough and Doucette (2003) provide an excellent discussion of the use of personal selling, a practice that can be very effective but often is not considered by pharmacists for a variety of reasons, including pharmacists' discomfort with this role.

Positioning

Positioning is "the act of designing the company's offering and image to occupy a distinctive place in the mind of the target market" (Kotler and Keller, 2006, p. 310). Positioning is about what a marketer can do to the mind of the target consumer; it is not about what marketers do to the product attributes per se. For example, Volvo's core positioning is safety and durability; this is what the company hopes its target market will think of when they think of a Volvo automobile. Because the target market for many pharmacies does not understand what MTM services are, pharmacists have a wonderful opportunity to position these services in the minds of consumers. These pharmacies can position themselves as innovators, medication experts, caring practitioners, or partners in meeting health-related needs (McDonough, Sobotka, and Doucette, 2003; McDonough et al., 1998b).

◾ REEXAMINING THE FIRST P: PRODUCT

To a marketer, the term *product* means more than just a physical good. In pharmacy, physical goods (e.g., drugs and durable medical equipment) usually are combined with a service. Indeed, Shepherd (1995, p. 53) observed that "pharmaceutical products require a service component." However, in pharmacy, it is not uncommon for a service to be provided without a physical good. Kotler and Keller (2006) described five categories of offerings that are distinguished based on how much the service component is part of the offering:

- *Pure tangible good.* The offering consists primarily of a tangible good, such as toothpaste, toilet paper, or napkins.
- *Tangible good with accompanying services.* The offering consists of a tangible good accompanied by one or more services; as the sophistication for use of the good increases, the more dependent its sale is on services.
- *Hybrid.* The offering consists of equal parts of goods and services, such as the purchase of a meal at a restaurant (consists of food and service).
- *Major service with accompanying minor goods and services.* The offering consists of a major service accompanied by other services and supporting goods, such as the purchase of airplane transportation (primarily a service accompanied by some tangibles such as food and drinks).
- *Pure service.* The offering consists primarily of a service, such as attending an orchestra performance or psychotherapy.

Christensen, Fassett, and Andrews (1993) differentiated among three types of services associated with pharmaceutical care. Although there are some differences, their classification scheme in many respects resembles Kotler and Keller's (2006) categories, which are applicable to all goods and services, not just those related to pharmacy.

- *Dispensing services.* These are services associated with dispensing a prescription that are obligatory under board of pharmacy regulations. These services include accurately filling a prescription order, clarifying orders, not dispensing an order that contains obvious errors that would be identified by a "reasonable and prudent" pharmacist, and communicating drug-use instructions as required by state statutes and regulations.
- *Dispensing-related value-added pharmaceutical services (VAPS).* These are services that extend beyond *routine* dispensing activities required by law. These services include activities such as conducting drug regimen reviews for patients receiving a medication, selecting appropriate drug products, monitoring refill behaviors, and consulting with other health providers about a patient's drug regimen (beyond routine clarification questions).
- *Nondispensing-related value-added pharmaceutical services (VAPS).* These are services that are not associated with the dispensing of a prescription and are not required by law nor inherent in the fee charged for a prescription. These services include screening programs (e.g., osteoporosis, lipids, and blood pressure), weight management programs, in-service training provided to health care providers, and discharge counseling in an inpatient setting.

The preceding discussion may lead one to ask: What is the difference between a physical good and a service? Several authors have attempted to define characteristics that distinguish goods from services. While there is some debate as to which characteristics best represent the fundamental differences, it is important to recognize that any list represents generalizations that may not be applicable to all services (Lovelock and Wright, 2002). The following list contains nine basic differences that can help to distinguish

services from physical goods (Lovelock and Wright, 2002)[§]:

- Customers do not obtain ownership of services.
- Service products are intangible performances.
- There is greater involvement of customers in the production process.
- People may form part of the product, including other patrons.
- There is greater variability in operational inputs and outputs, making it more difficult to standardize and control.
- Many services are difficult for customers to evaluate.
- There is typically an absence of inventories.
- The time factor is relatively more important.
- Delivery systems may involve both electronic and physical channels.

Each of these differences may affect the design of a marketing program. For example, a major consideration in service delivery is matching demand levels and capacity. This is so because services are perishable and cannot be inventoried. One mechanism that can be used to better match supply and demand is the use of reservations (e.g., hotel and airline industries) and appointments (e.g., physicians and other health care providers). As another example, because of the greater variability inherent in the production of a service, service organizations need to pay special attention to the standardization of the service-performance process or risk damaging the quality of the service provided. One mechanism that can be used is a service blueprint (see Chapter 21). In health care, protocols and practice guidelines are commonly used to standardize care to enhance quality.

The differences between services and physical goods contribute to the distinctive nature of service performances. This distinctive nature has led several authors to propose that the traditional four P's of the

---

[§] For an alternative view regarding the meaning and importance of these differences, see Vargo and Lusch (2004a).

marketing mix are insufficient as a set of marketing tools for service businesses (Booms and Bitner, 1981; Kotler, 2002; Lovelock and Wright, 2002).|| Additional elements must be included in the marketing mix, and our view of the tools that form the traditional components must be modified because of the fundamental differences between goods and services. Building on the work of Booms and Bitner (1981), Lovelock and Wright (2002) have proposed the "eight P's" of integrated service management: (1) product elements, (2) place, cyberspace, and time, (3) promotion and education, (4) price and other user outlays, (5) process, (6) productivity and quality, (7) people, and (8) physical evidence. Notice that the first four are closely related to the traditional four P's of the marketing mix, with some modifications because of the distinctive nature of services, the changing environment, and other enlightened recognitions by marketers. The last four variables deserve additional discussion.

Process

The creation and delivery of product elements require that special attention be given to the design, implementation, and evaluation of processes. A *process* is the method and sequence in which a service is created, produced, and delivered. The service blueprint (see Chapter 21) can be useful in understanding and designing processes. For a pharmacy, the focus may be on the entire process of dispensing a prescription starting with presentation of the prescription by a patient (or a telephone order from a nurse or physician) all the way through verifying patient understanding of the

---

|| Services marketing, coupled with other streams of marketing literature, such as relationship marketing, resource management, and market orientation, have led some (e.g., see Vargo and Lusch, 2004b) to argue that marketing, as an academic discipline and as a business practice, has shifted from a goods-dominant view, largely based on discrete transactions, to a service-dominant view, where relationships play a central role. One could argue that pharmacy has experienced a similar evolution.

medication (Holdford and Kennedy, 1999). Alternatively, a pharmacy may focus on a specific component of the process, such as what steps will be taken if one learns during a patient history that he or she smokes cigarettes.

Poorly designed processes may lead to ineffective service delivery, causing customer frustration and dissatisfaction, as well as employee frustration and dissatisfaction. For example, long waits at checkout lines in a retail environment caused by poorly designed systems that fail to anticipate customer flow are troublesome for customers in line as well as the few employees who are running registers.

Productivity and Quality

Productivity focuses on the efficiency in the transformation of service inputs into outputs, whereas *quality*, in this application, refers to the degree to which a service meets the needs, wants, and expectations of customers. Service firms must attempt to balance these elements. Improving productivity may help to keep costs down, but cuts in service levels may adversely affect perceptions of quality. Similarly, while service quality may be critical for building customer loyalty, investing in quality improvement without understanding the impact on incremental costs and revenues can have negative consequences for profitability. From a managed-care pharmacy perspective, efforts to increase efficiency by limiting the use of certain medications may lead to a significant decrease in quality perceptions not only by patients but also by network providers.

People

People provide most services; thus the selection, training, and motivation of employees are critical tasks for service firms. Interactions with employees can have a significant impact on perceptions of service quality. Pharmacy managers need to pay special attention to all members of the pharmacy staff, not just pharmacists and technicians. Clerks, maintenance staff, volunteers, students, and anyone else who has contact with customers need sufficient training. In addition, other patrons may form part of the service experience, and firms often need to take these individuals into consideration. For example, the behavior of other patrons at an amusement park may have a dramatic effect on the quality of one's experience and one's level of satisfaction.

Physical Evidence

The appearance of the physical environment where the service is delivered (including buildings, landscape, employees, and furnishings), signs, printed materials, and other visible and tangible cues may provide evidence to customers concerning the service quality of an organization. Pharmacy managers should ask such questions as: Do we have adequate parking? Is the appearance of the pharmacy neat, and does it imply a professional image? Is our signage consistent? Is our equipment up to date?

■ EXPECTATIONS, SATISFACTION, QUALITY, VALUE, AND LOYALTY

Several terms have been used repeatedly in the preceding sections of this chapter. Although exchange is considered the core concept in marketing, these other concepts (i.e., expectations, satisfaction, quality, value, and loyalty) also play a critical role in understanding what marketing is all about.

Expectations

Critical to understanding customer satisfaction and perceived service quality is a clear understanding of expectations. *Expectations* are internal standards used by customers when evaluating a product or service. While they may initially influence a decision whether or not to purchase a product and from whom, they also play a critical role in consumers' judgments of service quality and satisfaction. Conceptual models have suggested that expectations consist of several different elements: desired service level, adequate service level, predicted service level, and a zone of tolerance (Zeithaml, Berry, and Parasuraman, 1993; see also Parasuraman, Zeithaml, and Berry, 1994a).

The *desired service level* is defined as what customers hope to receive and reflects a combination of what customers believe can and should be delivered. As customers realize that they cannot always get what they desire, they hold another, lower level of expectation that reflects the minimum level of service they are willing to accept, called the *adequate service level*. The *zone of tolerance* represents the difference between adequate and desired levels and recognizes that customers are willing to accept some variation in service delivery. The range they are willing to accept is the zone of tolerance, suggesting that expectations are not a single level but are best characterized by a range of levels bounded by desired and adequate service levels. If a performance falls outside the range and below adequate levels, customers likely will be frustrated and dissatisfied. If performance exceeds desired levels, it likely will surprise and please the customer, leading to customer delight (Lovelock and Wright, 2002). Finally, there is a *predicted service level,* which reflects the level of service customers believe that they are most likely to get. This predicted service level directly affects how the adequate service level is defined for that occasion.

The desired service level can be elevated or lowered based on personal needs and enduring beliefs about what is possible. The adequate service level can be influenced by a number of factors, including the perceptions of service alternatives and situational factors (e.g., emergencies and catastrophes). Explicit and implicit promises made by the service provider, past experiences, and word-of-mouth communications are proposed to influence the desired service level directly and affect the adequate service level indirectly through the predicted service level (Zeithaml, Berry, and Parasuraman, 1993).

Marketers can have a significant role in influencing consumer expectations. Setting expectations in the mind of the consumer that are too high can create significant problems, such as possibly setting up the customer for frustration, disappointment, and dissatisfaction. On the other hand, setting expectations too low may lead to difficulties in attracting new customers. Indeed, a significant problem facing the profession of pharmacy is that many patients do not expect to receive MTM services. In planning their marketing communications effort and promotion mix, organizations (including pharmacies) must attempt to set a balance with respect to customer expectations.

Satisfaction and Quality

Some authors use the terms *quality* and *satisfaction* interchangeably. However, there are some notable differences. While there are different conceptualizations of satisfaction (Schommer and Kucukarslan, 1997), in marketing, the most common approach is based on the confirmation/disconfirmation of expectations model.[#] Thus Kotler and Keller (2006, p. 144) define *satisfaction* as "a person's feelings of pleasure or disappointment resulting from comparing a product's perceived performance (or outcome) in relation to his or her expectations." Thus, if performance is worse than expected (negative disconfirmation), the customer will be dissatisfied. If performance matches expectations (confirmation), satisfaction will result. If performance exceeds expectations (positive disconfirmation), the customer will be highly satisfied and possibly delighted.[**] There are vast differences between satisfied and completely satisfied customers (e.g., see Lovelock and Wright, 2002). For example, completely or highly satisfied customers are much more likely to remain loyal to a business and spread positive word of mouth about the company.

As with satisfaction, there is a rich history concerning the concept of quality. A broad definition of *quality* is superiority or excellence. Researchers note a difference between *objective quality* (i.e., measurable and verifiable superiority on some predetermined ideal standard) and *perceived quality* (Zeithaml, 1988). Perceived quality is a global assessment made by a consumer that is posited to exist at a higher level of abstrac-

tion from a consumer's perceptions of a product's specific attributes (Zeithaml, 1988). *Service quality* is defined as "customers' long-term cognitive evaluation of a firm's service delivery" (Lovelock and Wright, 2002, p. 87) and results from a comparison of expectations and perceptions of service performance (Parasuraman, Zeithaml, and Berry, 1988). Since service quality represents a global impression rather than an encounter-specific evaluation, consumers are posited to update their perceptions of service quality following their interactions with service providers.

Service quality has been conceptualized to contain multiple dimensions (Parasuraman, Zeithaml, Berry, 1985). One measure of service quality, the SERVQUAL scale (Parasuraman, Zeithaml, and Berry, 1988), identifies five such dimensions:

- *Tangibles*—the appearance of a firm's physical facilities, equipment, personnel, and communication materials
- *Reliability*—the ability of the firm to perform the promised service dependably and accurately
- *Responsiveness*—the willingness of the firm to help customers and provide prompt service
- *Assurance*—the knowledge and courtesy of employees and their ability to convey trust and confidence
- *Empathy*—the caring, individualized attention the firm provides to its customers

Another useful distinction made by service quality researchers is between technical quality and functional quality. *Technical quality* refers to customer perceptions about what is received from a service (e.g., Was the outcome of the service successful?), and *functional quality* refers to customer perceptions about how a service was performed (e.g., Did the service provider demonstrate concern and inspire confidence?) (Kotler, 2003). Perceptions of both functional and technical quality are important determinants of service quality, suggesting that service providers need to focus on being "high touch" as well as "high tech." In pharmacy, there is some evidence that functional quality has a greater impact on consumer perceptions of service

---

[#] For an interesting and somewhat alternative view of the concept of satisfaction, see Fournier and Mick (1999).

[**] For a provocative discussion of customer delight, see Oliver, Rust, and Varki (1997) and Rust and Oliver (2000).

quality than technical quality (Holdford and Schulz, 1999).

Both service quality and customer satisfaction are based on comparisons of expectations and performance. Are these really different constructs? There has been considerable debate in the marketing literature concerning this issue. One way that these two concepts have been distinguished is by examining the type of expectations that are used as the comparison. For service quality assessments, the focus is on desired and adequate service levels. For satisfaction evaluations, the focus has been on predicted service levels (Parasuraman, Zeithaml, and Berry, 1988; Spreng, MacKenzie, and Olshavsky, 1996; Zeithaml, Berry, and Parasuraman, 1993). Another way these concepts have been distinguished is that service quality is a global judgment or assessment, whereas satisfaction is transaction-specific (Parasuraman, Zeithaml, and Berry, 1988). This suggests that customer satisfaction leads to service quality. However, others have suggested that service quality leads to customer satisfaction. In an effort to work around this debate, Parasuraman, Zeithaml, and Berry (1994b), building on the work of Teas (1993), suggested that both service quality and customer satisfaction can be examined meaningfully at the individual transaction level and be thought of as global (or overall) assessments that are formed following numerous transactions.

Regardless of this theoretical debate, there is considerable evidence that enhancing customer satisfaction and service quality can lead to positive outcomes for the organization and the consumer. As mentioned earlier, highly satisfied customers are more likely to exhibit loyalty, which means a consistent stream of revenues over a period of years for the firm (Lovelock and Wright, 2002). These customers also may be more forgiving when there is a service failure and may make fewer demands and fewer mistakes as they gain experience as consumers of a company's products or services, thus reducing the firm's operating costs (Lovelock and Wright, 2002). Positive word of mouth is also a key effect of high levels of satisfaction and perceived service quality. This outcome is extremely important to providers of professional services such as pharmacists.

Satisfied customers also means less negative word of mouth, which can travel faster (and farther) than positive comments. All these behavioral impacts can help to improve the bottom line of the company, namely, profitability (Zeithaml, Rust, and Lemon, 2001).

Value

Many marketers believe that the fundamental role of marketing is to create value for customers (Lovelock and Wright, 2002). But what is *value,* and how is it different from perceived quality? When customers evaluate a product or a service, they consider the benefits it offers (i.e., what they get) relative to the costs (i.e., what they give up). The benefits of a product or service include fulfilling a functional need, making a process more convenient, and providing an emotional payout such as prestige or a boost to self-esteem. Costs to a consumer include not only monetary costs but also the nonmonetary outlays associated with the time, effort, and discomfort related to the processes of searching for, purchasing, and using the product (including costs associated with a product or service failure). *Value* is conceptualized as either the ratio (Kotler, 2003) or the difference (Lovelock and Wright, 2002) between the perceived benefits and the perceived costs (i.e., perceived sacrifice). Figure 20-1 is a useful approach to visualizing how a customer may calculate value.

To increase the value for a customer, marketers can increase the benefits derived from the core product, enhance or provide supplementary services, or reduce the monetary costs or nonmonetary outlays associated with acquiring and using the product (Lovelock and Wright, 2002). Alternatively, a marketer can increase costs to the customer as long as there is a corresponding greater increase in benefits or an offset to some other outlay. Consumers paying a premium price to save time or gain greater comfort are an example of the latter. Marketers still can enhance value for customers by reducing benefits, as long as there is a corresponding greater decrease in costs. It is important to recognize that a consumer's perception of the value of a product may be different before and after consumption, indicating that an individual's perceptions of benefits and

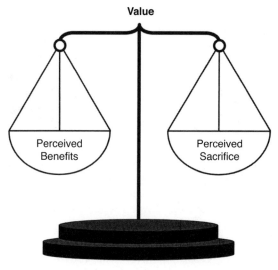

Figure 20-1. A conceptualization of value.

costs may be altered by product use and what happens after product use.

Quality and value are not the same thing. The concept of value is more individualistic and personal than quality and thus is theorized to exist at a higher level of abstraction in the mind of the consumer. In addition, quality is usually conceptualized as part of the "get" component, whereas value involves a trade-off of get and give components (Zeithaml, 1988). Because they are related, it is not surprising that efforts directed at increasing quality (or customer satisfaction for that matter) also can lead to increases in perceived value, which may contribute to increased consumer intentions and behaviors and ultimately to improved profitability, as discussed earlier. An important consideration is that perceptions of quality and value exist after as well as prior to service delivery or product use. These preuse perceptions may be based on word-of-mouth messages (e.g., what acquaintances have said) or may be based on the promotional message of the firm. For pharmacists, this suggests that both effective provision of MTM services and appropriate use of the promotion mix are necessary for communicating value to prospective members of the target market. Pharmacists must understand how to use both sides of the value equation if they want to both attract and retain customers.

Loyalty

Loyalty has received a considerable amount of attention from both marketing theorists and practitioners. Most would agree that there are positive consequences associated with a loyal customer base. However, there are other areas of disagreement associated with customer loyalty.

Part of the debate has been with respect to how loyalty should be conceptualized and subsequently measured. Historically, the concept has been thought of as a behavioral outcome, namely, repurchase or switching intentions and behaviors (Oliver, 1999). Others have argued that loyalty has psychological meaning. For example, firm adoration, identification with the firm, and willingness to assist the service provider and other customers are thought to be part of the loyalty construct (Oliver, 1999; Jones and Taylor, 2007). To better understand the concept, some have suggested viewing loyalty in service provider–consumer relationships in the same manner as pro-relationship behaviors that develop in friendships and even romantic relationships (Jones and Taylor, 2007).

In addition to issues of conceptualization and measurement, marketers also have debated the antecedents of loyalty. The role of satisfaction in the development of loyalty has received the most attention. While there is most likely a relationship between these two variables (satisfaction begets loyalty), the relationship is not perfect; many customers may be satisfied or even highly satisfied yet fail to display repurchase behaviors (Oliver, 1999). Others have demonstrated that it is not just the level of satisfaction that plays a role in determining loyalty, but the strength (degree of certainty) with which a customer expresses his or her satisfaction (Chandrashekaran et al., 2007).

Oliver (1999, p. 41) states that ultimate loyalty requires that "the consumable must be subject to adoration." The object or service must be lovable. The negative demand associated with most pharmaceutical products and services suggests that ultimate loyalty may be an elusive goal. This should not suggest that pharmacy cannot learn from the growing body of knowledge regarding loyalty. Because of its known relationship to firm performance, at the very least pharmacy should be concerned with customer retention and repurchase intentions, even if such conceptualizations fail to recognize the psychological dimensions of loyalty. Related to this issue is a useful recommendation based on the work of Reichheld (2003), who suggests that firms need to be aware of only a single-item measure when thinking about the concept of loyalty: "How likely is it that you would recommend [Company X] to a friend or colleague?" This single-item measure has been shown to be related to the revenue growth rate of firms in several industries.

The recipient of loyalty attitudes and behaviors should also be considered. As mentioned earlier, some have conceptualized service loyalty to be similar to loyalty in interpersonal relationships like friendships. This suggests that the pharmacist, rather than the pharmacy, may be the subject of loyalty attitudes and behaviors (pharmacist-owned loyalty).* Such loyalty can be beneficial to the firm if the specific pharmacist continues his or her tenure with the pharmacy. Pharmacy employers need to understand this concept and the importance of good human resources management; management and marketing do not exist in isolation.

Collecting Customer Data

To create, deliver, and communicate superior customer value requires that a company understands its target market's expectations as well as its customers' assessments of satisfaction, quality, and value. Relying on customer complaints (or a lack of them) as evidence that a business is satisfying needs and meeting expectations is notoriously flawed. Studies show that most dissatisfied customers never complain to the company; rather, they buy less or switch to another company (Lovelock and Wright, 2002). Therefore, companies need to take a more active approach in gathering data about improving their products or services. Some examples of how such an effort can be implemented include (Lovelock and Wright, 2002):

* Posttransaction surveys. The goal of this approach is to collect data concerning customer satisfaction and perceptions about the service experience immediately after (or within a few days of) the encounter. Questions usually are specific to the immediate past transaction or experience, although some more global questions may be included. You probably have been asked to fill out such a questionnaire at a recent visit to a restaurant or during a stay at a hotel. Doucette and McDonough (2002) provide an example of a survey used for a weight control and wellness program at a pharmacy.

* Overall evaluation surveys. While posttransaction surveys focus on consumer evaluations of the most immediate encounter, the focus when conducting an overall evaluation survey is on global impressions of a firm. This can include "customers'" overall satisfaction with the firm, as well as "their overall impressions of the firm's service quality, product quality, and price" (Parasuraman, Zeithaml, and Berry, 1994b, p. 122). These evaluations should reflect customers' accumulated experiences over time. For this reason, as well as the costs associated with conducting these studies, Lovelock and Wright (2002) recommend that these surveys be administered less frequently than posttransaction surveys. Larson and MacKeigan's work regarding a measure of patient satisfaction with pharmacy services (Larson and MacKeigan, 1994; MacKeigan and Larson, 1989) and with pharmaceutical care (Larson, Rovers, and MacKeigan, 2002) are examples of this approach. An example outside of pharmacy is the SERVQUAL scale (Parasuraman, Zeithaml, and Berry, 1988).

* Mystery shopping. This technique involves sending individuals posing as ordinary customers to gather information and provide feedback about service experiences. This technique allows for gathering information on individual employees and can be used to award superior performance or as an indication of the need for additional training. This approach may not be as useful for pharmacies that have few new customers because employees may be able to identify the mystery shopper. Consideration should be given to how employees might react to this deceptive practice. Suggestions include informing

---

* For an interesting application to sales representatives, see Palmatier, Scheer and Steenkamp (2007).

employees that this may be happening at some time, informing them on the criteria on which they will be assessed, and evaluating performance over a series of encounters rather than a single visit (Lovelock and Wright, 2002).

- *Noncustomer, new customer, and declining/former customer surveys.* Surveys of these groups may be useful for identifying unmet needs, expectations and image (e.g., noncustomer surveys), reasons for patronage (i.e., new customers), and information about a firm's deficiencies (i.e., declining and former customers).

- *Focus groups.* A more qualitative approach to gathering customer data is the use of focus groups, or groups of customers who are assembled by a researcher for an in-depth discussion on a specific topic. The group is led by a trained moderator who is responsible for keeping the group on task. Focus groups can be useful in learning about customers' needs and expectations, determining how customers evaluate a firm's performance, gathering in-depth information about service problems, or obtaining feedback about a proposed product or service. Pharmacists should be cautioned about projecting results from a focus group to an entire market segment. Bislew and Sorensen (2003) provide an example of how focus groups might be used in a pharmacy setting.

- *Employee data.* Companies should not discount the value of the information that can be obtained from talking and *listening to* employees. Employees have first-hand experience with customers that may lead to improvements in the product or service delivery. Surveys, focus groups, and one-on-one interviews all can be used to collect data from employees.

▨ RELATIONSHIP MARKETING

While the concepts inherent in relationship marketing are not new, it has only been within the past 25 years that the practice and science of marketing have grown aware of the relevance of relational exchanges. The concepts discussed throughout this chapter have significant meaning in a relationship-marketing paradigm. Indeed, an understanding of many of these concepts, such as expectations, satisfaction, perceived quality,

value, and loyalty, may be even more critical in a relationship-marketing paradigm because they are key to maintaining long-term collaborations and retaining customers. So what is relationship marketing? There has been considerable debate in the marketing literature concerning an appropriate definition of relationship marketing (e.g., see Parvatiyar and Sheth, 2000). One useful definition has been provided by Lovelock and Wright (2002, p. 102), who define *relationship marketing* as "activities aimed at developing long-term, cost-effective links between an organization and its customers for the mutual benefit of both parties."

Key to understanding relationship marketing is appreciating the distinction between discrete transaction-based exchanges and relational exchanges. Weitz and Jap (1995, p. 305) note that ". . . the growing interest in relationship marketing suggests a shift in the nature of general marketplace transactions from discrete to relational exchanges—from exchanges between parties with no past history and no future to exchanges between parties who have an exchange history and plans for future interactions." Thus, in the practice of transactional marketing, each transaction is viewed as a separate event, or a one-shot deal. The fact that one transaction has occurred does not predict that a future transaction will occur (Gummesson, 2002); the focus of both parties is to make the most of each individual transaction. However, a customer may use the same supplier repeatedly, possibly because of high switching costs, not because he or she is committed to that individual supplier (Gummesson, 2002).

While purely discrete transactions are rare, and while there are numerous benefits to both customers and producers who operate in a relationship-marketing paradigm, neither of these should imply that all forms of transactional marketing are inherently bad or wrong. Indeed, several authors have noted that transactional marketing can be a functional option for some marketers based on the characteristics of the situation and the players involved (Gummesson, 2002; Kotler, 2003; Sheth, Sisodia, and Sharma, 2000). These characteristics include the time horizon of the customer, the level of customer involvement, the costs associated with switching to another organization, the level of customer interest in establishing a relationship, and the ability of an organization to implement such an approach efficiently (i.e., the cost and revenue implications must be understood). In their synthesis of the relationship marketing literature, Palmatier and colleagues (2006) find that relationship marketing is more effective when relationships are more important to customers, such as in the context of service offerings and business-to-business relationships, and when relationships are established with individuals rather than with the firm as a whole.

Other authors have noted that transactional marketing still can be customer-centric, focusing on the needs, wants, and resources of individual consumers and customers rather than on those of mass markets or segments (Sheth, Sisodia, and Sharma, 2000). Sheth (2002) has argued that the future of relationship marketing includes the selective and targeted use of relationship marketing coupled with transactional marketing efforts depending on the characteristics of the customer segment.

The basic concepts of relationship marketing have historical roots dating back to the earliest merchants (Berry, 1995; Sheth and Parvatiyar, 1995). However, the concept of relationship marketing as we know it today gained popularity beginning in the early 1980s. Sheth (2002) described three antecedents for this increased interest:

1. *The economic environment.* Increased global competition was an outcome of the excess capacity and high raw materials costs that resulted from the energy crisis of the 1970s and the consequent poor economic conditions. For these reasons, a shift occurred that resulted in an increased focus on the retention of customers and a lessened focus on customer acquisition; ongoing relational exchanges became much more important that one-time transactional exchanges.
2. *The emergence of services marketing.* During this period, services marketing emerged as an area of study and practice. Indeed, the U.S. economy has evolved such that today it consists of a 70–30 services-to-goods mix (Kotler and Keller, 2006). The recognition that services were fundamentally different from physical goods suggested a different approach to marketing. Furthermore, service delivery often focuses on multiple transactions over time, implying the existence of relationships.
3. *Supplier partnering.* The success of the Japanese automobile industry (and other industries) in developing partnerships with suppliers led to the recognition that such an approach can improve quality while also lowering costs. This collaborative, rather than combative, approach to interacting with suppliers resulted in viewing exchanges as relational rather than transactional and set the stage for later developments in business-to-business marketing.

What Does Relationship Marketing Entail?

Gummesson (2002) outlines the fundamental values of relationship marketing:

- *Marketing management should be broadened into marketing-oriented company management.* This value is similar to the marketing concept's call for an integrated marketing orientation throughout an organization. Firms practicing relationship marketing must have an understanding of the importance of marketing throughout the whole organization, *not just for the marketing department.* Effective relationship marketing requires a customer-centric focus (Sheth, Sisodia, and Sharma, 2000).
- *Long-term collaborations and win-win.* A key to relationship marketing is a focus on collaboration, viewing suppliers, customers, and others as partners rather than as combatants. This belief implies that relationships will create mutual value, leading to an extension of the duration of the relationship. This also implies that relationship marketing encourages retention marketing over attraction marketing.
- *All parties should be active and take responsibility.* The producer is not the only player in a relationship. Indeed, in many business-to-business relationships, the customers initiate innovation and force suppliers to change their products or services. With respect to services, customers are often involved in the production of the service, suggesting a critical interactive role, depending on the situation.

- *Relationship and service values instead of bureaucratic-legal values.* This value does not suggest that laws should be broken but instead implies that flexibility rather than rigidity should guide the management of customer relationships. Customers are individuals and should be treated as such.

Service firms and other businesses use a variety of approaches to maintain and enhance customer relationships, such as treating customers fairly, offering service augmentations, and treating each customer as if he or she were a segment of one (Lovelock and Wright, 2002). Significant to maintaining relationships in the delivery of services is the fulfillment of promises made to customers. Bitner (1995) outlined three essential activities to attracting, building, and maintaining service relationships:

- *Make realistic promises in the first place.* Through the eight P's of integrated service management, an organization makes promises to its target market regarding what they can expect. As discussed previously, companies must strike a balance between setting expectations too high (possibly setting up the customer to be disappointed) and setting expectations too low (which may lead to a failure to attract customers). McDonough, Sobotka, and Doucette (2003, p. 217) suggest that "it is better to overperform than to overpromise."
- *Enable employees and systems to deliver on promises.* Process and people, two of the eight P's, are critical to the fulfillment of promises. Promises are easy to make, but without the right people using the right processes and tools, they are difficult to keep. Resources must be available, and people must have the training and motivation to serve customers.
- *Keep promises to customers when delivering services.* Every time a customer interacts with the organization (through its employees or a technological interface), an opportunity exists to keep or break a promise. These encounters, called *moments of truth,* form the basis for how a service relationship is built. Depending on the service and the situation, a single negative encounter (failure to meet a promise) can be enough to sever a relationship or at least cause a

weakening of the relationship, even a long-lasting relationship. A service-recovery plan is critical for dealing with these situations (see Chapter 11). On the other hand, a series of positive encounters (repeatedly meeting promises and exceeding expectations) can lead to customer trust in the organization and a feeling of commitment to the relationship with the organization (Morgan and Hunt, 1994).

What Are the Consequences of Relationship Marketing?

The definition of relationship marketing stresses that its practice is mutually beneficial for an organization and its customers. Benefits to the organization, such as customer loyalty, referrals, and profitability (Palmatier et al., 2006), are manifested through improvements in marketing productivity and by making the marketing function more effective and more efficient (Sheth and Parvatiyar, 1995). By focusing on individual customers (rather than on mass markets or market segments), and by increasing the involvement of the customer in the marketing effort, relationship marketing should be *more effective* in meeting customer needs and wants. Furthermore, focusing on customer retention, reducing some of the wasteful practices associated with mass marketing, and letting the customer become a more active participant in the production process (i.e., letting customers perform some of the tasks historically performed by marketers—think ATMs) may lead to increases in *marketing efficiency.*

The point with respect to customer retention may need some elaboration. Estimates suggest that at least 65 percent of the average company's business comes from its present satisfied customers (Schoell and Guiltinan, 1990). Other evidence indicates that attracting new customers is significantly more expensive than retaining existing ones (Kotler and Keller, 2006). There is empirical evidence that shows that as customers remain in relationships for longer periods, they are more profitable to the firm (Sheth and Parvatiyar, 1995). These findings lead to the conclusion that focusing on customer retention rather than customer acquisition should be a less expensive (and more profitable) way to conduct business.

Relationship marketing also has significant benefits to the customer (Bitner, 1995). Certainly customers benefit economically and receive higher value when a company consistently fulfills promises. Long-term relationships also can reduce both stress and risk for customers as the relationship becomes more predictable and trust in the service provider increases. Such relationships also reduce the need to change, an act that most humans prefer to avoid. Remaining in a relationship simplifies one's life, saving time and effort by lessening the need for information search and decision making. Finally, relationship marketing offers social benefits, such as being made to feel important and having a customer–service provider relationship develop into a friendship or part of a social support system. For years, pharmacists have recognized the importance of this last consumer benefit.

How Does Relationship Marketing Apply to Pharmacy?

Many of the applications of relationship marketing to pharmacy practice and health care are fairly self-evident. In many pharmacy settings, pharmaceutical goods and patient care services are provided to individuals who require attention and treatment over a long period of time because of their chronic conditions. The establishment of a provider-patient relationship is critical to the successful treatment of patients. Indeed, the nature of the therapeutic relationship between pharmacist and patient has been labeled as *foundational* to the conceptualization of pharmaceutical care (Cipolle, Strand, and Morley, 1998). Interestingly, the definition of a therapeutic relationship (Cipolle, Strand, and Morley, 1998, p. 344), "a partnership or alliance between the practitioner and the patient formed for the purpose of identifying the patient's drug-related needs," refers to several of the elements discussed throughout this chapter. Additionally, the discussion of a therapeutic relationship explicitly recognizes that not only does the practitioner have responsibilities but also the patient—a concept not inconsistent with relationship marketing. While the nature of the patient-provider relationship takes on additional ethical meaning within

the context of health care, many of the concepts discussed in this section (and throughout this chapter) have direct applications to the delivery of health care and pharmaceutical services.

A few additional points concerning relationship marketing and pharmacy practice are warranted. First, practitioners need to recognize that most pharmacies (and their computer systems) are full of data that can be used for one-to-one marketing and satisfying the unique needs of individual customers. These data can be used not only as part of the production and the delivery of the service but also to communicate with customers, prescribers, and other stakeholders. Second, it is important to consider individuals and organizations other than patients when implementing a relationship-marketing program within a pharmacy. The same principles can be applied to interactions with physicians and other providers, employer groups, third-party payers, computer vendors, wholesalers, and even others within your own firm. Establishing, developing, and maintaining relationships with these stakeholders have the potential to enhance or facilitate relationships with the ultimate customer, the patient. Third, building relationships does not happen overnight; relationships take time to establish and develop. However, practitioners should be encouraged to consider every service encounter as a relationship-building opportunity (Doucette and McDonough, 2002).

▓ REVISITING THE SCENARIO: A SUMMARY

At the beginning of this chapter we met Jim Smyth and Sue Davidson, who recognized that something needed to be done to enhance the financial position of their pharmacy. Many questions were raised during their impromptu brainstorming session with their employees, and most were related to the marketing function. To be effective (and efficient), health care providers and pharmacists (including Drs. Smyth and Davidson) need to wear a marketing hat as well as a clinical hat. They must understand how to integrate a marketing philosophy throughout their organizations. They must realize that focusing on customers' needs and learning how to translate those needs into wants and demands are critical steps. They must master the tools of the marketing mix, including the additional considerations required because of the distinctive nature of services. To stay in business, and to continue to reap the intrinsic benefits from helping patients, requires that pharmacists keep an eye on the bottom line, namely, the profitability of the organization (or at least its financial success measured in other terms when considering nonprofit firms). This means that pharmacists must understand the concepts of expectations, satisfaction, quality, value, and loyalty. Finally, while patient-centered pharmacy services already call for the establishment of a therapeutic relationship with patients, the practice of relationship marketing can help to enhance the level of service provided by pharmacists, potentially leading to improved outcomes for patients, improved financial performance for organizations, and rewarding practices for pharmacists.

▇ QUESTIONS FOR FURTHER DISCUSSION

1. What philosophical approach to marketing is most common in today's pharmacy practice environment? Do you think one is more appropriate than the others?

2. What role does marketing play in ensuring the success of pharmacist-delivered MTM services? How can and should the profession (rather than individual pharmacists and businesses) use marketing principles and practices?

3. How can the expectations of patients be changed regarding the delivery of pharmacist-delivered MTM services?

4. How have your perceptions of marketing changed after reading this chapter?

5. Should the application of marketing principles be different for health professionals (compared with other service providers)?

REFERENCES

Berry LL. 1995. Relationship marketing of services: Growing interest, emerging perspectives. *J Acad Market Sci* 23:236.

Bislew HD, Sorensen TD. 2003. Use of focus groups as a tool to enhance a pharmaceutical care practice. *J Am Pharm Assoc* 43:424.

Bitner MJ. 1995. Building service relationships: It's all about promises. *J Acad Market Sci* 23:246.

Booms BH, Bitner MJ. 1981. Marketing strategies and organization structures for service firms. In Donnelly JH, George WR (eds), *Marketing of Services,* p. 47. Chicago: American Marketing Association.

Chandrashekaran M, Rotte K, Tax SS, Grewal R. 2007. Satisfaction strength and customer loyalty. *J Market Res* 44:153.

Christensen DB, Fassett WE, Andrews GA. 1993. A practical billing and payment plan for cognitive services. *Am Pharm* NS33:34.

Cipolle RJ, Strand LM, Morley PC. 1998. *Pharmaceutical Care Practice.* New York: McGraw-Hill.

Day GS, Montgomery DB. 1999. Charting new directions for marketing. *J Market* 63:3.

Doucette WR, McDonough RP. 2002. Beyond the 4 P's: Using relationship marketing to build value and demand for pharmacy services. *J Am Pharm Assoc* 42:183.

Feldstein PJ. 1999. *Health Care Economics,* 5th ed. Albany, NY: Delmar Publishers.

Fournier S, Mick DG. 1999. Rediscovering satisfaction. *J Market* 63:5.

Gummesson E. 2002. *Total Relationship Marketing,* 2d ed. Oxford, England: Butterworth-Heinemann.

Hepler CD, Strand LM. 1990. Opportunities and responsibilities in pharmaceutical care. *Am J Hosp Pharm* 47:533.

Holdford D, Schulz R. 1999. Effect of technical and functional quality on patient perceptions of pharmaceutical service quality. *Pharm Res* 16:1344.

Holdford DA, Kennedy DT. 1999. The service blueprint as a tool for designing innovative pharmaceutical services. *J Am Pharm Assoc* 39:545.

Hunt SD. 1976. The nature and scope of marketing. *J Market* 40:17.

Hunt SD. 1983. General theories and the fundamental explanations of marketing. *J Market* 47:9.

Hunt SD. 2002. *Foundations of Marketing Theory: Toward a General Theory of Marketing.* Armonk, NY: ME Sharpe.

Jones T, Taylor SF. 2007. The conceptual domain of service loyalty: How many dimensions?. *J Serv Market* 21:36.

Keefe LS. 2004. What is the meaning of "marketing"? *Marketing News* 38:17.

Kohli AK, Jaworski BJ. 1990. Market orientation: The construct, research propositions, and managerial implications. *J Market* 54:1.

Kotler P. 2003. *Marketing Management,* 11th ed. Upper Saddle River, NJ: Prentice-Hall.

Kotler P, Keller KL. 2006. *Marketing Management,* 12th ed. Upper Saddle River, NJ: Pearson Prentice-Hall.

Larson LN, MacKeigan LD. 1994. Further validation of an instrument to measure patient satisfaction with pharmacy services. *J Pharm Market Manag* 8:125.

Larson LN, Rovers JP, MacKeigan LD. 2002. Patient satisfaction with pharmaceutical care: Update of a validated instrument. *J Am Pharm Assoc* 42:44.

Levitt T. 1960. Marketing myopia. *Harvard Bus Rev* 38:45.

Lovelock C, Wright L. 2002. *Principles of Service Marketing and Management,* 2d ed. Upper Saddle River, NJ: Prentice-Hall.

MacKeigan LD, Larson LN. 1989. Development and validation of an instrument to measure patient satisfaction with pharmacy services. *Med Care* 27:522.

Mathur A. 1996. Older adults' motivations for gift giving to charitable organizations: An exchange theory perspective. *Psychol Market* 13:107.

McAlister L, Bolton RN, Rizley R (eds). 2006. *Essential Readings in Marketing.* Cambridge, MA: Marketing Science Institute.

McCarthy EJ. 1960. *Basic Marketing: A Managerial Approach.* Homewood, IL: Irwin.

McDonough RP. 2003. Obstacles to pharmaceutical care. In Rovers JP, Currie JD, Hagel HP, et al. (eds), *A Practical Guide to Pharmaceutical Care,* 2d ed., p. 267. Washington, DC: American Pharmaceutical Association.

McDonough RP, Doucette WR. 2003. Using personal selling skills to promote pharmacy services. *J Am Pharm Assoc* 43:363.

McDonough RP, Sobotka JL. 2003. Reimbursement. In Rovers JP, Currie JD, Hagel HP, et al. (eds), *A Practical Guide to Pharmaceutical Care,* 2d ed., p. 222. Washington, DC: American Pharmaceutical Association.

McDonough RP, Sobotka JL, Doucette WR. 2003. Marketing pharmaceutical care. In Rovers JP, Currie JD, Hagel HP, et al. (eds), *A Practical Guide to Pharmaceutical Care,* 2d ed., p. 203. Washington, DC: American Pharmaceutical Association.

McDonough RP, Rovers JP, Currie JD, et al. 1998a. Obstacles to the implementation of pharmaceutical care in the community setting. *J Am Pharm Assoc* 38:87.

McDonough RP, Pithan ES, Doucette WR, Brownlee MJ. 1998b. Marketing pharmaceutical care services. *J Am Pharm Assoc* 38:667.

Morgan RM, Hunt SD. 1994. The commitment-trust theory of relationship marketing. *J Market* 58:20.

Narver JC, Slater SF, MacLachlan DL. 2004. Responsive and proactive market orientation and new-product success. *J Prod Innov Manag* 21:334.

Oliver RL. 1999. Whence consumer loyalty? *J Market* 63:33.

Oliver RL, Rust RT, Varki S. 1997. Customer delight: Foundations, findings, and managerial insight. *J Retail* 73:311.

Palmatier RW, Dant RP, Grewal D, Evans KR. 2006. Factors influencing the effectiveness of relationship marketing: A meta-analysis. *J Market* 70:136.

Palmatier RW, Scheer LK, Steenkamp JEM. 2007. Customer loyalty to whom? Managing the benefits and risks of salesperson-owned loyalty. *J Market Res* 44:185.

Parasuraman A, Zeithaml VA, Berry LL. 1985. A conceptual model of service quality and its implications for future research. *J Market* 49:41.

Parasuraman A, Zeithaml VA, Berry LL. 1988. SERVQUAL: A multiple-item scale for measuring consumer perceptions of service quality. *J Retail* 64:12.

Parasuraman A, Zeithaml VA, Berry LL. 1994a. Alternative scales for measuring service quality: A comparative assessment based on psychometric and diagnostic criteria. *J Retail* 70:201.

Parasuraman A, Zeithaml VA, Berry LL. 1994b. Reassessment of expectations as a comparison standard in measuring service quality: Implications for further research. *J Market* 58:111.

Parvatiyar A, Sheth JN. 2000. The domain and conceptual foundations of relationship marketing. In Sheth JN, Parvatiyar A (eds), *Handbook of Relationship Marketing,* p. 3. Thousand Oaks, CA: Sage.

Peter JP, Olson JC. 1983. Is science marketing? *J Market* 47:111.

Reichheld FF. 2003. The one number you need to grow. *Harvard Bus Rev* 81:46.

Rovers JP, Currie JD, Hagel HP, et al. 1998. *A Practical Guide to Pharmaceutical Care.* Washington, DC: American Pharmaceutical Association.

Rust RT, Oliver RL. 2000. Should we delight the customer? *J Acad Market Sci* 28:86.

Schoell WF, Guiltinan JP. 1990. *Marketing: Contemporary*

Concepts and Practices, 4th ed. Reading, MA: Allyn and Bacon.

Schommer JC, Kucukarslan SN. Measuring patient satisfaction with pharmacutical services. *Am J Health-Syst Pharm* 1997;54:2721.

Shepherd MD. 1995. Defining and marketing value added services. *Am Pharm* NS35:46.

Sheth JN. 2002. The future of relationship marketing. *J Serv Market* 16:590.

Sheth JN, Parvatiyar A. 1995. Relationship marketing in consumer markets: Antecedents and consequences. *J Acad Market Sci* 23:255.

Sheth JN, Sisodia RS, Sharma A. 2000. The antecedents and consequences of customer-centric marketing. *J Acad Market Sci* 28:55.

Siecker B. 2002. Principles of place, channel systems, and channel specialists. In Smith MC, Kolassa EM, Perkins G, Siecker B (eds), *Pharmaceutical Marketing: Principles, Environment, and Practice,* p. 219. New York: Pharmaceutical Products Press.

Smith MC. 1996. Pharmacy marketing. In *Effective Pharmacy Management,* 8th ed., p. 423. Alexandria, VA: NARD.

Smith MC. 2002. General principles. In Smith MC, Kolassa EM, Perkins G, Siecker B (eds), *Pharmaceutical Marketing: Principles, Environment, and Practice,* p. 3. New York: Pharmaceutical Products Press.

Smith MC, Kolassa EM. 2001. Nobody wants your products: They are negative goods. *Product Management Today* 12:22.

Spreng RA, MacKenzie SB, Olshavsky RW. 1996. A reexamination of the determinants of consumer satisfaction. *J Market* 60:15.

Teas RK. 1993. Expectations, performance evaluation, and consumers: Perceptions of quality. *J Market* 57:18.

Van Waterschoot W, Van den Bulte C. 1992. The 4P classification of the marketing mix revisited. *J Market* 56:83.

Vargo SL, Lusch RF. 2004a. The four service marketing myths: Remnants of a goods-based, manufacturing model. *J Serv Res* 6:324.

Vargo SL, Lusch RF. 2004b. Evolving to a new dominant logic for marketing. *J Market* 68:1.

Weitz BA, Jap SD. 1995. Relationship marketing and distribution channels. *J Acad Market Sci* 23:305.

Wilkie WL, Moore ES. 1999. Marketing's contributions to society. *J Market* 63:198.

Wilkie WL, Moore ES. 2003. Scholarly research in marketing: Exploring the "4 eras" of thought development. *J Public Policy Market* 22:116.

Zeithaml VA. 1988. Consumer perceptions of price, quality, and value: A means-end model and synthesis of evidence. *J Market* 52:2.

Zeithaml VA, Berry LL, Parasuraman A. 1993. The nature and determinants of customer expectations of service. *J Acad Market Sci* 21:1.

Zeithaml VA, Rust RT, Lemon KN. 2001. The customer pyramid: Creating and serving profitable customers. *Calif Manag Rev* 43:118.

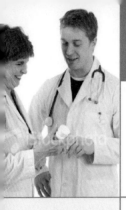

21

MARKETING APPLICATIONS

William Doucette

About the Author: Dr. Doucette is a Professor in the Division of Clinical and Administrative Pharmacy at the College of Pharmacy of the University of Iowa. He received a B.S. in pharmacy, an M.S. in pharmacy administration, and a Ph.D. in social and administrative sciences in pharmacy from the University of Wisconsin. He has managed several community pharmacies. His teaching interests are in pharmacy management and marketing of health care, whereas his primary research interest is evaluating pharmacy services and collaboration between pharmacists and other health care professionals. Dr. Doucette has published his work in many pharmacy journals.

■ LEARNING OBJECTIVES

After completing this chapter, students should be able to

1. Describe a marketing management process for pharmacies.
2. Illustrate how to evaluate a pharmacy market.
3. Discuss a market planning process for pharmacies.
4. Illustrate a marketing mix for a pharmacy service.
5. Describe promotional techniques for pharmacy services.
6. Discuss how to control and evaluate marketing activities.

■ SCENARIO

Debbie Butler, Pharm.D., is the manager of Feel Great Pharmacy, located in Church Cliff, a city of 152,000 people. She recently decided that Feel Great Pharmacy should offer pharmacist services to compete with the large retail chains that have opened pharmacies in her city. Her prescription volume and her net profit percentage have only grown slightly during the last 2 years.

She discusses her pharmacy's situation with other pharmacy managers that she knows. One of them suggests that she market her pharmacy's goods and services. She has heard of marketing but does not know much about it. And while she supports an expanded role for pharmacists, she has been unsure about how to add new pharmacy services into her own practice.

Dr. Butler decides to learn more about marketing by reading articles and talking with other pharmacists. In addition, she finds that there are several pharmacists in her area with experience in developing and marketing pharmacy services. With their encouragement, she decides to develop and implement a marketing plan for Feel Great Pharmacy.

CHAPTER QUESTIONS

1. Describe how a marketing management process can be used to influence decisions in a pharmacy practice.
2. How can a SWOT analysis be used in the marketing management process?
3. Describe the characteristics of attractive target markets.
4. What are the key decisions in creating a marketing mix for a pharmacy service?
5. What are the advantages and disadvantages of using each of the four primary promotional techniques?
6. Describe three ways in which a pharmacy could monitor the performance of its marketing activities.

INTRODUCTION

Intense competition and pressure on containing costs have pushed many pharmacy owners to seek new sources of revenue for their practices. While various approaches can be adopted, more and more pharmacy managers are choosing the path taken by Debbie in the scenario. That is, the marketing of pharmacy goods and patient care services is becoming more widespread.

Marketing principles were described in Chapter 20. This chapter focuses on applying these marketing principles to the goods (e.g., prescription drugs, over-the-counter products, and other tangible items) and services (e.g., patient counseling, disease-state management, and medication therapy management) offered by many pharmacy organizations. First, a marketing management process is described. Then ways to evaluate a market are discussed. Preparation of a marketing plan is addressed, including establishing a marketing mix. Techniques for promoting pharmacy goods and services are discussed. The chapter ends with sections on implementing a marketing plan and a discussion of how to monitor and control a pharmacy's marketing efforts.

To be effective, a marketing management process should be a basic component of any pharmacy practice. A marketing management process has three essential steps: (1) evaluating a market for opportunities, (2) planning and developing marketing strategies and tactics, and (3) implementing and controlling the marketing effort. A *market* typically can be viewed as the buyers and sellers that interact in a geographic area. With pharmacy markets, other parties such as insurers and prescribers are important players to consider.

EVALUATING MARKET OPPORTUNITIES

Evaluating a market involves consideration of both a macroenvironment and a microenvironment. A *macroenvironment* refers to forces that affect the parties in a market and encompasses five sectors: competitive, economic, technological, social, and regulatory (Achrol, Reve, and Stern, 1983; Doucette, Schommer, and Wiederholt, 1993). Competitive considerations such as a merger of pharmacy chains with outlets in the market can affect the demand for pharmacy goods and services at a pharmacy in that market. Similarly, the use of electronic prescribing by a local integrated delivery system can require investment in equipment for pharmacies associated with the delivery system. Social factors such as the presence of a large ethnic group can present opportunities for specialized services targeted to that group. A regulatory factor to consider is the inclusion of pharmacists as providers of medication therapy management (MTM) services under Medicare Part D.

SWOT Analysis

In addition to identifying important influences in the macroenvironment, the microenvironment should be evaluated (McDonough et al., 1998). This means that important stakeholders in the market should be identified and assessed. A *stakeholder* is anyone who can affect the success of the practice. Stakeholders include other health care providers, third-party payers, employers, community leaders, and public agencies. Stakeholders can influence a pharmacy practice by supporting or opposing new service ideas, assisting in marketing efforts, and affecting local norms of care. For example, a health department in one community might support pharmacists as providers of health screening services, whereas the same agency in another community might not.

For the planning process, pharmacy managers can scan their markets by assessing public sources of information about various stakeholders. For example, advertisements and Web pages can be informative. Also, interested parties such as pharmaceutical manufacturer representatives can provide useful information, which can be incorporated into a SWOT analysis. A SWOT analysis assesses the internal *s*trengths and *w*eaknesses of the pharmacy in context with the *o*pportunities and *t*hreats that may exist in its external environment (Kotler, 2001). While a SWOT analysis allows a pharmacy to improve its overall marketing management process, it is especially useful during planning (see Chapters 3 and 4). A SWOT analysis can help to identify likely opportunities, assist in eliminating poor opportunities, guide choices of marketing targets, and help in allocating scarce resources to marketing efforts.

Through a SWOT analysis, a pharmacy manager can identify areas where marketing efforts are likely to be successful. For example, a small group of patients with an unmet need may be more attractive target market for a new pharmacy service than a larger group that is already being served by several competitors. In addition, a SWOT analysis can help a pharmacy to focus on market opportunities that take advantage of the pharmacy's strengths.

Case: Market Evaluation

Consider the ways in which Dr. Butler can evaluate the market for Feel Great Pharmacy. She performed some market scanning and then prepared the following analysis of her pharmacy's environment:

There are 45 pharmacies in Church Cliff. They include chain pharmacies (16), mass merchandisers (8), grocery store pharmacies (12), and independent pharmacies (9). There are 4 hospitals and 12 clinics that support 200 physicians and staff. Of these, the Elvin Health System operates 2 hospitals and 4 medical clinics with 60 physicians practicing among their facilities. One of the large clinics has developed a diabetes care service that is run by an endocrinologist, with certified diabetes educators on site. Elvin Health System has recently incorporated an electronic patient record system linking its hospitals and clinics. Outside the Elvin Health System, there are two multispecialty clinics that each have about 20 physicians and a number of other clinics and private practitioners that have smaller numbers of physicians and fewer types of specialists. Of note is a small clinic operated by a group of three allergists.

The economy of Church Cliff is diverse, with a dozen large employers in manufacturing and service industries. A check of U.S. Census data for Church Cliff (www.census.gov) finds that while the majority of the population is Caucasian (75 percent), there has been rapid growth in the Hispanic (12 percent) and Asian (10 percent) populations over the past 10 years. The population generally is well educated, with more than 90 percent who have completed high school and 30 percent who have completed at least 4 years of college. About 16 percent of the population is over age 65.

In reviewing her pharmacy's prescription records and speaking with local physicians, Dr. Butler finds that there appear to be good numbers of patients with a wide variety of chronic conditions, including cardiovascular disease, hypertension, and diabetes. There is the usual mix of payers for care (i.e., 10 percent Medicaid, 20 percent Medicare, 60 percent private insurance, and 10 percent no insurance) with a high penetration of managed care (especially among the employees of the large manufacturers). Elvin Health HMO has 30,000 covered lives, whereas several smaller managed-care organizations cover an additional 60,000 lives. While most patients have some coverage for prescription drugs, they are used to paying fairly high copayments (e.g., $15 to $30 per prescription).

Church Cliff has one daily and three weekly newspapers. There are also eight radio stations, two TV stations, and a cable TV service. Approximately 70 percent of Church Cliff's households have Internet access.

Dr. Butler believes that medication safety has recently become a more visible issue in her community. That is, more people are thinking about how medi-

cations can be used safely. Her state allows collaborative practice agreements between physicians and pharmacists. She identifies two suppliers of extensive lines of nutritional supplements and herbal products. Both these suppliers have high-quality products, but only one has a promotional program.

Table 21-1 shows the highlights of the SWOT analysis for Feel Great Pharmacy. Dr. Butler recognized that certain groups of patients in her community with common chronic conditions could be targets for her pharmacy's goods and services, such as herbal products, disease-state management services, or a wellness service. She also talked with someone at one of the large medical clinics without a diabetes service and found out that the clinic was interested in adding this service. Knowing that well-educated people tend to use herbal

Table 21-1. SWOT Analysis for Feel Great Pharmacy

Strengths
1. Feel Great Pharmacy has loyal patients owing to high service quality.
2. Feel Great Pharmacy pharmacists have excellent clinical skills and knowledge and thus a good reputation among most local physicians.
3. The prescription volume at Feel Great Pharmacy is expected to be sufficient to support the incorporation of an automated dispensing system.

Weaknesses
1. One of the older pharmacists has stated a reluctance to provide new services.
2. Debbie and staff have limited experience in delivering pharmacy services other than dispensing.
3. May need to remodel somewhat to create space for new services.

Opportunities
1. Relatively large population with cardiovascular diagnoses, including hypertension and hyperlipidemia.
2. There are no bone health clinics or arthritis clinics currently offered in Church Cliff.
3. Consumers who prefer to self-treat with herbals and/or vitamins appear to be prevalent.
4. The older adult population of Church Cliff could have special needs.
5. Cardiovascular conditions tend to be managed by primary care physicians, with control rates typical of national figures.

Threats
1. The retail chain pharmacies are putting pressure on the dispensing business.
2. More and more pharmacies are using automated dispensing equipment.
3. A previous attempt to provide an asthma management service by a different pharmacy was considered an attack on physicians' turf by one of the clinics.
4. An independent pharmacy has developed a successful compounding service.

supplements and vitamins, she viewed that group as an opportunity. Finally, she knows that the older adult population in Church Cliff takes a lot of medications and could benefit from specialized services.

Dr. Butler identified four primary threats to Feel Great Pharmacy. A prominent threat is that the retail chain pharmacies (i.e., pharmacy chains, mass merchandisers, and grocery chains) are putting pressure on Feel Great's dispensing business. Also, she knows that the growth of the chains has resulted in a relative shortage of pharmacists in Church Cliff. Third, Dr. Butler talked with a friend about how the local allergist group was a vocal opponent of a pharmacist-run asthma management service. Those physicians saw the service as invading their turf. Finally, she noted that an independent pharmacy had developed a successful compounding service.

Dr. Butler identified three specific strengths of Feel Great Pharmacy. One is that Feel Great has loyal patients owing to the fact that it takes the time to get to know its patients personally and takes pride in counseling every patient about his or her medications. Also, the pharmacists at Feel Great have excellent clinical skills and current knowledge of drug therapy. This has created a good reputation for the pharmacy among most local physicians. Third, Feel Great installed an automated dispensing system 6 months ago. This system has freed up the pharmacists to spend more time with patients.

Dr. Butler also described three weaknesses of Feel Great. First, one of the older pharmacists has stated a reluctance to provide new pharmacy services. He said that he has always dispensed and wants to keep doing that. Also, Dr. Butler and other Feel Great staff have little experience providing pharmacy services other than dispensing. Such inexperience could result in mistakes as they develop new service offerings. Third, Feel Great may need to be remodeled to create more private space for a new service to be delivered. She wondered if Feel Great Pharmacy would be able to support an MTM service.

After evaluating Church Cliff as a market for new pharmacy services offered by Feel Great Pharmacy, Dr. Butler was ready to move on to the next step in the marketing management process: planning marketing strategies and tactics. An excellent way to organize such planning is to prepare a marketing plan.

PREPARING A MARKETING PLAN

A *marketing plan* describes what goods and services a pharmacy will offer, at which groups its marketing efforts will be targeted, and the specific marketing activities it will undertake. The marketing plan builds on the analyses done during the evaluation phase, especially the SWOT analysis. Included in the marketing plan should be a process to monitor the results of the plan so that necessary adjustments can be made. The elements of a marketing plan include (1) a SWOT analysis, (2) goals and objectives, (3) target markets, (4) marketing mix, and (5) control processes (McDonough et al., 1998; Schwartz and Sogol, 1987). The SWOT analysis performed in the market evaluation provides important information that can shape decisions about the other parts of the marketing plan.

Goals and Objectives

A marketing plan should contain a set of goal statements that lead to objectives that a pharmacy wants to accomplish. Goal statements are general and provide direction for the practice to meet the mission of the pharmacy. Each goal statement has its own specific objectives that are the outcomes needed to meet the goals. The objectives that are developed for the plan should be clearly stated, realistic, and measurable (Rothschild, 1987). It is through the objectives that pharmacists can determine the level of success of their marketing plan. A marketing plan with clear, quantifiable objectives can provide pharmacists with the feedback mechanism to change and refine specific components of the plan. To achieve the goals and objectives, one must accomplish specific tasks in accordance with a timeline that provides a reasonable period for completion of each task. Table 21-2 provides examples of a goal statement and associated objectives.

Once the goals and objectives are developed, time should be spent thinking about the groups of

Table 21-2. Goal and Objectives for Feel Great Pharmacy

Goal: To provide profitable pharmacist services to our patients.

Objective 1: By the end of 1 year, have 35 patients receive new pharmacy services for which payment is received.

Objective 2: Within 12 months, receive 8 referrals from physicians for patients to receive a new pharmacy service.

consumers (target markets) who could benefit from the goods and services offered by the practice. The goal of a pharmacy's marketing activities is to stimulate exchanges with patients who need and are likely to benefit from the services provided by the pharmacy.

Target Markets

Marketing activities should help people to recognize a benefit from the good or service being marketed. It is expected that people will vary in the degree to which they will believe purchase of the product will bring them benefit or value. Thus a key principle in marketing has been to direct marketing efforts toward groups of people expected to benefit from the product (Kotler, 2001). These groups toward which marketing activities are directed are called *target markets.* Focusing marketing efforts on such groups can bring efficiency to a pharmacy's marketing.

The identification of target markets involves *market segmentation.* This is the process of grouping consumers who have similar wants or needs into clusters so that a pharmacy can respond by tailoring its goods and services to those clusters (Holdford, 2003). Typically, one or more market segments are targeted and are considered to be target markets.

Target markets should possess several characteristics to be attractive. One characteristic is that the segment is *identifiable.* That is, what is the extent to which the group can be profiled? For example, the distribution of age, gender, or family size could be considered. A second characteristic of a target market is

its *accessibility,* or the degree to which individuals in the market can be reached via marketing. How are the individuals in a market segment dispersed geographically throughout the market? Is it likely that they can be reached via a common mass-media outlet such as a local newspaper?

An attractive target market consists of individuals willing and able to purchase the good or service being marketed. Willingness to pay is related to the value one expects to gain from purchase of the product. People's ability to pay for a pharmacy service can be influenced by their insurance coverage. In the absence of insurance coverage of a pharmacy service, the willingness and ability to pay out of pocket should be considered when evaluating a target market. Similarly, a target market's *profitability* is an attribute of interest. This means that the expected revenue from the group should exceed the expected costs in serving it. The final characteristic of a favorable target market is its *compatibility* with the pharmacy. The target market should fit with the other groups being served and be consistent with the pharmacy's image.

When identifying target markets for a pharmacy, information can be gathered from a variety of sources. A handy starting place is patient information stored in the pharmacy's computer system (Doucette and McDonough, 2002). For example, people who have had a statin drug dispensed at least twice during the past 6 months could be identified. These people could be further characterized by tabulating insurance status, age, gender, and presence of specific comorbidities such as hypertension or diabetes. Also, home addresses and physician clinics could be of interest as well. Table 21-3 describes two target markets for Feel Great Pharmacy.

Beyond a pharmacy's own records, useful information could be gathered about potential target markets from other sources. Knowledgeable people could be interviewed, such as other pharmacists, pharmaceutical representatives, physicians, and administrators. These people can help to identify unmet needs and opportunities, which will help in selecting target markets. Further, such discussions can help to eliminate potential target markets. To help quantify the size of a target market, Census data could be used (i.e., www.census.gov).

Table 21-3. Target Markets, Marketing Mix, and Control Process for Feel Great Pharmacy

Target markets

1. This target market consists of young (younger than 40 years old) people who are relatively healthy and interested in having a fit appearance. They are active in some forms of physical activity. These people may be single or have young families. Most are well educated and have incomes at or above average.

2. This target market is made up of people who are middle-aged and older and are taking at least four chronic prescription medications. They likely will have multiple chronic conditions such as diabetes, arthritis, hypertension, and hyperlipidemia. They are concerned about managing all their medications and being healthy. Generally, they are not very physically active. Their families are older; few have children at home. Most are well educated. Those working have incomes at or above average, but about half this market is retired.

Marketing mix

Products

Stay Fit Program Aimed at target market 1, this program provides clients with key measures to allow them to judge the effects of their health and fitness activities. Body fat analysis and resting metabolic rate will be performed in the pharmacy with equipment that will be leased. A 20-minute nutritional counseling session will focus on selecting proper nutrition that will assist clients in achieving goals. The pharmacy will add a line of high-quality nutritional supplements to be available on appropriate recommendation. The services in this program are

1. Body-fat analysis
2. Assessment of resting metabolic rate
3. Nutritional counseling

Med Check Program Aimed at target market 2, this MTM program helps patients have safe and effective drug therapy. This program addresses prescription medications, over-the-counter medications, and herbal products taken by a patient. Patients will receive a comprehensive review of all their medications, with a written report and patient education about each drug-related problem identified for their medications (e.g., dosing issues and duplication). A pharmacist will work with the patients and their physicians to develop a plan to address the drug-related problems. The services in this program are

1. Comprehensive medication regimen review and patient education
2. Development of a plan to manage any drug-related problem in coordination with the patient and physicians

Place: Both the Stay Fit Program and the Med Check Program will be provided in the pharmacy.

Price: Each service will be available as a complete program or as separate service components. The complete Stay Fit Program will cost $130, which includes one of each of the three services. Separate component costs are as follows: body-fat analysis, $65; resting metabolic rate, $60; and nutritional counseling, $35. The basic Med Check Program will cost $95, which will include one evaluation of all the patient's medications (including a written report), patient educational for identified drug-related problems, and communication with physicians to address drug-related problems. Additional follow-up visits are available for $45 each.

(Continued)

Table 21-3. Target Markets, Marketing Mix, and Control Process for Feel Great Pharmacy *(Continued)*

Promotion: The following promotional methods will be used.

1. Body-fat analyses and resting metabolic rate assessments will be performed at a local fitness club during special event.
2. Separate newspaper ads will promote the Stay Fit Program and the Med Check Program. The Stay Fit ads will be put in the sports section and the Med Check ads will be in the health section.
3. Flyers about the Stay Fit Program will be posted in fitness clubs and recreation centers.
4. A brochure describing the Med Check Program will be sent to all local physicians.
5. A brochure about the Med Check Program will be mailed to patients using at least four medications regularly.
6. An op-ed piece on patients proactively managing their medications will be written and submitted to a local newspaper.
7. Pharmacy staff will be trained and given incentives to personally sell the programs in the pharmacy. Such opportunities will arise during routine interactions with patients, especially for the Med Check Program.

Process management: An appointment system will be used to provide the new services. Initially, the services will be available during specific blocks of time a day or two a week. These times will be expanded to meet demand. During the "program time" extra staff will be present to provide the necessary services. Pharmacists will rotate through as service providers in a regular manner.

Personnel: Pharmacists will be the primary service providers. They will provide the medication review and patient education for the Med Check Program. Also, pharmacists will provide the nutrition counseling for the Stay Fit Program. All pharmacists will be trained in nutrition and supplements, performing medication regimen reviews, communicating with physicians about drug-related problems, and personal selling techniques. A medical technician will be hired and trained to perform the body-fat analysis and the resting metabolic rate assessments. A dietitian will be identified to assist with the nutritional training and to serve as a consultant if needed. All pharmacy staff will be trained to be familiar with the processes for the two new programs.

Physical facility: A patient service area distinct from the dispensing area will be created. The space will use cubicle dividers to allow privacy to perform the tests and to allow the education and counseling sessions. The space will be large enough to fit the equipment, a desk or table, chairs, and a computer. A patient record system that can interface with the dispensing software will be used.

Control process

Service quality: Service providers will be debriefed about their impressions of the quality of their first three service episodes for each program and periodically thereafter. A brief report card will evaluate the quality of the written report of the medication reviews.

Patient/client satisfaction: An annual survey of patient satisfaction will be performed on all service recipients. Satisfaction with the service process and with outcomes will be assessed.

Financial performance: An income statement will be developed for the new programs. This will include service revenue, actual or estimated costs of providing the services, and any net profit.

Service growth: Each month the number of service clients and the number of service episodes will be tabulated.

After target markets have been chosen, planning can proceed to consideration of the marketing mix.

Marketing Mix

The *marketing mix* is the set of decisions that the pharmacy makes to market its goods and services. The marketing mix for services can be viewed as eight P's: product, place, price, promotion, process, personnel, physical facilities, and productivity and quality (see Table 21-3). Product decisions focus on what is available for purchase. A *product* may be a good only or a service only or a combination of a good and service. *Place* involves considerations about where the product can be purchased or received. *Price* decisions determine how much customers or patients must pay for the product. *Promotion* involves how a pharmacy informs people about its goods and services. *Process management* deals with getting a fit among goods and services offered in a pharmacy. Decisions also need to be made about which *personnel* will provide particular pharmacy services. *Physical facility* decisions address the need for changes in pharmacy layout and equipment needed to deliver the goods and services. Finally, the *productivity* of the service providers, such as the number of patients served in a day, needs to be monitored and managed.

Products are anything that is capable of satisfying a patient want or need. They can include goods, services, places, and ideas. *Goods* are physical objects that can meet a consumer's needs and include prescription drugs, over-the-counter (OTC) products, and other goods typically found in pharmacies. On the other hand, *services* are activities performed by one party for another and are essentially intangible. Services available from pharmacies include MTM, diabetes management, asthma management, blood lipid management, immunizations, and anticoagulation management. Hospital pharmacists have developed services that they provide to patients, as well as to physicians, such as pharmacokinetic dosing and drug information services.

Services have four major characteristics that affect marketing decisions made about them: intangibility, inseparability, variability, and perishability (McDonough, Sobotka, and Doucette, 2003). Unlike goods, services cannot be seen, tasted, or felt before they are purchased. Such *intangibility* makes it difficult for patients to decide the value of a service. For example, a patient who has experienced an asthma management service may have difficulty in determining if he or she got "his or her money's worth." This could be addressed by incorporating something tangible into the service, such as a written report or form.

Inseparability of services refers to the situation that services typically are produced and consumed at the same time. This means that the service provider and the patient are both part of the service experience. Thus provider–patient interactions are an important facet of pharmacy services. Service interactions can go more smoothly if both the provider and the patient are ready to perform their respective parts. Some effort, such as using brochures, can be made to "train" patients to help a service episode go as planned.

Because a service experience depends a lot on who provides it, such experiences are variable. *Variability* can be addressed by hiring and training personnel who consistently provide a high-quality service. For pharmacy services, this often means that pharmacists need to possess proper clinical knowledge. In addition, all personnel involved in providing the service need to be thoroughly knowledgeable about the service process. This includes service providers, as well as support personnel who may not actually interact with patients.

The fourth major characteristic of services is *perishability*, which refers to the inability to store services. Since providers and patients must be present, the pharmacy needs to be able to provide a service when demanded by the client. This situation can create problems because demand often fluctuates for pharmacy services. One approach that has been used to better match demand and supply of pharmacy services is an appointment system. That is, patients make appointments with pharmacists for future services, similar to scheduling a clinic visit with a physician. Although services present marketing challenges, most can be managed in some way.

Another marketing-mix component is *place*. Most pharmacy products are available only at pharmacies. However, because some patients cannot visit the pharmacy, goods and services can be provided beyond the pharmacy. A traditional service of delivering prescription drugs to a patient's home is one example. Another version of a service delivered outside a pharmacy is to have a pharmacist provide a service at the patient's home. For example, such home visits may be made available to patients with disabilities. Some pharmacies also offer their services in the workplace. For example, disease-state management and immunization services have been delivered by pharmacies to employees at their workplaces (Wilson et al., 2003). Hospital pharmacists may provide goods and services in a pharmacy or in patient care areas.

Price is a marketing-mix variable. Setting an appropriate price is important to the successful marketing of any new service. Important considerations in setting fees for pharmacy goods and services include the estimated cost of providing the service (i.e., salary and benefits, materials, and overhead), demand for the service, and competition from other providers. In addition to costs, a reasonable profit should be covered by the price of a pharmacy offering. Demand for pharmacy goods and services will be related to the value that patients expect to receive from purchase. Patients who pay for a service are likely to be satisfied if they receive value similar to what they expected. The presence of competitors can influence prices by providing a standard to which

patients can compare a pharmacy's prices. If insurers are involved, then a discounted contract price probably will be determined. The pricing for services should be firmly established before any promoting begins.

Promotion is a vital marketing-mix component that is intended to inform people in a target market about the availability of goods and services that could meet their needs. Multiple promotional methods can be used in a pharmacy's promotional mix, including advertising, sales promotion, publicity, and personal selling (Rothschild, 1987). See Table 21-4 for a comparison of promotional methods. Advertising is paid, nonpersonal promotion by a sponsor, usually using mass media. It provides good control of a message because the sponsor is paying. However, advertising, especially through broadcast media (e.g., TV and radio), can be expensive. The choice of a specific medium depends on the message, the target market, and the pharmacy's budget. Various media can provide information describing the readership or audience for specific publications or programs. Figure 21-1 shows a print ad for herbal products available at Feel Great Pharmacy.

Targeted direct mailing can be an efficient approach to advertising. A mailing list can be built from pharmacy records, membership rosters of service and support groups, phone directories, and information collected during special events. These mailings

Table 21-4. Comparison of Promotional Methods

	Type of Communication	Relative Cost	Control of Message	Examples
Advertising	Mass	$$$	High	Newspaper Magazine Radio Cable TV Direct mail
Sales promotion	Mass	$$	High	Coupon Sample Trial
Publicity	Mass	$	Low	News release
Personal selling	Personal	$$	Moderate	Pharmacist offering services

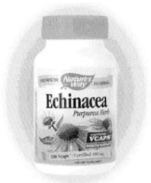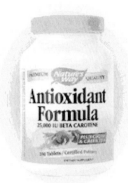

**Stay Healthy Naturally with
Herbal Products**

Echinacea—Supports the immune system & promotes health during the
cold/flu season

Antioxidants—Protect many body systems by fighting free radicals that
can damage cells

See our complete line of herbal & nutritional products

Feel Great Pharmacy
294 W. Main Street
Church Cliff, VA 22022

703-458-3210
www.feelgreatpharmacy.com

Figure 21-1. Print advertisement for herbal products.

typically include a letter and often a promotional print piece (e.g., brochure). The mailing should be tailored to deliver a specific message to a selected audience. The cover letter should be simple and written at the appropriate level for the audience. For example, a mailing announcing a new asthma management service with an accompanying brochure could be mailed to all patients receiving asthma medications from the pharmacy. Overall, the direct mailing should balance providing information about a good or service with persuading members of the target market to try it or find out more about it. Table 21-5 shows content for a brochure about the Med Check Program at Feel Great Pharmacy.

Sales promotion refers to the use of short-term incentives to stimulate the purchase of goods or services. Sales promotion methods include coupons, samples, and trials. The intent is to lower the cost to patients so that they try a good or service. Such an approach could

be useful when introducing a new service. A low-cost trial would allow patients to judge the value of the service to them. A concern with sales promotions is that people can come to expect a discounted price. That is, they only want to purchase the good or service when a sales promotion is present. The judicious use of sales promotions in the presence of other promotional techniques can limit this problem. See Fig. 21-2 for an example of a coupon for a service discount.

Publicity is nonpersonal information about a product or organization that is not paid for by the organization. Because publicity is not paid for by a pharmacy, it can contain positive information or negative information. That is, the control of the message in publicity is much less than with advertising. However, publicity typically is viewed as more credible that advertising. Calling a local news medium (e.g., TV or radio station or a newspaper) about a special event or achievement by the pharmacy can stimulate publicity. Table 21-6

Table 21-5. Content of Flyer for the Med Check Program

Med Check Program

The Med Check Program provides you with peace of mind regarding the medications you are taking. We will answer all of your questions about your medications. You will gain confidence that you are taking the medications that are best for you. Our pharmacists will work with you and your doctors to avoid any problems with your medications.

Med Check Provides Three Services in One

1. Medication review
2. Education about medications
3. Coordination of therapy changes

Medication Review

Our pharmacists will evaluate all your medications to make sure they are right for you. Helps:

- Avoid duplication of therapy
- Eliminate harmful drug interactions
- Find the least expensive therapy
- Recognize any side effects
- Adjust doses to fit you

After reviewing your medications, our pharmacists will discuss their recommendations about any changes. Also, they will contact your doctors to discuss recommended changes in your medications.

Education about Medications

Our pharmacists will help you to understand why you are taking each medication and learn how to monitor the effects of them. This will help you:

- Be informed about all your medications
- Watch for side effects
- Take control of your medications

Coordination of Therapy Changes

Our pharmacists will work with you and your doctors to make any changes in your medications. This will:

- Address any problems with your medications
- Make sure that you and your doctors are involved in any changes
- Assure you that your mix of medications is best for you

Feel Great Pharmacy

Feel Great Pharmacy has developed services that help you improve your health. Our pharmacists will work with you and your doctor to help you reach your health goals. Our expertise in medications can help you make informed choices for what is best for your health.

Our Pharmacy Services

Med Check Program   Focuses on having the best medication therapy for you.

Stay Fit Program   Helps you to reach your fitness goals while maintaining good nutrition.

Herbal & nutritional products   We have a full line of herbal and nutritional products to help you stay healthy naturally.

Pharmacists

Debbie Butler, Pharm.D.

Jennie Dobson, Pharm.D.

Ralph Townes, R.Ph.

Jean Stangel, R.Ph.

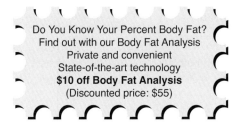

Figure 21-2. Coupon for discounted body fat analysis.

shows a news release about the importance of a medication review.

The fourth promotional method is *personal selling*. Personal selling is interpersonal communication about a good or service. One model of personal selling of pharmacy services describes a dialogue between a pharmacist and a patient containing five steps: (1) assessing patient information, (2) asking probing questions, (3) presenting features and benefits of the service, (4) addressing concerns, and (5) offering the service (McDonough and Doucette, 2003). The early steps in such an interaction involve collecting information on patient health care needs to identify concerns about their health. Once important patient health needs are identified, the pharmacist determines if a pharmacy service can help the patient. If so, the pharmacist proceeds to describe the service's features (i.e., specific components) and benefits (i.e., how it helps to meet the patient's health needs). Pharmacists may need to address

patient objections through further dialogue. Once the patient's questions or objections have been addressed satisfactorily, the pharmacist can offer the service. That is, the pharmacist asks the patient to commit to using the service, such as by making an appointment (Table 21-7). Pharmacies should use a combination of promotional techniques to deliver messages about the goods and services available to their target markets.

Another marketing-mix component is *managing the processes* of providing multiple goods and services within a pharmacy. These decisions deal with how a pharmacy's good or service fits with other activities being performed in the pharmacy. Most pharmacies have a well-established process for dispensing. When a new pharmacy service is being planned, decisions need to be made to ensure a good workflow for both dispensing and the new service. For example, how will staffing be adjusted? Perhaps extra staff will be on duty when the new service will be provided, although some trial and error is likely. Some pharmacies rotate their staff through dispensing roles and pharmacy service roles in which dispensing is not the primary activity. Such rotation can help with coordination among the various activities within the pharmacy. As mentioned previously, training personnel to provide consistent, high-quality services is needed.

Decisions about personnel are another area of the marketing mix. Personnel should possess appropriate knowledge, skills, and attitudes to provide what is

Table 21-6. News Release on the Importance of Having a Medication Review

Adverse Drug Events Are Common and Costly

Adverse drug events (ADEs), defined as any injury owing to a medication error, happen often. The Institute of Medicine has reported that at least 1.5 million preventable ADEs occur each year in hospitals and in people's homes. You can reduce your risk of having an ADE by having all your medications reviewed by your doctor or pharmacist.

If you think you need a medication review, talk with your doctor or pharmacist about having all your medications reviewed. Dr. Debbie Butler from Feel Great Pharmacy says, "Having a comprehensive medication review is easy. Give us a call, and we can schedule an appointment for you. Our Med Check Program can identify potential problems with your medications. Then we can work with you and your doctor to make changes to give you the best medications for you."

You can find out more about medication safety and ADEs by visiting the Web site of the Institute of Medicine at www.iom.edu.

Table 21-7. **Dialogue for Offering Med Check Program to a Patient**

Pharmacist Jennie Dobson is preparing to counsel 60-year-old Mr. Jack Barton, who has refilled two of his five prescription medications: chlorthalidone 25 mg and albuterol inhaler. This dialogue illustrates how Dr. Dobson identifies Mr. Barton's potential need for the Med Check Program and how Dr. Dobson offers the service to Mr. Barton.

Pharmacist: Hi, Mr. Barton. Here are your chlorthalidone and your albuterol inhaler. Have you been having any problems with your medicines?

Patient: No, I've been taking them regularly and can't complain.

Pharmacist: How has your asthma been for you this spring?

Patient: You know, it has been difficult lately. I think the pollen is getting me.

Pharmacist: I see that the last albuterol inhaler lasted you about 2 weeks. How often are you taking it?

Patient: I have been taking a couple of puffs four or five times a day. I can't seen to shake this cough, though my wheezing does improve somewhat after I take the inhaler. I'd like to get my asthma under control without bothering my high blood pressure or high cholesterol.

Pharmacist: It sounds like you want to learn how to better manage your asthma without creating other problems.

Patient: Yes, I'd like to get the right mix of medications.

Pharmacist: We have a service called the Med Check Program that does a comprehensive review of all your medications. The pharmacist can work with you and your physicians to address any problems she finds with your medications. The pharmacist will coordinate any changes in your medications and make sure that you understand how you should be taking each one of them.

Patient: That sounds good, but how much does the program cost?

Pharmacist: The Med Check Program costs $95, which includes the medication review, a written report, a visit to go over your report, and communication with your doctor, if needed.

Patient: Oh, that sounds expensive. I don't know if I can afford it.

Pharmacist: I know that it may seem costly. But after talking with you, it sounds like you have concerns about how to control your asthma while avoiding problems with your other medications. Is that correct?

Patient: Yes, I do want to get a better handle on my asthma in a safe way.

Pharmacist: In our Med Check Program, our pharmacist will consider all your medications while evaluating ways to improve control of your asthma. She will talk to you about it, as well as your doctor. She'll develop a plan that can work for you to safely manage your asthma better. Also, we can set up a payment plan that will allow you to pay for the program in several payments.

Patient: Well, that sounds like it could work.

Pharmacist: May I schedule a time for you to come in later this week for the Med Check Program?

Patient: Yes, that would be good. How much time will we need?

Pharmacist: We should be done in about 30 minutes. Please bring along a list or bottles of any nonprescription medications you take regularly. After the review, we can schedule a time to go over the written report.

Patient: Well, I could come on Friday morning. Would that work for you?

Pharmacist: Yes, I will put you down for 10:30. I'll see you then.

needed. Knowledge of therapeutics and the pathophysiology of a disease would be needed for a disease-state management service. In addition, physical assessment skills such as taking accurate blood pressure readings could be required. Investment in specialized training may be needed. For example, Dr. Butler likely would have to get her staff educated about herbal and nutritional products prior to adding a focus in that area.

A pharmacist also is likely to make use of interpersonal communication skills when interacting with patients and other practitioners such as physicians. Training in these skills is essential. For example, pharmacists may need practice and critical feedback in writing effective SOAP (subjective, objective, assessment plan) notes to be sent to physicians. It is important that pharmacy personnel develop confidence in their ability not only to provide new pharmacy services but also to market their services to all groups of consumers (i.e., patients, health care providers, and payers).

The next marketing-mix variable is the *physical facility*, which refers to the setting where the service will be delivered. Usually this is somewhere within the pharmacy. A question is, "Does this setting make the patient ready to receive the service?" For example, does the patient perceive sufficient privacy to participate in a health care service? Private or semiprivate consultation areas can create the environment needed to provide pharmacy services satisfactorily. Also, consideration should be given to space and workflow. A new pharmacy layout may be needed to accommodate a new pharmacy service because new equipment or space may need to be put in place.

The last marketing-mix variable is *productivity and quality*. One issue here is creating efficiency in pharmacy service activities. This means that monitoring and feedback of service encounters should be performed. Then pharmacists can be trained to be efficient in the time spent with patients when providing services. Time benchmarks can be established for various service offerings. Nonpharmacist personnel should be used where appropriate, such as in scheduling appointments and billing payers.

Manufacturers generally maintain the quality of goods, but this can be an issue for some types of prod-ucts, such as generics or herbals. For these products, the quality and dependability of goods should be evaluated when selecting vendors. In contrast, the quality of services is maintained primarily within the pharmacy. Pharmacies need to establish accurate patient expectations for what will happen during a service encounter. Thus promotional messages should not overpromise what the pharmacy will provide. Also, service quality can be improved through a continuous quality improvement approach. For example, a sample of service encounter notes in patients' charts could be evaluated for quality. A report card could be used to grade the quality of care recorded in the note. Feedback to pharmacists about their performance can be focused on areas where service quality improvements are needed.

The decisions for the marketing mix are interrelated. For example, the decision to include a blood test as a monitoring component of a disease-state management service has implications for other marketing-mix components such as physical facilities, personnel, and pricing. Because of this, it is likely that an iterative process will be needed in establishing the marketing mix. Thus initial decisions should be viewed as tentative until other factors are considered. It can be useful to start with product and work from that point. Several cycles through the marketing-mix decisions may be needed to arrive at a satisfactory plan.

Another consideration in marketing for pharmacies is relationship marketing, in which the pharmacy seeks to establish a relationship with a patient (see Chapter 20). Such an approach is especially pertinent for patients with chronic conditions because it supports appropriate care as the condition progresses. Pharmacies can use their patient record systems to identify people with whom they want a long-term relationship. In addition, the patient records can be used to maintain a customized file of information about the patient. Such information can be used to inform staff when interacting with patients. For instance, a pharmacist could recognize that a patient had changed her hypertensive medication recently when preparing to counsel her on a refill for an arthritis drug. Then, in addition to counseling about the arthritis medication, the pharmacist could ask a patient about her experience with the new hypertensive therapy. This tailoring contributes to a lasting bond between the patient and the pharmacy.

Control Process

The final part of a marketing plan is a control process that will allow assessment of performance in comparison with selected objectives. When such monitoring is combined with feedback and adjustments, then the success of a pharmacy's marketing efforts will be enhanced. This approach can be viewed as a quality improvement process that is linked to marketing objectives (Gronroos, 2000). The scope of such a process could include the quality of care, financial performance, patient satisfaction, and service growth.

A control process will be more likely to be successful if it is part of the operational routine in the pharmacy. That is, regular collecting and reporting of performance will mean that such information will receive more attention from pharmacy personnel. Such attention will assist in early identification of performance problems and can help to improve implementation of solutions. To increase the likelihood that performance data will be collected on a regular basis, a limited set of key indicators should be developed. For example, an annual patient satisfaction survey could be performed. Also, the number of patients receiving services and the number of services provided should be tracked. A marketing budget is another useful performance-improvement tool. Actual spending on the service can be compared regularly with budgeted figures, allowing for adjustments to be made in the future (e.g., increasing money spent on specific promotional strategies based on where customers learned about the service). For improving the quality of care, a report card could be used to assess the quality of care as recorded in the patient records. A focused approach to controlling marketing activities should raise the likelihood of marketing success.

Case: Preparing a Marketing Plan

Dr. Butler has built on the previous SWOT analysis and objectives to generate a marketing plan for Feel

Great Pharmacy. As shown in Tables 21-3 and 21-5 to 21-7 and Figs. 21-1 and 21-2, she has identified two target markets. Target market 1 is made up of active young people (younger than 40 years of age) who are interested in being and looking fit. This group is working and has above-average household incomes. Target market 2 consists of people middle-aged and older people who use at least four chronic prescription medications. They likely will have multiple chronic conditions such diabetes, arthritis, hypertension, or hyperlipidemia. They are concerned about managing all their medications and being healthy. This group is not very physically active, and about half are retired.

Two bundles of pharmacy services have been developed: a Stay Fit Program aimed at target market 1 and a Med Check Program for target market 2. The Stay Fit Program, intended to assist clients achieve their fitness goals, contains three services: a body-fat analysis, an assessment of resting metabolic rate, and a 20-minute nutritional counseling session. Each of these services can be performed in the pharmacy. A complement to this program is a new line of herbal and nutritional products that will be added to the pharmacy. Dr. Butler believes that people interested in the Stay Fit Program will be interested in such goods.

The Med Check Program will help patients to improve the safety and effectiveness of their drug therapy, including prescription medications, OTC medications, and herbal products. Patients will receive a comprehensive review of all their medications, with a written report and patient education about each of their drug-related problems. A pharmacist will work with the patients and their physicians to develop a plan to address these problems.

Each service will be available as a complete program or as separate service components. The complete Stay Fit Program will cost $130, which includes one of each of the three services. Separate component costs are body-fat analysis ($65), resting metabolic rate ($60), and nutritional counseling ($35). The basic Med Check Program will cost $95, which will include an evaluation of the patient's medications (including a written report), patient education for identified drug-related problems, and communication with physicians to address drug-related problems. Additional follow-up visits are available for $45 each.

The promotional mix will include advertising, publicity, and personal selling. The Stay Fit Program will be promoted through a special event at a fitness club, a coupon for a discounted body-fat analysis, flyers posted at fitness clubs, newspaper ads, and personal selling by pharmacy staff in the pharmacy. The Med Check Program will be promoted through newspaper ads, a direct mailing to physicians and patients taking at least four chronic medications, publicity via an op-ed piece in the local newspaper about the benefits of patients proactively managing their medications, and personal selling by pharmacy staff in the pharmacy.

The services will be provided in a new service area in the Feel Great Pharmacy. The service area will contain testing equipment, a computer, chairs, and a workspace. It will be made private through the use of cubicle dividers. Pharmacists will provide most of the services, except the body-fat analysis and resting metabolic rate assessments, which will be provided by a medical technician. An appointment system will be used so that extra staff can be present during delivery of the new services.

A control process will address four areas: service quality, patient/client satisfaction, financial performance, and service growth. Service quality will be assessed by using a brief report card to evaluate the quality of a sample of the written reports of medication reviews. An annual survey of patient/client satisfaction with the service processes and outcomes will allow evaluation of patient satisfaction. The pharmacy's income statement will be developed to monitor the financial performance of the new programs. This will include service revenue, associated costs, and any net profit. Service growth will be tracked by tabulating the number of service clients and the number of service episodes each month.

On completing the marketing plan, Dr. Butler is ready to take the next steps. That is, she is ready to begin to make the changes in Feel Great Pharmacy necessary to develop and provide the new goods and services. She will work toward the day when she will go "live" with the services at Feel Great Pharmacy.

▆ IMPLEMENTING A MARKETING PLAN

Once a marketing plan has been created, the next challenge is to put the plan into action. The goods and services described in the plan must fit into the pharmacy practice, which is an ongoing combination of people, equipment, and information. Putting a new service into practice means that the pharmacy will be disrupted in some way. Ideally, such disruption will be limited in time and done in a manner that minimizes problems for staff and customers. A couple of tools that can support a coordinated practice change are a service blueprint and an action plan.

Service Blueprint

A *service blueprint* is a picture or map of a service that permits a better understanding of all the processes involved in its delivery (Holdford and Kennedy, 1999). It details the activities that need to occur to deliver the service. Developing a service blueprint forces pharmacy personnel to describe each of individual behaviors needed to deliver the service, from the clerk who makes the appointment to the pharmacist who provides the service to the technician who bills the payer. A service blueprint brings the details together into an integrated picture of patient and pharmacy personnel interacting during the service episode. Because such a fine level of detail is used, a service blueprint can help to identify problems that can be addressed prior to or during implementation. For example, pharmacy staff can discuss workflow and service responsibilities to ensure coordination.

A service blueprint specifically considers the patient perspective. That is, a patient's experience during the delivery of the service is described. In so doing, a service blueprint illustrates three types of activities performed by pharmacy personnel: onstage activities, backstage activities, and support processes. *Onstage activities* are those which are visible to the patient during the service encounter. Conversely, *backstage activities* are service activities that are not visible to the patient but still are essential to delivery of the service. *Support processes* are activities that support the employees in contact with the patients before, during, and after service delivery.

Consider Fig. 21-3, which is a service blueprint of Feel Great's Med Check service. The blueprint is divided by three lines: line of interaction, line of visibility, and line of internal interaction. The *line of interaction* separates patients from contact employees. It signifies interactions that occur between the patient and the contact employee, such as taking a medication history. The *line of visibility* separates onstage employee actions from backstage employee actions. Above this line appear the actions that the patient can see, whereas below it are actions that the patient does not see. In Fig. 21-3, the patient sees the pharmacist take a medication his-

tory but does not see her work up the drug therapy plan and generate the written report. The *line of internal interaction* separates the contact employees from support processes. For example, when working up the drug therapy plan, a pharmacist may consult drug literature or contact a physician. Mapping these actions can identify steps that need support, such as having access to a drug literature database.

A service blueprint can be created in a systematic manner once a service to be blueprinted has been determined. A starting point would be to map the service process from the patient's view. Consider the patient's actions and choices as the patient proceeds through the service process. Think about how the patient is likely to perceive the service experience. For example, will adequate privacy be present?

The next step in developing the service blueprint is to map the actions of contact employees. One point

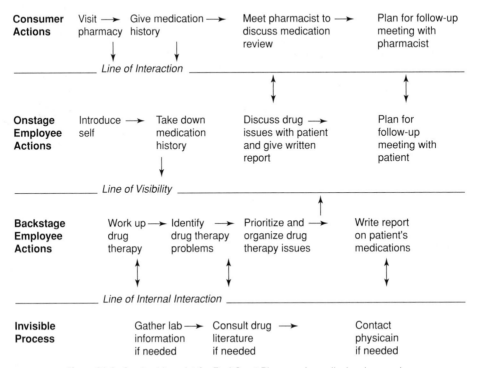

Figure 21-3. Service blueprint for Feel Great Pharmacy's medical review service.

here is to distinguish between onstage and backstage activities. It can be useful to discuss these activities with the staff that will be expected to perform them. This will identify responsibilities and roles and can help to resolve problems that may arise. A next step is to map internal support processes. This will help to identify external interactions that may be needed to support the delivery of the service, such as contacting a patient's physician.

The last step in creating a service blueprint is to add evidence of service where appropriate. This means that tangible components are incorporated into the service. Such evidence can be used by patients to evaluate a service. For example, the written report for the medication review gives a patient something that helps him or her put a value on the service. Tangible evidence should have a natural fit with the service.

Action Plan

Another tool that can help to organize the implementation process is an action plan. An *action plan* is a listing of the tasks that need to be performed to start a service, when they should be completed, and who is responsible for completion (Hagel, 2003). The action plan should address important issues such as facility redesign, workflow and staffing, staff training, marketing materials, and documentation. An action plan can encompass time spent developing a marketing plan, or it can focus on activities after a marketing plan has been developed.

Table 21-8 shows a 12-month action plan for implementing the Med Check Program at Feel Great Pharmacy after the marketing plan has been completed. This action plan shows the main task categories with little detail within each category. Greater detail can be added to list more tasks. For example, lines can be added under "Prepare Promotional Materials" for each promotional activity: newspaper ads, brochure and cover letter to physicians, personal selling training, and the op-ed piece for the newspaper. Another piece that should be added to Table 21-8 is a column listing the individual who is responsible for the action in each line.

Table 21-8. Action Plan for Med Check Program at Feel Great Pharmacy

Month	1	2	3	4	5	6	7	8	9	10	11	12
Remodel service area	XXX	XXX	XXX									
Set workflow and staffing	XXX	XXX	XXX									
Develop medication history and report forms	XXX	XXX	XXX									
Prepare promotional materials (ads, brochure)		XXX	XXX	XXX								
Train staff for medication review process			XXX	XXX								
Promote service (MD letter, newspaper ads)					XXX	XXX	XXX	XXX	XXX	XXX	XXX	XXX
Go live with service					XXX							
Provide medication review services					XXX	XXX	XXX	XXX	XXX	XXX	XXX	XXX
Debrief pharmacists on service encounters and overall process						XXX	XXX	XXX		XXX		XXX
Adjust service process as needed							XXX	XXX	XXX		XXX	

An action plan can be used to monitor the progress toward a service start date. An action plan makes apparent that any delays in early actions could push back other activities and, ultimately, implementation of the service. Any late activities should be addressed immediately to limit delays. Also, sometimes actions can take longer than expected owing to an underestimate of time needed for completion. Updated versions of the action plan are likely to be needed, especially in pharmacies with little experience in implementing new services.

Once service delivery has begun, the control process goes into action. A goal is to make the performance monitoring, evaluation, and feedback activities routine. Intensive monitoring of the quality of initial service encounters provides important feedback on problems that need to be addressed.

Financial performance (i.e., revenue from services and sales of new herbal and nutritional products) and service growth should be monitored closely during initial implementation. Patient satisfaction should also be monitored with surveys or interviews of early service clients.

▥ REVISITING THE SCENARIO

Dr. Butler has created a service blueprint for the Med Check Program at Feel Great Pharmacy. She will also create a service blueprint for each of the Stay Fit Program components. These documents will help her to implement the new services in her pharmacy. Similarly, she has an action plan for one part of her new programs. Dr. Butler can add more details to the current action plan and later expand it to encompass both programs. This approach allows her to coordinate all the tasks that need to be completed for Feel Great Pharmacy to offer the new goods and services.

Working through the marketing management process has put Dr. Butler and Feel Great Pharmacy in a position to generate new revenue. Dr. Butler intends to accomplish this by selling new herbal and nutritional goods and by providing new professional services that fit both within the community and with the strengths of her pharmacy. A systematic approach to marketing the pharmacy's goods and services will increase the likelihood of success for pharmacies that choose to expand their practices.

▥ QUESTIONS FOR FURTHER DISCUSSION

1. What other target markets might Dr. Butler have selected for Feel Great Pharmacy? Why?
2. How do you feel about asking pharmacists to personally sell their services to patients?
3. Marketing a pharmacy service at a chain pharmacy may differ from marketing one at an independent pharmacy. Discuss expected differences and similarities.
4. What do you believe to be the biggest obstacles to marketing pharmacy services successfully?

REFERENCES

Achrol RS, Reve T, Stern LW. 1983. The environment of marketing channel dyads: A framework for comparative analysis. *J Market* 47:55.

Doucette WR, McDonough RP. 2002. Beyond the 4 P's: Using relationship marketing to build value and demand for pharmacy services. *J Am Pharm Assoc* 42: 183.

Doucette WR, Schommer JC, Wiederholt JB. 1993. The political economy of pharmaceutical marketing channels: A conceptual framework. *Clin Ther* 15:739.

Gronroos C. 2000. *Service Management and Marketing: A Customer Relationship Management Approach,* 2d ed. West Sussex, England: Wiley.

Hagel HP. 2003. Developing a practice implementation plan. In Rovers JP, Currie JD, Hagel HP, et al. (eds), *A Practical Guide to Pharmaceutical Care,* p. 287. Washington, DC: American Pharmaceutical Association.

Holdford DA. 2003. *Marketing for Pharmacists.* Washington, DC: American Pharmaceutical Association.

Holdford DA, Kennedy, DT. 1999. The service blueprint as a tool for designing innovative pharmaceutical services. *J Am Pharm Assoc* 39:545.

Kotler P. 2001. *A Framework for Marketing Management.* Upper Saddle River, NJ: Prentice-Hall.

McDonough RP, Doucette WR. 2003. Using personal selling skills to promote pharmacy services. *J Am Pharm Assoc* 43:363.

McDonough RP, Sobotka JL, Doucette WR. 2003. Marketing pharmaceutical care. In Rovers JP, Currie JD, Hagel HP, et al (eds), *A Practical Guide to Pharmaceutical Care,* p. 203. Washington, DC: American Pharmaceutical Association.

McDonough RP, Pithan ES, Doucette WR, Brownlee MJ. 1998. Marketing pharmaceutical care services. *J Am Pharm Assoc* 38:667.

Rothschild ML. 1987. *Marketing Communications: From Fundamentals to Strategies.* Lexington, MA: D.C. Heath.

Schwartz A, Sogol E. 1987. Developing a marketing plan. *Drug Top* 6:69.

Wilson J, Osterhaus M, Currie J, et al. 2003. A cost analysis on the implementation of a cardiovascular wellness program from the pharmaceutical care provider's perspective. *J Am Pharm Assoc* 43:291.

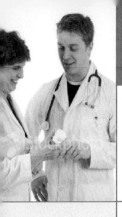

22

PURCHASING AND INVENTORY MANAGEMENT

Donna West

About the Author: Dr. West is an Associate Professor at the University of Arkansas for Medical Sciences College of Pharmacy. She received a B.S. in pharmacy and a Ph.D. in pharmacy administration from the University of Mississippi. She coordinates the community pharmacy management course and teaches pharmaceutical policy in the health care system. Dr. West serves as a pharmacy consultant for the Arkansas Foundation for Medical Care and the Arkansas State Employee Insurance Group and is the faculty liaison for the National Community Pharmacists Association student chapter. Her research interests pertain to understanding provider and patient behavior to improve medication use and advance community practice.

▨ LEARNING OBJECTIVES

After completing this chapter, students should be able to

1. Explain the importance, both financially and operationally, of purchasing and inventory management to a pharmacy.
2. List purchasing objectives and inventory management objectives for a pharmacy.
3. Describe procurement and carrying costs for a pharmacy.
4. Calculate inventory turnover rates and use this information to make purchasing and inventory control decisions.
5. Describe three methods of inventory management.
6. Describe the role of technology in improving inventory management in pharmacies.

▨ SCENARIO

It's 5:00 p.m. on a Monday at Community Mental Health Center pharmacy, and for the fifth time today, Marie Parker, Pharm.D., does not have the medication she needs to fill a prescription. She has had to explain to each patient that he will have to come back tomorrow to pick up his medication or take his prescription elsewhere. What a day! Meanwhile, the wholesaler delivery person just arrived with today's order—4 hours late! The chief executive officer (CEO) of the mental health center is questioning how much the pharmacy has been spending on medications and pressuring Marie to find a less expensive vendor. Marie decides that she will look into using another vendor. Fortunately, a representative from XYZ Wholesale Drugs dropped off her card last week. XYZ Wholesale Drugs is a large national company with a good reputation. Marie contacts the XYZ representative and describes her current situation. She is constantly running out of products, and with her

pharmacy's gross margins shrinking, she needs to obtain drug products at the best price possible. The level of service provided by her current wholesaler seems to be decreasing (e.g., the order is frequently late, and she seldom sees a customer service representative to discuss these issues). Marie asks the XYZ representative some questions and uses this information to compare XYZ Wholesale Drugs with her present wholesaler (Table 22-1). Now that she has all this information, she is not sure what to do.

■ CHAPTER QUESTIONS

1. Why is balancing supply and demand important to inventory management?

Table 22-1. Scenario Wholesaler Comparisons

I. Price on two drug products

Product (No. of Bottles per Month)	XYZ Wholesale Drug		Current Wholesaler	
	Unit Price	Ext. Price ($US)	Unit Price ($US)	Ext. Price ($US)
Paxil 20 mg 100s (9)	210	1,890	215	1,935
Atacand 8 mg 30s (19)	50	950	60	1,140
Total		2,840		3,075

	XYZ Wholesale Drug	Current Wholesaler
II. Cash discounts	Weekly EFT: 1.25% Weekly prepay EFT: 1.50%	EFT every 7 days: 1.25% EFT every 15 days: 1.00%
III. Inventory management systems	Perpetual inventory system, Internet accessible; provide inventory management reports	Perpetual inventory system; provide inventory management reports
IV. Return-goods policy	If the merchandise is salable and returned within 180 days of purchase date, wholesaler will provide a 100 percent credit. If it is returned after 180 days, only 85 percent credit will be given. Partial bottles, products that are 3 months after date of expiration, and other selected products are nonreturnable.	Merchandise that is returned within 30 days of invoice date will be credited 100 percent of original invoice amount (assuming it is in salable condition). If the merchandise is returned after 30 days and is in salable condition, 75 percent of the original invoice amount will be credited. Partial bottles, controlled/schedule II products, and other selected merchandise cannot be returned.

2. What are the advantages of joining a group purchasing organization?
3. How does inventory management affect a pharmacy's profit margins and cash flow?
4. How does the inventory turnover rate indicate how efficient the pharmacist is at managing the inventory investment?
5. How has technology improved the pharmacist's ability to manage inventory?

▓ INTRODUCTION

Inventory usually represents a pharmacy's largest current asset. Inventory also is the least liquid current asset, given that it generally cannot be turned to cash until it is sold to a consumer. The value of inventory to all pharmacies continues to rise owing to the increased variety and expense of pharmaceutical products. Therefore, proper management of inventory has a significant impact on both the financial and the operational aspects of any pharmacy (Huffman, 1996; West, 2003).

Acquisition, procurement, carrying, and stock-out or shortage costs are the four general "costs" associated with inventory. Acquisition, procurement, and carrying costs can be calculated accurately and are an important financial consideration in pharmacy management. These three types of inventory costs generally place little direct stress on busy pharmacy staff but can depress the organization's operating margins if not monitored appropriately. Shortage costs represent failures in customer service and therefore lost sales. These costs may be difficult to quantify but definitely have an impact on any pharmacy.

From a financial perspective, effective inventory management decreases the cost of goods sold and operational expenses, resulting in increased gross margins and net profits. For example, saving $100 on the purchase of prescription drugs will increase the gross margin and net profit by $100 (assuming that operational expenses remain constant). Moreover, having less money invested in inventory improves cash flow (West, 2001). A pharmacy that has merchandise that is not selling or an oversupply of product sitting on the shelf has less cash available to pay expenses and/or invest in other business operations. A pharmacy that is able to reduce its inventory by $100 has that much more cash to spend on day-to-day operations, invest in new services, or place in a savings or checking account.

From an operational perspective, effective inventory management is important in meeting consumer demands for both goods and services (Carroll, 1998). Not having a product when needed may cause the pharmacy to lose a sale and potentially a customer. Furthermore, not having a needed product at the right time may cause physical harm to a patient, especially in settings (e.g., hospitals) where lifesaving emergency drugs are needed routinely at a moment's notice.

Inventory management means minimizing the investment in inventory while balancing supply and demand. People use inventory management in their everyday lives. For example, when people shop for groceries, they think about what they would like to eat (i.e., needs and wants) and what items they have on hand (i.e., current inventory). From this, they create a grocery list. This list is revised depending on how much money they have, grocery store specials, storage space, and how quickly the food will spoil. They may compare products and shop at various grocery stores. They eventually make purchases and evaluate how well those purchases satisfy their needs and wants. The process is repeated and reevaluated on a continuous basis. This is similar to how pharmacies purchase their inventory. Pharmacists or their staff create lists of products they need, revise the list based on current inventory, determine how much money they have to purchase these goods, evaluate any specials from their vendors and their available storage space, and then finally make and evaluate their purchases.

To effectively accomplish the purchasing process, it is important for pharmacy managers to be aware of both purchasing and inventory management objectives (West, 2003). These are distinct yet interrelated functions. Having the right product at the right time at the right price is essential to meeting consumer demand. At the same time, pharmacy managers desire to minimize inventory investment. This chapter will discuss first the purchasing functions and then the inventory management functions.

▪ PURCHASING

Some pharmacists perceive that purchasing is just a routine function necessary to keep inventory on the shelf. However, since most pharmacies literally spend millions of dollars every year to acquire medications and other goods, purchasing is actually a substantial investment process. It involves buying the *right products* in the *right quantity* at the *right price* at the *right time* from the *right vendor* (Tootelian and Gaedeke, 1993), as listed in Table 22-2. Many pharmacies, especially in hospitals and other health care facilities, have a designated person or purchasing agent whose responsibility is to order and receive products.

Right Product

Having the right products is an essential purchasing objective. To determine the product mix, the pharmacy manager should consider how much space is available to stock products and how much money is available to invest in products. Having products on the shelf that are not selling because they are not needed in the institution or wanted by pharmacy customers is a waste of resources and leads to obsolescence costs. Opportunity costs are realized because this space and money could be used to supply products that are more likely to be needed and wanted by consumers. Space should be allocated to items generating the greatest sales, and items that are not selling frequently should be given a lower priority.

Deciding what products to stock is also a marketing question. Determining the real and perceived needs of the pharmacy's patients, patrons, and prescribers

---

Table 22-2. Purchasing Objectives

1. To obtain the right products
2. To obtain products in the right quantity
3. To obtain products at the right time
4. To obtain products at the right price
5. To obtain products from the right vendor

Source: Tootelian and Gaedeke, 1993.

---

is an important consideration when deciding what to purchase. The pharmacy manager should evaluate the following factors when deciding what products to order (Huffman, 1996; Tootelian and Gaedeke, 1993; West, 2003):

- *Past usage.* Pharmacy managers should review drug usage reports and new and refill prescription orders to determine what to stock.
- *Target market.* The market where the pharmacy is located will affect product selection. A pharmacy located in a children's hospital will need different products than a pharmacy located in a mental health facility. Likewise, a community pharmacy located next to a pediatric clinic likely will need more liquid antibiotics than other pharmacies. Prescribing behaviors of area physicians can provide insight into what drug products are needed.
- *Pharmacy image and goals.* Pharmacy managers should consider the pharmacy's image and business goals. Product selection should complement the pharmacy's image. For example, a pharmacy that is attempting to establish itself as a diabetes care center should maintain a greater inventory of specialty diabetes products. Similarly, pharmacies that promote high levels of service and never being out of needed medications will need to maintain higher inventory levels or obtain more frequent deliveries from vendors.
- *Formularies.* In hospitals and other health care institutions, formularies can drive the decision of what goods to stock (Carroll, 1998). A formulary is essentially a list of preferred drugs for use in that institution that are selected based on a combination of clinical and economic benefits. Pharmaceutical products that are placed on a formulary should be well stocked because these are the products that prescribers will be encouraged to use. Alternatively, products that are not on the formulary may not need to be stocked at all. Nonformulary items generally can be special ordered if needed. Pharmacy managers also must consider intravenous tubing, needles, and other supplies that may be needed at their institutions. Formularies may also influence drug purchasing

decisions in the retail pharmacy setting. Products that are more prominent on third-party payer formularies may need to be stocked to a higher degree than products that are not paid for by third-party payers in the area.

- *Industry data.* Pharmacy journals and magazines contain a wealth of information that can be used to provide insight into what drug products should be selected. Pharmacists commonly use "top 200 prescribed drug product lists" to monitor trends in prescription drug use. Additionally, these publications commonly alert pharmacy managers to new products or product changes that may affect patron and prescriber needs in the future.
- *Industry representatives.* Both drug company and wholesaler representatives can provide valuable information about available products. These representatives often have industry trend data and are familiar with prescribing habits in the local geographic area. Moreover, industry representatives have information about new and soon-to-be-released products.
- *Consumer information.* Asking patrons, prescribers, and employees is another way to determine what to stock. Monitoring consumer requests for products is also helpful.

Right Quantity at the Right Time*

As stated previously, having too much product ties up a pharmacy's money without providing an adequate return on investment. On the other hand, having too little product may result in lost sales and profits when the product is not available when consumers want to make a purchase. Not having enough product available also inconveniences pharmacy staff and customers and may result in the loss of customers in the future. Thus, not only is having the right product critical to inventory

management, but also having the right quantity at the right time is also essential.

The right quantity means having just enough product on hand to cover consumer demand at any given time. Determining the right quantity for any given product is difficult, if not impossible, given that demand may fluctuate unexpectedly. However, it is still important for pharmacy managers to track consumer demand for their products and monitor trends that may affect their use. While managers may not always have the right quantity on hand, use of this information helps them to anticipate fluctuations in demand (e.g., increasing the supply of antibiotics and certain over-the-counter medications during winter months).

In general, there are three types of stock to consider. *Cycle stock* is the regular inventory that is needed to fulfill orders. *Buffer,* or *safety, stock* is additional inventory that is needed in case of a supply or demand fluctuation. *Anticipatory,* or *speculative, stock* is inventory that is kept on hand because of expected future demand or expected price increase (e.g., flu vaccine in the fall and winter months). Buying anticipatory stock is risky, and therefore, pharmacists usually do not carry much anticipatory stock and place higher markups on such anticipatory stock. These types of stock are important to consider when deciding how much to order and when to order (Silbiger, 1999).

In order to estimate the minimum quantity of goods needed to meet demand, the pharmacy manager or purchasing agent should know the following information for each item stocked:

1. How much is on hand
2. At what point to reorder
3. How much to order

How do pharmacy managers determine *stock depth* (i.e., the point where it is reasonably certain that the item will be available on demand)? Establishing stock depth (product quantity) involves consideration of

1. An item's rate of sale (average demand)
2. The length of time between stock checks (review time)

---

*Parts of this section are excerpted with permission from West DS. Purchasing and inventory control. In Jackson R (ed), *Effective Pharmacy Management CD-ROM,* 9th ed. Alexandria, VA: National Community Pharmacists Association Foundation, 2003, Sec. 17.

3. The period of time between placing and receiving an order (lead time)
4. A safety stock to account for variations in average demand during the buying time (review time plus lead time)

Thus the formula to set the *reorder point* is

Reorder point = [(review time + lead time) × average demand] + safety stock

This basic formula has been used to develop an *economic order quantity* (EOQ) model (Carroll, 1998; Huffman, 1996; Silbiger, 1999; Tootelian and Gaedeke, 1993). While the EOQ model may be difficult to derive and calculate, it is often incorporated into computer software used by many pharmacies to manage their inventory and make purchasing decisions. The EOQ model describes the level of inventory and reorder quantity at which the combined costs of purchasing and carrying inventory are at a minimum. The formula is

$$Q = \sqrt{\frac{2(c)(D)}{(I)(UC)}}$$

where

Q = economic order quantity
c = procurement cost per order
D = demand for the product expressed either in dollars or physical units
I = inventory carrying costs
UC = unit cost of the item

Another factor determining how much to order is the budget. Hospital pharmacy directors may estimate this year's budget by increasing last year's budget by a certain percent (e.g., 5 or 10 percent). This budget estimate will provide a guide for how much money can be spent each month to order product. Community pharmacy managers also evaluate the profit-and-loss statement to determine whether too much product is being bought compared with the amount of sales.

Using an open-to-buy budget helps to control the total dollar investment in inventory (Carroll, 1998;

West, 2003). It limits the manager to a set predetermined dollar amount of purchases during a given time period. The basic steps of this purchase technique are listed below (Huffman, 1996; West, 2003). This procedure is repeated on a monthly basis.

Step 1. Forecast purchase budget for each month in the next fiscal year based on sales and cost of goods sold (COGS) data from the preceding year.
Step 2. Each month's forecasted sales are then multiplied by the COGS percent to calculate the monthly unadjusted purchase budget.
Step 3. At the end of each month, the month's actual sales and purchases are recorded. Next month's purchases are then adjusted based on the past month's actual sales and purchases. If sales were greater than predicted, then next month's purchase budget may be increased to accommodate for the increased sales. Alternatively, if the sales were lower than expected, then the purchase budget for the next month would be decreased.

Right Price

Once the right product is selected, it is important to acquire it at the right price. Purchasing pharmacy products (especially prescription drugs) is not unlike purchasing a car in that the "list" or "sticker" price is often different from the final price that pharmacies actually pay. For pharmacy products, the list price and the terms of sale have an impact on the overall acquisition cost. *Terms of sale* pertain to discounts and dating (Huffman, 1996; West, 2003).

Discounts
Discounts describe the reduction(s) in price, whereas *dating* pertains to the period of time allowed for taking the discounts and the date when the invoice becomes payable. Although there are a number of discounts, three main discounts are described below.

QUANTITY DISCOUNTS Quantity discounts traditionally have been offered as an incentive for purchasing large quantities of single products or a special grouping of specific products offered by a manufacturer (West, 2003). For example, a wholesaler may sell one bottle of a drug for $100. A quantity discount may apply so that if the pharmacy orders a dozen bottles at one time, a 2 percent discount is given. Thus the pharmacy that orders 12 bottles will acquire each bottle at a cost of $98, resulting in a total savings of $24. These discounts based on a quantity of the same product being purchased on the same order are described as *noncumulative quantity discounts* (Huffman, 1996; Tootelian and Gaedeke, 1993; West, 2003).

The purchasing agent or pharmacy manager should be aware of these special discounts and adjust ordering to take advantage of them. Assuming that the product purchased is salable in the pharmacy, quantity discounts can decrease the actual acquisition cost of the drug product. However, managers should also balance the savings generated by quantity discounts with the costs of storing and carrying excess inventory, the risks of not being able to sell the extra products, and the opportunity costs that come with spending money on inventory that could have been used in other ways.

Some vendors offer quantity discounts to pharmacies if their total purchases reach a target monetary amount during a specific time period. These discounts involving a variety of products on separate orders over a period of time are termed *cumulative quantity discounts* or *deferred discounts* (Huffman, 1996; Tootelian and Gaedeke, 1993; West, 2003). For example, generic drug manufacturers often offer rebates to pharmacies that are based on the amount of generic product purchased during a given time period (e.g., quarterly or yearly). Similarly, hospital pharmacies, retail pharmacies, and others negotiate discounts based on volume purchasing. The pharmacy receives a discount based on the volume purchased in a specified time period. A hospital or institutional pharmacy may be able to negotiate lower prices because a pharmaceutical product is placed on its formulary. The pharmacy can estimate that a certain amount of volume will be purchased or the product will get a percent of the market share. In exchange for this market share or volume purchasing, a discounted price is negotiated.

CASH DISCOUNTS Cash discounts are small discounts offered for the prompt payment of invoices (Huffman, 1996; Tootelian and Gaedeke, 1993; West, 2003). The discount is stated as a percentage of the amount remaining after all other discounts have been deducted from the bill. A common discount is "2/10 EOM, net 30," which translates into a 2 percent discount if the invoice is paid within 10 days of the date of the invoice; otherwise, the net amount is due in 30 days.

Pharmacy managers should be aware of these discounts and take advantage of them, especially because they are not required to purchase excess inventory to do so. Many managers state that they do not take advantage of cash discounts because they do not have enough cash on hand to pay their invoices quickly. One thing that these managers could do is take out a short-term loan or line of credit to obtain the cash needed to take advantage of the discount. In most cases, the savings provided by the cash discount more than makes up for the interest expense on the borrowed money.

Electronic funds transfer (EFT) is now being used by pharmacies to take advantage of cash discounts and even prepay for purchases. An example of this is displayed in Table 22-1 (West, 2003). Prepayment requires the pharmacy to pay a week or month ahead of actual purchases based on its average weekly or monthly purchases over the last 3 to 6 months. In exchange for prepayments, vendors offer pharmacy managers additional cash discounts, allowing them to reduce their COGS further. Vendors offer Web-based systems that allow pharmacy managers to view their account information and invoices online in real time. This allows accounts payable to be monitored closely and invoices to be paid quickly online in real time. Additionally, these systems reduce procurement costs for the pharmacy by decreasing personnel time and bookkeeping expenses.

SERIAL DISCOUNTS Serial discounts occur when multiple discounts are applied at the same time. Serial discounts accumulate as shown in Table 22-3. In this example, the pharmacy manager is able to obtain the product at approximately $12 less than the original list price by taking advantage of both quantity and cash discounts.

Table 22-3. Example of Serial Discount

Invoice price	$100
10% Quantity discount	$100.00 × 0.1 = $10.00
	$100.00 − $10.00 = $90.00
2% Cash discount	$90.00 × 0.02 = $1.80
	$90.00 − $1.80 = $88.20

Dating

The other purchase term that needs to be considered is the dating of the invoice. *Dating* refers both to the time before the specified amount of discount may be taken and to the time at which payment becomes due (Huffman, 1996; West, 2003). There are three general types of dating: (1) *prepayment,* where the pharmacy pays for the merchandise before it is ordered and delivered, (2) *collect on delivery* (COD), where there is no time before a discount may be taken and payment becomes due, and (3) *delayed* or *future dating,* where the invoice is due sometime in the future (West, 2003). When no specific dating has been placed on the invoice, it is usually assumed that payment is due 10 days from the last day of the month in which the purchase was made. Two other terms related to the dating of invoices and statements for merchandise include *AOG,* meaning "arrival of goods," and *ROG,* meaning "receipt of goods." For example, "2/10 ROG, net 30" means deduct 2 percent within 10 days after receipt of goods or otherwise pay net within 30 days after receipt of goods.

Right Vendor

Being able to obtain the right product at the right time at the right place depends on the vendor. Pharmacy managers should be careful when selecting a vendor. Although a pharmacy can select a single vendor or multiple vendors, it is advised that pharmacies have a primary vendor and a secondary vendor. Establishing a positive relationship with a vendor can be helpful because it may lead to prompt delivery, special buying opportunities, special pricing information, and prompt resolution of problems. A secondary vendor is advised for times when product is not available from the primary vendor owing to drug product shortages and to obtain special pricing opportunities.

Among the many effective mechanisms used by vendors to market their products to pharmacies are salespersons, service representatives, and account representatives. These individuals try diligently to maintain good communications with their clients. Many wholesaler representatives, for example, visit or telephone major purchasers every 2 to 4 weeks. The salesperson or representative serves as an important source of market information; consequently, many pharmacy managers make it a practice to talk with salespersons and representatives who call on them. Additionally, talking with the representative keeps them aware of new programs and services offered by the vendor.

While favorable pricing and purchase terms are important considerations when selecting vendors, additional criteria should also be used (Tootelian and Gaedeke, 1993; West, 2003)(Table 22-4). Selecting a vendor with a good reputation is desirable. Accuracy and fill rates are also important considerations. Pharmacy managers should select vendors that provide quality products and services and have few out-of-stock situations. It is important to select vendors with prompt and reliable delivery. An inconsistent delivery service likely will result in the pharmacy not having the right products at the right times. Moreover, it is suggested that pharmacy managers evaluate their vendors periodically to ensure that they are receiving competitive prices and discounts. Many pharmacies seek bids from wholesalers periodically (e.g., every 3 years) to ensure competitive pricing and quality service.

Types of Vendors[†]

The most common type of vendor for pharmacies is the wholesaler. Wholesalers or distributors are often

---

[†] Parts of this section are excerpted with permission from West DS. Purchasing and inventory control. In Jackson R (ed), *Effective Pharmacy Management CD-ROM,* 9th ed. Alexandria, VA: National Community Pharmacists Association Foundation, 2003, Sec. 17.

Table 22-4. Criteria to Select Vendors

- Are they reliable and dependable? What is their order accuracy? Do they have a good reputation?
- Will they provide drug pedigree information and certify that the drug is not stolen, diverted, or counterfeit?
- Will they negotiate price and purchase terms with the pharmacy? Will they help to ensure contract compliance when ordering?
- What is their delivery schedule?
- Are they innovative?
- Do they provide financing and credit options?
- Do they have good customer relations? How often will a representative call on the pharmacy? Can I develop a positive business relationship with this supplier?
- Do they offer any value-added services? Will they help with advertising and promotion, provide inventory reports and analyses, or assist with pharmacy layout and design? Do they offer a private-label line of products?
- What technology do they offer to help with purchasing and inventory management?

known as *middlemen*. They search the marketplace and buy a wide assortment of products from thousands of different manufacturers and vendors. They then sell the products to pharmacies for use and resale. Most present-day wholesalers can be described with the term *full-service wholesalers* (Huffman, 1996; West, 2003).

The full-service wholesaler's most important function for the pharmacy manager is to serve as a buying agent. This means that the wholesaler anticipates the pharmacy's needs, goes into the market to obtain the necessary goods, and has them available at the appropriate time (West, 2003). This assembling of merchandise is a gigantic task involving thousands of different items that wholesalers store until the goods are wanted by a pharmacy. From a pharmacy manager's standpoint, it is much more efficient to do business with a full-service wholesaler that carries many products from many different vendors than to have to purchase products from each vendor separately. Most wholesalers offer just-in-time (JIT) delivery that allows for next-day delivery, thereby reducing the pharmacy's risk and improving the pharmacy's cash flow.

In addition to assembling various product lines, full-service wholesalers render other valuable programs and services that may be offered complementary or for a fee. The account representative may provide information on marketing and merchandising techniques, assist with pharmacy layout and design, and provide customized inventory management reports and information on the availability of new products.

Programs offered by wholesalers include offering private-label products, repackaging services, and back-order programs to improve inventory management for the pharmacy. A backorder program means that the pharmacy can order a product on backorder, and as soon as the wholesaler receives the product, the pharmacy's backorders get top-priority filling status and are shipped before the day's regular orders. Some wholesalers offer programs where products are delivered on consignment, meaning that the pharmacy does not have to pay until the product is sold. This reduces the amount of money the pharmacy has invested in inventory. Some wholesalers also offer pharmacy ownership programs and third-party assistance services. Ownership programs assist people with buying a pharmacy by providing special financing for the initial inventory, store layout design consulting, and other services. Third-party assistance services include third-party contracting, pharmacy benefit management audit assistance, and tools to help with other third-party reimbursement issues.

Some large pharmacy chains perform many of the wholesaler's service functions within their own organizations. These chains must assume wholesaler functions, such as purchasing, storing, financing, and delivering products to each of their units. While these chains serve as their own primary "vendor," they often still use full-line wholesalers as secondary vendors to obtain selected products or in special circumstances.

Pharmacies in practically every practice setting participate in some type of group purchasing organization (GPO) or central purchasing organization (Carroll, 1998; West, 2003). The purpose of a GPO is to pool the buying power of pharmacies together to obtain better prices and discounts from vendors. With profit margins being squeezed and drug budgets being scrutinized, pharmacies are looking for ways to decrease the cost of goods. A GPO negotiates with wholesalers and manufacturers for better pricing. One caveat to remember is that participating pharmacies must order products according to the terms of their GPO contract to receive special pricing and drug cost savings. If the pharmacists or technicians are not cognizant of the contract when they order, they may select the needed product at random from the list of potential sources. If the selection is not compliant with the contract, the pharmacy will not receive any negotiated prices.

Hospitals and hospital pharmacies are commonly members of GPOs, using the purchasing power of hundreds of hospitals to negotiate the best acquisition costs through competitive bidding. These hospital GPOs typically "bid out" almost every type of good used within the hospital, including equipment, supplies, and drugs. GPOs may also contract wholesaler services to select the wholesaler with the best combination of services, dependability, and costs. The GPO's central office organizes these bids and contracts through formal processes. Highly skilled representatives and professionals within these member hospitals represent the buying groups in the bidding and selection process. For example, GPOs commonly seek the advice of clinical pharmacists regarding comparative drug efficacy and future trends in drug therapy.

A *pharmacy buying group* is defined as a pharmacy organization whose purpose is to seek better drug prices for its members (e.g., community pharmacies, hospital pharmacies, and long-term care facilities) based on their collective buying power. Most, if not all, wholesalers are connected with one or more buying groups. The wholesaler will work with the pharmacy to find the best buying groups to join. Also, the pharmacist may identify a buying group with competitive pricing and then select a wholesaler that has a relationship with that buying group. Most buying groups charge a monthly or annual fee to members.

Another option used by pharmacies is to purchase directly from a pharmaceutical manufacturer. However, many manufacturers have substantial minimum purchase requirements, making it less favorable to buy from the manufacturer. Pharmacies may be receiving discounts based on volume purchased from the wholesaler; thereby giving an incentive to the pharmacy to buy most of its products from one wholesaler. Wholesalers also offer next-day delivery and other value-added services that help pharmacy managers minimize inventory costs. Thus most pharmacies do not purchase products from manufacturers very often.

Pharmacies, particularly those with formularies (e.g., hospital pharmacies), that purchase large volumes of select drug products may negotiate prices directly with manufacturers. Bids for these products are sought from manufacturers, and then a contracted price is agreed to between the pharmacy and the manufacturer. While the contract involves a pharmacy and a manufacturer, distribution of the product usually involves a wholesaler (Carroll, 1998). The pharmacy will order the product from the wholesaler and receive the price that has been negotiated with the manufacturer. The wholesaler then bills the manufacturer the difference between the list price and the negotiated price (often called a *chargeback*), and in return, the manufacturer credits the wholesaler's account.

▉ PURCHASING PROCESSES

Usually, a designated person (e.g., purchasing agent or pharmacy technician) will submit an order via telephone, fax, or computer and receive order confirmation. It may seem that the purchasing function ends when the order is made and the merchandise arrives at the pharmacy; however, this is not the case. The products need to be counted, checked for damage, and stocked on the shelves (West, 2003). When an order arrives, a pharmacy technician or other designated individual should physically count each item in the shipment and compare it with the invoice. Handheld devices that use barcoding technology are being used to facilitate this process. The designated person can scan the barcodes of all items in the tote to create a list of exactly what is in the tote. This list then can be compared to the invoice. The products should also be checked for any damage or short expiration dates. The vendor should be notified immediately if there is any discrepancy or any damaged products. On receipt, the products need to be moved to a temporary storage area or stocked on the shelves. Proper storage of inventory is vital. Improper storage can result in product that no longer can be sold, resulting in losses of inventory, sales, and profits. When new products are added to the shelves, the technician should rotate the stock, placing the newest stock behind the older stock bottles. This will ensure that the oldest stock is used first, hopefully before it becomes outdated. As discussed later in this chapter, within most community and hospital pharmacy software systems, options are available for the software to count incoming and outgoing products and automatically order product to replenish stock based on models such as the economic order quantity. However, it is important to remember that these systems only work as good as the inputting of information, including the reduction of inventory through all channels including theft and obsolescence.

INVENTORY MANAGEMENT

Inventory refers to the stock of products held to meet future demand. Pharmacies hold inventory to guard against fluctuations in demand, to take advantage of bulk discounts, and to withstand fluctuations in supply (e.g., late deliveries) (West, 2003). There are four costs associated with having inventory: acquisition costs, procurement costs, carrying costs, and stock-out costs (Carroll, 1998; Huffman, 1996; Silbiger, 1999; Tootelian and Gaedeke, 1993; West, 2003).

The *acquisition cost* is the price the pharmacy pays for the product. *Procurement costs* are the costs associated with purchasing the product: checking inventory, placing orders, receiving orders, stocking the product, and paying the invoices. *Carrying costs* refer to the storage, handling, insurance, cost of capital to fi-

nance the inventory, and opportunity costs. Another carrying cost is the cost of loss through theft, deterioration, and damage. Procurement and carrying costs must be balanced. For example, increasing the average order size and decreasing the number of orders placed decrease procurement costs but increase carrying costs. The fourth cost is the *stock-out cost,* which is the cost of not having a product on the shelf when a patient needs or wants it. This is frustrating to the pharmacist who has to explain why the product is not available and is an inconvenience to the patient and prescriber (Carroll, 1998).

Inventory management is the practice of planning, organizing, and controlling inventory so that it contributes to the profitability of the business (Huffman 1996; West, 2003). The goals of inventory management are to minimize the amount invested in inventory and the procurement and carrying costs while balancing supply and demand (Huffman, 1996; Tootelian and Gaedeke, 1993; West, 2003). Inventory management is a key factor to success in a pharmacy because efficient inventory management can keep costs down, improve cash flow, and improve service. Alternatively, inventory mismanagement results in increased operating and opportunity costs.

Evaluating Inventory Management

The most common ratio used to determine how well a pharmacy is managing its inventory is the *inventory turnover rate* (ITOR). It can be calculated for the entire pharmacy, for departments (e.g., prescriptions or OTC products), and even for individual products. The ITOR is expressed as a ratio and is calculated by using the following formula (Tootelian and Gaedeke, 1993; West, 2003, 2006):

ITOR = cost of goods sold ÷ average inventory
value (at cost)

ITOR = cost of goods sold ÷ [(beginning inventory
value + ending inventory value) ÷ 2]

The cost of goods sold (COGS) can be found on the pharmacy's income (profit-and-loss) statement for a given period of time. The average inventory value can be found by obtaining the pharmacy's balance sheets for both the beginning and the end of the period represented on the income statement. The balance sheets should contain the value of the pharmacy's inventory at each point in time. The ITOR indicates the efficiency with which inventory is used. It measures how quickly inventory is purchased, sold, and replaced. Two advantages of increasing the ITOR are that reducing the investment in inventory frees capital for other business activities and increases the return on investment in inventory.

Table 22-5 provides an example of how to calculate ITOR. In this example, the pharmacy's overall annual ITOR is 10. This means that this pharmacy, on average, sells all the inventory that is typically kept in the pharmacy a total of 10 times over the course of a year. This is similar to the national average for independent pharmacies (West, 2006), indicating that the pharmacy manager probably is managing inventory efficiently. Comparing the current year's ratio with last year's ratio also indicates that the manager is improving her efficiency in managing inventory because the ITOR has increased over time. Note that if the COGS remained constant for the year and the average inventory increased, the ITOR would have decreased. This would have indicated that inventory was sitting on the shelf and not selling. The pharmacy manager

then would want to determine if she was ordering too much product or the wrong products.

Overall, pharmacy managers need to make sure that the ITOR is not too high. This may indicate that out-of-stocks may be occurring too frequently. Alternatively, if the ITOR is too low, then the pharmacy may be carrying too much inventory that is not salable or not being used. Hence cash is being spent to purchase the product, but cash is not flowing in from the sale of the product. Deciding what is too high or too low is pharmacy-dependent. The pharmacy manager should consider national or regional benchmarks as well as the pharmacy's trends when interpreting the ITOR. The ITOR is one indicator that should be considered when managing inventory, but it must be interpreted given the context of the pharmacy. For example, an ITOR of 30 may be acceptable if the pharmacy can order and receive items quickly from the vendor and there have not been complaints of shortages. It may be more helpful for the pharmacy manager to look at the ITOR within product lines or departments to facilitate decision making.

As gross margins have continued to shrink in retail pharmacies and drug budgets have gotten tighter in hospital pharmacies, pharmacy managers have been forced to become more efficient in their operations. One way to increase efficiency is to manage inventory properly. Trends have shown that pharmacy managers in various practice settings are making efforts to manage their inventories more efficiently. For example, independent pharmacy owners have increased their overall ITOR from 6.3 in 1995 to 10.4 in 2005 (West, 2006). Moreover, prescription inventory usually turns faster than the overall turnover of merchandise. The ITOR in 2005 for independent pharmacies was 10.4 for all merchandise and 11.8 for prescription inventory (West, 2006). Hospital pharmacies should be striving for an ITOR of at least 14 (Alverson, 2003). JIT deliveries and computerized inventory systems have facilitated this increased efficiency in inventory management, especially prescription inventory.

Another indicator of a pharmacy manager's ability to manage the investment in inventory efficiently is the net-profit-to-average-inventory ratio. This ratio

---

Table 22-5. ITOR Example

ITOR for Smith Pharmacy for FY 2005 = 8.2

ITOR for Smith Pharmacy for FY 2006 = 9.5

Data for Smith Pharmacy for FY 2007

Sales: $2,000,000	Cost of goods sold: $1,500,000
Gross margin: $500,000	Total expenses: $450,000
Net profit: $50,000	Average inventory: $150,000

ITOR = cost of goods sold/average inventory

ITOR = $1,500,000/$150,000

ITOR = 10

indicates whether the inventory is being used efficiently to make a profit. Pharmacy managers desire to have a ratio greater than 20 percent.

Factors to Consider in Inventory Management

Pharmacy managers must consider multiple factors when evaluating their inventory:

- *Selection of generic products.* Generic drug products usually have a lower acquisition cost, and therefore, by stocking generic products, the amount of money invested in inventory is reduced (Carroll, 1998). For example, a pharmacist may decide not to stock brand-name Lasix because generic furosemide is less expensive, thereby reducing the amount of money invested in inventory.
- *Reduction of inventory size.* A pharmacist may decide to have a small front end in his or her store to reduce the amount invested in inventory. He or she may carry only basic product lines (i.e., a smaller numbers of brands and items) as opposed to full product lines (i.e., every brand and every item).
- *Returned-goods policies.* One critical component is the evaluation of returned-goods policies. Many manufacturers and wholesalers have established policies regarding merchandise that may be returned. In exchange for returning unsalable goods, these vendors may provide credit on future purchases, replacement goods, or even cash back to the pharmacy. An example of wholesaler returned-goods policies is provided in Table 22-1. Pharmacy managers should monitor products closely that qualify for the various returned-goods policies, making certain that such returns are made on a regular, periodic basis before time limitations take effect. It is advised to have a staff member responsible for checking the shelves periodically for out-of-date items or items that are not selling. Because the management of return goods is critical, some pharmacies use returned-goods service companies to assist them with managing their returned goods. These companies will evaluate the pharmacy's inventory, return the appropriate products, and often return money from the returned products within 30 to 60 days. These companies

charge a fee based on the amount of returns. One major advantage to these companies is that they are aware of each manufacturer's and wholesaler's specific policies and can quickly identify product to be returned.

- *Management of unclaimed prescriptions.* Approximately 1.5 percent of all prescriptions received and/or filled in community pharmacies remain unclaimed (McCaffrey et al., 1998). A pharmacist must be aware of the amount of inventory that has been used to fill these unclaimed prescriptions. It is important for pharmacists to monitor these unclaimed prescriptions and after a specified period (e.g., 14 days) return the stock to the shelf.
- *Monitoring shrinkage.* Inventory shrinkage includes losses owing to shoplifting, employee theft, and robbery. It is estimated that 0.7 to 4.5 percent of sales are lost to shrinkage (Garner, 1994). The largest source of shrinkage for most retailers is employee theft. It is important to recruit honest personnel and monitor their activities, especially those working in the prescription area of a pharmacy, because theft of controlled substances in pharmacies is increasingly problematic. Equally important; however, is for the pharmacy staff to be observant, say hello to customers, keep displays neat, install security mirrors and cameras, and remove high fixtures to minimize shoplifting. Some pharmacies use technologies such as inventory-control bars to prevent loss of product from theft.
- *Use of formularies.* As stated previously, institutional pharmacies commonly use formularies to facilitate inventory management (Pearce and Begg, 1992). A formulary allows the pharmacy manager to carry one therapeutic equivalent within a class of drugs instead of each drug product within the class. This allows pharmacy managers to lower their overall investment in inventory.

Methods of Inventory Management

Three methods are used commonly in pharmacy to manage inventory: the visual method, the periodic method, and the perpetual method (Carroll, 1998;

Tootelian and Gaedeke, 1993; West, 2003). The *visual method* requires the pharmacist or designated person to look at the number of units in inventory and compare them with a listing of how many should be carried. When the number falls below the desired amount, an order is placed. The *periodic method* requires the pharmacist or designated person to count the stock on hand at predetermined intervals and compare it with minimum desired levels. If the quantity is below the minimum, the product is ordered.

Usually, a designated person is responsible for checking the shelves and placing orders. The pharmacy manager may have a specific checklist, indicating that the person should conduct a stock review weekly or look for expired products monthly, in addition to placing orders and keeping inventory orders to a specific level. This purchasing person will learn the turnover rates for specific products and will develop a skill for purchasing for the pharmacy. This method allows the purchasing person to account for fluctuations in supply and demand. Today, the purchasing person is likely to use a hand-held electronic device into which item numbers and quantities are entered or a hand-held scanning device that scans the barcodes on the product packaging or shelf labels (Carroll, 1998; West, 2003). These devices then can be used to submit an order electronically.

Although the visual and periodic methods are still used today, *perpetual inventory systems* are common in all pharmacy settings. These perpetual systems are computerized inventory management systems. Perpetual inventory management systems are the most efficient method to manage inventory. This method allows the inventory to be monitored at all times. The entire inventory may be entered into the computer, and with the filling of each prescription, the appropriate inventory can be reduced automatically. A perpetual system can tell precisely the amount of inventory on hand for any product at any time. Moreover, the pharmacy manager can quickly assess the value of current inventory.

Computer systems can be used to calculate the EOQ and reorder point so that a product is reordered automatically when the inventory falls below a mini-

mum standard (West, 2003). This type of system reduces procurement costs significantly. Although the computer can be programmed to order products automatically, it is important for pharmacy staff to monitor inventory daily and to make corrections for variances owing to fluctuations in supply and demand.

To maintain a perpetual inventory system, all purchases and sales must be entered into the computer system (Carroll, 1998; West, 2003). A clerk can enter data from purchases, or the computer dispensing system can be interfaced with the computer order system. The interface allows for the inventory to be reduced when a product is dispensed. The sales data can also be entered at the point of sale by devices that use optical scanning and barcode technology. Point-of-sale (POS) devices are advantageous in that they improve the accuracy of pricing and inventory data. They eliminate the need for price stickers, reduce the frequency of pricing errors, and automatically track inventory.

Regardless of which method is used, most pharmacies also conduct a physical inventory at least annually. This encompasses counting or scanning every item in the pharmacy. Pharmacy staff then can compare the product on-hand quantities in the computer or the value of inventory on the financial statements with what is actually on the shelves. It is important to conduct a physical inventory to verify periodically the accuracy of the pharmacy's financial records. Additionally, pharmacy managers should follow state board of pharmacy regulations with respect to inventory counts and control with respect to controlled substances, especially narcotics.

Role of Technology

Based on the preceding description of the purchasing process and perpetual inventory systems, one can recognize the value of technology in inventory management. Thus computerized inventory management systems are common today in pharmacies in all practice settings. Technology enables pharmacists to manage inventory faster and more accurately.

These computer systems can integrate the management of inventory, information, and costs. The ability to integrate inventory and cost data allows for the generation of a wide array of reports and analyses. Pharmacists use these management reports to identify high- and low-turnover items and determine stock levels for better allocation of shelf space. Examples of inventory management reports include

- *Purchase-trend report*—describes the quantity purchased of OTC products or prescription drug products by month or by quarter.
- *Sales-analysis report*—features a rolling 12-month statement that includes order quantity, shipped quantity, unavailable quantity, returns, credits, and dollars spent.
- *Item-movement report*—lists which items are selling the best.

Many wholesalers will provide the hardware and software for the inventory management system. The most current trend is Web-based systems. These allow pharmacy managers to view in real time the quantity on hand at the wholesaler, the list price, the manufacturer backorder status, and the online catalog. These Web-based systems also enable pharmacy staff to check purchase orders, invoices, and account information in real time. Another advantage is that the pharmacy staff can place orders and view account information from other locations besides the pharmacy.

Pharmacy staff can also order inventory via the Internet, which is termed *e-procurement*. e-Procurement allows the pharmacy to receive immediate item allocation and order confirmation. These sophisticated systems drastically cut down on the time and effort spent on procurement. Prices can be updated daily or weekly by using electronic invoice transmission, and returns and credits can be completed electronically. Invoices are then paid by electronic funds transfer (EFT).

It is important to note that Class II (C-II) controlled substances now can be ordered electronically. Pharmacies must first enroll with the U.S. Drug Enforcement Agency (DEA) to acquire a digital certificate. The C-II orders are created using a computerized inventory system, electronically signed using a password-protected digital certificate, and then submitted electronically to the wholesaler.

Clearly, technology is being used to facilitate ordering, receiving, managing, and paying for products. As newer technologies are available, pharmacies will adopt these to improve their inventory management efficiencies. Currently, there is much focus on the use of radiofrequency identification (RFID) microchips to improve product distribution from manufacturer to wholesaler to pharmacy (FDA, 2007). At the factory, an RFID microchip, or "tag," will be attached to a product. The tag will contain data on where the product was manufactured, when it arrived at the warehouse, and when it was stocked on the shelf. The tag will also allow the retailer to track the item through manufacturing and distribution. For example, when a product arrives at the store, sensors can update the store inventory. The sensor can also detect the product leaving the shelf and automatically reorder the product from the manufacturer. RFID tags are different from barcodes in that they have larger memory capacity, allow for data to be added and changed, and do not have to be physically swiped on a scanner to access the stored information. Data can be sent through the air and can penetrate clothing. Hence RFID tags provide a chain of custody for the pharmacy and may help to protect against theft. As manufacturers and wholesalers adopt the use of this technology, pharmacists also will be evaluating the value of the technology for the pharmacy.

DRUG DISTRIBUTION SAFETY

This chapter has focused mainly on purchasing and inventory management from the pharmacy's business perspective—having the right products available to sell while reducing the investment in inventory. Yet the distribution of pharmaceuticals from the manufacturer to the pharmacy is being closely scrutinized to ensure medication safety. Thus pharmacy staff also must focus on the supply-chain integrity. It is estimated that worldwide drug counterfeiting is a $32 billion business, and 1 to 2 percent of drugs in North America are fraudulent (National Association of Boards of Pharmacy, 2007). It is even possible that drugs dispensed by reputable pharmacies could be counterfeit (National Association of Boards of Pharmacy, 2007).

Pharmacy staff must be aware of the potential for purchasing and dispensing counterfeit products. To ensure that drug products are authentic, pharmacists should choose a reputable vendor with a reliable delivery system. There are large national and regional wholesalers that are considered "authorized distributors" that buy directly from manufacturers. There are thousands of secondary wholesalers that purchase products from other wholesalers or repackagers that may or may not be legitimate. If a lesser-known vendor calls with a special deal on a product that appears to be too good to be true, that probably is the case. When a package arrives, the staff person should look for problems such as old or worn packaging, a faded label around the expiration date, missing overt packaging marks, or product or packaging appearance that is different from normal. Pharmacists who suspect that they have purchased counterfeit drugs should contact the Food and Drug Administration (FDA) Medwatch program, the manufacturer of the drug product, their state board of pharmacy, and their local law enforcement authorities.

To guarantee the integrity of drug distribution in the United States, the FDA is requiring drug distributors to provide documentation of the chain of custody for drug products, especially for products at higher risk of being counterfeit (e.g., Lipitor, Celebrex, Nexium, Crestor, Viagra, and other common, expensive brand-name drug products). The FDA Counterfeit Drug Task Force recommends the use of electronic track and trace technology to provide an accurate drug pedigree, which is a chain of custody for the product as it moves through the supply chain from manufacturer to pharmacy (FDA, 2007). RFID tags would create an electronic pedigree for each drug bottle. This would make it more difficult for counterfeit products to enter the distribution system. Additionally, this pedigree would allow for more efficient and targeted drug recalls. Pharmacies could quickly and accurately withdraw recalled products from their shelves.

■ REVISITING THE SCENARIO

Referring back to Marie's predicament, it is easy to see that a number of factors may be influencing her pharmacy's purchasing and inventory control mechanisms. It is apparent that Marie has minimized her investment in inventory to an extent that it may be hurting sales. The pharmacy appears to be having frequent out-of-stock situations, resulting in decreased sales, loss of goodwill, loss of patrons, and possibly harm to patients. Regardless of which wholesaler is selected, Marie should evaluate her purchasing policies and decisions. She should talk with her wholesaler representative and evaluate the inventory management reports to determine which products have a high turnover rate and which products have a low turnover rate. Knowing this should facilitate ordering decisions.

Meanwhile, it appears that Marie is becoming dissatisfied with her current wholesaler. Seeking bids from wholesalers or evaluating other wholesalers periodically is suggested to ensure competitive pricing and quality service. If a new wholesaler is selected, Marie should develop a relationship with the customer representative and examine the services and programs offered by the wholesaler. Marie may also want to select a secondary wholesaler.

Buying goods at the lowest price is another concern. It is difficult to compare prices because price often depends on (1) purchasing volume, (2) rebates and discounts earned, and (3) membership in a GPO. Additionally, certain pharmacies, such as disproportionate share (DPS) hospital pharmacies, qualify for other pricing considerations. (*Note:* DPS hospitals qualify for special pricing because they provide a significant amount of care to low-income patients.) Regardless of which wholesaler Marie selects, she should work with her purchasing and accounting personnel to ensure that appropriate discounts are earned. Taking advantage of discounts is one way to reduce costs and improve cash flow for the pharmacy. Marie should also consider participating in a GPO. One of the most significant factors that affect pharmaceutical costs, other than discounts and rebates, is participation in a GPO or a buying group.

These are just a few of the parameters that Marie should consider. There are other purchasing and inventory management activities that Marie could evaluate. For example, she may want to contract with a return-goods company to assist with the return of goods. Another example would be to purchase and dispense more generic drugs because these products reduce the amount of money invested in inventory. Developing a formulary for the community mental health center may be another possibility. Overall, Marie constantly must be aware of the purchasing and inventory management activities. These activities can have a significant impact on both the financial and operational health of the pharmacy.

■ QUESTIONS FOR FURTHER DISCUSSION

1. What can a pharmacist do to reduce the amount of money invested in inventory in a community pharmacy? In a hospital pharmacy?
2. Describe how you think technology in the future will facilitate purchasing and inventory management in a pharmacy.
3. Discuss the various factors that affect the cost of goods in a pharmacy.
4. What are the current trends in the pharmacy wholesale industry?

■ ACKNOWLEDGMENT

I would like to acknowledge the National Community Pharmacists Association for releasing copyright on West DS. Purchasing and inventory control. In Jackson R (ed), *Effective Pharmacy Management CD-ROM,* 9th ed. Alexandria, VA: National Community Pharmacists Association Foundation, 2003, Sec. 17.

REFERENCES

Alverson C. 2003. Beyond purchasing-managing hospital inventory. *Manag Healthcare Exec,* November 1; available at www.managedhealthcareexecutive.com/mhe/content/printContentPopup.jsp?id=75802&searchString=purchasing; accessed on March 20, 2007.

Carroll NV. 1998. *Financial Management for Pharmacists,* 2d ed. Baltimore: Williams & Wilkins.

Food and Drug Administration (FDA). 2007. FDA Counterfeit Drug Task Force Report: 2006 Update; available at www.fda.gov/oc/initiatives/counterfeit/report6_06.html; accessed on March 20, 2007.

Garner DD. 1994. Pharmacy security. In *Effective Pharmacy Management,* 7th ed., p. 415. Alexandria, VA: National Association of Retail Druggists.

Huffman DC. 1996. Purchasing and inventory control. In *Effective Pharmacy Management,* 8th ed., p. 355. Alexandria, VA: National Association of Retail Druggists.

McCaffrey DJ, Smith MC, Banahan BF, et al. 1998. A continued look into the financial implications of initial noncompliance in community pharmacies: An unclaimed prescription audit pilot. *J Res Pharm Econ* 9:33.

National Association of Boards of Pharmacy. 2007. Drug Counterfeiting Fact Sheet; available at www.dangerouspill.com/identifying_reporting/fact_sheet.html; accessed on March 20, 2007.

Pearce MJ, Begg EJ. 1992. A review of limited lists and formularies: Are they cost-effective? *Pharmacoeconomics* 1:191.

Silbiger S. 1999. *The Ten-Day MBA,* rev. ed. New York: Quill William Morrow.

Tootelian DH, Gaedeke RM. 1993. *Essentials of Pharmacy Management.* St. Louis: Mosby.

West DS. 2001. *Managing Efficiencies in Pharmacy Cash Flow,* Vol. 6. Birmingham, AL: Mylan Institute of Pharmacy, Continuing Education Series.

West DS (ed). 2006. *2006 NCPA-Pfizer Digest.* Alexandria, VA: National Community Pharmacists Association.

West DS. 2005. Purchasing and inventory control. In Jackson R (ed), *Effective Pharmacy Management CD-ROM,* 9th ed., Sec. 17. Alexandria, VA: National Community Pharmacists Association Foundation.

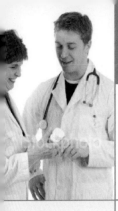

23

MERCHANDISING

Edward Cohen

About the Author: Dr. Cohen received a B.S. in pharmacy from the University of Illinois at Chicago (UIC) and a Pharm.D. from Midwestern University Chicago College of Pharmacy (MWU). After owning an independent pharmacy for many years, he moved into the corporate sector as Director of Pharmacy for Dominick's Finer Foods (a division of Safeway), and today, he serves as a Director in Clinical Services at Walgreen's Health Services. Dr. Cohen has been recognized nationally for his role in bringing pharmaceutical care to the forefront of community pharmacy practice. He holds adjunct faculty positions at UIC and MWU, as well as serving on both colleges' advisory committees. Dr. Cohen has served as Chair of the Administration Section of the American Pharmacists Association–Academy of Pharmacy Practice and Management and on the Board of Directors of the Illinois Pharmacists Association.

▥ LEARNING OBJECTIVES

After completing this chapter, students should be able to

1. Describe the evolution of merchandising in pharmacy from the beginning of the twentieth century to current practices used today.
2. Identify merchandising techniques that enhance the awareness and use of the pharmacy department as a health care destination for patients.
3. Explain how pharmacy layout and merchandising techniques affect consumers' senses.
4. Identify and discuss the implications of ineffective merchandising in a pharmacy.
5. Evaluate the impact of merchandising on the financial success of a pharmacy.

▥ SCENARIO

Mary Quint, a third-year doctor of pharmacy student, was home recently to attend a family gathering. There was much ado about Mary's progress in pharmacy school. Her family was asking numerous questions about school, her classes, her job, and her future. As the conversation continued, Mary found the family involved in a discussion about the different pharmacies in town. The family had a full range of opinions that addressed everything from the location of the store, to the pharmacist, to the store hours.

Mary was impressed with the conversation. She had never thought much about the issues being discussed by her family. It seemed that her pharmacy, Middletown South Pharmacy, is the least liked by her family. They said that the staff generally is unfriendly and unhelpful and that the store is dark and messy. The store always has a "talk radio" program playing on the speakers throughout the pharmacy. Her family complained that items never seem to be arranged in a logical order, making it just about impossible to find the products they were looking for. Customers always have to ask for assistance in finding items, and the employees working in the pharmacy always seem too busy to help.

Her family's favorite pharmacy in town is the new chain pharmacy (Healthway Pharmacy). Healthway Pharmacy is bright and open, making it easy to find items. The staff is friendly and is always doing something to make the store look nice. As people shop, they often find and buy items that they need and that they had not even planned on purchasing that day. Healthway Pharmacy has many new products, making it enjoyable to shop in the store. The pharmacy department is large and open with a comfortable waiting area and a private booth to talk with the pharmacist. The store is easy to access from the major streets in the area and has a large parking area. The store also has a drive-through window by the pharmacy, an in-store medical clinic, and an electronic kiosk to order prescriptions without having to be at the prescription counter and is open 24 hours a day, 7 days a week. Everyone encouraged Mary to visit Healthway Pharmacy and inquire about getting a job there.

CHAPTER QUESTIONS

1. What are the most prominent merchandising features that drive customers to shop in a particular pharmacy?
2. How does merchandising affect consumer senses?
3. What is the impact of merchandising on the overall operation and profitability of a pharmacy?
4. What are the goals of effective merchandising methods for a pharmacy?
5. Which factors should be considered in the design of the exterior of a pharmacy? In the design and layout of the interior?

INTRODUCTION

The scenario demonstrates the effects of some "invisible" principles of merchandising. The lack of effective merchandising in one pharmacy was enough to send Mary's family to another pharmacy to do business. Many of the physical features of community pharmacies frequently are taken for granted. The exterior design is important to create an identity with customers. The colors and shapes of the outdoor signage add to the pharmacy's identity. Pharmacy managers can plan the ease of entry into the store and everything seen and felt by consumers inside the pharmacy. Merchandising activities used by pharmacy managers can attract customers and make their shopping experience more enjoyable.

Almost every retail store (including community pharmacies) is designed for selling merchandise (Hilditch, 1981). Given the decline in profit margins in the prescription department, the success of a pharmacy's "front end" is crucial to the total financial success of the business.

Drug stores traditionally have been retail establishments where customers can find staple items, basic health care needs, and a pharmacy. Larger chain pharmacies have expanded this definition by promoting and selling large varieties of merchandise that often are well beyond the basic mixture of products found in a traditional drug store (Francke, 1974). Today, pharmacies are also found in hospitals, clinics, grocery stores, and even large discount stores. The location of the pharmacy within these often very large buildings, as well as the mix, location, and condition of the goods and services the pharmacy offers, is important to the pharmacy's success.

Attracting customers into a pharmacy and inviting them to make purchases while they are there are the main objectives of all merchandising efforts. Pharmacies must consider their design, layout, and merchandise to draw shoppers who will then make purchases. It is important to keep in mind that most of the items sold in a pharmacy can also be purchased in other retail outlets or on the Internet. The proper mix of convenience, price, and service will add to the appeal of the pharmacy.

Pharmacies are working to establish their business as customers' total health care destination. Many pharmacies are expanding their offering of professional activities the pharmacist can perform, increasing the offerings of healthier foods, carrying more professional products (e.g., durable medical equipment, blood glucose and other diabetes specialty items, and expanded vitamin and herbal offerings), and adding in-store medical clinics for treatment of minor ailments.

Customers respond to what they see, hear, and feel. Designing a pharmacy to address the everyday needs of our on-the-go society will make the store successful. Merchandising tools are used in every aspect of the pharmacy business, drawing customers to the location, making it easy and comfortable to shop in the stores, and building customer loyalty.

PHARMACY MERCHANDISING TRENDS THROUGH THE 1900s

Early in the last century, people came to drug stores for relief from their ailments. Pharmacists had a handful of drugs, sold mostly in compounded mixtures, and did what they could to ease their patients' discomfort. Drug stores were not merchandised as they are today. Drug stores contained low-cost traditional items that people used every day. Some of the traditional items found in drug stores were cosmetics, magazines, tobacco, stationery, and candy. The prescription business was a small portion of the total sales of the store. Each pharmacy owner built his or her reputation on individual achievements with his or her customers.

With Prohibition during the 1920s, the drug store fountain replaced the tavern as the new socially acceptable gathering place. Pharmacists and their clerks were busy making milkshakes and other soda fountain creations. During Prohibition, pharmacies became the only legitimate place to purchase alcohol products because they were only available with a doctor's prescription. When Prohibition was lifted in the 1930s, many pharmacies continued to sell liquor, having developed a reputation as legitimate outlets (Higby, 1997).

After World War II, many new medications came to the market. Pharmacies began filling more prescriptions using prefabricated convenient dosage forms and thus spent less time compounding medications. Pharmacists began to spend most of their time dispensing prefabricated prescription drug products, making sure the patient received the medication in an efficient manner, with the focus on providing product not information. The front end of the store took on a new look and feel as well. Pharmacies began to stock many perfabricated staple items. As a result of filling an increasing number of prescriptions, pharmacists had less time to manage the front ends of their pharmacies. Prescriptions were becoming another commodity in the store, much to the dismay of pharmacists. Pharmacists were looking to transition their practices to have patient safety as their primary concern. By the late 1960s, the profession had taken a firm stand to change and regain the professional stature of the pharmacy (Higby, 1997).

PHARMACY DESIGN, LAYOUT, AND MERCHANDISING

Most consumer purchases in pharmacies are not planned very far in advance. Pharmacy managers use pharmacy design, layout of fixtures, and merchandising of products to affect the purchasing behaviors of their customers. Studies have shown that more than 80 percent of all purchases are made by people who less than a week before their purchases were not planning to buy these particular items (Eisenpreis, 1983). The primary reasons why consumers make unplanned purchases are emergencies (running out of a needed item), latent buying interests brought on by a good price or a new product, and impulse purchases (buying on a whim to try something new or different).

An important contribution to sales success is the store design and layout of merchandise. Getting people into a pharmacy, making it easy to find and purchase both needed and wanted items, and increasing the number of return visits consumers will make to a pharmacy all can be influenced by design and layout factors. The design and layout of a pharmacy must allow for customer convenience, ease of shopping, and an exciting atmosphere that will promote the selling of both goods and services.

Pharmacy Design

Today's consumers demand convenience, service, and ambience. While pharmacies have not always been known for these attributes, consumers have come to expect a certain atmosphere and comfort level from any retail establishment.

From the 1940s to the 1960s, pharmacy store design and decor did not highlight merchandise or professional activities. Most pharmacies carried a mix of staple items, tobacco, and liquor; had soda fountains; and gave little thought to where the best place might be to locate these items in the store. During the 1970s and 1980s, pharmacy designs transitioned to highlight the products to be sold, resulting in simpler decor and allowing the merchandise to become part of the pharmacy's design.

It is important to select the most appropriate design aspects for a pharmacy without becoming too trendy or rapidly outdated. The target of today's pharmacy designs is the shopper. To determine a pharmacy design, managers first must determine the characteristics and needs of the customers to be served. Customers want pharmacies that are convenient, well organized, and in supply of the goods and services they desire when they need them. Pharmacies that frustrate, disappoint, or waste consumer time searching for items will not be patronized.

Studies indicate that women make most pharmacy purchase decisions (Raven, 1984). Other findings regarding consumer behavior in pharmacies include

- Customers spend more money per trip when they have less time to shop.
- The average time spent in a pharmacy is 13.6 minutes per trip.

- Only 42 percent of all pharmacy purchases are planned by consumers before their arrival at the store. More than half of pharmacy purchase decisions are made after the consumer has entered the store.
- Pharmacies that are perceived as being "fun to shop" and "well merchandised" experience up to 15 to 20 percent higher average purchases than pharmacies that are not rated highly for these attributes (Raven, 1984).

The size of a pharmacy or pharmacy department commonly is determined by industry averages or by evaluating the sales per square foot of various pharmacy departments. Store managers can obtain industry information on the ideal size for their pharmacies from wholesalers and other vendors, as well as from their professional associations (e.g., National Community Pharmacists Association or National Association of Chain Drug Stores).

Managers can calculate the ideal size of a department (an area within a pharmacy that contains related goods or services) by estimating the total dollar amount of sales from that department and dividing by their expected sales per square foot. While this method is simple to use, it should be applied with care and common sense. Estimates of sales are not always accurate indicators of the need for space for particular types of goods and services. The characteristics of space inside the store (e.g., walls, lighting, and fixtures) and the physical characteristics of the goods and services to be sold in a department both should be considered when allocating space within a pharmacy (Rodowskas, 1996).

Another key point when designing a pharmacy is to make sure that prescription dispensing and counseling sections are in step with the profession. With pharmacists providing an array of patient counseling and pharmaceutical care services, additional space for pharmacists to talk privately with patients may be needed. Setting aside and designing an appropriate consultation area and a patient waiting area are important. Many pharmacies also sell items that do not require a prescription, but they often sell better if a pharmacist is available to explain their use to patients (e.g., durable medical equipment, blood glucose monitors, or natural products). These departments often are placed near the prescription department for the convenience of both the patient and the pharmacist.

The Americans with Disabilities Act (ADA) of 1990 has affected almost all businesses, including pharmacies. This federal mandate prohibits discrimination based on any form of disability. To comply with the ADA, pharmacies may be required to adjust counter heights, aisle widths, telephone equipment, doorways, and almost any other physical aspect of their operations. The act allows for reasonableness in designing stores without undue hardship on daily operations. The design goal is to have a store that offers equal access to all products and services for all customers (Laskoski, 1992).

The Heath Insurance Portability and Accountability Act (HIPPA) is a federal mandate designed to protect the confidentiality of patient information. HIPPA considerations in the design and layout of a pharmacy are to ensure that disclosure of protected health information is minimized. Pharmacy managers are to make reasonable efforts to protect the privacy of their patients. Some of the efforts made by pharmacy managers include installation of a partition extending the height of the pharmacy counter, redesigned storage areas for prescriptions that are waiting to be picked up by customers, designated staging areas for patients waiting to be served by pharmacy staff, and private patient consultation areas.

Internal and external environmental factors play a major role in the design and layout of a pharmacy. The age, race, sex, and income levels of consumers are important characteristics that should be addressed. Addressing the needs of a predominant ethnic or age group is beneficial in attracting these potential patrons to a pharmacy. For example, elderly people may be more likely to patronize a pharmacy that has a large section of durable medical equipment.

Designing the exterior of a pharmacy is just as important as design and layout of the interior. When designing the exterior of a pharmacy, one must consider legal requirements, local codes or ordinances that govern materials, the number and sizes of windows,

external signage, and the number and placement of doorways.

The exterior design of a pharmacy may need to complement other stores in a shopping center. Many shopping centers place restrictions on the exterior designs of their stores. Pharmacies commonly will try to add defining features (e.g., signage and lighting) that allow their stores to be recognized easily.

The placement of entrances and exits to the shopping center is key to the ease of getting to the pharmacy. The traffic patterns and placement of traffic signals on the roads adjacent to the shopping center affect the convenience of shopping in the pharmacy. Pharmacy managers often negotiate with local officials to have traffic signals at or near the entrance and exit of the center.

The traffic pattern of a shopping center will influence the placement of entrances and exits of the pharmacy. Pharmacy managers wish to maximize the number of patrons that find their store once they are in the shopping center. Pharmacies often desire to be located next to a grocery store or other high-traffic stores to attract cross-shoppers.

Pharmacy Layout

A pharmacy's layout contains numerous cues, messages, and suggestions that communicate to shoppers. A pharmacy manager's goal is to create a mood that welcomes customer traffic, increases time spent browsing (yet not wasting time searching for needed items), encourages customers to make more purchases than originally planned, and invites them to return to the pharmacy in the future.

The layout or arrangement of in-store fixtures should be designed to move patrons around the pharmacy to obtain the items they need or desire. Ideally, customers should visit as many areas of the pharmacy as possible to increase the probability of impulse purchases.

Pharmacy layout should capitalize on the strengths of the prescription department and pharmacist because they are what make pharmacies unique from other retail outlets. Pharmacy layout should have the prescription department very prominent and visible to

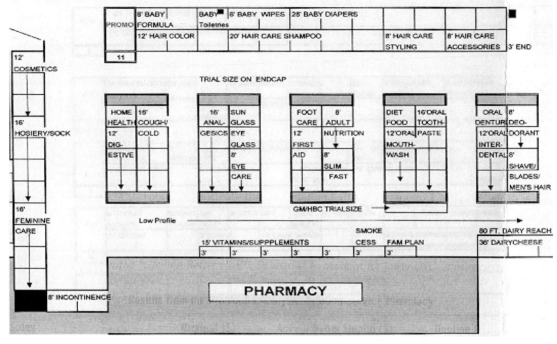

Figure 23-1. Store aisle design.

patrons in any part of the store (Fig. 23-1). Ideally, consumers should travel past a variety of merchandise on their way to the prescription department. This explains why many prescription departments are located in the rear of a pharmacy. While this layout is popular with pharmacy managers, it is not always popular with consumers. For example, some elderly patrons may find it difficult to walk through the entire store to get to the prescription counter. They may choose to use the drive-through window or frequent a pharmacy that has the prescription counter in the front of the store. The demographics of the population that shops the pharmacy will be very influential to the design of a pharmacy and prescription counter (Walker, 1996).

Gaedeke and Tootelian (1993) discussed two types of store layouts: grid and free flow. In a *grid layout,* all the counters and fixtures are at right angles to one another. Merchandise is displayed in straight, parallel lines, encouraging maximum travel time in the aisles and maximum product exposure. The *free-flow layout* groups merchandise and fixtures into patterns that al-

low for an unstructured flow of customers. Many of the fixtures are irregularly shaped circles, arches, and triangles. This design is used often in gift and specialty stores, mostly encouraging browsing and impulse buying.

Grid layouts are more common in community pharmacies than free-flow layouts. Aisles are set in straight-line grid arrangements with key departments or service areas located to encourage shoppers to visit the four corners of the store. Departments are arranged to place high-demand items in the rear of the store, promoting traffic past lower-demand and impulse-purchase items. In grid layouts, the prescription department often is located in the back of the store, adjacent to high-demand over-the-counter (OTC) items and other items that may sell better if accompanied by a recommendation from a pharmacist (e.g., durable medical equipment or natural products).

Department placement is done with the intent to entice customers to purchase more than they had intended originally. Some locations in a pharmacy tend to attract more traffic. High-traffic areas are a good place to generate additional sales with placement of new product displays or impulse items. In pharmacies, placement of impulse items near or on the prescription counter may increase sales of these items owing to the increased traffic in that area of the store.

In almost any retail business, the risk of theft of merchandise (both by shoppers and by employees) is always present. Pharmacy managers can use store design and layout to minimize losses from theft. High-cost and other items that may be liable to theft generally are placed in open areas where store personnel can observe both the items and shoppers easily. Pharmacies are increasingly using locked cabinets to store items that are liable to theft (e.g., smoking-cessation products and weight-control products). Most states also have enacted laws that require products containing psuedoepherine be kept behind the pharmacy counter despite the fact that it technically has OTC drug status. This has been done to decrease the theft and inappropriate use of psuedoepherine, particularly in the production of methamphetamine. Efforts should be taken not to place high-cost and high-theft items in corners (which are more difficult for personnel to see) or near exits (where it would be easier for shoppers to steal an item leave without being noticed). Many pharmacies use store security personnel, video surveillance equipment, one-way mirrors, and even sensors embedded in products to detect and prevent losses of merchandise.

Pharmacy Merchandising

Merchandising involves the proper placement of goods on pharmacy shelves. The space a pharmacy has for goods to be displayed is limited by the size and design of the store. Pharmacies commonly separate their space into departments or sections that contain major categories of products (e.g., prescription area, cough and cold, headache, and first aid).

Merchandise in a pharmacy tends to flow from one department to the next. This flow is accomplished by placing related departments next to or near each other. *Cross-selling* is the process of selling across departments to facilitate customers purchasing more items than they may have intended originally. Arranging departments in a logical transition from the front to the back of the store will guide shoppers to areas where they may find additional items to purchase. Cosmetics, hair-care products, and health and beauty aids commonly are located near toiletries and feminine hygiene products because consumers who come to a pharmacy to purchase the former products also tend to need the latter (see Fig. 23-1).

Pharmacy aisles are of various lengths and heights. For the convenience of shoppers, aisles tend not be more than 50 feet in length (Raven, 1984). If an aisle is longer, cross aisles should be provided. Cross aisles are a break in a long run of shelving creating an aisle that allows customers to move easily across the store. Cross aisles provide for smooth traffic flow and increase visible space for item placement.

Many pharmacies use the space at the beginnings and ends of the aisle runs. These spaces often are referred to as *end caps.* End caps often feature displays of promotional and seasonal items, bulk items, impulse items, and new products designed to gain shoppers' attention (Fig. 23-2).

Aisle heights also vary among pharmacies (Raven, 1984). Some smaller pharmacies use a lower aisle height of 54 in. This allows store personnel to see across the entire pharmacy. Larger pharmacies often use fixtures with heights of 60 to 72 in. Higher shelves provide additional space for merchandise and storage. Higher shelves also help consumers to keep eye contact with products in the aisles. Not allowing visibility across aisles is a tool used by retailers to keep the shopper's eye on the items in that section.

When deciding what items and how many of each item to place in a section or a department, pharmacy managers strive for balance between variety and duplication. This balance will vary by and within categories of merchandise. The two considerations to be addressed in achieving such a balance are an understanding of the customers and an analysis of current market trends. Both these considerations address the placement of merchandise to respond to demographics, the type of customer and his or her needs, or market trends, responding to a new or very popular item.

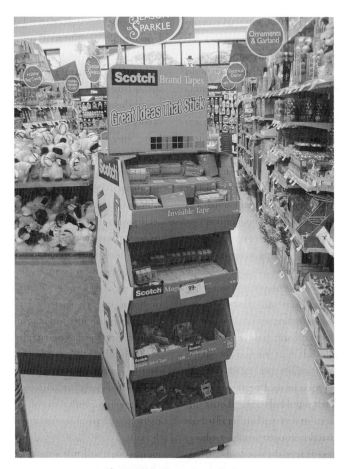

Figure 23-2. Floor stand display.

To assist with proper placement of items on shelves, many pharmacy managers use *plan-o-grams*. Plan-o-grams are diagrams that show the placement, space, and management of each item in a particular section of shelves. Plan-o-grams may be produced by manufacturers, wholesalers, corporate pharmacy offices, or the pharmacy staff itself. Plan-o-grams should be based on current sales and market information, as well as on the size and physical characteristics of the items themselves. A properly planned and executed plan-o-gram enables pharmacies to maximize sales and profit opportunities for a given section of space.

Plan-o-grams should arrange products to increase their visibility to consumers. Manufacturers strive to make the fronts and tops of their packaging clearly visible to consumers. A product *facing* is the arrangement of a product one package wide on a shelf. Placement of items on shelves so that these package facings are visible to consumers allows for maximum exposure and increases the likelihood of sales. By increasing the facings of a single product from two to four, pharmacies have found that sales of that product will increase by 36 percent (Portner, 1996).

When viewing a section in a pharmacy, the most popular items will be placed at eye level for the majority of shoppers (approximately 60 in high). Items placed very high or very low in a section traditionally will be slower-selling items. Customers in North

American pharmacies typically scan from left to right when looking at items on a shelf. Items on the shelf should be set vertically, from top to bottom, allowing the customer's eye to scan the shelf across as he or she goes from top to bottom. Pharmacy managers use this concept to cross-merchandise and add items for impulse purchasing. Additionally, most customers are right-handed and will grab the item to the right. Consumers commonly find larger-sized products (which generate higher sales and profit margins) kept to the right of smaller-sized products.

Pharmacy managers will place some items in more than one department. Fast-moving, high-profit items can be displayed in various departments throughout the pharmacy using a technique known as *cross-merchandising*. For example, displaying facial tissues not only with the paper products but also in the cough and cold section will increase impulse sales of these items.

In addition to placing items in designated sections or departments, pharmacy managers commonly use displays throughout a pharmacy to highlight specific products. Displays often are set in an aisle in front of a shelf to showcase new items or those with special pricing. Floor-stand displays are used to place large quantities of an item on display, making the products easily accessible to consumers. Manufacturers often supply these displays and other promotional materials to pharmacies to highlight their products (Fig. 23-3).

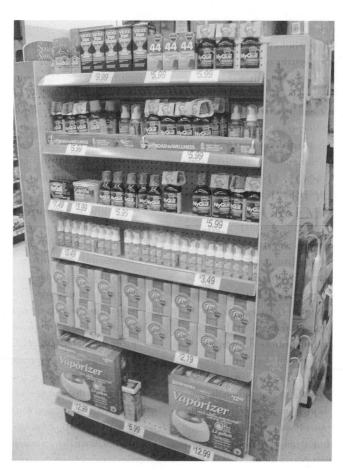

Figure 23-3. End cap.

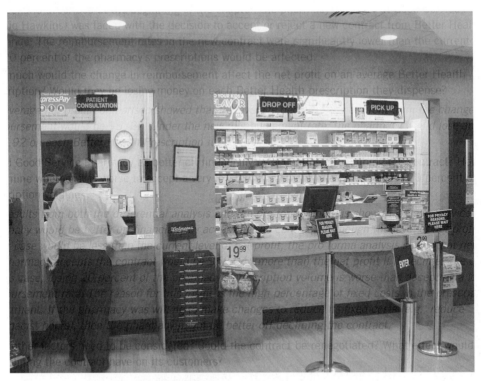

Figure 23-4. Prescription department.

Point-of-purchase materials (signage) also are used to highlight items. Header cards, banners, and price signs are all examples of point-of-purchase materials. These sales aids give product information, demonstrate features, reinforce a sale or special price, and have the ability to generate sales. Other methods used to highlight products are shelf extenders. These are small trays that are attached to a shelf and extend out several inches to highlight an item. Shelf talkers are signs that extend outward from the shelving and "speak" to customers about items or services found in the store.

Merchandising the Prescription Department

The prescription department is the one area that distinguishes a pharmacy from other retail stores that sell similar merchandise. The prescription department should be given a position of prominence in the store. This department usually takes up 300 to 600 square feet of space, having 18 to 24 feet across the front of the department. The prescription department usually is identified with prominent signage or decor to make it easily identifiable to customers to see and use (Fig. 23-4).

Consumers typically view the prescription department as a professional area. When they are able to view the interior of the pharmacy, they should see that this department is clean and well organized. Pharmacy personnel need to exhibit a friendly and professional demeanor because individual attention can distinguish one pharmacy from another.

The front of the prescription department traditionally is used to highlight vitamins and herbal remedies, products that commonly require the advice of a pharmacist for proper use (e.g., glucose monitors), or high-priced specialty items that may be at risk for theft if stocked in a less visible section (e.g., smoking-cessation products). The areas where prescriptions are dropped off or picked up are good places to display new products or impulse-purchase items (e.g., new OTC medications, Chap-Stick, or pill reminders). These areas are also natural spots for small displays of new OTC items that previously were prescription items (e.g., Prilosec or Claritin). The pharmacist's recommendation is one way to increase purchases of these items.

Designing prescription departments with the pharmacist–patient relationship in mind is a merchandising technique intended to have an impact on prescription sales, OTC purchases, and purchases of professional services (e.g., patient education programs, screenings, or immunizations). When pharmacies design prescription departments to be open, patrons feel more comfortable approaching the pharmacy staff with questions. Having the prescription department near other health care items makes the pharmacist's recommendation more likely to result in increased sales of these goods and services.

Some prescription departments are built elevated from the rest of the pharmacy, giving the department an appearance of prominence to the customer. Special lighting may also be used to highlight the pharmacy. The use of brighter lighting in and around the department highlights the pharmacy and draws customers to that area of the store.

Pharmacy design should also include a patient waiting area, a patient consultation area, and in some locations a drive-through window. The patient waiting area provides patients with space away from the sales floor to wait comfortably for their prescriptions. As prescriptions are being filled, customers have an opportunity to view health information or learn more about specific goods or services the pharmacy may offer (Fig. 23-5).

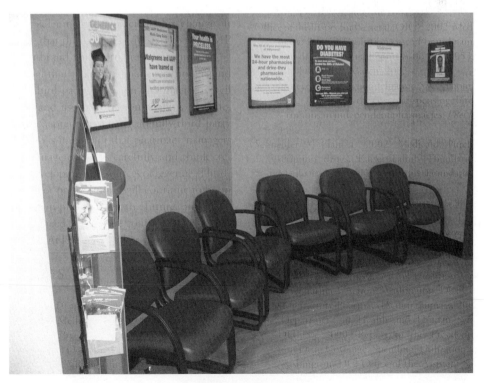

Figure 23-5. Patient waiting area.

The patient consultation center of the prescription department provides an area for patients and the pharmacist to discuss medications and related patient questions. The consultation center may be as small as an 18-inch window built into the prescription counter or as large as a freestanding patient care center. Patient care centers provide pharmacy staff with a place to offer counseling and medical information and provide screenings for various disease states, therapeutic drug monitoring, and immunizations.

Drive-through windows are a patient convenience item seen today in many pharmacies. Patients are able to purchase prescriptions and limited OTC items without having to leave their cars. Industry measurements have shown that drive-through windows are viewed by customers as an added convenience, increasing stores sales by as much as 7 percent over stores without this convenience (Laskoski, 1992) (Fig. 23-6).

Pharmacies are continually looking for new and better ideas to differentiate themselves from other retail outlets and to offer additional health care services to their customers. The addition of in-store medical clinics allows customers to receive medical care that is quick, inexpensive, and convenient (Fig. 23-7). Staffed by nurse practitioners and physician assistants that have prescribing authority, patients can choose from a posted list of services provided, receive treatment, and be on their way in less time than at a medical clinic or emergency room. Patients who need OTC or prescription items can pick up these items right in the store.

Retail clinics provide greater access to medical care for common problems. Physicians generally are not happy about this trend and would like to see more regulations governing in-store medical clinics. Clinics are not intended to replace primary care, and patients

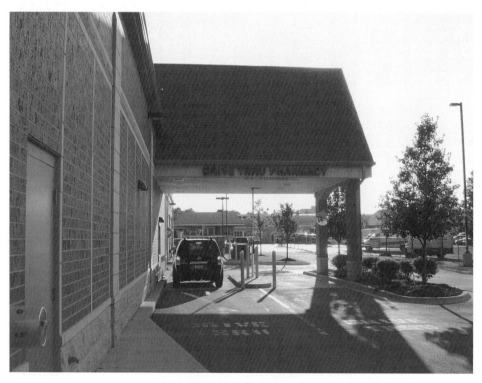

Figure 23-6. Drive-through window.

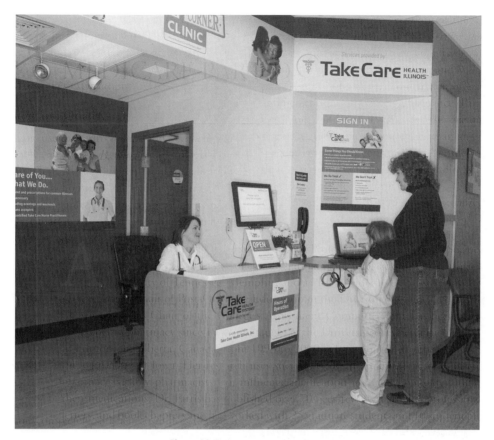

Figure 23-7. In-store medical clinic.

who need a higher level of medical attention need to be referred to doctors in a timely manner.

■ REVISITING THE SCENARIO

Mary Quint, our third-year doctor of pharmacy student, recently visited Healthway Pharmacy. She took some time to understand the factors that made her family so happy to shop there. The pharmacy manager indicated that the store's goal is to create an environment for shoppers that will make the pharmacy easy, fun to shop, and the health care destination of choice for its customers. He explained that the store attempts to satisfy customers' needs by appealing to their senses. What customers see and hear throughout the store is influential to their shopping experience.

Customers are assisted by merchandising techniques to find what they need and experience items and services they may not have thought of purchasing. The location is easily accessible to the wide variety of consumers who shop there. All this made Mary think long and hard about continuing to work at Middletown South Pharmacy.

REFERENCES

Eisenpreis A. 1983. How today's customers shop: What it means to drugstores. *American Druggist* 188:92.

Francke DE. 1974. Accepting things as they are. *Drug Intel Clin Pharm* 8:221.

Gaedeke R, Tootelian D. 1993. *Essentials of Pharmacy Management.* St. Louis: Mosby–Year Book.

Higby GJ. 1997. Pharmacy in the American century: 100 years of change. *Pharmacy Times* 63:16.

Hilditch J. 1981. Maximizing the value of the sales area. *Pharm J* 227:638.

Laskoski G. 1992. Design: Good, the bad, and the ugly. *American Druggist* 205:38.

Nannery M. 1999. Chain drug stores' image problem. *Chain Store Age* 209:41.

Portner T. 1996. *Effective Pharmacy Management: A Compre-hensive Presentation of Practical Management Techniques for Pharmacy,* 8th ed. National Community Pharmacists Association. Alexandria, VA.

Raven M. 1978. K-D furniture. *Drug Top* 122:43.

Raven M. 1984. Drugstore design and layout: Looking at the right angles. *Drug Top* 128:44.

Rodowskas C. 1996. Space allocation and profit maximization. *Pharmacy Times* 62:70.

Walker G. 1996. Debacle of OTC. *Pharm J* 256:775.

SECTION VI

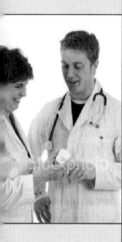

MANAGING VALUE-ADDED SERVICES

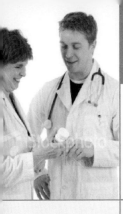

24

APPRAISING THE NEED FOR VALUE-ADDED SERVICES

David P. Zgarrick

About the Author: Dr. Zgarrick is the John R. Ellis Distinguished Chair of the Department of Pharmacy Practice and Professor of Pharmacy Administration at Drake University's College of Pharmacy & Health Sciences. Dr. Zgarrick received a B.S. in pharmacy from the University of Wisconsin and an M.S. and Ph.D. in pharmaceutical administration from The Ohio State University. He has practice experience in both independent and chain community pharmacy settings. Dr. Zgarrick teaches courses in pharmacy operations management, business planning for professional services, and drug literature evaluation. His research interests are in pharmacist compensation and workforce issues, professional service development, and the use of evidence-based medicine (EBM) by pharmacists.

■ LEARNING OBJECTIVES

After completing this chapter, students should be able to

1. Identify factors that should drive the development of value-added pharmacy services.
2. Describe how the business planning process applies to value-added pharmacy services.
3. Evaluate the market for value-added pharmacy services:
   a. Consumer characteristics and needs
   b. Impact of the internal and external environments
   c. Services already available in the market
   d. Market potential
   e. Consumer willingness and ability to pay for services
4. Evaluate the ability of a pharmacy to provide services that meet consumer needs.

■ SCENARIO

By all accounts, Alan Brouchard, Pharm.D., is a great pharmacist. He graduated at the top of his class in pharmacy school and started a successful career with a pharmacy chain in suburban Chicago. While he enjoyed working with all his patients, he especially liked counseling children and their parents. He had a reputation for being good with kids and informative with their parents, which resulted in many referrals to the pharmacy where he worked.

Last year Dr. Brouchard's wife was offered a job opportunity in Phoenix. While he loved his job in Chicago, his wife's opportunity was too good to pass up, and he knew that there were plenty of pharmacist jobs in the Phoenix area. He arranged a transfer to another pharmacy in his chain that was located in Sun City (a suburb just northwest of Phoenix). When he arrived, he was anxious to further develop the pediatric services he had started in Chicago. He convinced his pharmacy manager to purchase special equipment to teach children how to monitor their asthma, to remodel the pharmacy to include a private counseling area, and to spend money promoting these services in the local community.

After 3 months, Dr. Brouchard was very disappointed in how his service had been received. On a good week, only one or two people would come in for his services, and these often were older customers seeking advice for their grandchildren. The pharmacy manager began using the private counseling area to store diabetes supplies (which always seemed to sell as fast as the pharmacy could get them in). Dr. Brouchard did not understand why his services, which were so successful in Chicago, were not nearly as well received in Sun City. He often wondered what he could do to increase the appeal of his services to a larger number of the pharmacy's customers.

■ CHAPTER QUESTIONS

1. How does an organization's strategic plan affect the kinds of goods and services it offers?

2. In what ways is business planning useful in the development of value-added pharmacy services?
3. In addition to patients, who else should be considered consumers of value-added pharmacy services?
4. What information should be gathered before making a decision to offer a value-added pharmacy service? Where and how can this information be gathered?

■ "BUILD IT AND THEY WILL COME"?

One of the most popular films of the 1980s was *Field of Dreams,* starring Kevin Costner. Costner's character, Roy Kinsella, had moved from a large city to rural Iowa to become a farmer. While working on his farm, he kept hearing a voice that said, "Build it and they will come." At first Roy couldn't figure out what he should be building or who would come if he did. As the plot progressed, Roy plowed under his cornfield, built a baseball field, and waited for a group of baseball players to come and play. Most of the people in his town thought he was crazy, plowing under valuable corn. Even his wife and family had doubts when they had trouble paying their bills. However, a group of deceased baseball players from the distant past (some Hall of Fame legends, others practically unknown) started coming out of the cornfield every night to play on the field. Roy and his family enjoyed watching these players, but the people in his town still doubted their existence. Eventually, Roy's deceased father showed up to play, and they had a father and son game of "catch" that they both regretted they had not had in the past. By the end of the movie, the players had begun using the field during the day, the people of the town came to see them play, and Roy started charging admission, saving the family farm. Talk about a "Hollywood ending"!

What could *Field of Dreams* possibly have to do with pharmacy in the twenty-first century? On the one hand, if you ask some pharmacists why they offer the goods and services they do, they might just give you an answer similar to if you had asked Roy Kinsella why he built a baseball field in an Iowa cornfield. Maybe it was a voice inside their heads that told them to offer a pediatric asthma consulting service. They may have figured that if they "built" an herbal medicine section in their pharmacy, people would naturally come and purchase these items. Many pharmacists develop goods and services based primarily on their own desires or the needs of their organizations. They may have a personal interest in a particular area or have learned how to provide a specialized service during pharmacy school, residency, or on the job. While offering a good or service based primarily on personal interests or skills may sound like a good thing to do, one very important principle of marketing is being overlooked.

In the real world, Hollywood endings are quite rare. Businesses that develop goods and services based primarily on their own interests, skills, or needs usually end up regretting they had invested their time, money, and other resources. Many of these businesses fail after a short period. This is so because one of the fundamental principles of marketing that is often overlooked by marketers is that the purchase of any good or service or the acceptance of any idea is driven by the *needs of consumers,* not those of the marketer (Kotler, 1997). Contrary to what some people may believe, marketers cannot force consumers to purchase or accept products they do not need. Consumer needs exist regardless of a marketer's products. Successful marketers start by identifying their consumers, evaluating their needs, and developing products (i.e., goods, services, and ideas) designed to meet consumer needs better than their competitors.

All pharmacists and pharmacy organizations are marketers of goods (e.g., prescription and over-the-counter medications, durable medical equipment, candy, greeting cards, and a wide variety of other items) and value-added services (e.g., dispensing prescriptions, delivery, drug utilization evaluation/review, disease-state management, and medication therapy management). A major challenge for any pharmacist or organization is to identify its consumers and evaluate their needs. Pharmacists and pharmacies then must develop products that meet consumer needs, as well as

their own personal, professional, and organizational needs. This can be a daunting task, and there is no guarantee of success.

■ REVISITING THE SCENARIO

At Dr. Brouchard's annual performance review, his pharmacy manager let him know that he would not be allowed to continue to offer pediatric services at the pharmacy. While he was disappointed, he understood why, given the few people who had used the service and the amount of time and money his organization had invested for seemingly little in return. At the same time, he saw that the rest of the pharmacy continued to be successful. Prescription volume was up over 10 percent in the past year, and sales of medications for arthritis, diabetes, and heart disease were increasing even faster. Several of the customers he had counseled about their grandchildren had told the pharmacy manager that they were very pleased with Dr. Brouchard's professional manner and advice. He was happy to hear this and thought to himself that if only there were some way he could continue to offer this level of service to a larger group of patients.

■ APPLYING THE BUSINESS PLANNING PROCESS TO PHARMACY SERVICES

One way that many pharmacists identify consumer needs, develop new ideas for new goods and services, and manage the risks involved in any business venture is by using the business planning process (see Chapter 4). Business planning helps decision makers evaluate their markets and environments. It gives managers the freedom to explore new ideas without having to invest their resources in actually developing and offering the product. Using the business planning process does not guarantee that consumers will accept a product or that the product will meet organizational goals. However, business planning does help managers identify risks and assess the likelihood that a new product will be successful.

Many administrators require their pharmacists to develop written business plans to justify offering a new good or service. This helps administrators decide whether to allocate scarce resources (especially money, time, and personnel) to the development of a new good, service, or idea. One important aspect to keep in mind about business planning is that administrators and pharmacists are under no obligation to implement a plan. If the research done in the planning process indicates that a product will not meet consumer or organizational needs, that it would not be feasible to offer, or that the risks involved are greater than the organization cares to take, a decision can be made simply not to move forward with the plan. While it takes an investment of time to develop a business plan, not implementing a plan that is likely to fail consumes far less time, money, and other resources than developing a new good or service that does in fact fail.

Applying the business planning process to the development of value-added pharmacy services is not that different from how the process is used to evaluate any other good, service, or idea. One of the first steps when starting the business planning process should be to identify the organization's strategic plan and mission statement. Since these documents represent the road map for what the organization wishes to become and how it plans to get there, it is important that the development of any new good or service bears these in mind. One question that almost all administrators will want to have answered is how the implementation of any new value-added service will help their organization achieve the goals set out in the strategic plan.

It is important to recognize that mission statements and strategic plans vary among types of organizations, especially within health care. The mission statement and strategic plan of a not-for-profit children's research hospital likely will be different from that of a for-profit pharmacy chain (Table 24-1). The aspects of a professional service that will need to be emphasized in a business plan will vary as well. The not-for-profit children's research hospital may want to see how a new professional service will result in enhanced clinical outcomes or benefit the greatest number of children at the lowest possible cost. On the other

| Table 24-1. Mission and Vision Statements |

St. Jude Children's Research Hospital Mission Statement

The mission of St. Jude Children's Research Hospital is to advance cures, and means of prevention, for pediatric catastrophic diseases through research and treatment. Consistent with the vision of our Founder Danny Thomas, no child is denied treatment based on race, religion, or a family's ability to pay (St. Jude, 2007).

Walgreen's Mission Statement

We will treat each other with respect and dignity and do the same for all we serve.

We will offer employees of all backgrounds a place to build careers.

We will provide the most convenient access to healthcare services and consumer goods in America.

We will earn the trust of our customers and build shareholder value (Walgreen's, 2007).

hand, a for-profit pharmacy chain may want to see how the service will expand its market share or enhance its shareholders' value of owning the company.

The next step of the business planning process is to explore the prospects for various types of value-added services. At this point it is helpful to have several ideas for value-added services that could be implemented. One of the best ways to do this is to observe and speak with pharmacy department customers. This is essential to learn more about their needs and can help business planners learn more about their environments (which will be important later in the process). Other sources for ideas about value-added pharmacy services include colleagues, professional organizations, pharmacy magazines and journals, professional meetings and seminars, the Internet, consultants, books, and full-service wholesalers.

The next step in exploring the prospects for value-added pharmacy services is to learn more about the potential services that have been identified. Many pharmacists start this process by performing a literature review about potential services using electronic databases such as PubMed (National Library of Medicine, 2007) or International Pharmaceutical Abstracts (IPA) (Thomson Scientific, 2007). These databases can identify primary and secondary literature that provides additional information about services, descriptions of services implemented by others, and research studies that evaluate the outcomes of similar services. Nonmedical Internet search engines such as Google (www.google.com) also may be helpful, but users should be cautioned that finding valuable information can be difficult given the vast amount of information available on the Internet (see Chapter 6).

Professional pharmacy and medical organizations [e.g., the American Pharmacists Association (APhA), the American Society of Health-System Pharmacists (ASHP), the National Community Pharmcists Association (NCPA), and the American Medical Association (AMA)] and health care organizations [e.g., the American Diabetes Association (ADA) or the American Heart Association (AHA)] also provide valuable information about many health conditions and value-added services. This information is important not only in the development of a service but also in justifying the need for a service with consumers and administrators. These organizations also provide treatment guidelines and additional resources that can be used when developing an operations plan for a service (see Chapter 25).

While learning more about potential value-added pharmacy services, it is a good idea for business planners to speak with others about their ideas. Many pharmacists who have already developed value-added services will gladly share what they have learned. Visiting a setting where value-added pharmacy services are already in place not only provides evidence of how these services actually work but also will answer many questions pharmacists may have later in the planning process. Other pharmacists, technicians, and pharmacy employees may have experienced value-added services in their prior practice experiences and may provide insights into how they work. Other health care professionals can provide feedback about additional services that they or their patients may need. Payers [e.g., insurance companies, health maintenance organizations (HMOs), employers, and governments] may be willing to share ideas about value-added pharmacy services that may improve the health of their constituents while saving them money.

Most administrators and organizations do not like to be surprised to learn that their pharmacists are working on proposals for new value-added pharmacy services. It is important to work with administrators and organizations early in the business planning process not only to keep them informed but also to learn what they desire from an administrative standpoint. Taking the views of administrative and organizational personnel into account throughout the process increases the likelihood that administrators will support and provide the resources necessary to implement value-added pharmacy services in the future.

■ REVISITING THE SCENARIO

Dr. Brouchard began to think about what the chain he worked for might want in a professional service. The chain's mission statement said that it was dedicated to providing patients with high-quality customer service while using modern technology. The chain also was open to developing innovative ways to attract new customers and serve its existing customers. The chain's strategic plan stated that it had a rapid expansion plan and that it expected new services to contribute a 15 percent return on investment (ROI) after 3 years. After reading this, Dr. Brouchard knew that his chain was open to developing new services but that he also would need to show that such services could contribute to profitability in a relatively short time.

With this in mind, Dr. Brouchard thought of some ideas for value-added pharmacy services that he could pursue. While his pediatric asthma service was not successful, perhaps he could offer the same service to an adult population. He had seen a report on the local news mentioning that the prevalence of asthma had increased greatly in their area over the last several years. Like many other pharmacies serving patients of the "baby boom" generation and older, his pharmacy dispensed many prescriptions for hypertension and hyperlipidemia. And while diabetes was not a specialization he had considered previously, it was difficult to ignore the number of prescriptions the pharmacy filled for diabetes medications and the amount of related supplies the pharmacy sold. Dr. Brouchard had even read in a pharmacy journal that insurance companies and government agencies were paying pharmacists to provide diabetes education services. He decided to research these ideas and then approach his pharmacy manager to get her thoughts.

■ EVALUATING THE MARKET FOR PHARMACY SERVICES

In evaluating potential professional services, it is essential to consider the characteristics of the market where they will be offered. Since any service first must satisfy consumer needs before a pharmacist's personal, professional, or organizational goals can be met, evaluating potential consumers of a service should be the first aspect of the market that is considered.

When pharmacists think of potential consumers of their value-added services, the first (and often only) group they think about is patients. After all, pharmacists interact with patients on a daily basis. While patients are essential to the success of most value-added pharmacy services, pharmacists must remember that groups of consumers other than patients may benefit from pharmacy services as well.

When planning for value-added pharmacy services, pharmacists often classify consumers into one of the three P's. These three groups are patients, physicians and other health care professionals, and payers (Table 24-2). Pharmacists should consider carefully the characteristics and needs of each of these groups in the business planning process.

While almost all patients that pharmacists interact with have some type of medication-related need (e.g., a drug product, advice about an adverse drug effect, etc.), not all patients may need the same level of service that pharmacists can provide to patients (Hepler and Strand, 1989). It is important for pharmacists to identify subgroups of patients who may benefit more directly from their services. For an asthma service, pa-

Table 24-2. Types of Consumers of Value-Added Pharmacy Services

Patients and caregivers
   Patients with particular disease states
   Patients who have multiple disease states
   Patients who are not well controlled on existing therapy
   Caregivers of children, elderly, and invalid
Physicians and other health care professionals
   Primary care physicians (e.g., family medicine, general medicine, internal medicine, and pediatricians)
   Specialists (e.g., cardiology and endocrinology)
   Physician assistants, nurse practitioners, and nurses
   Dentists, podiatrists, and veterinarians
Payers
   Private insurance companies
   HMOs
   PPOs
   Government programs (i.e., Medicare, Medicaid, and state and local assistance programs)
   Employers

tients with asthma and other pulmonary conditions likely would have a much higher need for the service than others without these conditions. For a diabetes education service, there are different categories of patients with diabetes on which one may focus (e.g., type I versus type II). In addition to the patients themselves, caregivers (e.g., parents, adult children of the elderly, etc.) should be identified and their needs evaluated. The primary need of patients is health care, the purpose of which is to allow them to live a longer, healthier life. Pharmacists who can convince their patients and caregivers that their services will improve their quality of life will be on their way to developing a successful service.

Pharmacists desiring to implement new professional services must develop relationships with other health care professionals such as physicians, nurses, therapists, and other specialists. For these relationships to be successful, all parties much recognize the others' needs and be prepared to describe how each would benefit from their interactions (Doucette and Mc-Donough, 2002). For example, a pharmacist starting an anticoagulation monitoring service needs patient referrals from cardiologists, internal medicine specialists, vascular surgeons, and other health professionals who prescribe anticoagulation therapy. The pharmacist also will need information about these patients and perhaps even support from the professionals in billing for their services. On the other hand, the health care professionals need information not only about their patients but also about drug therapy. Physicians also are faced with challenges in today's managed-care environment and often need to see many patients per day to maintain their financial viability. Physicians are seeking ways in which they can use other health care professionals to extend their services while maintaining high-quality patient care. Chapter 25 will describe ways in which pharmacists can develop and enhance these relationships with other health care professionals.

One group of consumers whose needs often are overlooked by pharmacists is payers. Today, almost all pharmacy goods and services are paid for by someone other than the patient. These third-party payers include insurance companies, managed-care plans, employers, and local, state, and national government agencies. While pharmacists often do not enjoy interacting with third-party payers, most of them have needs that pharmacists are in a unique position to satisfy. Payers generally want to obtain high-quality goods and services at the lowest possible costs. Payers also recognize that they may not always be getting optimal benefits from their expenditures, especially those related to drug therapy. Pharmacists, given their expertise in drug therapy and proximity to their enrollees, are in an ideal position to help payers improve the quality of care while controlling costs, especially through their value-added services. Pharmacists who can demonstrate the value of their services to payers often find that payers are willing to encourage their enrollees to use pharmacy services (Cranor, Bunting, and Christensen, 2003; Kepple, 1998).

Another aspect of the market for any value-added pharmacy services that must be considered is the competition. When identifying competitors, it is important to acknowledge exactly what services the pharmacy will pursue. When identifying competitors for value-added services, pharmacists often limit their search to other pharmacies and pharmacists. While this may be appropriate for traditional pharmacy goods and services (e.g., dispensing drug products), pharmacists considering new value-added services must cast a much broader net. Many value-added services offered by pharmacists are still at the introductory point of their product life cycles. Few, if any, other pharmacies may offer these services in a particular market. On the other hand, other competitors may be very well established. For example, while diabetes education services currently are not offered in many community pharmacies, physicians and certified diabetes educators (who can be physicians, nurses, pharmacists, and other health care professionals) have provided this service for a number of years (Zrebiec, 2001).

Recognizing and evaluating competitors is an important part of the business planning process (see Chapter 4). While competitors have an established clientele and represent a potential threat to the success of a new pharmacy service, much can be learned from observing how they provide their services. If a large number of competitors are present in a market, it may be daunting to think about how a new value-added pharmacy service can compete successfully for customers. Competitors represent a challenge, but with proper research and planning, many pharmacists find that these challenges can be overcome. One way is by positioning a value-added pharmacy service in the market such that consumers see it as different from the others. This is often referred to as *niche marketing* (Doucette and McDonough, 2002). A pharmacy that hopes to establish a smoking-cessation service may find that there are a number of established competitors in the market (e.g., physicians, psychologists, support groups, and over-the-counter medications). However, if the pharmacy can provide its service in such a way that consumers recognize that it is more convenient or has higher quality or a lower price than competitors, the pharmacy and its smoking-cessation service still can be successful in the market.

For any value-added pharmacy service to be viable, there must be a sufficiently large number of consumers in the market who may be willing to purchase the service. Investing too many resources into a service that benefits a small number of consumers ultimately will lead to the demise of any business venture. Several sources can be used to determine the size of a market for a professional service. The easiest place for a business planner to start is to review a pharmacy's patient profiles, purchasing and financial records, and other internal data. Knowing how many prescriptions are filled for different classes of medications will help the planner to determine which conditions are the most prevalent among the pharmacy's patients. The only downfall of this method is that the information is limited to the pharmacy's current clientele. Many pharmacies would like to provide value-added pharmacy services that attract new patients.

Reviewing the literature to learn the potential size of a market can be helpful, especially epidemiologic studies that describe the incidence and prevalence of a condition. Unfortunately, most of these studies are done on a state, national, or even international level and may not provide information about the prevalence of a condition in a specific geographic location of interest. This disadvantage can be offset in part by combining a literature review with interviews of other health care professionals in the pharmacy's market area. They may be able to provide specific information about the number of patients they and others professionals treat.

Perhaps the best way to determine the size of a market for a value-added pharmacy service is to perform a market research study. Survey research methods can be used to gather information from potential customers. Not only can this information be used to determine the number of potential consumers in a specific area, but it also can provide additional information about consumers that can be useful in developing a value-added pharmacy service (e.g., if/where they currently obtain this service, their level of satisfaction with the service, and their willingness to obtain the service from a pharmacist). Some of the drawbacks of market research

include the specialized knowledge and skills needed to carry out a study properly, the amount of time involved, the relatively high cost of performing this type of research, and the potential biases that are inherent in any type of survey research. Several studies have been published that used market research to determine the size and characteristics of potential consumers of value-added pharmacy services (Larson, 2000; MacKinnon and Mahrous, 2002; Zgarrick and Cohen, 2000).

Even if there are a large number of consumers who might be interested in obtaining a value-added service from a pharmacist, the ultimate question that must be answered is whether these consumers are willing and able to make this purchase. Some consumers (especially patients) may be very interested in obtaining a health service from a pharmacist and actually may say on a survey that they would be willing to pay for this service. However, saying that one is willing to pay does not always result in an actual payment for the service. The consumer may not have the means to pay the price being charged by the pharmacist or may be able to obtain the service from another provider (e.g., a physician) for only a small insurance copayment.

Other groups of consumers also may be interested in obtaining a value-added pharmacy service and often have the financial resources to do so (e.g., other health care professionals, insurance companies, employers, and government agencies). However, pharmacists often find that these groups may not be willing to pay for these services until the pharmacist can demonstrate the value of the services (Poirier, Buffington, and Memoli, 1999). This has created a "chicken and egg" problem for many pharmacists. Pharmacists state that they cannot show the value of the service unless they are given the opportunity to provide it. At the same time, pharmacists state that they cannot afford to provide the service unless they are paid to do so. Several demonstration projects have been performed to show the value of professional services to various groups of consumers (Bluml, McKenney, and Cziraky 2000; Singhal, Raisch, and Gupchup, 1999). Medicare has begun to provide opportunities for pharmacists to receive payment for medication therapy management (MTM) services through the Part D program (see Chapters 17 and 26).

Several methods can be used to learn more about consumers' willingness and ability to pay for value-added pharmacy services. Getting to know consumers and observing their habits (e.g., what services they will pay for, how much they will pay, and what they expect to receive in return) can be done relatively quickly and easily in most practice settings. Market research and the pharmacy literature also can be used, but it is important to remember that what a consumer says he or she will pay for a value-added pharmacy service on a survey may not represent what he or she actually will pay when presented with the service in the pharmacy. The only way to truly determine what a consumer will pay for a value-added pharmacy service is to offer the service, charge a price, and observe whether the consumer actually makes the purchase. Unfortunately, this can occur only after the decision has been made to offer the service.

REVISITING THE SCENARIO

Dr. Brouchard's research into asthma and diabetes services provided him with a great deal of information. The initial data he gathered from Internet searches and the primary and secondary literature showed him that each service had a great deal of potential. He visited other pharmacies in the Phoenix area that offer these services and came away impressed with the level of service that was being provided and the pharmacists' willingness to share their ideas.

He started looking into the market for each of these services. After checking the pharmacy's dispensing records, he found that there were a large number of patients using asthma medications and even more on lipid-lowering and cardiac medications, but the largest proportion of patients was using oral hypoglycemic drugs. The local physicians he spoke with said that they were having a difficult time keeping up with all the new cases of diabetes they were seeing. Several of them stated that they employed nurses who were certified diabetes educators (CDEs) to educate their patients about their disease (especially since Medicare was now paying them to do so) but that it took more than 6 months from the time they made the initial diagnosis until they could get a patient into an education

program. Dr. Brouchard imagined that at least some of these patients might be willing to pay out of their own pockets to get this service sooner than to wait more than 6 months to get this education from a nurse. Besides, how well could the nurse explain all the mediations that are being used to control this disease?

CAN A PHARMACY MEET THE NEEDS OF CONSUMERS?

Assuming that there is a consumer need and a market for a particular value-added pharmacy service, business planners must ask themselves a very serious question before moving forward. The question is whether they actually can meet the needs of consumers. The answer to this question is not always as easy as it might appear and requires a great deal of introspection on the part of the pharmacist and the organization.

One way that business planners can begin to answer this question is to perform a SWOT analysis, as described in Chapters 3 and 4. SWOT analysis (i.e., *s*trengths, *w*eaknesses, *o*pportunities, and *t*hreats) has applications in both strategic and business planning. In strategic planning, managers perform this analysis on a broad level, looking at the entire organization. In business planning, strengths, weaknesses, opportunities, and threats are evaluated only at the level of the service being considered. Strengths and weaknesses are considered to be internal to an organization and are the easiest to *initially* evaluate. They are also within the control of the organization, such that aspects that initially may be considered a weakness can be addressed and perhaps even become strengths of the organization in the future. Opportunities and threats generally exist external to an organization. Given that they are part of the external environment, they often are more difficult to control. At the same time, they can exert just as much influence over the success or failure of a value-added pharmacy service as internal strengths and weaknesses.

The first internal factor that an organization planning to offer a value-added pharmacy service should evaluate is the resources necessary to provide the service. This starts with the abilities and interests of the staff to provide the service. Many value-added pharmacy services require knowledge and skills beyond those used in traditional dispensing functions. Staff members may need to attend educational or training programs to gain the appropriate knowledge and skills. Some value-added services require that pharmacists become certified to demonstrate their knowledge and skills in an area before the service may be offered. States that allow pharmacists to administer immunizations often require that they become certified before providing this service (APhA, 2007). Medicare and many insurance companies require that pharmacists become CDEs before they will compensate them to provide diabetes education services. Becoming a CDE involves completing a series of exercises, gaining experience in providing diabetes education to patients, and passing an examination. This process generally takes about 2 years to complete. As of 2007, about 1,000 pharmacists had successfully completed the CDE requirements (NCBDE, 2007).

It may go without saying that pharmacists should be interested in providing value-added services if they are to be successful. It is important to match the skills and interests of a pharmacy's personnel with the services the pharmacy intends to provide. If a pharmacist is not interested in providing a service, can he or she be provided with an incentive that may motivate him or her to do so? If not, can another pharmacist be hired who has the interest and skills needed to be successful?

Pharmacies need a number of physical resources to provide most value-added services. This usually begins with the layout of the pharmacy. Many value-added pharmacy services require at least some degree of privacy. Unfortunately, pharmacies that were designed to maximize the efficiency of the dispensing process often do not have a private office or classroom space necessary to provide patient care services. Other physical resources that may be needed to provide a professional service include computer hardware and software, testing devices, medical supplies, and office supplies.

Pharmacies must be willing to commit financial resources to the development of a new value-added service. Working capital is needed to support the purchase of equipment, supplies, and marketing before the service can be offered. Since most services do not bring in enough income initially to cover their costs, money also will be needed to pay employees and continue to purchase needed resources. Business planners must consider how much working capital they will need to start a service and how long they are willing to support the service before it is expected to cover its costs and contribute to organizational profitability.

Another internal resource that cannot be overlooked is support from administrators within the organization. Administrators who "buy in" to the concept of providing value-added services are much more likely to support their development and provide the resources needed to get them off the ground. Pharmacists hoping to gain this support generally work to convince administrators how implementation of value-added services will help the organization reach its overall goals.

Many external factors, such as patient demographic trends, can be viewed as both a threat and an opportunity for the development of a value-added service. The aging of the population and the increased reliance on drug therapy as a medical treatment have greatly increased the number of prescriptions filled in pharmacies (NACDS, 2007). This can be seen as a threat, in that pharmacy staff may not have as much time to provide other nondispensing services. On the other hand, these trends also present opportunities for pharmacists to implement new services that meet the increased patient needs for health information and drug therapy monitoring.

Other external factors that may influence the success or failure of a value-added service include laws and regulations affecting practice (both of pharmacists and of other health care professionals), reimbursement and compensation policies of third-party payers, competition from other pharmacies and health care providers, technology, and the ever-changing needs of health care consumers themselves. While these factors may be difficult for business planners to influence, they are manageable. Pharmacists willing to take a proactive stance regarding these issues (especially though involvement in professional organizations and other groups) often are able to have their voices heard and help to shape the policies that affect their futures.

■ REVISITING THE SCENARIO

After assessing the market for a diabetes education service, Dr. Brouchard took a closer look at his environment. Within his pharmacy and organization, the outlook appeared to be fairly positive. While he was not a diabetes expert, he spoke with another pharmacist in his chain who had become a CDE. The chain had supported his training and even helped to pay part of the certification fee. Dr. Brouchard always had been willing to learn more, so he decided that he would start the certification process on his own.

The pharmacy already had a private counseling area, and he figured that he could use some of the resources he had obtained for the pediatric asthma service for a diabetes service. When he told his pharmacy manager about his idea, she seemed excited, especially given the potential for the service to attract new customers to the pharmacy. She did stress that her budget to support this service was limited and that he would have to provide more financial projections that she could share with her district manager before she could commit to support the service.

There were threats that could have an impact on the service, but none that he felt could not be overcome. There always seemed to be more prescriptions to be filled, and the current shortage of pharmacists was not helping matters. However, he knew that his chain was developing new technologies that would speed the dispensing process and that his state had just changed its pharmacy practice act to allow pharmacy technicians to perform more functions. He figured that these changes should help to free up some time that would be needed to develop, market, implement, and ultimately provide a diabetes education service to patients.

■ CONCLUSION

Pharmacies, like any other business or organization, cannot build new value-added services with the hope that consumers will adopt them. Pharmacy managers can use business planning as a tool to evaluate consumer needs, the market, and their own resources before deciding whether to offer value-added services and which services would be most likely to succeed. While using business planning does not guarantee that a new value-added pharmacy service will be successful, the process helps pharmacy managers manage the risks involved in this increasingly important area of their organizations.

■ QUESTIONS FOR FURTHER DISCUSSION

1. What are the dangers of the "build it and they will come" approach to developing professional services?
2. Compare and contrast the types of value-added pharmacy services that most likely would be accepted at St. Jude's Children's Research Hospital and Walgreen's (see Table 24-1).
3. How would have developing a business plan before he implemented the pediatric asthma service in Arizona have helped Dr. Brouchard?
4. Given what you now know, what other professional services also may be viable for Dr. Brouchard to offer at his new pharmacy?

REFERENCES

American Pharmacists Association (APhA). 2007. Pharmacy-Based Immunization Delivery Certificate Program; available at the APhA Web site, www.pharmacist.com; accessed on October 2007.

Bluml BM, McKenney JM, Cziraky MJ. 2000. Pharmaceutical care services and results in Project ImPACT: Hyperlipidemia. *J Am Pharm Assoc* 40:157.

Cranor CW, Bunting BA, Christensen DB. 2003. The Asheville Project: Long-term clinical and economic outcomes of a community pharmacy diabetes care program. *J Am Pharm Assoc* 43:173.

Doucette WR, McDonough RP. 2002. Beyond the 4 P's: Using relationship marketing to build value and demand for pharmacy services. *J Am Pharm Assoc* 42:183.

Hepler CD, Strand LM. 1989. Opportunities and responsibilities in pharmaceutical care. *Am J Pharm Educ* 53:7S.

Kepple SR. 1998. Pharmacists in Asheville, North Carolina, pick up city paychecks for diabetes services. *Am J Health-Syst Pharm* 55:10.

Kotler P. 1997. *Marketing Management: Analysis, Planning, Implementation, and Control,* 9th ed. Upper Saddle River, NJ: Prentice-Hall.

Larson RA. 2000. Patient willingness to pay for pharmaceutical care. *J Am Pharm Assoc* 40:618.

MacKinnon GE, Mahrous H. 2002. Assessing consumers' interest in health care services offered in community pharmacies. *J Am Pharm Assoc* 42:512.

National Association of Chain Drug Stores (NACDS). 2007. *The Chain Pharmacy Industry Profile: 2006.* Alexandria, VA: National Association of Chain Drug Stores.

National Certification Board for Diabetes Educators (NCBDE). 2007. NCBDE Web site; available at www.ncbde.org; accessed on October 2007.

National Library of Medicine. 2007. Pub Med Web site; available at www.ncbi.nlm.nih.gov/sites/entrez; accessed on October 2007.

Poirier S, Buffington DE, Memoli GA. 1999. Billing third party payers for pharmaceutical care services. *J Am Pharm Assoc* 39:50.

St. Jude Children's Research Hospital. 2007. Mission Statement, St. Jude's Web site; available st www.stjude.org; accessed on October 2007.

Singhal PK, Raisch DW, Gupchup GV. 1999. The impact of pharmaceutical services in community and ambulatory care settings: Evidence and recommendations for future research. *Ann Pharmacother* 33:1336.

Thomson Scientific. 2007. International Pharmaceutical Abstracts Web site; www.thomson.com/content/scientific/brand_overviews/ipa; accessed on October 2007.

Walgreen's. 2007. Mission Statement, Walgreen's Web site; available at www.walgreens.com; accessed on October 2007.

Zgarrick DP, Cohen E. 2000. Consumer demand for disease management services in a chain of grocery store community pharmacies. *J Am Pharm Assoc* 40:158.

Zrebiec J. 2001. A national job analysis of certified diabetes educators by the National Certification Board for Diabetes Educators. *Diabetes Educ* 27:694.

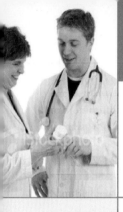

25

IMPLEMENTING VALUE-ADDED PHARMACY SERVICES

Randal McDonough

About the Author: Dr. McDonough is co-owner and Director of Clinical Services at Towncrest and Medical Plaza Pharmacies in Iowa City. He is also an Adjunct Professor (Clinical) at the University of Iowa College of Pharmacy. Dr. McDonough received a B.S. in pharmacy, an M.S. in pharmacy administration, and a Pharm.D. from the University of Iowa College of Pharmacy. At his community practice in Iowa City, he has developed and implemented several pharmacy services, including pharmaceutical case management (PCM), medication therapy management (MTM), immunization services, and health screenings. He is board certified in geriatrics and pharmacotherapy. He serves as faculty for the American Pharmacists Association's certificate programs for diabetes and hyperlipidemia. He is invited frequently to speak about practice development and implementation and has published numerous articles and book chapters on these topics.

▨ LEARNING OBJECTIVES

After completing this chapter, students should be able to

1. Describe the types of value-added services that pharmacists have implemented in their practices.
2. Discuss the components of a value-added service to consider before implementation.
3. Recognize the key components of a policies and procedures manual.
4. Discuss management of the marketing mix during service implementation.
5. Describe the role that collaborative practice agreements have in developing value-added services.

SCENARIO

Carol Smith, the pharmacist-owner of Care-Rite Pharmacy, is interested in expanding her clinical services. Her pharmacy is located in a city with a population of approximately 100,000 people. Although she has not implemented any specific value-added services in the past, patients and other health care providers recognize her practice as customer-friendly and service-oriented. She has two full-time pharmacists and two part-time pharmacists who have been working at the pharmacy for a number of years (range 5 to 15 years). Recently, they have completed a strategic plan, a SWOT analysis, and a survey of their patients. The results of the patient survey identified their key target market as women 50 years of age and older. Initially, they had wanted to implement a diabetes educational program, but their market research determined that a local hospital sponsored an American Diabetes Association (ADA)-recognized program. The hospital is a strong presence in their community, and the hospital's diabetes educators were not interested in collaborating with local pharmacies. Also, they looked into developing a community-based anticoagulation service, but after some checking into the reimbursement for this type of service, they realized that this service would not be feasible financially. Their market research did show that there was a need in their community for a medication therapy management (MTM) program. They already had a large percentage of high-risk patients who were taking four or more chronic oral medications and had several chronic medical conditions. Many of these patients expressed a need for assistance with medication management issues. Also, they noted that there was not a similar program elsewhere in the community.

CHAPTER QUESTIONS

1. What are the different types of value-added services that pharmacists have implemented in their practices? Describe the medication management process for each.
2. What are the components of a value-added service that pharmacists should consider and plan before implementation?
3. Why is a policies and procedures manual important to successful service implementation?
4. How should pharmacists manage the marketing mix during the implementation of value-added services?
5. How can a collaborative practice agreement help pharmacists implement value-added services?

INTRODUCTION

As discussed in previous chapters, implementing value-added pharmacy services requires a comprehensive strategic plan that includes a mission statement, SWOT analysis, goals and objectives that the practice hopes to achieve, and strategies to achieve the objectives. This plan provides direction for the practice and guides the allocation of resources and efforts. As the scenario demonstrates, the planning process helped Carol, the pharmacist-owner, to identify a service that fits with the pharmacy's strategic plan and yet has a niche in the marketplace. Pharmacists can implement many types of services in their practices, but it is essential that they do some market research to determine the opportunities and threats in the marketplace to ensure the success of the new service. Also, it is important to assess the pharmacists' motivations and abilities to provide a service. Ultimately, the success of any service depends both on market opportunities and the pharmacists' ability to provide the service.

TYPES OF VALUE-ADDED SERVICES

Value-added services can be thought to exist along a continuum (Fig. 25-1). On one end of the continuum, pharmacists are more narrowly focused on drug therapy issues that occur during the dispensing functions (i.e., point of care). On the other end of the continuum, pharmacists provide ongoing drug therapy management services for select individuals who have multiple comorbidities requiring complex therapies (i.e., case management). Other types of services fall between these two ends of the continuum. For example, disease-state management programs, clinical services such as anticoagulation or lipid clinics, and

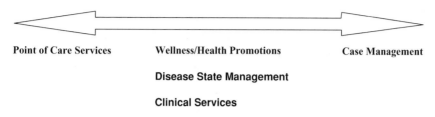

Point of Care Services   Wellness/Health Promotions   Case Management

Disease State Management

Clinical Services

Figure 25-1. Value-added services continuum.

health screening services fall somewhere in the middle of the value-added service continuum.

Regardless of the service being provided, the clinical activities and process of medication management provided by pharmacists implementing value-added services are similar along the continuum. These clinical activities or patient workups have been described elsewhere (McDonough, 1996; Strand, Cipolle, and Morley, 1988, 1992). The medication management process includes collection of pertinent patient data regarding the patient's medical and medication histories, evaluation or assessment of this information, identification of a problem occurring with the patient's medication, development of a plan of action to resolve the problem, and implementation of the plan, including follow-up as needed. Implementing a plan to manage drug therapy typically involves communication with the patient (i.e., patient education), as well as with practitioners (e.g., physicians). Appropriate documentation of patient care activities is an integral component of value-added services.

A number of studies have examined the impact that pharmacists can have delivering drug therapy management services at the point of care during the dispensing process (Christensen et al., 1999; Dobie and Rascati, 1994; Knapp et al., 1998; Rupp, 1988, 1992; Smith, Faussatt, and Christensen, 1999). The information that needs to be collected at the point of care may not be as comprehensive as for other services along the continuum. For example, during the dispensing process, it may be determined that the patient has an allergy to a specific medication. By focusing efforts on resolving this problem, the data collected pertain to this allergy, an alternative is identified, the physician is called, the pharmacist's recommendation is made, the medication is changed, and the pharmacist documents

a quick patient note (in the patient dispensing record) to complete the process. While the clinical process in this scenario is narrowly focused, this is an essential and clinically relevant service commonly performed by pharmacists.

Pharmacist' monitoring/screening services and wellness/health-promotion programs are the next level of value-added services along the continuum. These types of services, although relatively narrowly focused, require more patient data collection and may be delivered over an extended period. Documentation may be more comprehensive, with a patient chart being created in addition to the dispensing record. The clinical process remains the same as the point-of-care service but occurs separate from the dispensing function. Examples of ongoing monitoring services include pharmacist-managed anticoagulation services (Ansall et al., 1997; Davis and Sczupak, 1979; Knowlton et al., 1999; McCurdy, 1993; Norton and Gibson, 1996; Reinders and Steinke, 1979) and lipid management services (Furmaga, 1993; Simpson, Johnson, and Tsuyuki, 2001; Tsukuki et al., 1999). Health-promotion/screening programs also have been developed in community pharmacies in areas of smoking cessation (Kennedy et al., 2002), osteoporosis screening (Elliott et al., 2002), and lipid screenings with cardiovascular assessment (Madejski and Madejski, 1996; Tice and Phillips, 2002).

The next types of clinical services along the continuum are those which pertain to disease-state management. These services occur separately from the dispensing function over an extended period but have an added feature of ongoing patient education and an extensive review of drug therapy as it relates to attainment of the patient's therapeutic goals. A comprehensive patient chart is created, patient sessions may last from 15 to

60 minutes, and pharmacists may review the entire medication profile, although their efforts are focused more on the disease state they are following. Pharmacist-managed hypertension (Hawkins et al., 1979; McKenney et al., 1973, 1978; Reinders and Steinke, 1979), diabetes (Baran et al., 1999; Berringer et al., 1999; Coast-Senior et al., 1998; Jaber et al., 1996; Schilling, 1977; Swain and Macklin, 2001; Tiggelaar, 1987), and asthma (Grainger-Rousseau et al., 1997; Herbog et al., 2001; Kneoll et al., 1998; Pauley, Magee, and Cury, 1995; Rupp, McCallian, and Sheth, 1997) disease-state management programs have been cited frequently in the literature.

The most comprehensive of drug therapy management services is that of case management. In this situation, pharmacists are responsible for complete patient workups. A thorough patient history needs to be taken, a comprehensive review of all medications is done, and the patient is followed for an extended period. These services also occur separate from dispensing and can be the most challenging for pharmacists. Patients' medical problems can be complex, and multiple physicians often are involved. Several studies have investigated the impact of pharmacists' reviews in high-risk patients in the community setting. (Cowper et al., 1998; Hanlon et al., 1996; Petty et al., 2002).

▓ COMPONENTS OF A VALUE-ADDED SERVICE

Once it is determined which service is to be implemented, it is important to put some thought into what the service will look like and how it will be delivered at the practice. As discussed previously, regardless of the type of service (i.e., diabetes, lipids, asthma, etc.), the medication management processes used by pharmacists remain relatively the same. Some component of the service will require the pharmacist to collect patient clinical information, including laboratory data. The pharmacist also needs to assess the patient information that has been collected and make a clinical decision regarding the appropriateness of the therapy. Patient education is a component of each type of service but may be emphasized more so with certain services (e.g.,

wellness programs and services focused on disease-state management). Lastly, some consideration should be given to the clinical outcomes that the pharmacists want to achieve when implementing the service.

Data Collection

Patient data collection is an extremely critical component of a value-added service. The information collected provides pharmacists with important baseline and monitoring parameters for patients. The amount and type of information needed from the patient or other health care providers may differ depending on the service, but nonetheless, this information is the foundation on which the other components of the service are built. Forms can be developed to help pharmacists collect this information (see Figs. 25-2 through 25-4). In addition, some consideration should be given to how this information will be stored (e.g., paper charts or electronic patient database). The information that should be collected from the patient includes demographic information, medical history, family history, and medication history. Since some of the information may need to be collected from other providers and health care institutions, an authorization to release medical information should be signed by the patient and kept as part of the chart (see Fig. 25-5). Lastly, pharmacists should ensure that their site is in compliance with the Health Insurance Portability and Accountability Act (HIPPA) and reinforce to their patients that the information they provide is confidential and secure at the pharmacy.

Pharmacy-Based Laboratory Monitoring/Screening Services

Although pharmacists can receive objective patient data from local laboratories or from physicians, it may be decided that it is more convenient for the patient and pharmacist if a laboratory monitoring/screening service is performed at the point of care. Several types of monitors and equipment can be purchased by pharmacists and integrated into their practices. For example, pharmacists who implement a wellness program may purchase a body-fat analyzer, a weight scale, or a monitor that measures the lipid and glucose levels of

Patient History Form

Name: _____   Phone: (H) _____ (W) _____

Address: _____   City: _____   State: _____

Date of Birth: _____   Height: _____   Weight: _____   Gender: _____

Marital Status: _____   Pregnancy Status: _____

Medical Alerts (examples; hearing aids, prosthesis, heart valves, eyeglasses, artificial hips): _____

_____

Allergies/reactions:

_____   _____

_____   _____

Smoking History: **Caffeine Hostory:**

_____ Never Smoked   _____ Never Consumed

_____ Packs Per Day for_____Years   _____ Drinks Per Day

_____ Stopped_____ Years Ago   _____ Stopped _____ Years Ago

Alcohol History: **Dietary History:**

_____ Never Consumed   _____ Number of Meals Per Day

_____ Drinks Per Day   _____ Food Restrctions (explain)

_____ Stopped _____ Years Ago   Other: _____

Since health information may change periodically, I will notify the Pharmacist, to the best of my ability, of any new medications (prescription and non-prescription), any changes in directions of medicines, any new allergies, drug reactions or health condition changes. I authorize any releases of information and insurance benefit payments to the above pharmacy on my behalf.

_____   _____

Signature   Date

This information is requested by your Pharmacist as required by state regulations so that he/she can provide appropriate pharmacy services to you. This information will be kept confidential.

I do not wish to complete this form and WILL NOT HOLD THE PHARMACY RESPONSIBLE FOR ADVERSE SIDE EFFECTS I MAY INCUR.

_____   _____

Signature   Date

Figure 25-2. Patient history form.

Care-Rite Pharmacy
Patient Medical History Form

Medical History: Have you or any of your blood relatives had (mark all that apply)

Disease State	Self	Relative
High Blood Pressure		
Asthma		
Cancer		
Depression		
Lung Disease		
Diabetes		
Heart Disease		
Stroke		
Kidney disease		
Mental Illness		
Substance Abuse		
Other		

Medical Problems: Have you experienced or do you have any of the following?

Disease	Yes	No	Disease	Yes	No
Frequent urinay infections			Sores on legs or feet		
Difficulty with urination			Known blood clot problems		
Frequent urination at night			Leg pain or swelling		
Known liver problems			Unusual bleeding or bruising		
Trouble with certain foods			Anemia		
Nausea/Vomiting			Thyroid Problems		
Constipation/Diarrhea			Known hormone problems		
Bloody or black stools			Arthritis or joint problems		
Abdominal pain or cramps			Muscle cramps or weakness		
Frequent heartburn/cramps			Memory problems		
Stomach ulcers			Dizziness		
Shortness of breath			Hearing or visual problems		
Coughing up phlegm or blood			Frequent headaches		
Chest pain or tightness			Rash or hives		
Fainting spells or passing out			Change in appetite/taste		
Thumping or racing heart			Walking or balance problems		

Figure 25-3. Care-Rite Pharmacy patient medical history form.

Care-Rite Pharmacy
Medication History and Medical History

Collected by: _____ Date: _____

Patient Name: _____ Sex _____ Birth Date _____ Ht _____ Wt _____ LBW _____ Race _____

Prescribed Medications (Rx and OTC)					
Name/Strength	Dose/Sig	Duration	Indication	Dr	Comments

Past Medications Not Currently Taking (Rx and OTC)					
Name/Strength	Dose	Duration	Indication	Dr	Reason for Stopping

Figure 25-4. Care-Rite Pharmacy medication history and medical history.

AUTHORIZATION TO RELEASE MEDICAL INFORMATION

Date: _____   Date of Birth: _____

SSN: _____

Patient Name: _____

Address: _____

I, the undersigned, do hereby grant permission for the above named pharmacy to ☐obtain from or
☐release to:

_____ _____

_____ (Name of person or institution the information will be coming from)

_____ _____

_____ (Address of person or institution the information will be coming from)

The following information from the patient's clinical record:

_____ _____

_____ _____

_____ _____

_____ _____

_____

I understand that this information will be used for the purpose of:

☐   Providing information to allow pharmaceutical care to be provided to the patient
☐   Providing information to the physician regarding the care provided by the Pharmacist
☐   Supporting the payment of an insurance claim
☐   Other: _____

This authorization will be valid for the period of twelve months unless otherwise specified below.

I understand that I may revoke this consent at any time by sending a written notice to the above named pharmacy. I understand that any release which has been made prior to my revocation which was made in reliance upon this authorization shall not constitute a breach of my rights to confidentiality. I understand that I may review the disclosed information by contacting the above named pharmacy.

_____
_____   _____

Stignature of Patient or Patient's Authorized Representative/Date   Relationship of Authorized
Representative

_____

Pharmacy Representative/Date

Specific authorization for release of information protected by state or federal law - I specifically authorize by writing my initials beside the category and signing below the release of data and information relating to:

☐ Substance abuse

☐ Mental Health

☐ AIDS/HIV

_____

Signature and date of Patient or Patient's Authorized Representative

☐   Release mailed or information sent _____
                                        Signature/Date

Prohibition on Rediclosure
This form does not authorize rediclosure of medical information beyond the limits of this consent. Where information has been disclosed from records protected by federal law for alcohol/drug abuse, by state law for mental health records or HIV/AIDS related records, federal requirements (42 CFR Part 2) and state requirements (Iowa Code chs..228/141) prohibit further disclosure without the specific written consent of the patient, or as otherwise permitted by such law and/or regulation. A general authorization for the release of medical or other information is not sufficient for these purpose. Civil and/or criminal penalties may attach for unauthorized discloure of alcohol/drug abuse, mental health or HIV/AIDS information.

Figure 25-5. Authorization to release medical information.

patients. Alternatively, pharmacists who develop a diabetes program may obtain a device that measures the glycosylated hemoglobin (A_{1c}) of patients. Also, some pharmacists may decide to develop a women's health program and purchase a bone densitometer that measures bone mineral density to determine fracture risk owing to osteoporosis.

Pharmacies implementing monitoring/screening services must become familiar with the Clinical Laboratory Improvement Amendments of 1988 (CLIA). CLIA was enacted to ensure that all medical laboratories meet quality standards. These amendments are administered by the Centers for Medicare and Medicaid Services (CMS), which is responsible for laboratory registration, certificate generation, surveys, and surveyor guidelines for development and training. Tests typically performed by pharmacists in pharmacies [e.g., glucose, lipid panels, hemoglobin A_{1c}, and international normalization ratio (INR) tests] are considered *CLIA-waived* tests. CLIA-waived tests are considered by the Centers for Disease Control and Prevention (CDC) and the Food and Drug Administration (FDA) to be simple to administer and have little risk of error. Currently, 40 tests have been approved for certificate of waiver (COW) (Centers for Medicare and Medicaid Services, 2003).

If a pharmacy is interested in performing waived tests as part of its service, it must complete a certificate of waiver (COW). Instructions for how to obtain a COW can be found at www.cms.hhs.gov/CLIA. The COW should be sent to the local CMS office. CMS will assign the pharmacy with a CLIA number and send the pharmacy a CLIA fee-remittance coupon. Pharmacies must pay a nominal fee for the COW ($150 in 2007), and the COW must be renewed every 2 years. After receiving the CLIA number, the pharmacy may start providing the service. Pharmacists providing waived tests agree to follow good laboratory practices, which include following the manufacturer's instructions on instrument operation and maintenance, performing quality-control procedures, appropriately documenting test data, and storing the monitoring equipment and its reagents properly (Rosenthal, 2000).

In addition to CLIA, pharmacists should be knowledgeable about the Occupational Safety and Health Act (OSHA), which regulates workplace safety. In particular, pharmacists who perform laboratory tests that require finger sticks are at risk from exposure to blood-borne pathogens. Pharmacies who perform these tests should have a blood-borne pathogen exposure control plan (BPEPC) that describes who should be trained about the hazards of blood-borne exposure, precautions that need to be taken to prevent exposure, and what to do when an exposure incident occurs (Rosenthal, 2000). More information regarding OSHA and an example BPEPC can be found at the OSHA Web site (www.osha.gov).

Medication Management Protocols

The next component of the value-added service is the medication management that pharmacists will provide once they have collected the patient's clinical information and laboratory data. During this component of the service, pharmacists will assess patients, determine if they are reaching their goals of therapy, identify and resolve any drug therapy problems, and develop a care plan that helps to guide the pharmacists' follow-up and monitoring of the patients. For some services, protocols may be developed to help guide the pharmacists' therapeutic decisions (e.g., anticoagulation clinic protocols). For others, general decision pathways may be used to guide the pharmacists depending on the clinical situation that may occur during the patient assessment (e.g., lipid management programs). The protocols may be specific (e.g., adjustment of warfarin given a specific target INR) or more general without specific drug therapy recommendations regarding patients' therapy. For example, in case of management services, a protocol may be developed to describe what clinical activities the pharmacists will perform at each patient visit, but it is left to the pharmacists' discretion on how they will resolve a drug therapy problem. The protocols and clinical decision pathways should be evidence-based and supported by national guidelines and/or the primary literature.

Patient Education

Patient education is a component of each type of value-added service. The comprehensiveness of the education differs, though, depending on the service being implemented. For example, pharmacists implementing lipid screenings may see patients for a limited time (during the screening) and provide them with baseline education to help them understand their cardiovascular risk factors, fasting lipid panel results, and lifestyle-modification strategies. On the other hand, pharmacists providing diabetes educational services may provide more comprehensive education by determining the patients' educational needs, providing ongoing educational services to help them achieve their self-management goals, and assessing if the patients are achieving their therapeutic end points. In this situation, there usually will be multiple educational sessions with patients, including comprehensive documentation. In both examples, patient education is a well-defined and integrated component of the service.

Pharmacists can create or identify existing patient educational resources (e.g., patient brochures, educational fliers, and flip charts) to help reinforce important educational messages. These resources should be screened for accuracy and completeness. Also, reading difficulty should be assessed to make sure that difficult technical terms are replaced with more patient-friendly language (e.g., instead of blood glucose, use the term *blood sugar*). Another consideration is that some patients may not be able to read at all, especially if English is not their primary language. Therefore, it is not appropriate to simply hand out educational materials without first assessing the patient's understanding and reading ability. Once the educational resources are selected, it should be determined how they will be used as part of the service. Also, adequate copies should be ordered or created, and these should be inventoried periodically to make sure that there are sufficient supplies to meet patients' demands.

■ OUTCOME MEASUREMENTS

Outcome measurements are covered in more detail in Chapter 27, but pharmacists should determine what outcomes they will be assessing to evaluate the effectiveness of their service. These measures help pharmacists decide if certain aspects of the service need review-

ing and altering if outcomes are not being achieved. Clinical outcomes are the most readily apparent and easiest outcomes to assess. These outcomes include objective parameters such as blood pressure, lipid panels, blood glucose, hemoglobin A_{1c}, and weight. Clinical outcomes usually are part of the patient chart and so are easily accessed. Humanistic outcomes (e.g., health-related quality of life and patient satisfaction) can be collected from surveys that become part of the service delivery. If such surveys do become a component of the service, then it should be determined how frequently patients fill out the surveys and how the data will be stored and used. Economic outcomes may require other types of data that pharmacists do not always collect, such as hospitalizations, emergency room visits, or physician visits. If economic outcomes are of interest, then a data-collection tool can be created that routinely requests these types of data. Patient knowledge also may be of interest to pharmacists who are providing comprehensive educational services. For this type of outcome, before and after knowledge-assessment quizzes/tests can be used.

■ REVISITING THE SCENARIO: CARE-RITE PHARMACY AND SERVICE DEVELOPMENT

Data Collection

After performing a SWOT analysis and some baseline market research, Carol and the other pharmacists at Care-Rite Pharmacy have decided to develop a Pharmacy Check-up Service (MTM). One of Carol's pharmacists volunteered to put together a prototype patient chart that will be used by the pharmacists to document their activities. The patient chart contains several forms, including a patient history form that requests some basic demographic information (see Fig. 25-2), medical and medication histories forms (see Figs. 25-3 and 25-4), and an authorization to release medical information that is signed and dated by the patient (see Fig. 25-5). Also, a communication form was created to fax clinical information and pharmacists' recommendations to the physician (Fig. 25-6).

Care Rite Pharmacy

Physician Communication Form

Physician: _____ Fax: _____   _____

☐ Initial   ☐ Follow-up   ☐ New Problem   ☐ Preventative   ☐ Other

Patient Name: _____

Birth date: _____ Gender: _____

Pharmacist: _____ Date: _____

Subjective Findings:

Objective Findings:

Assessment:

Plan:

Recommended Pharmacist Follow-up Assessment: ☐ 4 weeks   ☐ 8 weeks   ☐ 6 months   ☐ Other

Pharmacist Signature: _____

Physician: _____ Date: _____

☐   I agree with the above recommendations:

☐   Proposed modified plan:

Pharmacist Follow-up   ☐ As recommended   ☐ Other: _____

Physician Signature: _____

Figure 25-6. Physician communication form.

Several copies of each individual form will be kept in separate folders in a file cabinet located in the patient care area of the pharmacy. One of the pharmacists will be responsible for making sure that enough copies are always on hand. Completed charts will be kept in a filing cabinet that is arranged in alphabetical order by patient last name.

Pharmacy-Based Laboratory/Monitoring Service

The pharmacists at Care-Rite Pharmacy decided to purchase a Cholestech LDX portable analyzer to measure the lipid profiles of their patients. They realized that many of their patients who they were targeting for the Pharmacy Check-up Service had cardiovascular disease. By purchasing the Cholestech LDX analyzer, they are able to assess lipid profiles and glucose levels for those patients who are willing to pay for this additional service. The system was chosen for its ease of use, quick results, and wide range of tests that it offers (i.e., lipid profile, glucose, and ALT). The Cholestech LDX lipid profile is considered a CLIA-waived test. Also, the pharmacists sent in their completed application for a certificate of waiver (COW), paid the biennial fee, and received their CLIA number. All the pharmacists were trained in use of the Cholestech and how to perform quality-control procedures. The pharmacists were taught how to do finger sticks, appropriate procedures on how to minimize exposure to blood-borne pathogens, and proper disposal of used supplies. Each pharmacist was required to perform a test on another pharmacist to demonstrate his or her competency in using this analyzer. Lastly, a cardiovascular risk assessment form was created. The results from the test are added to the form and reviewed with the patient during the 5-minute test (see Table 25-1).

Medication Management Protocols

Owing to the complexities of the patients that the Care-Rite pharmacists were targeting for their Pharmacy Check-up Service, they determined that there was not one single type of protocol that they could use to assess and manage a patient. For patients who did have cardiovascular disease requiring lifestyle modifica-

tions and/or lipid-lowering therapy, however, a general protocol using data from the ATP III guidelines was developed (see Table 25-2). The protocol provided a clinical decision pathway to determine treatment strategies depending on the patients' low-density lipoprotein (LDL) concentration and risk factors. To help in their assessment of patients, the pharmacists used the cardiovascular risk assessment form. The protocol, although providing direction for pharmacists, did not give specific recommendations regarding which medications to choose if the patients need LDL-lowering medications in addition to therapeutic lifestyle changes (TLCs). By using this protocol, the pharmacists still had some discretion regarding medication options based on patient-specific factors.

Patient Education

The pharmacists of Care-Rite Pharmacy also developed patient educational tools to be used during the patient assessment and patient education components of the Pharmacy Check-up Service. Because many of the targeted patients have similar medical conditions, education materials were developed for specific disease states, including hypertension, ischemic heart disease, diabetes, asthma, chronic obstructive pulmonary disease (COPD), etc. Also, educational materials were developed for certain therapeutic classes of medications. The Care-Rite pharmacists also determined that many patients needed individualized education materials, so they implemented a drug information/educational service as part of the MTM service. With this service, patients can ask questions regarding their medical conditions and/or drug therapies. The pharmacists will research and provide an individualized written response for each patient.

Outcome Measures

The main patient outcome measures of interest to the pharmacists at Care-Rite Pharmacy are clinical outcomes, patient knowledge, and patient satisfaction. Also, the pharmacists were interested in monitoring physician response to their clinical recommendations. The information collected would be kept in the patient chart. An electronic database was created to store

Table 25-1. Cardiovascular Risk Factors

Positive risk factors

+ 1   Female ≥55 years old, or premature menopause without estrogen replacement therapy
+ 1   Family history or premature CHD:
      MI or sudden death of father or first-degree male relative (i.e., father, brother, son)<55 years old
      MI or sudden death of mother or first degree female relative (i.e., mother, sister, daughter) <65 years old
+ 1   Current cigarette smoking
+ 1   Hypertension (>140/90 mm Hg on multiple measurements on several occasions), or currently taking antihypertensive medications
+ 1   Low HDL cholesterol (<40 mg/dL), confirmed by multiple measurements

Negative risk factors

− 1   High HDL cholesterol (>60 mg/dL), confirmed by multiple measurements

Total risk factors = _____(positive risk factors + negative risk factor)

Risk Factors	LDL Goal
Without CHD, and 0–1 risk factors	<160 mg/dL
Without CHD, and 2 or more risk factors	<30 mg/dL
With CHD or CHD risk equivalents	<100 mg/dL

CHD and CHD risk equivalents

• CHD = myocardial infarction (MI), significant myocardial ischemia (angina), history of coronary artery bypass graft (CABG), history of coronary angioplasty, angiographic evidence of lesions, carotid endarterectomy, abdominal aortic aneurysm, peripharal vascular disease (claudication), thrombotic/embolic stroke, transient ischemic attack (TIA)
• Diabetes mellitus
• Multiple risk factors that confer a 10-year CHD risk of > 20%

and collate outcome data. One of the pharmacists is responsible for periodically entering data. The information garnered from these efforts would be used to identify areas needing improvement, to market the program to other providers, and to ensure payment from third-party payers.

POLICIES AND PROCEDURES

To help provide an organized approach to service delivery, a policies and procedures manual should be created to guide pharmacy staff during program implementation. The policies and procedures manual is a comprehensive road map to the service, providing information regarding the purpose of the service, patient eligibility, how patients will be evaluated, what happens during each clinic visit, and the documentation that will be kept. Also, a copy of all forms, patient educational tools, patient assessments, and protocols are included in the manual. The policies and procedures manual is a dynamic document that must be updated and changed as new information becomes known or as the program is modified.

The policies and procedures document should be kept at the pharmacy, used as a training tool for pharmacists and other personnel, and referred to as needed during the patient care process. It should be easy to access information in the manual. A table of contents should be included, sections tabbed, and an appendix created containing the forms that will be part of the

Table 25-2. Medication Management Protocol Example

1. Perform fasting lipoprotein analysis and risk factor assessment.
   a. If the patient has 0 to 1 risk factor (10-year risk usually < 10%)
      (1) If LDL < 130 mg/dL
         (a) Provide education on healthy life habits and risk factor reduction strategies.
         (b) Repeat fasting lipoprotein analysis and risk factor assessment in 5 years.
      (2) If their LDL = 130–139 mg/dL
         (a) Provide education on healthy life habits and risk factor reduction strategies.
         (b) Repeat fasting lipoprotein analysis and risk factor assessment in 1 year.
      (3) If LDL ≥ 160 mg/dL
         (a) Initiate therapeutic lifestyle changes (TLCs) for 3 months.
            (1) Reduce intake of saturated fats and cholesterol
            (2) Weight reduction
            (3) Increased physical activity
         (b) After 3 months, reassess LDL.
            (1) If LDL < 160 mg/dL, continue TLCs.
            (2) If LDL = 160–189 mg/dL, continue TLCs and consider LDL-lowering medications in certain high-risk patients.
            (3) If LDL ≥ 190 mg/dL, continue TLCs and consider adding LDL-lowering medications.
   b. If the patient has multiple (2+) risk factors and the 10-year risk is 10–20%
      (1) If LDL < 130 mg/dL
         (a) Provide education on healthy life habits and risk factor reduction strategies.
         (b) Repeat fasting lipoprotein analysis and risk factor assessment in 1 year.
      (2) If LDL ≥ 130 mg/dL
         (a) Initiate TLCs for 3 months.
            (1) Reduce intake of saturated fats and cholesterol.
            (2) Weight reduction
            (3) Increased physical activity
         (b) After 3 months, reassess LDL.
            (1) If LDL < 130 mg/dL, continue TLCs.
            (2) If LDL ≥ 130 mg/dL, continue TLCs abd consider LDL-lowering medications.
   c. If the patient has multiple (2+) risk factors and the 10-year risk < 10%
      (1) If LDL < 130 mg/dL
         (a) Provide education on healthy life habits and risk factor reduction strategies.
         (b) Repeat fasting lipoprotein analysis and risk factor assessment in 1 year.
      (2) If LDL ≥ 130 mg/dL
         (a) Initiate TLCs for 3 months.
            (1) Reduce intake of saturated fats and cholesterol.
            (2) Weight reduction
            (3) Increased physical activity

(Continued)

Table 25-2. Medication Management Protocol Example *(Continued)*

    (b) After 3 months, reassess LDL.
        (1) If LDL ≤ 160 mg/dL, continue TLCs.
        (2) If LDL ≥ 160 mg/dL, continue TLCs and consider LDL-lowering medications
  d. If the patient has CHD or CHD risk equivalents
    (1) If LDL ≥ 130 mg/dL
      (a) TLCs
      (b) LDL-lowering medications
        (1) If LDL < 100 mg/dL, continue these therapeutic interventions.
        (2) If LDL = 100–129 mg/dL, consider other therapeutic options.
      (c) If LDL = 100–129 mg/dL
        (1) TLCs
        (2) Therapeutic options
      (d) If LDL < 100 mg/dL
        (1) TLCs
        (2) Control other risk factors

program. Also, published medical guidelines and key articles from the primary literature should be included in the manual.

▮ REVISITING THE SCENARIO: POLICIES AND PROCEDURES FOR THE CARE-RITE PHARMACY CHECK-UP SERVICE

The Care-Rite pharmacists created a comprehensive policies and procedures document for their Pharmacy Check-up Service. They determined that the purpose of their program is to

- Manage the drug therapy of high-risk patients. The criteria chosen to define the target population for the program were patients who used four or more chronic oral medications and had at least one chronic medical condition.
- Assess patients for drug therapy problems.
- Resolve drug therapy problems by working collaboratively with patients, physicians, and other prescribers.

- Provide comprehensive and ongoing education to patients and/or family members about common drug therapy problems, therapeutic goals, and the importance of becoming informed consumers of their own health care.

Next, they developed their policies for the program. The policies contained information regarding the evaluation of patients. The initial evaluation will occur after the patient is enrolled into the Pharmacy Check-up Service by either a physician or self-referral. A patient chart will be created containing the patient's demographic information and medical and medication histories. The patients will sign an authorization to release medical information form and a lipid clinic contract that outlines the patient's responsibilities in the program. To be eligible for the program, patients must meet the eligibility criteria. Patients must be able to attend clinic appointments, must agree to come in for scheduled follow-up visits at the pharmacy, and should have the capacity to understand their health condition and the implications for therapy. Also, patients must be willing to be active participants in their health maintenance.

It was decided that there will be an initial visit and one to three follow-up visits within a 12-month period. All sessions will include a comprehensive review of medications, vital signs and laboratory values (as needed), patient education (as needed), and physician communication.

The initial session will last approximately 45 to 60 minutes, and the follow-up visits will last approximately 20 to 30 minutes. The follow-up visits will occur at 3-month intervals depending on the clinical situation. Pharmacists will assess the following information at each visit:

- Patient vital signs
- Dietary considerations
- Patient laboratory values
- Family history
- Medication history
- General activity
- Social history, including alcohol use and smoking
- Health problems
- Compliance with therapy
- Signs and symptoms of intolerance to a drug

Medication and/or dosage changes will be made, if necessary, based on the pharmacists' assessment, and patients will be counseled on these changes. The physician communication form will be used to communicate clinical recommendations regarding drug therapy. Also, patient education will be reinforced and documented. Patients will be instructed on when to return to the clinic, and referrals to physicians will occur as needed. The referrals are based on patient complications of therapy or condition and patient resistance to therapy.

The documentation will occur via a patient chart. Subjective patient information and objective laboratory data will be stored in the chart. Assessments of patients during the clinic visit will be documented in pharmacy progress notes contained in the chart. Acceptance of pharmacy recommendations by physicians will constitute an order change, and this will be documented in the patient record as well. Lastly, patient

outcomes (i.e., clinical, knowledge, and satisfaction) will be documented in the patient record.

The other components of the policies and procedures manual include the medication management protocol and detailed instructions on use of the Cholestech LDX analyzer. The appendix of the policies and procedure manual contains copies of the forms and patient educational tools used in the program.

PHARMACIST TRAINING

As with any successful implementation of a pharmacy service, education and training of pharmacy staff prior to the implementation of the service are essential for success. Pharmacists should achieve proficiency in providing the service before the start date of the service. The time needed to train pharmacy staff depends on the complexity of the service and the experience of the staff. Not only do the pharmacists need to be knowledgeable about the service, but they also may need to practice some of the skills required for some services (e.g., giving a flu shot or completing a lipid panel). Therefore, there should be sufficient practice and a demonstration of competence before they work with actual patients. To help illustrate how the education and training can occur, the preparation of pharmacists at Care-Rite Pharmacy for their Pharmacy Check-up Service will be discussed.

REVISITING THE SCENARIO: PHARMACIST TRAINING FOR THE CARE-RITE PHARMACY CHECK-UP SERVICE

Care-Rite Pharmacy developed a comprehensive pharmacist educational/training program for its Pharmacy Check-up Service. This educational program had multiple components and activities that the pharmacists needed to demonstrate knowledge of or proficiency in before they were ready for service implementation. Initially, it was determined that a general knowledge of pharmaceutical care, types and categories of drug therapy problems, and how to perform a patient assessment should be the foundation for the rest of the education. To help improve pharmacists' knowledge of this topic, the pharmacists were responsible for reading several articles on pharmaceutical care delivery from the primary literature, a general overview of patient medication assessment from a therapeutics textbook, and articles on how to communicate to physicians and other prescribers. The readings were standardized so that the pharmacists were all learning from the same materials. They were given 4 weeks to read all the material and also given 10 standardized patient cases to work up to demonstrate their knowledge. At the end of the 4 weeks, a 3-hour review of the material and cases was scheduled so that the pharmacists could discuss their cases and ask any questions regarding the material.

Carol had hired a local clinical pharmacist who had expertise in ambulatory care as a consultant to assist with the pharmacists' education and skills development. The clinical consultant facilitated the case discussions. The cases that were developed for this program required pharmacists to assess and modify patients' dietary habits and activity levels. Also, they needed to identify and develop plans for resolving drug therapy problems. They practiced writing recommendations to physicians on the physician communication form.

The next component of the pharmacists' education was demonstrating their abilities to perform a finger stick and a lipid panel. The pharmacists first watched a video provided by Cholestech that demonstrated these two activities. Also, a component of the training included information regarding CLIA, the importance of good technique when performing a test, OSHA requirements, and discussions about the reduction of exposure to blood-borne pathogens. The pharmacists were given adequate time to practice using the Cholestech LDX analyzer. Once the practice was over, pharmacists were assessed on their competency to perform the test. A checklist with required activities that needed to be completed during a lipid panel was used as the grading criterion. Once the pharmacists were capable of providing the test, their proficiency with the Cholestech LDX analyzer was documented and stored in their personnel files.

■ MANAGING THE MARKETING MIX

Once the service is ready for implementation, recruiting patients into the program becomes the next activity. This requires a basic knowledge of marketing principles that were covered in Chapters 20 and 21. The marketing mix is viewed commonly as the eight P's of marketing: product, place, price, promotion, process management, personnel, physical facilities, and productivity. Successful implementation of a value-added service requires that pharmacists manage the marketing mix. An illustration of how Care-Rite Pharmacy managed its marketing mix is provided below.

■ REVISITING THE SCENARIO: MARKETING THE CARE-RITE PHARMACY CHECK-UP SERVICE

The product that Care-Rite Pharmacy is marketing is its Pharmacy Check-up Service. As discussed throughout this chapter, much attention has been given to developing each component of the service and planning for its implementation so that it is perceived as a quality service by patients and other providers. Also, pharmacists updated their knowledge regarding pharmaceutical care and medication assessments and developed proficiency for testing patients' lipid panels. They hope to be perceived as knowledgeable and competent when providing the service. Lastly, protocols, policies and procedures, and standardized forms were all created to ensure consistency in service delivery among the providers.

The next marketing-mix variables that need careful consideration are the place and physical facility. Care-Rite Pharmacy will be providing the Pharmacy Check-up Service on site. Therefore, pharmacy staff need to consider patient privacy and space to provide the service. In preparation for this service, Carol did some remodeling of her pharmacy. She created two semiprivate patient areas using office partitions. One area was designated as the area where lipid testing would be performed. The Cholestech LDX analyzer and its supplies were stored in this area. Also, CLIA and OSHA guidelines were kept there as well. The second patient care area was created in case there were multiple appointments at the same time. Both areas had a small table, three chairs, and a computer terminal as standard equipment. Price is the third marketing-mix variable. Carol and the pharmacy staff spent considerable time discussing the price of their service. They estimated the length of the time for each session, estimated the costs to provide the service, researched the price of office visits for other providers, and determined the profit level they needed to help them develop a pricing structure for their service. While no local pharmacies provided a pharmacy check-up service, Carol decided to price the service to be competitive with similar services offered by physicians. The pricing structure for the service is as follows:

- Initial visit: $75
- Follow-up visits: $40 each
- Fasting lipid panel: $50

The pharmacists will monitor patient responses to these prices and their profitability before making any adjustments.

The next marketing-mix component is promotion. Care-Rite has selected several promotional strategies to market its services. Also, Carol has created a marketing budget for the practice. The pharmacists will use press releases in the local newspaper to announce the new service. Next, they decided to run an advertisement in the local newspaper twice per month promoting this service. They chose Sunday and Mondays as the days they would place the ads in the newspaper. Sunday was chosen because of the large readership of the newspaper, and Monday was chosen because the newspaper had a special health section on that day. Also, they purchased airtime on their local cable TV to promote the service. They selected channels that had a viewership of consumers whose demographics matched with their target markets (e.g., women over age 50). They placed an ad for the program in a local magazine that was directed toward women, and they created a new ad for their pharmacy in the local telephone directory.

One of the pharmacists began to call on physicians so that he could promote the services face to face. The pharmacist met with some of the local pharmaceutical company representatives to find out which physicians should be identified as key targets for the promotional efforts. Also, the pharmacy created a physician newsletter entitled, "Progress Notes," that would be sent every other month to key physicians. The format of the newsletter includes sections on new drug updates, clinical pearls, and message updates about Care-Rite Pharmacy. The first newsletter was dedicated to the Pharmacy Check-up Service.

In-store signage and patient brochures were created to help market the program to current pharmacy patients. Pharmacists were instructed to market the program to patients they encountered who were receiving four or more chronic oral medications. A mailing list was created from the pharmacy's computer system from patients taking four or more chronic oral medications. A brochure describing the program was sent to each of those patients. Lastly, bag stuffers and monthly patient billing statements included information about the new program.

Process management, the next marketing-mix variable, refers to how Care-Rite Pharmacy incorporated the new Pharmacy Check-up Service into its existing practice. Workflow decisions were made regarding patient flow during the service. It was decided that the service would be by appointment only to minimize disruption of the other aspects of the practice. Schedules for pharmacists were created so that one pharmacist was responsible for clinic services while another covered the dispensing area.

The last marketing-mix variable that needs addressing is personnel. Care-Rite's pharmacists and staff were trained and assessed to ensure that they had adequate knowledge and skills regarding all aspects of pharmacotherapy management. Also, pharmacists need to take responsibility for the success or failure for the program. This means that they should continue to identify patient candidates for the lipid management program, use various promotional strategies to increase the community's awareness of the program, and ensure that they have the knowledge and skills to provide quality care to patients. Carol changed the format of her annual evaluations of pharmacists to include reviewing their impact on the Pharmacy Check-up Service. As a reward for their efforts, she has agreed to cover the costs of their continuing education each year and attendance at one national pharmacy meeting of their choice.

ONGOING MONITORING OF VALUE-ADDED SERVICES

Once the service is implemented, several strategies should be in place to provide ongoing monitoring to ensure program quality and success. Regularly scheduled staff meetings should be considered, especially early during the implementation phase. These meetings should be used to discuss the number of patients who have enrolled, patient and physician acceptance of the service, feedback that has been received, and areas that need improvement. Staff can provide their own feedback on how they perceive the program's effectiveness and how it can be improved. These meetings can be used as educational offerings for the pharmacists to keep their therapeutic knowledge up to date. It is important to keep a time limit on these meetings to minimize disruption of the practice.

Another strategy to ensure program quality is to monitor the outcomes of the service of interest to the practice itself. One of the goals for service implementation is to create new business and generate a profit for the pharmacy. The goals should be realistic and challenging to ensure economic viability for the practice. Pharmacists need to be held accountable for their efforts to help the practice reach its goals. Service outcomes that may be of interest to pharmacy staff are number of patients enrolled, revenue generated from the service, number of physician referrals, and profitability of the service (revenues minus expenses). If the service is not profitable, then it needs to be either eliminated or altered (price increases or improved service delivery efficiencies).

An additional continuous quality improvement strategy is to request feedback from patients who have completed the program and physicians who have referred patients to the pharmacy. The feedback could be as simple as a one-page questionnaire asking open-ended questions to provide more qualitative comments about the service. The information that is gathered from these surveys and/or questionnaires can be used to improve patient and physician perception of the service. Furthermore, the request for feedback gives the impression that the practice is proactive toward meeting the needs of patients and other providers.

REVISITING THE SCENARIO: CARE-RITE PHARMACY'S CONTINUOUS QUALITY IMPROVEMENT STRATEGIES

Carol decided to schedule pharmacy staff meetings twice monthly on the second Tuesday and fourth Thursday of each month. Those days were selected to ensure that all staff members had the opportunity to attend at least one meeting monthly. The meetings were scheduled at 11:00 a.m. because this usually is the least busy time for the pharmacy. The time limit for the meetings was 1 hour. The format of the meetings were as follows:

- Review of service outcomes (i.e., patient enrollment, revenue generation, and physician referrals): 5 minutes
- Pharmacists' discussion of program improvements: 15 to 20 minutes
- Review of feedback from patients and/or physicians: 5 to 10 minutes
- Miscellaneous issues: 5 to 10 minutes
- Therapeutic updates for pharmacists: 20 to 25 minutes

Carol is tracking the service outcomes over time and documenting pharmacists' activities to ensure successful program implementation. She informed the staff about the change in their annual evaluations to include reviews of their impact on the program. Also, she developed a patient satisfaction survey that patients are given after completing the program. A one-page physician questionnaire has been developed and is sent to physicians who have had patients enrolled in the service.

COLLABORATIVE PRACTICE AGREEMENTS

Collaborative practice agreements (CPAs) are a strategy that pharmacists can use to integrate their value-added services with physicians (Ferro, 1998). CPAs are used to formalize relationships between providers. They spell out the responsibilities of each provider and the acceptance of mutually agreed-on drug therapy management protocols. Although CPAs are an important aspect of service implementation, they require that pharmacists develop working relationships with physicians. The development of collaborative working relationships (CWRs) between providers is a four-stage process, with the final stage usually representing the time when physicians are most comfortable signing off on a CPA (McDonough and Doucette, 2001).

Although physicians and pharmacists may be aware of one another in a certain community, they may not be collaborating, and they may communicate only during discrete episodes of care (stage 0: professional awareness). Pharmacists who are interested in developing services that require the sharing of patient information and regular communication with physicians and other providers will need to increase their interaction with these other providers. For example, the owner of Care-Rite Pharmacy could meet with physicians in her community and discuss her desire to start an MTM service. During these meetings, she could provide the physicians with preliminary protocols and communication forms and request their feedback. By increasing her communication and face-to-face interactions, she moves into the next stage of the collaborative working relationship (stage 1: professional recognition).

In the professional recognition stage, physicians not only are aware that a pharmacy exists, but they also recognize that something is different about the practice. Since not all pharmacies are providing MTM services, Carol has set herself and her practice apart from other pharmacies in her community. Although

attainment of stage 1 is important early in the working relationship between providers, not much information sharing is occurring yet. Therefore, pharmacists need to develop closer and stronger professional relationships with other providers. In Carol's situation, she requested and received feedback from one physician group regarding her protocol. The physicians in this practice, although initially skeptical of this new service, believed that some of their patients might benefit from the pharmacy's education regarding risk factors, medications, and lifestyle modifications. Therefore, it was agreed that they would refer one or two patients to Care-Rite's Pharmacy Check-up Program (stage 2: exploration and trial).

The exploration and trial stage is one in which physicians are ready to try the service. It is important that pharmacy staff are ready to perform at a high level because the physicians will be monitoring their patients' progress closely. Following along with the chapter's scenario, Carol's staff was fully prepared to provide high-quality services for the two patients that were referred to the program. They worked up the patients, performed the medication management services, provided the patient education, and communicated back to the physicians after each patient appointment. After the patients completed several appointments with the pharmacists, Carol met with the physicians to seek their input regarding the program. The feedback was positive, and the physicians' recommendations to improve the program and communication flow were integrated into the program. The physicians agreed to refer more patients to the Pharmacy Check-up Service (stage 3: professional relationship expansion).

If physicians and other provides are satisfied with the quality and efficiency of a pharmacy service, they may be willing to increase their referrals. It is during this stage that communication between providers becomes more bilateral, and physicians and pharmacists are exchanging information more equally. Also, physicians begin to develop expectations about the pharmacists and the service. It is important during this stage that pharmacists maintain or increase the quality of the service so that physicians see a benefit to referring patients. If pharmacists perform consistently and at a

Management by Care-Rite Pharmacists

1. Care-Rite pharmacists will complete lab orders and coordinate the draw (finger stick) to fit the patient's schedule.
2. The patient's fasting lipid panel, cardiovascular risk factors, and dietary and exercise habits will be assessed.
3. Care-Rite Pharmacists will follow the protocol mutually agreed to by the physician to manage the patient's lipid therapy.
4. Care-Rite Pharmacists will communicate their assessment and recommendations to the physician via fax.
5. The physician will communicate via fax with their response to the pharmacists' recommendations within 24 hours.
6. If the physician agrees to the recommendations, their signature should constitute a new order and the pharmacists will carry out thier orders.
7. Pharmacists will schedule patients for follow-up visits at the designated times discussed in the policy and procedures manual.
8. Ultimately, the physician is responsible for the care of the patient and at anytime can discontinue the patient's involvement in the program.

_____   _____
              Physician Signature   Date

_____   _____
              Pharmacist Signature   Date

Figure 25-7. Collaborative practice agreement for the Pharmacy Check-up Program.

high level, they may earn the right to develop a CPA with the physicians (stage 4: collaborative working relationship).

In the final stage, the collaborative working relationship, pharmacists have proven their clinical abilities, performed reliably and consistently, and gained the trust of physicians. Because of this trust, physicians are now willing to sign a CPA. This is the case with Care-Rite Pharmacy. Carol and her pharmacists consistently helped the physicians' patients reach their goals of therapy. The patients became more compliant with lifestyle changes, and they spoke positively of their experience working with the pharmacists. At Carol's next meeting with the physicians, she discussed developing a CPA, and the physicians agreed to sign it and refer patients regularly to her practice.

The components of the CPA include the information contained in the policies and procedures manual, drug therapy management protocols, and pharmacist/physician responsibilities. Pharmacists should seek input from physicians regarding patient eligibility criteria and drug therapy management protocols. Once this information is agreed to, then physicians and pharmacists should sign an agreement form. A copy of the CPA should be kept at the pharmacy and at the physician practice. An example of a CPA for Care-Rite Pharmacy is shown in Fig. 25-7.

CONCLUSION

Pharmacists are implementing several types of value-added services in their practices. It is important that they follow a systematic process during development and implementation of these services so that the services are of high quality. Regardless of the service being implemented, the process remains the same. First, pharmacists need to determine the essential components of the service (e.g., data collection, medication management, patient education, etc.). Next, they should develop a policies and procedures manual that provides the purpose of the service, patient selection, and a description of each patient visit. Also, it is important that pharmacists are trained to provide quality and efficient care. For a pharmacy to be successful, management will need to manage the marketing mix (the eight P's of marketing) and develop collaborative working relationships with other providers.

Pharmacists can ensure their success with program implementation if they follow these steps. By preplanning and preparing before service initiation, pharmacists can minimize the challenges with any new startup program. As part of their preparation, the development of documentation tools, protocols, and physician communication forms is essential. Lastly, as they develop a trusting relationship with other providers and begin to receive regular referrals, a CPA may need to be created. With this document, pharmacists and physicians will know each other's roles, and an efficient exchange of information begins to occur.

■ QUESTIONS FOR FURTHER DISCUSSION

1. This chapter emphasized that the process of implementing value-added services remains the same regardless of the service. What may be some differences in the forms used, protocols, and CPAs if the service were a diabetes educational program instead of a medication management service?
2. Discuss how the eight P's of marketing may be similar/different from the scenario used in this chapter and a pharmacist implementing a heart failure clinic.
3. Think about a value-added service that you have an interest in implementing. What are the components of the service?

REFERENCES

Ansell JE, Buttaro JL, Thomas OV, Knowlton CH. 1997. The anticoagulation guidelines task force: Consensus guidelines for coordinated outpatient oral anticoagulation therapy management. *Ann Pharmacother* 31:604.

Baran RW, Crumlish K, Patterson H, et al. 1999. Improving outcomes of community-dwelling older patients with diabetes through pharmacist counseling. *Am J Health-Syst Pharm* 56:1535.

Berringer R, Shibely MC, Cary CC, et al. 1999. Outcomes of a community pharmacy-based diabetes monitoring program. *J Am Pharm Assoc* 39:791.

Centers for Medicare and Medicaid Services. 2003. What is waived testing? Available at www.fda.gov/cdrh/ clia; accessed on June 14, 2003.

Christensen DB, Holmes G, Fassatt WE, et al. 1999. Influence of a financial incentive on cognitive services: CARE project design/implementation. *J Am Pharm Assoc* 39:629.

Coast-Senior EA, Kroner BA, Kelley CL, Trilli LE. 1998. Management of patients with type 2 diabetes by pharmacists in primary care clinics. *Ann Pharmacother* 32:636.

Cowper PA, Weinberger M, Hanlon JT, et al. 1998. The cost-effectiveness of a clinical pharmacist intervention among elderly outpatients. *Pharmacotherapy* 18:327.

Davis FB, Sczupak CA. 1979. Outpatient oral anticoagulation: Guidelines for long-term management. *Postgrad Med* 66:100.

Dobie RL, Rascati KL. 1994. Documenting the value of pharmacist interventions. *Am Pharm* 34:50.

Elliott ME, Meek PD, Kanous NL, et al. 2002. Osteoporosis screening by community pharmacists: Use of national osteoporosis foundation resources. *J Am Pharm Assoc* 42:101.

Ferro LA, Marcrom RE, Garrelts L, et al. 1998. Collaborative practice agreements between pharmacists and physicians. *J Am Pharm Assoc* 38:655.

Furmaga EM. 1993. Pharmacist management of a hyperlipidemia clinic. *Am J Hosp Pharm* 50:91.

Grainger-Rousseau TJ, Miralles MA, Hepler CD, et al. 1997. Therapeutic outcomes monitoring: Application of pharmaceutical care guidelines to community pharmacy. *J Am Pharm Assoc* NS37:647.

Hanlon JT, Weinberger M, Samsa GP, et al. 1996. A randomized, controlled trial of a clinical pharmacist intervention to improve inappropriate prescribing in elderly outpatients with polypharmacy. *Am J Med* 100:428.

Hawkins DW, Fiedler FP, Douglas HL, Eschbach RC. 1979. Evaluation of a clinical pharmacist in caring for hypertensive and diabetic patients. *Am J Hosp Pharm* 36:321.

Herborg H, Sondergaard B, Froekjaer B, et al. 2001. Improving drug therapy for patients with asthma: 2.

Use of antiasthma medications. *J Am Pharm Assoc* 41: 551.

Jaber LA, Halapy H, Fernet M, et al. 1996. Evaluation of a pharmaceutical care model on diabetes management. *Ann Pharmacother* 30:238.

Kennedy DT, Giles JT, Chang ZG, et al. 2002. Results of a smoking cessation clinic in community pharmacy practice. *J Am Pharm Assoc* 42:51.

Knapp KK, Katzman H, Hambright JS, Albrant DH. 1998. Community pharmacist interventions in a capitated pharmacy benefit contract. *Am J Health-Syst Pharm* 55:1141.

Knoell DL, Pierson JF, Marsh CB, et al. 1998. Measurement of outcomes in adults receiving pharmaceutical care in a comprehensive asthma outpatient clinic. *Pharmacotherapy* 18:1365.

Knowlton CH, Thomas OV, Willamson A, et al. 1999. Establishing community-based anticoagulation education and monitoring programs. *J Am Pharm Assoc* 39:368.

Madejski RM, Madejski TJ. 1996. Cholesterol screening in a community pharmacy. *J Am Pharm Assoc* NS36:243.

McCurdy M. 1993. Oral anticoagulation monitoring in a community pharmacy. *Am Pharm* 10:61.

McDonough RP. 1996. Interventions to improve patient pharmaceutical care outcomes. *J Am Pharm Assoc* NS36:453.

McDonough RP, Doucette WR. 2001. A conceptual framework for collaborative working relationships between pharmacists and physicians. *J Am Pharm Assoc* 41:682.

McKenney JM, Brown ED, Necsary R, Reavis HL. 1978. Effect of pharmacist drug monitoring and patient education on hypertensive patients. *Contemp Pharm Pract* 1:50.

McKenney JM, Sliining JM, Henderson HR, et al. 1973. The effect of clinical pharmacy services on patients with essential hypertension. *Circulation* 1973;48:1104.

Norton JL, Gibson DL. 1996. Establishing an outpatient anticoagulation clinic in a community hospital. *Am J Health-Syst Pharm* 53:1151.

Pauley TR, Magee MJ, Cury JD. Pharmacists-managed physician-directed asthma management program reduces emergency department visits. *Ann Pharmacother* 29:5.

Petty DR, Zermansky AG, Raynor DK, et al. 2002. Clinical medication review by a pharmacists of elderly patients on repeat medications in general practice: Pharmacist interventions and review outcomes. *Int J Pharm Pract* 10:39.

Reinders TP, Rush DR, Baumgartner RP, Graham AW. Pharmacist's role in management of hypertensive patients in an ambulatory care clinic. *Am J Hosp Pharm* 32:590.

Reinders TP, Steinke WE. 1979. Pharmacist management of anticoagulant therapy in ambulant patients. *Am J Hosp Pharm* 36:645.

Rosenthal W. 2000. Establishing a pharmacy-based laboratory service. *J Am Pharm Assoc* 40:146.

Rupp MT. 1988. Evaluation of prescribing errors and pharmacist interventions in community practice: An estimate of "value added." *Am Pharm* NS28:766.

Rupp MT. 1992. Value of community pharmacists' interventions to correct prescribing errors. *Ann Pharmacother* 26:1580.

Rupp MT, DeYoung M, Schondelmeyer SW. 1992. Prescribing problems and pharmacist interventions in community practice. *Med Care* 30:926.

Rupp MT, McCallian DJ, Sheth KK. 1997. Developing and marketing a community pharmacy–based asthma management program. *J Am Pharm Assoc* NS37:694.

Schilling KW. 1977. Pharmacy program for monitoring diabetic patients. *Am J Hosp Pharm* 34:1242.

Simpson SH, Johnson JA, Tsuyuki RT. 2001. Economic impact of community pharmacist intervention in cholesterol risk management: An evaluation of the study of cardiovascular risk intervention by pharmacists. *Pharmacotherapy* 21:627.

Smith DH, Fassatt WE, Christensen DB. 1999. Washington State CARE project: Downstream cost changes associated with the provision of cognitive services by pharmacists. *J Am Pharm Assoc* 39:650.

Strand LM, Cipolle RJ, Morley PC. 1988. Documenting the clinical pharmacist's activities: Back to basics. *Drug Intell Clin Pharm* 2:63.

Strand LM, Cipolle RJ, Morley PC. 1992. Pharmaceutical care: An introduction. In *Current Concepts,* p. 1. Kalamazoo, MI: Upjohn Company.

Swain JH, Macklin R. 2001. Individualized diabetes care in a rural community pharmacy. *J Am Pharm Assoc* 41:458.

Tice B, Phillips CR. 2002. Implementation and evaluation of a lipid screening program in a large chain pharmacy. *J Am Pharm Assoc* 42:413.

Tiggelaar JM. 1987. Protocols for the treatment of essential hypertension and type II diabetes mellitus by pharmacists in ambulatory care clinics. *Drug Intell Clin Pharm* 21:521.

Tsukuki RT, Johnson JA, Teo KK, et al. 1999. Study of cardiovascular risk intervention by pharmacists (SCRIP): A randomized trial design of the effect of community pharmacist intervention program on serum cholesterol risk. *Ann Pharmacother* 33:910.

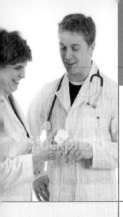

26

COMPENSATION FOR VALUE-ADDED PHARMACY SERVICES

Kathleen Snella

About the Author: Dr. Snella is the Assistant Dean of the University of Missouri–Kansas City School of Pharmacy and Vice Chair and Associate Professor for the Division of Pharmacy Practice in Columbia, Missouri. Her pharmacy education includes a B.S. in pharmacy from the University of Iowa and a Pharm.D. from the University of Texas–Austin/University of Texas Health Sciences Center, San Antonio. She also completed a specialty residency in primary care at the William S. Middleton Veterans Hospital in Madison, Wisconsin. Dr. Snella has been working in the area of compensation for pharmacist services for over 10 years. She has provided value-added services in both private physician offices and hospital outpatient clinics. She is invited frequently to speak regarding pharmacist service compensation and has authored several articles and book chapters on this topic.

▓ LEARNING OBJECTIVES

After completing this chapter, students should be able to

1. Describe the difference between compensation and reimbursement.
2. Identify different reimbursement strategies that are available to various pharmacy environments.
3. Describe how pharmacist–insurance payer relationships influence the choice of compensation strategies.
4. Identify the advantages and disadvantages of various compensation strategies.

▓ SCENARIO

Now that Alan Brouchard (see Chapter 24) had his diabetes education clinic outlined, he wants to explore how to make the service financially viable. He has designed a service that would offer comprehensive diabetes education. Since patients with diabetes are at increased risk for heart disease, his patients might benefit from cholesterol education/monitoring, smoking cessation, and blood pressure monitoring. To offer both these types of services, he needs a way to check blood glucose and hemoglobin A_{1c} levels, cholesterol levels, and blood pressure in addition to having a variety of diabetes education materials available.

Before Dr. Brouchard can begin providing these services, he wants to make sure that his program is financially feasible. To do this, he needs to explore ways to be compensated for his services. He is familiar with being compensated for durable medical equipment, so he knows the pharmacy can bill for blood glucose meters, but he has never tried to bill third-party payers or patients for other types of services.

CHAPTER QUESTIONS

1. Why should compensation rather than reimbursement be the goal for payment for value-added services?
2. What types of costs should be considered when determining a compensation fee?
3. How does being viewed as a provider influence the ability to be compensated?
4. How can compensation be optimized within various pharmacy settings?

INTRODUCTION

Pharmacists offer many types of value-added services, including education, preventive health services, laboratory monitoring, and management of medication-intensive health conditions. Chapter 25 reviewed several examples of value-added services that can be provided, including medication therapy management (MTM) services, anticoagulation and hyperlipidemia monitoring, smoking cessation, osteoporosis screening, and cardiovascular risk assessment. For these services to be successful over the long term, each should be feasible financially. This chapter will focus on compensation for value-added services from both patients and third-party payers.

When first exploring compensation strategies, it is important to understand the terminology used in direct patient care billing. Throughout this chapter, terminology will be introduced, such as compensation, reimbursement, provider status, Clinical Laboratory Improvement Amendments (CLIA)-waived testing, Current Procedural Terminology (CPT) codes, and International Classification of Diseases (ICD-9-CM) codes. Understanding the language of compensation is important, especially when discussing compensation strategies with health insurance companies. This chapter will review the strategies that can be used to bill patients and third-party payers for direct patient care services. The specific strategy that can be used may depend on the practice location, the specific third-party payer involved, and in some cases the type of service offered.

COMPENSATION

The difference between compensation and reimbursement is one of the first concepts that require further explanation. One of the goals of value-added services is to receive *compensation* for services. This means that the patient, insurance company, or some other entity has paid for the direct cost of the service *plus* the perceived value of that service. *Reimbursement,* on the other hand, is payment for only the direct cost of the service *without* any payment above that (Hogue, 2002). In order to have a profitable service, compensation should be targeted instead of reimbursement. If only reimbursement is targeted, then only the direct costs of providing the service, such as payment for supplies, is recovered, and the net revenue may be minimal.

Compensation can come from many different types of services. Examples include weight-loss counseling, education/management of asthma, lipid and osteoporosis monitoring, and general MTM. Pharmacists may also receive compensation for procedures that support these services, such as the collection of blood cholesterol panels via CLIA-waived tests or heel ultrasounds. Another example is the provision of immunizations, such as influenza and pneumonia vaccinations. All these services can be grouped into direct patient care services (e.g., smoking-cessation counseling), laboratory services (e.g., CLIA-waived testing), procedures (e.g., bone mineral density assessments), and immunization services.

COSTS ASSOCIATED WITH OFFERING VALUE-ADDED SERVICES

When providing value-added services, there are always costs involved. Costs in providing direct patient care may include salaries, space, office equipment (e.g., computer, fax machine, and software), photocopying, postage (to mail letters to patients and/or physicians), advertising, patient care equipment (e.g., blood pressure cuffs and scales to check patient weights), and educational material. If laboratory services are going to be offered, then the cost of the license to perform tests, laboratory equipment (e.g., laboratory devices, testing cartridges or strips, and quality-control devices), sharps containers, lancets, gloves, alcohol pads, and biohazard waste removal services also need to be included. The cost to perform procedures such as a heel ultrasound or spirometry can include the cost of the device and any supportive equipment that may be needed. If vaccinations are offered, the cost of the vaccines, gloves, syringes, alcohol pads, and bandages should be considered. Many pharmacies may have some of this equipment on hand already, so it does not need to be purchased specifically for the new service.

To calculate the total costs to provide a service, consider how much pharmacist and supportive personnel time will be involved in offering the service, as well as fixed costs and per-patient costs. One way to estimate how much time will be spent on providing direct patient care is to consider the time spent with each patient and how many patients will be targeted. The pharmacy's computerized database may be able to be supply the number of clients on a specific medication or with a specific health condition. This may help to estimate the number of potential patients for the service. This step is important because one of the first targets for a new value-added service can be the pharmacy's existing clientele. This will also ensure that there is an adequate population of patients to support such a service. Of course, one of the goals of offering a new service may be to increase the number of clients attracted to the pharmacy and therefore to increase prescription volume or prescription-related purchases. A search of the pharmacy database can identify the most common insurance carriers serving these patients and also may help to identify potential referring physicians.

Fixed costs are costs that must be considered regardless of the number of patients enrolled in the service. These may include office equipment, patient care equipment (e.g., blood pressure cuffs and weight scales), and laboratory costs (e.g., licensing costs, laboratory machines, quality controls, and sharps containers). Variable costs typically are those which can be calculated on a per-patient basis, such as the cost of the individual patient laboratory test cartridges/strips, postage, syringes, and gloves. With the estimated number of patients seen, the per-patient costs can be calculated. Together with the salary estimates, the fixed and variable costs can be used to help establish what fee will be charged for the service.

REVISITING THE SCENARIO

Dr. Brouchard has outlined what he would like to offer with this new service. He decides to target patients with type 2 diabetes and to offer comprehensive diabetes self-management education. He wants to educate patients on how to control their diabetes not only with medications but also with healthy eating habits, weight loss, and exercise. He also wants to discuss blood glucose monitoring, management of low blood sugar, and how to manage diabetes during acute illnesses. He also wants to help his patients avoid diabetes complications by helping them to quit smoking, control their blood pressure, and better manage their cholesterol.

To estimate the costs of offering this service, Dr. Brouchard has made a worksheet of all the costs necessary to provide the service. He has reviewed the pharmacy database and has found that there are at least 800 patients who are taking at least one oral agent for diabetes or on insulin therapy and who have been seen in the last 12 months. He realizes that this is just an estimate of the total number of potential patients because some patients may be controlling their diabetes with diet and exercise, but he also knows that he wants to target patients who currently have uncontrolled blood glucose levels.

Dr. Brouchard calculates how much time he can devote to offering these services. He estimates that if he has his patients come into the pharmacy during times when the pharmacy is traditionally slower and when he has another pharmacist assisting in the pharmacy, he can begin by offering appointments for 2 hours each weekday, or 10 hours per week. He also estimates that he would like to reserve 45 minutes for a patient's first visit and 30 minutes for all follow-up visits. Therefore, he estimates that initially he could see one to two new patients and one to four follow-up patients each day. If he recruits from his existing clientele and also targets a few physicians who have been receptive to pharmacist education in the past, he believes that he has enough patients to support this service.

In his fee calculations, he adds the amount of time he will be spending directly with patients into the cost analysis. In addition to using his hourly salary rate, he includes the cost of his fringe benefits into these salary calculations. Because he also anticipates that his pharmacy technician will assist him with paperwork and phone calls, he considers adding a small percentage of a technician's time into the salary calculations.

Dr. Brouchard's next step is to inventory the equipment and supplies he already has available in the pharmacy and what he would need to purchase. There is already space to see patients, and the pharmacy already has a photocopier, fax machine, and computer. He has already located free high-quality diabetes educational brochures from several pharmaceutical companies that can be used to teach his patients. Additional equipment that he needs includes two blood pressure cuffs (one regular- and one large-sized) and an accurate scale for patient weights. He also would like to have two types of finger-stick laboratory testing devices, one that measures hemoglobin A_{1c} levels and one to perform cholesterol panels. He plans to teach each patient how to use his or her blood glucose meter. If they do not already have a meter, the patient will be able to purchase one from the pharmacy.

Additional costs include the finger-stick laboratory testing devices, which require a licensing fee (a CLIA waiver), gloves, bandages, and sharps containers. He assumes for his cost analysis that he will check each patient's hemoglobin A_{1c} an average of three times a year and fasting lipids approximately twice a year. He plans on printing computerized notes to document the education provided, the patient's progress, results of any laboratory tests performed, and goals for the next appointment at the pharmacy. He plans on sending each patient's physician a copy of these reports following each visit.

◼ STRATEGIES FOR COMPENSATION

There are several ways to approach compensation depending on the type of insurance, the pharmacy environment, and the types of services offered. The type of insurance a patient has will have an important influence on the compensation strategy selected. A pharmacy that serves primarily Medicare patients may have different strategies than a pharmacy that serves patients belonging to a health maintenance organization (HMO). The physical location of the service is also a factor that should be considered when seeking compensation. At first glance, the compensation strategies for patient care would seem the same regardless of the location. However, there are several practice locations that have very specific billing practices that can only be used in that particular setting. Strategies that can be used by a pharmacist working in a physician's office may not be the same as those used by pharmacists in a community pharmacy or a hospital-based outpatient clinic. The type of service offered may also influence the compensation strategies (e.g., there may be specific strategies for certain services such as diabetes education and CLIA-waived laboratory testing).

Compensation Based on Type of Payer

First-Party Payers

Compensation traditionally is provided by a patient (e.g., first-party payer) or by an insurance carrier (third-party payers). With first-party payers, the fee for the service is requested directly from the patient. There are advantages and disadvantages to charging patients directly for a clinical service. Advantages include the fact that the pharmacist can ask directly for and immediately receive payment for the service. This eliminates the lag between submitting claims to a third-party payer and the time when compensation is received. Another advantage of billing a patient directly is that all services are theoretically covered. For example, not all third-party insurance carriers cover all types of services, or they may limit the number of times a patient can be seen for a particular health condition. Regardless of whether a patient is a first-party payer or has third-party insurance, the pharmacist always should make sure that the patient understands that there is a charge for the service and how much that charge will be before providing or enrolling the patient in the program. If the patient does not agree to payment or does not see the value of the service, it may be difficult to receive successful compensation for that service.

Third-Party Payers

With third-party payers, compensation is requested from the insurance carrier. The pharmacist or pharmacy typically submits a *claim form* to the insurance carrier describing the service provided and requesting payment for services. Owing to the number of insurance carriers and the types of insurance plans that exist (e.g., fee-for-service, HMO, etc.), each company may have specific requirements regarding this process and different payment strategies. For example, an HMO insurance plan may compensate the pharmacist based on a uniform fee per client regardless of the number of times the pharmacist sees the patient. In contrast, a fee-for-service insurance plan may compensate a pharmacist following each specific patient visit. Despite the differences with each fee-for-service insurance carrier, all patients should be charged the same fee for the same service. In other words, the pharmacist should not charge a patient with insurance more or less than a patient who is paying cash. If these fees are not consistent, the practice may be considered fraudulent (Hogue, 2002; Snella et al., 2004).

Each third-party payer may or may not routinely compensate for pharmacist services. Each third-party payer may also have different processes for submitting claims. In general, there are three methods for requesting compensation, including becoming *creden-*

tialed, requesting prior authorization, and blind submission. Medicare and Medicaid are also examples of third-party payers, but because of their specific nuances regarding compensation, they are addressed separately.

CREDENTIALING Third-party payers typically compensate health care professionals who are enrolled as providers with their health care plan. To do this, the health care professional goes through a *credentialing* process. For example, a third-party payer may have specific criteria that must be met for a pharmacist or any another health care professional to become credentialed (Snella, 1999). If a health care professional meets all the credentialing criteria for an insurance carrier, that professional can be considered a *provider* for the carrier's plan. Being considered a provider means that the carrier has approved that specific professional to be compensated for seeing clients on its plan.

A pharmacist or any other professional does not necessarily have to become an official provider with each insurance carrier. However, an insurance carrier can restrict compensation to only those professionals considered to be providers (e.g., Medicare) or require that the patient be responsible for a larger portion of the bill if an "out of network" or nonapproved provider is seen.

To be credentialed, health care professionals usually are required to submit specific information to the insurance carrier, such as license numbers, malpractice insurance information, board certifications, and copies of diplomas. Health insurance plans may have specific requirements, such as requiring physicians and other health care professionals to have specific credentials, carry a specified amount of malpractice insurance, or be board certified. The health care professional typically submits this information along with an application (Snella, 1999).

When contacting an insurance company to become a provider, it is not unusual for the carrier to be unfamiliar with value-added pharmacist services. Explaining the goals of the service, what is included in the service, the benefits to the client and to the insurance carrier, and the pharmacist's unique capacity to offer such services will help to establish the value of the service to the insurance carrier (Snella, 1999; Snella et al., 2004). Relating your service to published literature that demonstrates the impact of this type of service on decreasing health care costs or improving patient outcomes may be especially motivating to the insurance carrier. Becoming a provider can be a process that requires persistence and perseverance, but when it is successful, it is one of the most potent strategies for compensation.

PRIOR AUTHORIZATION Another way to receive compensation from traditional third-party payers is to contact the payer for *prior authorization.* When using prior authorization, the pharmacist contacts the insurance company with information regarding the referral and requests approval for compensation before seeing the patient. With prior authorization, the insurance company may indicate how many visits will be approved and which billing codes may be used (Snella et al., 2004).

BLIND SUBMISSION Blind submission describes requesting compensation from a third-party payer by submitting a claim and waiting to see if the claim is approved (Snella et al., 2004). There is typically no contact with the insurance carrier prior to submitting the claim. One disadvantage of this method is the risk of having a claim rejected and needing it to be resubmitted to the insurance carrier. It also requires the pharmacist to take the time and effort to provide the service without prior knowledge that he or she will receive any payment for the service. Contacting the insurance carrier prior to submitting a claim should increase the success rate of compensation because the insurance carrier is already familiar with the claim, and the pharmacist may have clarified any questions regarding the claim prior to its submission.

Medicare

Medicare is a government-administered insurance program that is offered to people who are older than 65 years of age, have specific disabilities, or have kidney failure (DHHS, 2002a). The Centers for Medicare and Medicaid Services (CMS) oversees the Medicare program. For services provided in the outpatient setting,

there are two different types of Medicare plans that may influence compensation strategies: Medicare Part B and Medicare Part D. Medicare Part B describes the Medicare insurance that covers outpatient and physician services (CMS, 2007d). Medicare Part D describes the prescription drug coverage that was enacted under the Medicare Modernization Act of 2003 (see Chapter 17). The Medicare Modernization Act also contained language describing MTM for patients with Medicare Part D benefits. Within this act, Medicare Part D recipients who meet criteria based on their medications and medical conditions are eligible to receive MTM by a pharmacist who would help to optimize drug therapy and help to decrease the risk of adverse events (One Hundred Eighth Congress, 2007). All goods and services compensated through Medicare Part D are adjudicated through prescription drug plans (PDPs), which are administered by nongovernmental third-party payers such as insurance companies, HMOs, and pharmacy benefit managers. To receive compensation for MTM and other clinical services provided to eligible Medicare Part D beneficiaries, pharmacists must follow the policies and procedures established by each PDP, which may include the credentialing and prior authorization processes described earlier.

PHARMACISTS AS MEDICARE PROVIDERS CMS recognizes specific groups of health care professionals as providers of Medicare services. Examples of these professionals are physicians, nurse practitioners, physician assistants, nurse midwives, and clinical social workers (Social Security Administration, 2007). Each of these professionals may apply to become a provider with Medicare. Unfortunately, if a health care provider is not recognized within the Social Security Act, then he or she cannot be recognized as a provider (Snella et al., 2004).

In 2003, the Medicare Modernization Act included pharmacists as providers of MTM services for Part D-eligible clients. Although this was an important step forward in obtaining recognition, the Medicare Modernization Act did not recognize pharmacists as providers for Medicare Part B clients. This is an important distinction in that CMS does not currently recognize patient care services provided by pharmacists outside of MTM and other services stipulated in the Medicare Part D regulations.

There are several additional instances when Medicare does recognize pharmacists or pharmacies as providers. One example is when a pharmacist or pharmacy becomes a *mass immunizer*. Another example is when a pharmacy becomes a provider of durable medical equipment (Snella et al., 2004). Pharmacists also may submit claims to Medicare for CLIA-waived laboratory tests, but this recognition is specifically as a CLIA-waived laboratory and not for any other direct patient care or MTM services.

Medicaid

Medicaid is supervised by CMS but is administered by each individual state. In Medicaid, each state determines the list of health care professionals who can be considered as providers. For pharmacists to be considered providers of patient care services for Medicaid, the state can develop a Medicaid demonstration project (Snella, 1999). One example of a demonstration project is the Mississippi Medicaid project in which pharmacists were compensated for services such as asthma, diabetes, and hyperlipidemia management (Anonymous, 1998; Landis, 1998).

REVISITING THE SCENARIO

When Dr. Brouchard estimated the number of patients with type 2 diabetes, he also took note of their insurance carriers. Since Sun City, Arizona, is a major retirement community with strict age requirements for its residents, it was not surprising that most of the people served by the pharmacy were elderly (Northwest Valley Chamber of Commerce, 2007). Most of the patients with type 2 diabetes had Medicare insurance, followed by a variety of third-party insurance carriers. Because Medicare was the main insurance carrier for his patients, Dr. Brouchard knew he would have to consider compensation strategies for those patients with and without Medicare Part D coverage.

For those patients with Medicare Part D coverage, Dr. Brouchard planned on becoming an MTM service provider with several of the PDPs contracting with Medicare. For patients who did not have Medicare Part D coverage, he would be unable to bill Medicare for those claims. Therefore, he would request compensation directly from the patient. He would do the same for patients without any third-party insurance. When he provided CLIA-waived laboratory services, he planned on submitting claims to Medicare and the other third-party payers for the appropriate tests. If the patient had no insurance, he would also request compensation for these laboratory tests directly from the patient.

Compensation Based on the Pharmacy Setting

Most of the strategies discussed thus far can be applied to community pharmacy settings. However, this is not the only setting in which pharmacists offer value-added services. There are two specific practice settings that offer unique compensation strategies for ambulatory care pharmacists: the physician office and the hospital-based outpatient clinic.

Physician Office–Based Practices

Pharmacists who work within a physician office practice share the same compensation strategies as community pharmacies (i.e., billing patients directly and billing third-party payers for services). However, these pharmacists also have an additional avenue for compensation for Medicare Part B patients via the Incident to Physician Services Regulations (DHHS, 2002a). These guidelines allow physicians to bill for a nonphysician's services as long as they are performed while the physician is physically located within the office suite and the nonphysician is offering a service that is an integral part of care and commonly furnished. While there must be physician supervision, the physician does not have to see the patient physically (DHHS, 2002a). If these criteria are met, the physician, not the pharmacist, can request compensation for the service provided by the pharmacist. Only the lowest level of billing (and therefore the lowest level of compensation) is allowed via the Incident to Physician Services Regulations because a physician is not personally seeing the patient. Medicare only allows the Incident to Physician Services

Regulations to be applied to follow-up visits and not to new patients (i.e., those who have not been seen previously by the physician). Since the compensation goes from Medicare to the physician or the clinic, pharmacists may develop a contractual arrangement with the provider or clinic to be compensated for the incident to physician services (e.g., an hourly or per-patient fee) (Snella, 1999).

Hospital-Based Outpatient Clinics

The Outpatient Prospective Payment System (OPPS) is the method for compensation for hospital-based outpatient facilities (DHHS, 2000a). With this system, there is a *professional* component (e.g., for physician providers) and a *technical* component (e.g., for non-physician health care professionals) to billing that describes the various contributions of the health care team during the specific patient encounter. Ambulatory Payment Classification (APC) codes are used within this system to describe the type and complexity of the patient visit to the insurance company. When pharmacists provide services within a hospital-based clinic, the compensation for the service goes to the hospital facility instead of directly to the provider. The revenue generated should be able to be tracked internally as to which department or health care professional was involved in the care of the patient (Snella and Sachdev, 2003).

Compensation Based on Type of Service

Another item that influences compensation is the specific type of service that is provided. For example, compensation can be requested for laboratory services, procedures (e.g., immunizations), and specific health conditions (e.g., diabetes or preventive health counseling). Laboratory testing can offer a way to monitor drug therapy but can also become a source of compensation. The CLIA waiver allows low-complexity tests to be performed in a pharmacy or other setting. If moderate- or high-complexity laboratory testing is performed, the pharmacy or clinic must *register* with CLIA as a *laboratory* (Snella, 1999).

Once a site has received its CLIA waiver, the pharmacy or office can apply to become an indepen-dent laboratory with Medicare. The pharmacist completes an application to Medicare to become a *provider*. The provider number allows the pharmacist to submit claims to Medicare for laboratory tests. The provider number is not used to bill for patient care because it specifically represents the site as an independent laboratory. Other third-party payers may also be billed for laboratory tests, but the pharmacist should become familiar with insurance carriers, such as HMO plans, that have contracts with specific laboratories and restrict compensation to these laboratories (Snella, 1999).

Procedures such as heel ultrasounds and immunizations also can be sources of compensation. When providing immunizations, the state board of pharmacy may have additional restrictions, regulations, or training programs that must be met before a pharmacy or pharmacist can offer immunizations. Pharmacists also can bill Medicare for immunizations after filling out an application (Snella, 1999). This process is similar to becoming an independent laboratory, but the pharmacy or the pharmacist is applying to become a *mass immunizer*. Once the application is accepted, the mass immunizer will receive a provider number specifically for immunizations (CMS, 2007a).

The type of education or management service offered may also influence compensation. For example, not all third-party payers cover preventive health education services such as weight-loss counseling or smoking cessation. If the service is not covered, the patient is personally responsible for the fees associated with the program. If it is not already known if the insurance carrier will or will not consider these services under the health plan, it would be prudent to contact the carrier before providing the service to a specific patient. In this way, the patient is aware of whether the services will be covered or if the patient will be responsible for the charges.

Another specific condition that has its own compensation strategies is diabetes education or diabetes self-management education. For example, CMS has unique guidelines on who can receive compensation for diabetes self-management education. Diabetes education frequently is offered within a *diabetes program* consisting of an interdisciplinary team of health care professionals. As of 2007, only *providers* who are certified by a CMS-approved organization [such as the American Diabetes Association (ADA) and Indian Health Service (IHS)] can be compensated by Medicare (DHHS, 2001b, 2002b). In this case, the term *provider* also includes hospital outpatient clinics, dialysis centers, and durable medical equipment (DME) providers. DME providers who are enrolled with the National Supplier Clearinghouse can be compensated for diabetes self-management education as long as they are also recognized by a CMS-approved entity to provide diabetes education (DHHS, 2001b). To become an ADA-recognized diabetes education program, the program must include a registered nurse and dietician, as well as an advisory panel (American Diabetes Association, 2007; Mensing et al., 2007). Pharmacists practicing in a hospital-based clinic or in a physician's office may have more access to these other health care professionals, but other sites can apply to become a program as long as all the criteria are met. Once approved, a copy of the certificate should be included with the first claim submitted (DHHS, 2000b). Medicare also has regulations defining who can receive diabetes education and how many hours of education can be provided (DHHS, 2001a; Snella, 1999).

REVISITING THE SCENARIO

Dr. Brouchard decides to offer diabetes education services and purchases several CLIA-waived devices for the clinic. To offer these services, he began to gather materials to pursue compensation for both diabetes self-management education and CLIA-waived tests. Since most of his patients have coverage through Medicare, his options for billing for diabetes education include (1) billing the first- or third-party payers directly, (2) becoming recognized by a CMS-approved entity through the pharmacy's DME provider number, (3) billing as a CLIA-waived laboratory, or (4) a combination of approaches. Dr. Brouchard explores the option of becoming an ADA-recognized program. Together with his pharmacy manager, he decides that it may not be feasible for the pharmacy to become ADA-recognized at this time. He and his manager decide to focus on

billing first- and third-party payers directly and billing for CLIA-waived tests.

CODING TERMINOLOGY

Once the value-added service has been designed, fees established, and the method(s) for compensation selected, the pharmacist must learn how to submit claims. When providers submit claims to Medicare, Medicaid, or any other third-party payers, the claim typically is submitted on the CMS Form 1500. One exception to this is the hospital outpatient clinic, which uses CMS Form 1450. On CMS Form 1500, information regarding the submitting entity, referring physician, type of services offered, and related health condition is included. To convey this type of information, CPT codes and ICD-9-CM codes are used. These coding systems provide detailed information regarding the types of services provided and the specific health condition in a numerical format. Example CMS 1500 and 1450 forms are available on the CMS Web site (www.CMS.hhs.gov).

CPT Coding

CPT codes are numerical codes that are used to describe specific types of patient visits, procedures, and laboratory tests that are performed. By using a numerical scheme, these codes can convey a great deal of information with a single five-number code. Following an outpatient visit, this CPT code can indicate whether a patient is new or has been seen previously (established), whether the physician saw the patient, and the complexity of the office visit. For example, CPT codes 99211 to 99215 describe office visits provided to established patients, indicate the complexity of the visit (e.g., the higher the code in the series, the more complex), and may indicate if the patient was seen by a nonphysician (i.e., a physician is not required to see the patient personally with the 99211 code) (AMA, 2006).

Recently, CPT codes for MTM services were approved by the American Medical Association CPT Editorial Panel. These codes can be used by pharmacists to submit MTM claims pursuant to Medicare Part D beneficiaries through their PDPs as well as to other third-party payers. The 99605 code (formerly 0115T) is used for the initial patient encounter, and the 99606 code (formerly 00116T) is used for each follow-up visit. A third code, 99607 (formerly 0117T), is added to each of these codes to indicate that an additional 15 minutes of care was provided. For example, for a 45-minute initial visit, the insurance claim would include the codes 99605 (units = 1) and 99607 (units = 2) to represent the entire 45-minute visit (AMA, 2006; APhA, 2007).

The diabetes self-management codes for certified diabetes education programs include the Healthcare Common Procedural Codes (HCPC) G0108 and G0109. These two codes specifically describe diabetes education by a recognized provider. The G0108 code describes a 30-minute individual education session, whereas the G0109 code describes a 30-minute group education session (CMS, 2006). Each of these standardized codes is used on the billing form, and each code is associated with a specific compensation rate.

In general, the provider determines which CPT code best describes the service that was provided. The specific insurance carriers may have restrictions on which CPT codes can be used. For example, Medicare does not allow pharmacists to use CPT codes 99211 through 99215 but will allow a physician to bill for the nonphysician services (e.g., the pharmacist) using the 99211 code. This can be done if billing using the Incident to Physician Services Regulations described earlier in this chapter (Snella, 1999).

CPT codes also indicate which laboratory procedures were offered. On the billing claim form, each laboratory test or laboratory panel performed is coded separately. An example of a CPT laboratory code is 83036, which corresponds to a hemoglobin A_{1c} determination (AMA, 2006). The CPT code 83036QW indicates a hemoglobin A_{1c} determination was performed using a CLIA-waived device. A complete list of CLIA-waived tests and their CPT codes is located on the CMS Web site (CMS, 2007b, 2007c).

Immunizations also are coded according to CPT codes. When providing immunizations, the CPT codes used include the medication provided (e.g., 90658 for the influenza vaccination, split virus, and 90732 for the pneumococcal polysaccharide, 23-valent vaccine) and the physical vaccine administration (e.g., CPT code 90471 for one vaccine and 90472 for each additional vaccine) (AMA, 2006).

ICD-9-CM Coding

ICD codes are also standardized codes that convey information to the insurance carrier regarding the specific health condition addressed by the provider. These codes are three to five digits and not only describe the general type of health condition addressed but also may indicate whether the patient is stable or is having an exacerbation and the reason for the disorder. The ICD-9-CM code uses this digital code to provide a general description of the condition. The code uses the first three digits to globally classify a health condition and two additional numbers following the decimal to further identify the specific disorders. For example, the code 733 describes several bone and cartilage disorders. Osteoporosis is represented by 733.0, postmenopausal osteoporosis by 733.01, and idiopathic osteoporosis by 733.02 (Buck and Lockyear, 2007).

Some patients will be seen for multiple reasons; therefore, the pharmacist may need to record more than one ICD-9-CM code to fully describe the patient visit. For example, if a client with coronary artery disease (CAD) is referred to a pharmacist, it may not be uncommon that the physician requests education on lowering cholesterol through both diet and medications and education on weight loss and smoking cessation. All three conditions (CAD, obesity, and tobacco use) can be coded to represent the health conditions discussed. Example ICD-9 codes for these conditions include 414.01 (native-vessel disease), 272.2 (mixed hyperlipidemia), and 305.1 (tobacco-use disorder) (Buck and Lockyear, 2007). The specific ICD-9 code used on the claim form should be the same code used by the physician to decrease the risk of claim rejection owing to mismatched codes. Therefore, the ICD-9 code should be requested on the referral form from the physician (Snella et al., 2004).

CLAIM SUBMISSION

Following the patient visit, a claim form (CMS 1500 or CMS 1450) is filled out and submitted to the insurance carrier. The insurance carrier may want other items before approving the claim, such as a statement of medical necessity from the referring provider and a copy of the physician's referral. A *statement of medical necessity* is a statement signed by the provider that states that the referral to the pharmacist (or other provider) is necessary medically (Snella et al., 2004, Poirier et al. 1999). This type of statement can be incorporated into the physician referral form (Snella, 1999).

Before filling out the claim form, it is also useful to gather all the required information for the CMS forms, such as the physician's provider number, the ICD-9-CM code assigned by the provider, the CPT code that will be used to describe the client visit, and the client's insurance information. The referral form can also help to organize this information because the referral form can include areas for the physician's office to include its provider number and areas to mark or select the appropriate ICD-9-CM codes (Poirier, Buffington, and Memoli, 1999; Snella et al., 2004). Additionally, a copy of the client's medical insurance card should be made (Snella et al., 2004). This card typically contains phone numbers needed for prior authorization and for questions regarding claims submissions. If the patient has Medicare Part D benefits, it would be prudent to document the specific prescription drug plan the patient is enrolled in and the contact information for that plan as well.

REVISITING THE SCENARIO

Dr. Brouchard develops a referral form for his service and has included fields for the physician's office to complete regarding the type of insurance, the policy number, the ICD-9 codes, and the physician's provider number. He plans on requesting that referring physicians complete a referral form for each patient they send to the service. If a patient approaches him directly for the service, he plans on contacting his or her physician to fill out a referral form. In an effort to keep the referral form as simple as possible, he has provided check boxes to indicate which service the physician would like performed, the frequency of testing, and the ICD-9-CM codes. He includes sections to mark for diabetes education, insulin injection technique, laboratory monitoring, and additional space for the physician or nurse to include any unique or special instructions. With this information, he will know if the physician wants education only or also wants laboratory monitoring (e.g., hemoglobin A_{1c} and fasting cholesterol panels) and how often these tests are to be done.

The referral form also includes check boxes for the physician to mark the appropriate ICD-9-CM codes. For diabetes education, he includes the common ICD-9 codes 250.00 (i.e., uncomplicated type 2 diabetes, controlled), 250.02 (i.e., uncomplicated type 2 diabetes, uncontrolled), and an "Other" field with room for the physician to add a more specific code (Buck and Lockyear, 2007). For the hyperlipidemia component, he has also included the common codes used to describe these conditions. Within the referral form is the statement of medical necessity and contact information for the physician and patients to reach the pharmacy to make appointments. Although Dr. Brouchard likes the form that he has created, he plans on revising the form based on his experience and input from the physician's office after a few months of use. He wants to make sure that the referral form is as easy to use as possible and that it contains most of the information he needs to submit claims successfully.

CONCLUSION

While value-added services can enhance existing pharmacy services, to be maintained long term, they also must be financially feasible. Adequate compensation for these services is essential. Numerous compensation strategies are available, but they vary based on the insurance carrier and the physical setting where the service is provided. In addition to payment for direct patient care, compensation can also occur for laboratory tests and procedures. One continuing challenge for the profession is wider recognition of pharmacists as providers of direct patient care. One of the most powerful ways to recognize the value of pharmacist services is through direct payment for services and by granting provider status to pharmacists.

QUESTIONS FOR FURTHER DISCUSSION

1. What type of compensation strategies have you seen in practice? Are there any additional services that your pharmacy offers that would qualify for compensation? How do you think these strategies can be enhanced?

2. What types of compensation strategies would work in your anticipated practice site?

3. How would you adapt Dr. Brouchard's strategies for compensation for a different type of service, such as asthma education and monitoring, weight-loss, or osteoporosis counseling?

4. What information would you want on a referral form for an asthma education and monitoring, weight-loss, or osteoporosis counseling service?

5. How would you convince a third-party payer or a patient to pay for your services?

6. How would you convince a legislator or government regulator to expand current compensation for patient care services to include those provided by a pharmacist?

REFERENCES

American Diabetes Association (ADA). 2007. Education Recognition Program. Available at www.diabetes.org/for-health-professionals-and-scientists/recognition/edrecognition.jsp; accessed on May 2007.

American Medical Association (AMA). 2006. *CPT® 2007 Standard Edition.* Chicago: AMA.

American Pharmacists Association (APhA). 2007. CPT codes for MTM made permanent. Available at www.pharmacist.com/AM/Template.cfm?Section=Newsroom&TEMPLATE=/CM/HTMLDisplay.cfm&CONTENTID=14126; accessed on November 2007.

Anonymous. 1998. Medicaid to pay Mississippi pharmacists for disease management. *Am J Health-Syst Pharm* 55:1238.

Buck CJ, Lockyear KD. 2007. *Saunders 2007 ICD-9-CM,* Vols. 1, 2, and 3. St. Louis: Saunders.

Centers for Medicare and Medicaid Services (CMS). 2006. Guidelines for Payment for Diabetes Self-Management Training (DSMT); February 6, 2006. Available at www.cms.hhs.gov/ContractorLearningResources/Downloads/JA5433.pdf.

Centers for Medicare and Medicaid Services (CMS). 2007a. Adult Immunizations, Provider Resources. Available at www.cms.hhs.gov/AdultImmunizations/02_Providerresources.asp; accessed on May 2007.

Centers for Medicare and Medicaid Services (CMS). 2007b. Clinical Laboratory Improvement Amendments (CLIA), Tests Granted Waived Status under CLIA. Available at www.cms.hhs.gov/CLIA/10_Categorization_of_Tests.asp; accessed on May 2007.

Centers for Medicare and Medicaid Services (CMS). 2007c. List of Waived Tests—Updated April 1, 2007. Available at www.cms.hhs.gov/CLIA/downloads/CR5484.waivedtbl.pdf.

Centers for Medicare and Medicaid Services (CMS). 2007d. Medicare Program—General Information, Medicare Part B. Available at www.cms.hhs.gov/MedicareGenInfo/03_Part%20B.asp; accessed on May 2007.

Department of Health and Human Services (DHHS), Office of the Inspector General. 2000a. Medicare program, prospective payment system for hospital outpatient services. *Fed Reg* 65:18433; available at www.gpoaccess.gov/fr/.

Department of Health and Human Services (DHHS). 2000b. Program Memorandum Intermediaries/Carriers, Transmittal AB-00-67; July 20, 2000. Available at www.cms.hhs.gov/transmittals/downloads/ab0067.pdf.

Department of Health and Human Services (DHSS). 2001a. Medicare Intermediary Manual, Vol. 3: Claims Process, Transmittal 1836; June 15, 2001. Available at www.cms.hhs.gov/transmittals/downloads/R1836A3.pdf.

Department of Health and Human Services (DHHS). 2001b. Program Memorandum: Carriers, Transmittal B-01-40, Expanded Coverage of Diabetes Outpatient Self-Management Training; June 15, 2001. Available at www.cms.hhs.gov/Transmittals/downloads/B0140.pdf.

Department of Health and Human Services (DHHS). 2002a. Medicare Carrier's Manual, Vol. 3: Claims Process, Transmittal 1764; August 28, 2002. Available at www.cms.hhs.gov/transmittals/downloads/R1764B3.pdf.

Department of Health and Human Services (DHHS). 2002b. Medicare program: Approval of the Indian Health Service (IHS) as a national accreditation organization for accrediting American Indians and Alaska native entities to furnish outpatient diabetes self-management training. *Fed Reg* 67:13345; available at www.gpoaccess.gov/fr/.

Hogue MD. 2002. *The Pharmacist's Guide to Compensation for Patient-Care Services.* Washington, DC: American Pharmaceutical Association.

Landis NT. 1998. Mississippi moves forward with disease specific credentialing. *Am J Health-Syst Pharm* 55:2452.

Mensing C, Boucher J, Cypress M, et al. 2007. National standards for diabetes self-management education. *Diabetes Care* 30:S96.

Northwest Valley Chamber of Commerce. 2007. Sun City. Available at www.northwestvalley.com/sun_city.php; accessed on May 2007.

One Hundred Eighth Congress of the United States of America. 2007. Medicare Prescription Drug, Improvement,

and Modernization Act of 2003. Available at www.cms.hhs.gov/EmployerRetireeDrugSubsid/Downloads/MMAStatute.pdf; accessed on May 2007.

Poirier S, Buffington DE, Memoli G. 1999. Billing third-party payers for pharmaceutical care services. *J Am Pharm Assoc* 39:50.

Snella KA. 1999. Specific billing scenarios. In *How to Bill for Clinical Pharmacy Services.* Kansas City: American College of Clinical Pharmacy.

Snella KA, Sachdev GP. 2003. A primer for developing pharmacist-managed clinics in the outpatient setting. *Pharmacotherapy* 23:1153.

Snella KA, Trewyn R, Hansen LB, et al. 2004. Pharmacist compensation for cognitive services: Focus on the physician office and community pharmacy. *Pharmacotherapy* 24:372.

Social Security Administration. 2007. Compilation of the Social Security Laws, Part D: Miscellaneous Provisions (Sec. 1861s). Available at www.ssa.gov/OP_Home/ssact/title18/1861.htm, accessed on May 2007.

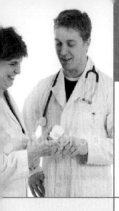

27

EVALUATING THE OUTCOMES OF VALUE-ADDED PHARMACY SERVICES

Michelle A. Chui

About the Author: Dr. Chui is currently an Assistant Professor at the University of Wisconsin in Madison, Wisconsin. She earned a B.A. in biological sciences from the University of California, Davis, a Pharm.D. from Creighton University, and an M.S. and Ph.D. in pharmacy administration from Purdue University. Her areas of research focus on identifying and disseminating evidence to prove the worth of community pharmacists in the overall health care system and improving the work life for community pharmacists so that they can focus on patient care.

▨ LEARNING OBJECTIVES

After completing this chapter, students should be able to

1. Discuss the different facets of the ECHO model.
2. Describe the differences among the five types of economic analyses.
3. List the advantages and disadvantages of the various methods of measuring humanistic outcomes.
4. Identify the objectives of the service and determine what types of outcomes a pharmacist would need to measure in a value-added pharmacy-related service.
5. Identify the advantages and disadvantages of the various methods used to collect data when evaluating value-added services.
6. List and describe the uses of outcomes evaluation.

▨ SCENARIO

Cynthia Marshall is a pharmacist who works at a closed-staff-model health maintenance organization (HMO) pharmacy. Pharmacists at this clinic have access to patient charts that can be used to supplement information given by the patient to the pharmacy staff and what is written on the prescription. Cynthia enjoys working at this pharmacy because she feels that the added information is helpful when she is assessing and counseling her patients.

Cynthia sees a number of heart failure patients every month. These patients see their physicians only annually. She notices that these patients can improve or deteriorate quickly and that their health conditions frequently change from month to month. They occasionally complain that their symptoms get so bad that they have to go to the emergency room. She thinks that these patients could have better outcomes if they were better educated about their conditions and monitored more closely.

Cynthia approaches the cardiologists in her clinic with an idea that she could start a heart failure clinic to provide additional education and monitoring for these patients. While the physicians would oversee the clinic, she could conduct monthly educational seminars about heart failure for patients, order and assess laboratory tests, and order medications and adjust dosages under physician-approved protocols.

Given the HMO's patient load, Cynthia figures that she would have to spend 50 percent of her time with the heart failure clinic. Because the pharmacy is always busy, the HMO would have to hire an additional part-time pharmacist to take care of her dispensing duties.

CHAPTER QUESTIONS

1. Why is it important to measure baseline data for individual patients and/or a cohort of patients before starting a clinic?
2. How can outcomes be used to prove the value of your service?
3. How do pharmacists use outcomes measures to assess the success of their value-added services?
4. What type of economic analysis would be appropriate to evaluate the service described in the scenario? How should the costs and outcomes be measured?
5. Why is it important to choose a perspective prior to starting a project? How do perspectives differ?

INTRODUCTION

Pharmacists make many contributions that improve the lives of their patients on a daily basis. These contributions range from catching a drug interaction, counseling a patient about his or her medication, or even providing a new value-added service such as the heart failure clinic proposed by Cynthia Marshall in the scenario. While many pharmacists would like to offer these value-added services to their patients, they can have upfront costs that cannot be ignored. How can pharmacists provide these services and show that they both help their patients and actually decrease the overall cost of care? Many studies have been conducted that show that pharmacists can make a difference both in cost and in the quality of their patients' lives (Cranor and Christensen, 2003; Etemad and Hay, 2003; McLean, Gillis, and Waller, 2003). How can Cynthia Marshall do the same in her situation?

FRAMING THE QUESTION

How does one start documenting the value of a pharmacy service? The first step is to define the problem or research question being addressed. Stating the problem upfront seems rather obvious, but it is not always done. Many pharmacists waste time and energy trying to answer poorly defined questions. For example, one can start with a very broadly defined problem such as heart failure, which arises from a combination of factors and results in numerous health outcomes. Evaluating all the possible causes and effects of heart failure may be an overwhelming task, so the problem should be narrowed. One could evaluate the effect of medication compliance in patients with heart failure or even one particular outcome of heart failure (e.g., blood pressure or quality of life). The more narrow the problem, the easier it will be to address.

After the problem has been stated, the next step is to define the objectives. A very broad problem will result in broadly defined objectives. If heart failure is broadly identified as the problem, an objective could be to reduce the number of patients with heart failure.

However, no specific method of reducing heart failure is addressed, and heart failure itself has many potential outcomes. On the other hand, if the problem is addressed more narrowly, a more narrowly defined objective could be studied. For example, one may look to reduce the number of heart failure exacerbations related to noncompliance with medications. Additionally, other specific objectives may be included, such as increasing the quality of life of patients with heart failure, reducing the number of medications used by patients with heart failure, or making patients more aware of behavioral and dietary modifications related to heart failure.

All objectives, regardless of whether they are broad or narrow, actually must be measurable. While this also may seem obvious, many objectives (especially if they are broadly defined) can be difficult, if not impossible, to measure. The broad objective of reducing heart failure may be difficult to measure because so many factors must be considered when arriving at a diagnosis of heart failure. On the other hand, specific objectives such as reducing blood pressure or improving quality of life in patients with heart failure are much easier to quantify and measure using previously validated methods.

The third step is to establish a framework to evaluate the question. When establishing the framework, pharmacists need to know some basic facts about the programs and diseases they are studying. Pharmacists undertaking these projects first should prioritize their objectives by determining what interventions and outcomes most need to be evaluated. For example, Cynthia Marshall may wish to determine the effect of her monitoring program on cost of care (an economic outcome), blood pressure (a clinical outcome), and quality of life (a humanistic outcome).

▨ SELECTING THE VARIABLES TO MEASURE

Many health care organizations make the mistake of focusing on only one area of health care when trying to reduce the overall cost of health care. Evaluating the cost of a single aspect of patient care in isolation from all other aspects is commonly known as *component management.* Examples of component management include focusing on the costs of drugs or laboratory tests without looking at the impact of these costs on overall health care costs or outcomes. Unfortunately, many health studies have focused on just one type of cost without considering the overall care of patients. For instance, New Hampshire's Medicaid program sought to reduce its medication costs by imposing a cap of three prescriptions per month. This strategy did decrease overall drug costs, but there was an overall increase in the health care system owing to increases in hospitalizations and nursing home admissions (Soumerai et al., 1991, 1994). In a more recent example, Kaiser-Permanente of northern California compared the clinical and economic outcomes of beneficiaries whose annual drug benefit was capped at $1,000 with those with unlimited drug benefits. A cap on drug benefits was associated with lower drug consumption but poorer adherence and control of blood pressure, lipid levels, and glucose levels. Savings in drug cost was offset by increases in costs of emergency department visits and hospitalizations (Hsu et al., 2006).

Disease management strives to consider all individual components of health care for a specific disease with a view toward an outcome that is important for successful management of that disease. Instead of dealing with one element at a time (such as prescription costs only), disease management attempts to control the disease by integrating the components of health care to provide the best total patient outcomes at the most reasonable cost. As a result, the number of variables measured in this paradigm is greater and more global. When making changes to one component of health care, other components are considered as well (Armstrong and Langley, 1996; Patterson, 1995; Zitter, 1994).

When identifying economic, clinical, and humanistic variables to be measured, it is important to integrate elements from all components of health care. In our example, Cynthia is trying to manage her patients' heart failure medications. Because she is a pharmacist, she may identify only medication-related variables to measure, such as cost of the drug or number of prescriptions filled. When evaluating this project with an eye toward disease management, one could also measure hospitalizations, emergency department visits, laboratory costs, physician visits, and other factors related to the care of these patients if those variables are available to her.

At the point where one is determining which outcomes will be measured, one also should be keeping in mind the perspective of those to whom the outcomes of the intervention will be of value. While practically any disease management project can be evaluated from the perspective of the patient (e.g., Did the patient's health and quality of life improve? Did the patient save money?), there are other important perspectives whose outcomes could be considered as well (Drummond, Stoddard, and Torrance, 1986). These perspectives include that of the health care provider (e.g., Did the job satisfaction of the pharmacist improve as a result of providing the service?), the department (e.g., Did the program result in lower drug costs to the pharmacy?), the organization (e.g., Did the program result in decreased costs of caring for heart failure patients for the HMO?), and even society (e.g., Did the program reduce the prevalence of heart failure in the community?). Not every outcome from every perspective needs to be considered in each evaluation. Pharmacists should revisit their original research question, objectives, and framework when determining which variables from which perspectives should be measured.

IDENTIFYING CONFOUNDING VARIABLES THAT CAN AFFECT OUTCOMES

After identifying a research question, study objectives, and variables to evaluate, researchers also need to think about other variables that may affect the results of the study. For example, Cynthia Marshall may wish to evaluate the impact of her monitoring service on the cost of caring for these patients from the perspective of the HMO. Her results may show that patients who used her service had much lower costs of care compared

with those who did not. Based just on this finding, one might jump to the conclusion that the service is an effective way to reduce the cost of caring for heart failure patients. However, on further examination, it may be discovered that many of the patients receiving the service had mild to moderate heart failure and only had one to two other disease states. In comparison, those who declined to participate may have had moderate to severe heart failure and multiple disease states.

Does this mean that the service did not have a positive effect? Actually, it means that the results are unclear. The severity of heart failure and number of disease states may have clouded the results of the study. For example, the service may not have saved the HMO any money, but the fact that those who used the service (less severely ill patients) generally had lower costs of care than those who did not use the service (more severely ill patients) may have made it look that way. Any variable that also may have an impact on the results of study but is not one of the primary variables being evaluated is known as a *confounding variable.*

It is important to minimize or control for the impact of confounding variables in any study. In order to do so, it is imperative that all possible variables that may have an effect on the primary outcome be identified. These usually include demographic variables such as age, sex, income level, education level, and ethnicity. Health-related variables such as comorbidities and severity of illness should also be recorded. Variables also may be identified that cannot be measured. These may include outside education, changes in family structure or support system, and drastic changes in health status not related to the pertinent disease state.

REVISITING THE SCENARIO

Cynthia would like to implement a new service that would manage the medications taken by the HMO's heart failure patients. The questions that the HMO is asking include "How much will the service cost?" and "Will the interventions conducted by the pharmacist reduce hospitalizations and emergency department visits?" Cynthia has additional questions: "Will the interventions I conduct increase my patients' health-related quality of life?" and "Will my patients be better satisfied with the quality of pharmacist care than with the care they currently receive?"

Cynthia's objectives are to reduce hospitalizations and emergency department visits by increasing compliance with heart failure medications and educating patients about their disease state and how to make diet and behavioral modifications, as well as improve patients' health-related quality of life and satisfaction with care.

Her research into heart failure has given her some information about what types of variables she should collect. Patients with heart failure show symptoms of decreased exercise tolerance, shortness of breath, increased fatigue, and fluid buildup in the lungs and tissues. Patients with heart failure are also classified clinically by their level of disability so that they may be followed longitudinally and provide a reference point when compared with other patients. This classification system is the New York Heart Association (NYHA) Functional Classification system and ranges from functional class I (no limitation of physical activity) to functional class IV (unable to carry on physical activity without discomfort) (Criteria Committee, 1973).

Cynthia has also discovered that heart failure is the most common hospital discharge diagnosis in individuals over age 65. Median survival rate from the time of diagnosis is 1.7 years in men and 3.2 years in women (Ho et al., 1993). Cynthia knows that she will have to collect some demographic variables as well as the variables that directly address her objectives. Pertinent demographic variables may include age, gender, marital status, ethnicity, income level, and mental status.

ECHO MODEL

Outcomes research is defined as studies that attempt to identify, measure, and evaluate the end results of health care services. Outcomes research may evaluate not only the clinical effects of health care services but also the economic and humanistic impact of these services. Proponents of outcomes research believe that we should measure not only the clinical and cost impacts of health care but also outcomes that take factors such as quality of life and satisfaction into account (Bootman, Townsend, and McGhan, 1996).

Many have proposed that evaluation of drug therapy and pharmacists' value-added services should include assessments of economic, clinical, and humanistic outcomes. The economic, clinical, and humanistic outcomes (ECHO) model assumes that the outcomes of medical care can be classified along the three dimensions of economic, clinical, and humanistic outcomes (Kozma, Reeder, and Schultz, 1993). *Clinical outcomes* are defined as medical events that occur as a result of disease or treatment. *Economic outcomes* are defined as the direct, indirect, and intangible costs compared with the consequences of medical treatment alternatives. *Humanistic outcomes* are defined as the consequences of disease or treatment on patient functional status or quality of life. All three of these outcomes need to be balanced simultaneously to assess value.

Economic Outcomes

Traditional cost-containment measures are not always consistent with improved patient care. Thus attention has turned toward demonstrating the value of health care. A full evaluation of relevant costs and consequences differentiates outcomes research from traditional cost-containment strategies. *Costs* are defined as the value of the resources consumed by a program or treatment alternative. *Consequences* are defined as the effects, outputs, and outcomes of the program or treatment alternative (Eisenberg, 1989).

Direct costs are the resources consumed in the prevention, detection, or treatment of a disease or illness. These costs can be divided into direct medical and direct nonmedical costs. *Direct medical costs* are specific monetary transactions associated with paying for medical care, such as hospitalizations, drugs, medical supplies, and physician visits. *Direct nonmedical costs* involve monetary transactions for required items or services that do not involve purchase of medical care. Examples include transportation to medical facilities, special foods, and the time that family members miss work to care for others.

Indirect costs are the costs that result from morbidity and mortality. These costs are related to changes in work production, such as costs incurred from missing work (absenteeism), costs incurred from decreased productivity despite presence at work (presenteeism), or costs incurred owing to premature death. *Intangible costs* are the costs incurred that represent nonfinancial outcomes of disease and medical care and are not expressed in monetary terms. These include pain, suffering, and grief.

The economic evaluation of medical care may occur from many perspectives. These perspectives, or viewpoints, will influence the costs and consequences identified, measured, and compared for a program or treatment alternative. An economic evaluation can be conducted from a single perspective or multiple perspectives. Common perspectives are those of the patient, provider, payer/insurer, and society. There are subtle differences between perspectives. A patient may be extremely concerned with his or her quality of life, level of pain, ability to see health care providers, or how much time is spent in the hospital or nursing home, in addition to the actual direct costs of health care. However, a payer may be interested only in the direct costs of health care to its organization. In fact, while a patient who is at the end of his or her life may be interested in extending life as long as possible, a payer may see this as an expensive prospect.

There are also differences between the payer's and societal perspectives. Many payers assume that patients will not be covered on their plans throughout their lifetime, so expensive interventions that provide benefits in the very long term tend to be discouraged (i.e., screening programs for diseases that manifest in the elderly). However, from a societal perspective, these screenings may be appropriate because they identify patients at risk earlier. In the long run, such screenings are beneficial to society.

Types of Economic Evaluations

The basic task of economic evaluations is to identify, measure, value, and compare the costs and consequences of the alternatives being considered. Therefore, a full economic evaluation must have two features: a comparison of two or more treatment alternatives and both the costs and consequences of the alternatives

being examined. Five types of economic analyses can be used to examine treatment alternatives: cost of illness, cost-minimization analysis, cost-benefit analysis, cost-effectiveness analysis, and cost-utility analysis.

Cost-of-illness analysis involves identifying all the direct and indirect costs of a particular disease or illness from a particular perspective (e.g., patient, payer, or society). This method, often referred to as *burden of illness,* results in a total cost of a disease that can be compared with the cost of implementing a prevention or treatment strategy.

Cost-minimization analysis is a tool used to compare two or more treatment alternatives that are assumed to be equal in efficacy. It simply compares the direct and indirect costs of treatment alternatives in dollars and does not consider the outcomes of the treatments (because they are assumed to be the same). Examples could be to compare the costs of intravenous versus oral dosage forms of the same drug or hospital versus home administration of intravenous pain management.

Cost-benefit analysis is used when the outcome can be expressed in monetary terms, such as in the amount of money an HMO might save if it implements a new program. The direct and indirect costs of a program or intervention are measured as they occur, and the benefits accrued from the program or intervention are identified and converted into dollars in the year in which they occur. These two values are then expressed as a ratio of the dollar value of the costs of the program or intervention to the dollar value of the outcomes that arose as a result of the program or intervention. For example, if the cost associated with new heart failure monitoring service were $100 per patient and, as a result of the service, the HMO saved $1,000 in hospital care per patient, the cost-benefit ratio would be expressed as the benefit, $1,000, divided by the cost, $100, or as 10:1. This ratio would be interpreted such that the service produces $10 of benefits for every $1 that is spent. The results may also be interpreted by subtracting the costs from the benefits or, in our example, as a $900 net benefit per patient.

Cost-effectiveness analysis is used when the treatment alternatives are not therapeutically equivalent or when outcomes cannot be expressed in monetary units. Cost is measured in monetary units, and outcomes are expressed in terms of obtaining a specific therapeutic objective, such as cases cured, lives saved, or millimeters of mercury drop in blood pressure. Cost-effectiveness analysis allows researchers to summarize the health benefit and resources used by two or more competing programs so that policymakers can choose among them (Detsky and Nagiie, 1990; Doubilet, 1986). For example, drug A may cost $100 and produce a 10 mg/dL drop in low-density lipoprotein cholesterol (LDL-C), whereas drug B may cost $250 and produce a 20 mg/dL drop in LDL-C. Using cost-effectiveness analysis to calculate the ratio of costs to benefits of each alternative results in a cost of $10 per 1 mg/dL drop in LDL-C for drug A and a cost of $12.50 per 1 mg/dL drop in LDL-C for drug B. Based on this analysis, drug A could be said to be more cost-effective than drug B.

Cost-utility analysis is used when quality of life is the most important outcome being examined. This is common in disease states in which how one feels or what one can do is more important than a clinical laboratory value or economic outcome (e.g., chronic diseases such as heart disease, diabetes, arthritis, cancer, or HIV/AIDS). Cost-utility analyses compare the direct and indirect costs of an intervention with some measurable level of humanistic outcome, such quality of life or level of satisfaction. The direct and indirect costs of treatment alternatives again are expressed in monetary terms. The humanistic outcomes associated with each intervention can be expressed as an SF-12 or SF-36 health survey score for quality of life (Ware, 1997), as a satisfaction survey score (MacKeigan and Larson, 1989), or as quality-adjusted life-years (QALYs). QALYs represent the number of full years at full health that are valued equivalently with the number of years experienced. For example, a full year of health in a disease-free patient would equal 1.0 QALY, whereas a year requiring a patient to carry an oxygen tank to breathe might be valued significantly lower, perhaps as a 0.5 QALY.

REVISITING THE SCENARIO

In order to determine what type of analysis to conduct, Cynthia must identify all the costs related to her project. She created a table to identify all possible costs from every perspective (see Table 27-1).

When determining which method of economic analysis she should use, she eliminated cost-minimization analysis because the treatment alternatives (service versus no service) will not result in equivalent outcomes. A cost-effectiveness analysis would not be appropriate because she is only interested in one particular program. A cost-utility analysis is also not appropriate because quality of life, while included in the project, is not the focus of her project. A cost-benefit analysis could be appropriate. A cost-benefit analysis requires that both the interventions and outcomes be valued in monetary units. She can determine the direct medical and/or nonmedical costs for each patient from data captured by her HMO. The HMO is very interested in costs, both those to implement the service and those it may save as a result. Cynthia decides that the most understandable analysis to present to the HMO is a cost-benefit analysis.

Uses of Economic Outcomes

Many benefits can be realized by applying pharmacoeconomic principles and methods to evaluating pharmacy services. Economic assessments can assist in balancing cost and outcome when determining the

Table 27-1. Costs of Heart Failure			
Direct Medical Costs	**Direct Nonmedical Costs**	**Indirect Costs**	**Intangible Costs**
Medications	Special food	Missing work	Pain
Hospitalizations	Transportation	Lost productivity	Suffering
Physician visits	Burden on family	Premature death	Grief

most efficient use of health care goods and services. Economic assessments are helpful in optimizing clinical decision making. Decisions involving formulary management, practice guidelines, drug policy, individual patient treatment, and resource allocation are all amenable to economic assessments.

Decision analysis is a technique used in economic evaluations to structure the logical and chronologic order of the analysis. It is a systematic, quantitative method of describing clinical problems, identifying possible courses of action, assessing the probability and value of outcomes, and making a calculation to select the optimal course of action. A tool used in decision analysis is a decision table or decision tree. A *decision tree,* shown in Fig. 27-1, allows researchers to display graphically all treatment alternatives being compared, the relevant outcomes associated with these alternatives, and the probabilities of these outcomes occurring in a patient population. It can allow for the algebraic conversion of all these variables into one summary measurement, often a cost-effectiveness ratio, to allow for a meaningful comparison of two or more treatment alternatives (Barr and Schumacher, 1994; Crane, 1988).

In economic evaluations, there is a need to make assumptions about the variables in the analysis. For instance, assumptions that are made commonly include the incidence of adverse effects, the drug's efficacy (in clinical trials) and effectiveness (use in actual practice), and the costs of drugs or other direct medical costs. It is important to keep in mind that assumptions are simply *predictions* about what a researcher thinks might happen as a result of a program or intervention. To account for the variety of outcomes that may arise in any intervention, researchers should use a technique known as *sensitivity analysis.* Sensitivity analysis is a tool that tests the robustness or strength of economic evaluation results and conclusions by making different assumptions about outcomes over a range of plausible results. In a sensitivity analysis, the researcher identifies one parameter, holds other evaluation parameters constant, and recalculates the study results using a range of the chosen parameter. The results of a sensitivity analysis can determine if the outcome of the study is "sensitive" to ranges in the chosen parameter. If changing the values of specific variables does not substantially alter the results, there is more confidence in the original findings.

For example, when comparing two antibiotics, one with an efficacy of 80 percent and another with an efficacy of 95 percent, if costs are equal, it is clear that the second antibiotic is "better" because patients would receive a higher benefit for the same cost. In a sensitivity analysis, researchers might adjust the assumptions made about the efficacy percentages or the costs of the drugs to determine if the second antibiotic is still the "better" drug.

Clinical Outcomes

To health care professionals, the most obvious variables that should be addressed when evaluating any medical intervention are the clinical outcomes. Any value-added service can assert that patients will receive better care if given that service. Clinical outcomes vary with each disease state but should include any pertinent medications [e.g., prescription, over the counter (OTC), and herbal], any side effects or adverse effects from the disease state or medications, any laboratory values used, the documented physical state, and any use of other health care providers or services.

▧ REVISITING THE SCENARIO

At Cynthia's pharmacy, patients with heart disease are usually on several medications for their heart disease: a diuretic, a beta blocker, and an angiotensin-converting enzyme (ACE) inhibitor. Patients with more severe disease may also be on an aldosterone inhibitor such as spironolactone, digoxin, hydralazine nitrate, and/or an angiotensin-receptor blocker (ARB). Some patients are

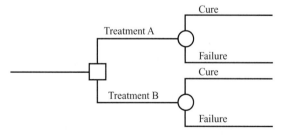

Figure 27-1. Decision tree.

also on oxygen. Patients are also required to submit to frequent laboratory testing for potassium and serum creatinine levels. They are assessed for blood pressure, weight, level of edema, and shortness of breath and then are assigned a NYHA classification (I, II, III, or IV). For the pharmacy's heart failure service, each of these pieces of clinical data would be recorded at baseline and at each subsequent visit by the pharmacist. Other clinical markers that Cynthia would like to measure include the incidence of medication side effects and adverse drug reactions.

Humanistic Outcomes

Quality of life refers to an evaluation of all aspects of our lives, including where we live, how we live, how we play, and how we work. Health-related quality of life (HRQL) encompasses only those aspects of life which are dominated or influenced significantly by personal health or activities performed to maintain or improve health. HRQL is defined as a multidimensional concept referring to a person's total well-being, including physical symptoms, functional ability, and perceptions. The first component, physical symptoms, includes disease-related symptoms and the impact of symptoms on functional ability and perceptions. The second component, functional ability, incorporates self-care activities, interpersonal areas, social support, sleep, and intellectual functioning, including coping and emotions. The third component, perceptions, involves judgments about one's own health status. Advances in medical science have encouraged attention to HRQL because medical care is no longer limited to providing only death-averting treatments (Coons and Kaplan, 1993).

Standardized questionnaires are used to capture HRQL data in a variety of settings. These standardized questionnaires may be self-administered or completed via telephone or personal interview, by observation, or by postal survey. Two basic approaches to HRQL measurement are available: generic instruments that provide a summary of health-related quality of life and specific instruments that focus on problems associated with individual disease states, patient groups, or areas of function.

Generic instruments apply to a wide variety of patients. Their broad applicability is derived from their coverage of the complete spectrum of function, disability, and distress that is relevant to HRQL. They are designed for use in a wide variety of conditions, but they may not focus on aspects of HRQL that are of interest to the investigator and may be unresponsive to small but clinically important changes. Some examples of generic instruments are the Sickness Impact Profile and the Medical Outcomes Study Short Forms 36 and 12 (SF-36 and SF-12) (Ware, 1991).

To evaluate aspects of HRQL that are specific to a particular disease or condition, specific measures also may be used. Specific measures include only important aspects of HRQL that are relevant to the patients being studied, such as the loss of function patients experience from asthma or the amount of pain they have from arthritis. Disadvantages of using specific measures are that they are not comprehensive and cannot be used to compare across conditions. They also cannot measure unforeseen side effects or conditions. Examples of specific instruments for heart failure are the Minnesota Living with Heart Failure Questionnaire and the Chronic Heart Failure Questionnaire (Guyatt et al., 1989; Rector, Kubo, and Cohn, 1987).

Another area of humanistic outcomes that may be important to measure is patient satisfaction. *Satisfaction* is defined as the extent to which individuals' needs and wants are met. This is linked with attitudes toward the medical care system, as well as expectations and perceptions regarding the quantity and quality of care received.

During the last decade, the health care industry has begun to recognize the importance of satisfaction with services as patients became increasingly recognized as consumers. Consumer or patient satisfaction surveys have evolved from marketing tools to measures of quality. In fact, the level of satisfaction with medical care has been shown to be associated directly with willingness to adhere to medical recommendations, rates of switching medical care providers, and disenrollment from prepaid health plans (Rossiter et al., 1989). In addition, the degree of patient satisfaction has been negatively correlated with a willingness to initiate malpractice lawsuits, meaning that people who are less satisfied with their health care are more likely to sue their health care professionals (Rubin et al., 1993).

Similar to HRQL surveys, patient satisfaction instruments are designed to be general or specific instruments. One of the most commonly used instruments is the Patient Satisfaction Questionnaire (PSQ). This survey measures global satisfaction, as well as the specific domains of technical quality, interpersonal manner, communication, financial aspects, time spent with the doctor, and accessibility of care (Fincham and Wertheimer, 1987; Larson and MacKeigan, 1994; MacKeigan and Larson, 1989).

Surveys specifically measuring outpatient pharmacy services have also been developed, notably the Satisfaction with Pharmacy Services Questionnaire. This is a 45-item survey that has been adapted from PSQs and tests for consideration, explanation, technical competence, financial aspects, and general issues. Table 27-2 shows a sample of these items (MacKeigan and Larson, 1989).

Although economic and humanistic analyses usually have been conducted using the perspective of the payer or insurance company, the perspective of the employer also has become more prevalent. To meet the evaluation needs of employers, work functioning can be measured as a humanistic outcome. Traditionally, work functioning has been measured as lost days from work (absenteeism). However, this measurement has become more specific and can be measured as reductions in productive capacity (presenteeism). Diseases that may cause reductions in work productivity include migraines, allergic rhinitis, and depression.

REVISITING THE SCENARIO

Cynthia has found that patients with heart failure report a number of physical symptoms that affect HRQL, such as dyspnea, fatigue, anorexia, cachexia, edema, sleeplessness, attention deficit, and memory impairment. Functional abilities such as problems with social interactions, depression, and poor psychosocial adjustment also may affect this patient population. Furthermore, perceived health status has been found to be lower in the heart failure population when compared with other patient populations with chronic disease states (Bohachick and Anton, 1990; Freedland, Carnet, and Rich, 1991; Grady et al., 1992; Kolar and Dracup, 1990; Rideout and Montemuro, 1986).

In addition to the analysis requested by the HMO, Cynthia is interested in measuring humanistic outcomes and thinks that it would be important to

Table 27-2.	Items from the Satisfaction with Pharmacy Services Questionnaire
General	The pharmacy services that I've received are just about perfect.
	I'm very satisfied with the pharmacy services that I receive.
Financial aspects	I am happy with the drug coverage provided by my medical insurance plan.
	The copayment that I am charged for prescription drugs is reasonable
Technical competence	The pharmacist is always thorough.
	I am confident that the pharmacist dispenses all prescriptions correctly.
Explanation	If I have a question about my prescription, the pharmacist is always available to help me.
	The pharmacist knows how to explain things in a way that I understand.
Consideration	The pharmacist spends as much time as is necessary with me.
	My prescriptions are always filled promptly.

Source: MacKeigan and Larson, 1989

collect information on her patients' HRQL, as well as clinical and economic measures. She chooses to use the SF-12 and the Chronic Heart Failure Questionnaire to assess HRQL. She also chooses to use some of the questions from the Satisfaction with Pharmacy Services Questionnaire to determine if patients are satisfied with her clinical services.

Cynthia is interested in measuring actual absenteeism from work as well as decreases in productivity owing to shortness of breath and fatigue. However, she acknowledges that these data would be difficult to obtain from patients and their employers, so she chooses not to collect data on these outcomes at this time.

DATA COLLECTION

Once the research question, objectives, variables, and methods of analysis have been identified, researchers must determine how they are going to collect data for each of their variables. While researchers can use a variety of sources and methods of data collection, health care professionals often can obtain most of their data from records they already maintain.

Partnerships with Other Health Care Entities

As pertinent variables are identified, it will become clear that some data will be easily obtainable, whereas information on other variables will be extremely difficult to acquire. Pharmacy-related data often are easily retrievable because much of the information can be obtained directly from the pharmacy's prescription computer program (and the patient profiles). Patient demographic information such as gender and age generally is also stored on the pharmacy computer. However, depending on the research question, data from other areas of the health care system may need to be collected as well. For instance, one hypothesis could be that a pharmacy service may result in a reduction in emergency department visits. Pharmacists often do not have access to data on emergency department visits in their own records.

To obtain disease-related health data, it is helpful to develop partnerships with physician groups and hospitals that serve patients participating in a clinical pharmacy service. A partnership with physicians may allow pharmacists access to patient charts to collect disease-related health data (with patients' permission). A patient chart contains progress notes, laboratory values, referrals to specialists, and any other pertinent information about the patient. A patient chart could provide a complete picture of the patient and serve to show how a patient has improved under a pharmacist's care.

Another partnership that would be helpful is with payers for health services. Insurance companies, HMOs, pharmacy benefits managers (PBMs), and government agencies such as Medicaid and the Veterans Administration generally maintain health care expenditure data for the patients for whom they pay for health services. Pharmacist interventions can be correlated with these health care expenditure data to determine the effectiveness of the intervention. For example, the numbers and costs of hospitalizations and emergency department visits for patients enrolled in a pharmacist-managed health program can be examined prior to the start of the program and again 1 year later.

ECONOMIC EVALUATION

Costs of goods and services seem intuitively simple to quantify. However, a number of potentially complicated issues must be considered. When identifying the goods or services, will the actual cost (wholesale cost) to the pharmacy or health care organization be measured, or will the charge to the patient or payer (retail cost) be measured? Sometimes access to cost data may be limited, or the data may be entirely unavailable. For instance, if Cynthia Marshall was using a hospital database to collect hospitalization and emergency department information for the HMO's heart failure patients, it may be impossible to isolate the actual costs related to heart failure, particularly if a patient was admitted for multiple reasons.

There are advantages and disadvantages to using different data sources. Primary data collection, in which data are collected solely for purposes of the project, are the best sources of data because the researcher can request and generate exactly the information that

Table 27-3. Characteristics of HMO Heart Failure Patients Prior to the Start of the Heart Failure Clinic

	Number	Cost	Average Length of Stay
Hospitalizations	5/year	$500/day	5.6 days
Emergency room	7/year	$1,000/visit	
Heart failure medications	3/month	$40/Rx	

is needed for the project. This is also helpful when it is important to see how a particular patient behaves or uses the health care system. For instance, if Cynthia changes a patient's drug regimen, she will want to collect data to determine if the patient becomes more compliant with his or her medications or has a better quality of life as a result. The disadvantage of primary data collection is that the data have to be collected manually as opposed to simply retrieving them from a database that already houses the information. Primary data collection can be time-consuming and expensive.

A secondary data source, such as a hospital or HMO database, can be a useful resource. Secondary data sources are particularly useful when gathering economic data because there is usually a direct correlation with how much an insurance company is charged and how much the product or service actually costs to provide. A researcher or clinician can also examine the data on a large pool of patients to see if an intervention actually affects a population of patients. A disadvantage of data such as these is that they are completely anonymous. There are no patient identifiers, and the data cannot be linked to individual patients. As a result, if one sample of patients patronizing one pharmacy is provided an intervention and another sample of patients is not, there is no way to detect economic change through the secondary data source.

■ REVISITING THE SCENARIO

Cynthia is using a secondary data source to conduct her cost-benefit analysis. After she has identified her variables of interest, she asks the HMO to provide her with baseline information on all heart failure patients prior to implementing her service. The HMO is able to stratify the data by diagnosis, so Cynthia asks for annual numbers and costs of hospitalizations, emergency room visits, and medications for their heart failure patients (see Table 27-3).

Cynthia forges ahead and starts her heart failure clinic. She successfully enrolls 250 patients in her service over the course of 1 year. At the end of the year, she conducts her cost-benefit analysis and asks the HMO for the same information that she collected at baseline (see Table 27-4).

Cynthia must also determine how much the clinic cost the HMO so that she can factor those costs into her analysis. She includes the salary and benefits of a part-time pharmacist to manage the service ($50,000) and the laboratory tests, supplies, and space costs necessary to monitor the patients ($72,000). Therefore, the direct cost of the clinic was $122,000 that year. The benefits of this service included decreases in the number of hospitalizations and average length of stay. Taken together, the total number of hospital days was reduced by an average of 7.2 days $[(5 \times 5.6) - (4 \times 5.2)]$ for each

Table 27-4. Characteristics of HMO Heart Failure Patients After the First Year of the Heart Failure Clinic

	Number	Cost	Average Length of Stay
Hospitalizations	4/year	$500/day	5.2 days
Emergency room	6/year	$1,000/visit	
Heart failure medications	4/month	$40/Rx	

of the 250 patients enrolled in the HMO and monitored by the service. If hospitalizations are assumed to cost the HMO $500 per day, the service saved the HMO $900,000 in hospitalizations (7.2 days × 250 patients × $500/day). The service also decreased the number of emergency department visits, resulting in savings of $250,000 ($1,000 × 1 visit × 250 patients). However, when Cynthia started to properly manage her heart failure patients, she found that they typically needed more medications to better manage their disease. The average number of prescription drugs for her patient population rose from three to four prescriptions per month, resulting in an increased expenditure of $10,000 ($40 × 1 prescription × 250 patients). When the costs and benefits are summed, the annual total cost of providing the service is $122,000, and the total benefits are $1,140,000 ($900,000 + $250,000 − $10,000). These results can be expressed as either a benefit-cost ratio of 9.3:1 ($1,140,000:$122,000) or a net benefit (cost savings) of $1,018,000. From this analysis, it appears that this service is valuable to the HMO.

Cynthia realizes that her analysis is only as strong as the variables that she has chosen to include. As a result, she decides to conduct a sensitivity analysis to ensure that her conclusions are sound. Some of the variables that she thinks may change the results of the project are the decreased number of hospitalizations, decreased length of stay, and decreased number of emergency department visits. She reexamines the data by taking half the difference in the number of hospital days and half the number of emergency department visits to see if the results change. The average number of hospital days per patient was decreased from 7.2 to 3.6 days, and the average of emergency department visits per patient was decreased from 1 to 0.5. As a result, hospitalizations cost savings were $450,000 (3.6 days × 250 patients × $500/day), and emergency department visits cost savings were $125,000 (0.5 visits × 250 patients × $1,000). This sensitivity analysis shows the total benefit to equal $565,000 ($450,000 + $125,000 − $10,000). The benefit-cost ratio drops to 4.6:1, and the net benefit is $443,000, but the service still clearly appears to be valuable to the HMO.

CLINICAL EVALUATION

Pharmacists have the ability to assess patients for general signs and symptoms of many disease states. In many states, pharmacists are also able to check blood glucose and lipid levels. They are able to measure peak flows in pulmonary patients and can assess minor skin abnormalities and wound care. All these clinical variables may be recorded at baseline and at each subsequent visit to chart changes and/or improvements in the patient's condition.

As with economic data, clinical information can be collected from primary and secondary data sources. Primary data can be collected at the point of care, when the pharmacist sees the patient. Primary data collection is the most reliable method of collecting clinical information because it provides the most control over the data collection process. The pharmacist can ask patients questions, perform necessary laboratory tests, conduct physical assessments, and record information either electronically or on paper.

Secondary data sources include hospital medical records, physician charts, and HMO databases. Medical records and charts traditionally are in paper form, but increasingly they are being computerized. Clearly, it would be easier to access the data electronically, but manual chart review, while time-consuming and tedious, may be necessary to gather all pertinent information. Again, one disadvantage of secondary data sources is that all the information needed may not be available. For instance, Cynthia may find that level of edema and blood pressure are recorded at each physician visit but not patient weight. The computer system being used by the HMO may not have a field or space to input the variable of interest. Cynthia's data would not be inclusive, and it will be more difficult to provide a complete longitudinal picture of her patients.

REVISITING THE SCENARIO

Cynthia has decided to collect information on each patient's level of edema, blood pressure, weight, NYHA classification, and shortness of breath. She also will record laboratory values where appropriate. When

Table 27-5. Changes in Clinical Outcomes of Heart Failure Clinic Patients After 1 Year

	Showed Improvement (%)	Remained Stable (%)	Symptoms Worsened (%)
Level of edema	45	35	20
Blood pressure	24	68	8
Patient weight	13	84	3
NYHA classification	15	79	6
Shortness of breath	67	19	14

patients are enrolled in her clinic, she records baseline values of the variables listed. She sees each patient every month for the first 3 months. Patients continue to be seen monthly until both Cynthia and the patient agree that the patient is stable, and then they will see Cynthia every 3 months thereafter. At each clinic visit, Cynthia recorded the same values in her electronic chart. At the end of the year, she complied the data to show that her medication management and education program have provided clinical benefits to her patients (see Table 27-5). She can also use statistical analysis to show if her clinic patients were statistically different.

HUMANISTIC EVALUATION

Humanistic outcomes generally are obtained directly from patients in the form of standardized questionnaires. There are two steps when collecting humanistic information. First is to identify the best and most appropriate survey or surveys to use (general or specific), and second is to decide how to administer the HRQL instruments or surveys. Usually, clinicians and/or researchers choose both general and specific HRQL instruments so that all elements related to a patient's quality of life are covered in the study. A patient satisfaction survey that has been used in a similar setting also may be administered. Clearly, the more information gathered, the more complete the picture will be. However, beware of *respondent burden,* or the time and energy it takes patients to complete the group of surveys. Patients who become tired may choose not to complete the survey or give false information in an effort to finish it quickly. This will not provide reliable data. The need for information must be balanced with patients' level of cooperation.

The next step is to determine how the survey will be administered. The four main ways to administer surveys are self-administered, face to face, mail, and telephone. When patients self-administer the surveys, they can answer the questions on their own. They are sometimes more willing to be truthful with sensitive information, such as income or sexual orientation. This method decreases the bias that can be introduced by an interviewer and also is the least expensive method. The downside of self-administered surveys is that patients sometimes do not finish the surveys and that some disease states make it difficult for patients to self-administer (e.g., glaucoma, rheumatoid arthritis, and Parkinson's disease).

Mail surveys generally have the same advantages as self-administered surveys and can effectively reach a large number of people. However, it often is difficult to motivate people to complete the survey and mail it back without some form of incentive, and it is also more logistically complicated for the researcher. Face-to-face interviews are effective in eliciting narrative responses and can be used with patients who lack good reading or writing skills, whose first language is not English, or who have difficulty seeing. The interviewer can gauge how the survey is going and can determine if the respondent is having difficulty understanding the items. On the flip side, interviews take more time, interviewers can introduce bias, and the process can be very costly.

Telephone surveys have the same advantages of face-to-face interviews but tend to be less expensive. Researchers can survey individuals from a large geographic area, and data can be linked to a record management system that can track respondents. Unfortunately, researchers cannot reach respondents who do not have a telephone and whose first language is not English, and they cannot verify the identity of the respondent. Multiple calls may be needed to contact the individual, and visual aids cannot be used unless they are mailed to respondents in advance.

The advantages and disadvantages of each method of administration are important as the study is designed and the patient population is identified. If an indigent population is being studied, the telephone format may not be appropriate because that population may not access to telephones. If a predominately Spanish-speaking population is being surveyed, face-to-face interviews with bilingual interviewers may be appropriate.

■ REVISITING THE SCENARIO

Cynthia feels that health-related quality of life and patient satisfaction are important aspects of her clinic. She thinks that these outcomes can serve to complement the economic and clinical outcomes that she is reporting to the HMO and can further prove her case that the clinic is a valuable service to the heart failure patients.

When patients enroll in the clinic, Cynthia assists them in completing the surveys. Most patients prefer to read the surveys and complete them at their own pace. Cynthia reads and records the survey information for those who are uncomfortable filling out the surveys individually. Through statistical analysis, she determines that there has been statistically significant change in all three quality-of-life measures over the course of the year (i.e., the SF-12, the Heart Failure Questionnaire, and the PSQ) and concludes that the clinic provides benefits from the patients' perspective.

■ DATA ASSESSMENT

After the data collection is completed, the data must be analyzed and assessed to interpret the results and reach meaningful conclusions. There are several ways to compile data so that they are easy to read and understand.

First, the service needs to be evaluated to determine if it provided a positive intervention for the patients. Prior to implementing the intervention, demo-graphic, clinical, and humanistic information should have been collected. These are called *baseline data* because collection is done at the beginning of the intervention, prior to any changes. Collecting baseline data is extremely important, a task that clinicians routinely forget to do prior to starting new programs or services.

After the program ends or has reached a predetermined point, the same pieces of information that were collected at baseline should be collected again. The data then are analyzed to determine if patient outcomes changed after enrolling in the clinic. Again, if baseline data were not collected, it becomes impossible to determine if changes in the values collected after the intervention were due to the intervention or to some other factor. For example, assume that a patient comes into a pharmacy and suggests that a new herbal remedy has caused her diabetes to get better. She says that she knows this because her blood sugar level is below 140 mg/dL. However, on further examination, she admits that she is not aware of what her blood sugar was prior to starting the herbal remedy. As a result, it is unclear whether the patient may have had blood sugar levels below 140 mg/dL prior to the remedy and to what extent, if any, the remedy provided any benefit.

Second, the financial impact of the service must be determined, keeping in mind the perspective of the analysis. For example, were the dollars saved from averted emergency department visit and hospitalization costs greater than the cost of implementing the clinic? Was the financial benefit to the patient worth the extra money he or she spent on the clinic? To perform these analyses, a sample of patients who participated in the clinic (intervention group) and a similar sample of patients (control group) who did not participate are needed. The total costs of health care between the two groups are compared to determine if there are differences. Total health care costs would include all hospitalizations, emergency department visits, physician visits, prescription medications, laboratory costs, and visits to the new clinic. To determine the benefit to the patient, various outcome variables are identified that measure change in patient status (e.g., humanistic outcomes such as HRQL and decreases in side effects) and increases in patient satisfaction and/or clinical outcomes (e.g., blood pressure, edema, and blood sugar levels). These variables can be evaluated separately or compiled to form an outcome measure.

USES OF OUTCOMES EVALUATION

Assessment of Success or Failure of a Service

After conducting an evaluation, the results may not be strongly in favor of a service. This does not necessarily mean that the service was a failure. There are many reasons why the results may be equivocal.

First, there may not have been enough patients in the analysis. If the changes that are sought are small but clinically and economically significant, a larger number of patients may have been needed to detect statistically significant changes. The number of subjects needed to detect the impact of the interventions should be determined prior to starting the clinic. In biostatistics, this concept is commonly referred to as *power*.

Second, many outcomes depend on how much time passes since the intervention. Many changes, particularly for clinical outcomes, take time to occur. A literature review of similar interventions may help to identify how much time may be needed to detect a clinically significant change. For instance, patients with asthma can see almost immediate relief when they are provided appropriate education and long- and short-acting medications to treat exacerbations. Conversely, comparisons between patients being educated with smoking-cessation classes and those not receiving education will be much more long term. Decades may be required to determine if some interventions provide economic, clinical, and humanistic benefits.

If the clinic was implemented and the analysis was conducted only to find that the outcomes were not as anticipated, what should a pharmacist do? While some outcomes can be disappointing, it is important to seek explanations for what was found in the results. Was the appropriate amount of time spent developing the clinic? Was there appropriate marketing to the patients? Was there buy-in by other employees in the pharmacy?

A Satisfaction with Pharmacy Services Questionnaire (SPSQ) may be used to determine what the patients think about the clinic. A focus group of patients also may be useful to learn what interventions they felt were beneficial and what was unnecessary.

Payment for Value-Added Services

To request compensation for value-added services, payers (i.e., patients and third-party payers) generally want to see that the service has value. In general, the better the outcome of a service, the more likely people will be willing to pay for the service. In the past, expanded pharmacy services could be justified simply by explaining to administrators that they were better for patient care. In today's cost-conscious environment, it is often necessary to objectively measure, compare, and analyze the cost and outcome differences to understand which programs or products provide the most value to consumers. By conducting these analyses, it is possible to decide whether the additional cost of a new treatment or clinic, in our case, is worth the additional benefits gained. This creates a rational way of understanding the value of a particular intervention.

It is important to present the results of these analyses in a clear and concise fashion. Most administrators will require that written and/or oral reports are presented on a regular basis. These reports should describe how the program is doing relative to stated objectives and goals.

Development of Additional Value-Added Services

Once a successful value-added service has been developed, it becomes easier to develop a new service in the future. The skills necessary to evaluate the outcomes of a service can be leveraged to start a new service. Perhaps a similar service with a different disease state would be a good next step. Be careful when thinking of starting new projects that are not directly similar to the one you have implemented. For instance, the skills gained with the heart failure clinic may not apply directly to starting a compounding specialty or wound care clinic.

To develop a new service, identify additional resources that will be required. More personnel, both for dispensing and for clinical functions, may be needed. More space for counseling, compounding, conducting classes, or placing diagnostic instruments or durable medical equipment also may be needed. Lastly, the way the pharmacy is perceived and marketed to the public may need some rethinking. If the pharmacy previously has dispensed only medications, the value-added services should be showcased, and the pharmacy can be marketed as a pharmacy with expanded patient care services.

Reassessing Your Service Objectives

As pharmacists who implement value-added services evaluate all they have accomplished, it is wise to do a little continuous quality improvement. They should identify the mistakes that they made along the way and think about how they can avoid making them again. They can also identify how they could have streamlined the process and created a better workflow for the service. Lastly, they may have conducted the project as a pilot project. These pharmacists will need to think about how they will expand the project in a seamless manner.

Pharmacists should seek the advice of those around them—their employees, supervisors, patients, and others affected by their services—to see if they have different viewpoints to share. Their input and constructive criticism may be as valuable as the economic, clinical, and humanistic results that were calculated.

REVISITING THE SCENARIO

After performing her analyses, Cynthia shared her results with her administrators at the HMO. They were very happy to see these results and asked Cynthia about other types of pharmacy services she might be able to develop. Cynthia said that she would look into expanding her heart failure clinic to become a more generalized cardiology clinic that included lipid management, anticoagulation management, and blood pressure management.

CONCLUSION

The objectives and goals of any value-added service should guide the outcomes data that are collected and how the data are analyzed. A common goal of any evaluation is to show the value of the value-added service. It must be remembered that value can have numerous meanings (e.g., clinical, economic, and humanistic) and can be measured from a number of different perspectives (e.g., patient, provider, organization, payer, and society). The desired outcomes and perspective of the analysis should drive the data-collection process and how the outcomes are assessed.

QUESTIONS FOR FURTHER DISCUSSION

1. What are some outcome measures that you can collect at your current practice?
2. How can you develop a relationship with a payer or physician group for the purpose of conducting economic analyses on your patients?
3. Based on Cynthia's objectives, did she forget to measure any variables?
4. List the direct and indirect and medical and nonmedical costs and outcome measures related to Alan Brouchard's diabetes education clinic and Carol's lipid management program?
5. What confounding variables should be measured in Alan Brouchard's diabetes education clinic and Carol's lipid management program?

REFERENCES

Armstrong EP, Langley PC. 1996. Disease management programs. *Am J Health-Syst Pharm* 53:53.

Barr JT, Schumacher GE. 1994. Applying decision analysis to pharmacy management and practice decisions. *Topics Hosp Pharm Manag* 13:60.

Bohachick P, Anton BB. 1990. Psychosocial adjustment of patients and spouses to severe cardiomyopathy. *Res Nurs Health* 13:385.

Bootman JL, Townsend RJ, McGhan WF. 1996. *Principles of Pharmacoeconomics*, 2d ed. Cincinnati: Harvey Whitney Books.

Coons SJ, Kaplan RM. 1993. Quality-of-life assessment: Understanding its use as an outcome measure. *Hosp Formu* 28:486.

Crane VS. 1988. Economic aspects of clinical decision-making: Applications of clinical decision analysis. *Am J Hosp Pharm* 45:48.

Cranor CW, Christensen DB. 2003. The Asheville Project: Factors associated with outcomes of a community pharmacy diabetes care program. *J Am Pharm Assoc* 43:160.

Criteria Committee, New York Heart Association, Inc. 1973. *Diseases of the Heart and Blood Vessels: Nomenclature and Criteria for Diagnosis,* 7th ed. Boston: Little, Brown.

Detsky AS, Naglie IG. 1990. A clinician's guide to cost-effectiveness analysis. *Ann Intern Med* 113:147.

Doubilet P. 1986. The use and misuse of the term "cost-effective" in medicine. *N Engl J Med* 314:253.

Drummond MF, Stoddart GL, Torrance GW. 1986. *Methods for the Economic Evaluation of Health Care Programmes,* p. 18. Oxford, England: Oxford University Press.

Eisenberg JM. 1989. Clinical economics: A guide to the economics analysis of clinical practices. *JAMA* 262:2879.

Etemad LR, Hay JW. 2003. Cost-effectiveness analysis of pharmaceutical care in a medicare drug benefit program. *Value Health* 6:425.

Fincham JE, Wertheimer AI. 1987. Predictors of patient satisfaction with pharmacy services in a health maintenance organization. *J Pharm Market Manag* 2:73.

Freedland KE, Carney RM, Rich MW. 1991. Depression in elderly patients with heart failure. *J Geriatr Psychiatry* 24:59.

Grady K, Jalowiec A, Grusk B, et al. 1992. Symptom distress in cardiac transplant candidates. *Heart Lung* 21:434.

Guyatt GH, Nogradi S, Halcrow S, et al. 1989. Development and testing of a new measure of health status for clinical trials in heart failure. *J Gen Intern Med* 4:101.

Ho KKL, Pinsky JL, Kannel WB, Levy D. 1993. The epidemiology of heart failure: The Framingham Study. *J Am Coll Cardiol* 22:6A.

Hsu J, Price M, Huang J, et al. 2006. Unintended consequences of caps on Medicare drug benefits. *N Engl J Med* 22:2349.

Kolar JA, Dracup K. 1990. Psychosocial adjustment of patients with ventricular dysrhythmias. *J Cardiovasc Nurs* 4:44.

Kozma CM, Reeder CE, Schultz RM. 1993. Economic, clinical, and humanistic outcomes: A planning model for pharmacoeconomic research. *Clin Ther* 15:1121.

Larson LN, MacKeigan LD. 1994. Further validation of an instrument to measure patient satisfaction with pharmacy services. *J Pharm Market Manag* 8:125.

MacKeigan LD, Larson LN. 1989. Development and validation of an instrument to measure patient satisfaction with pharmacy services. *Med Care* 27:522.

Mayou R, Blackwood R, Bryant B, et al. 1991. Cardiac failure: Symptoms, and functional status. *J Psychosom Res* 35:399.

McLean W, Gillis J, Waller R. 2003. The BC Community Pharmacy Asthma Study: A study of clinical, economic and holistic outcomes influenced by an asthma care protocol provided by specially trained community pharmacists in British Columbia. *Can Respir J* 10:195.

Patterson R. 1995. Disease management. *Case Rev* 1:59.

Rector TS, Kubo SH, Cohn JN. 1987. Patients' self-assessment of their heart failure: II. Content, reliability and validity of a new measure—the Minnesota Living with Heart Failure Questionnaire. *Heart Failure* 3:198.

Rideout E, Montemuro M. 1986. Hope, morale, and adaptation in patients with chronic heart failure. *J Adv Nurs* 11:429.

Rossiter SL, Langwell K, Wan TTH, et al. 1989. Patient satisfaction among elderly enrollees and disenrollees in Medicare health maintenance organizations: Results from the National Medicare Competition Evaluation. *JAMA* 262:57.

Rubin HR, Gandek B, Rogers WH, et al. 1993. Patients' ratings of outpatient visits in different practice settings: Results from the Medical Outcomes Study. *JAMA* 270:835.

Soumerai SB, McLaughlin TJ, Ross-Degnan D, et al. 1994. Effects of limiting Medicaid drug-reimbursement benefits on the use of psychotropic agents and acute mental health services by patients with schizophrenia. *N Engl J Med* 331:650.

Soumerai SB, Ross-Degnan D, Avorn J, et al. 1991. Effects of Medicaid drug-payment limits on admission to hospitals and nursing homes. *N Engl J Med* 325:1072.

Ware JE. 1991. Conceptualizing and measuring generic health outcomes. *Cancer* 67:774.

Ware JE. 1997. *SF-36 Health Survey: Manual and Interpretation Guide.* Boston: Health Institute, New England Medical Center.

Zitter M. 1994. Disease management: A new approach to health care. *Med Interface* 7:70.

SECTION VII

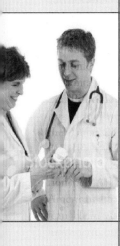

MANAGING RISKS IN PHARMACY

PRACTICE

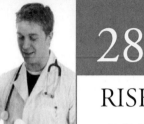

28

RISK MANAGEMENT IN CONTEMPORARY PHARMACY PRACTICE

Kevin Farmer and Donald Harrison

About the Authors: Dr. Farmer is Associate Professor of Pharmacy Administration at the University of Oklahoma Health Sciences Center College of Pharmacy. He received a B.S. in pharmacy and Ph.D. in pharmaceutical sciences from the University of Missouri–Kansas City. Dr. Farmer has experience in retail and hospital pharmacy practice settings and marketing research in the pharmaceutical industry. He teaches courses in U.S. health care systems and policy, financial management, and pharmaceutical marketing. Dr. Farmer's research is focused on issues related to medication adherence and health and economic consequences of health and medication health care policies.

Dr. Harrison is Assistant Professor of Pharmacy Administration at the University of Oklahoma Health Sciences Center College of Pharmacy. He received a B.S. in pharmacy from the University of Missouri–Kansas City. He received an M.S. in pharmacy and a Ph.D. in pharmaceutical sciences from the University of Arizona. Dr. Harrison has experience in many areas of pharmacy operations—retail, institutional, and research. Dr. Harrison teaches courses in research design, biostatistics, and pharmacoeconomics. Dr. Harrison's research interests are in the economic analyses of pharmaceutical services, outcomes research, and strategic planning by pharmacy institutions and businesses.

▪ LEARNING OBJECTIVES

After completing this chapter, students should be able to

1. Describe the role of risk management in pharmacy practice.
2. Identify critical components that constitute pure risk.
3. Describe the criteria for determining an insurable risk.
4. Discuss how risk management techniques can be used to manage emerging risks that may pose a threat to community pharmacy practice.

5. Describe how increased reliance on information technology and automation may exacerbate certain risks.
6. Describe the factors that affect performance risk of an information technology system used in pharmacies.
7. Characterize the risk of loss associated with the use of information technology in pharmacy operations.

■ SCENARIO

Bill Halsey, Pharm.D., has spent the past 2 years since graduating from pharmacy school working as a staff pharmacist for a well-respected community pharmacy to refine his skills as a clinically oriented community pharmacist. Bill's dream is to someday return to his hometown and purchase the pharmacy that had inspired him to pursue this career. That day seemed to arise even sooner than Bill expected when he learned that Mr. Simmons, the long-time owner of Corner Drug in his hometown, had suffered a minor heart attack. Mr. Simmons would like to sell Corner Drug and move to a retirement village. Bill quickly scheduled a trip back home to visit with Mr. Simmons and inspect the pharmacy to see what it might be worth. He also evaluated the current state of the pharmacy for providing specialized services in diabetes and geriatrics. Bill was somewhat surprised to see that the pharmacy was essentially in the same condition that it was when he worked there during high school. Mr. Simmons had always enjoyed chatting with his customers, so the pharmacy counter was very small with wide openings on both sides so that he and his employees could easily move in and out of the pharmacy department to interact with customers. The desk where the clerk took care of the insurance claims paperwork and charge accounts was in the corner of the customer waiting area. The computer appeared to be somewhat ancient, and Mr. Simmons joked that the high school students he hired as clerks often had to help him when the computer would start "acting up." Bill was understandably concerned. The delivery car could best be described as a "beater." He had been serving as the Health Insurance Portability and Accountability Act (HIPAA) compliance officer for his current pharmacy and was wondering what, if any, security and privacy measures were in place at Corner Drug. Bill also remembered Mr. Simmons lecturing him on his philosophy of the unnecessary reliance on insurance and wondered how well the pharmacy was protected from harm or loss or liability. Mr. Simmons always told him, "Your customers will never sue you if they love and respect you, so treat them well." Bill was beginning to question himself as to what may lie in store for him if he bought Corner Drug, as he now contemplated several emerging unresolved issues that could threaten the ability of the pharmacy to exist and prosper.

■ CHAPTER QUESTIONS

1. What is the primary difference between a speculative risk and a pure risk for an individual?
2. What are the common risk threats that pharmacies share with any type of retail business?
3. Is it possible for a community pharmacy to avoid all risks? If not, how should risk be handled?
4. How might HIPAA privacy rules affect a pharmacy's liability insurance coverage and costs?
5. What are four areas of risk that arise when pharmacies increase their reliance on information technology and automation?
6. What potential risk factor is considered the increased risks brought about by the moral and legal issues of the interaction of information technology and the safety and health hazards information technology poses to employees in the workplace?
7. Which six factors characterize the operational risk associated with information technology and automation in pharmacies?

INTRODUCTION

An element of risk exists in every human activity. One can become injured in an automobile accident on the way to work, become ill from food poisoning eating at a favorite restaurant, or lose thousands in retirement savings when the value of a company's stock declines significantly owing to an unexpected product recall. Pharmacists who own or operate pharmacies always must deal with the risk of business declines or even failure. There are always threats from the economy and the competition, as well as the potential for damage caused by a tornado, fire, flood, or hurricane. Indeed, a degree of risk is inherent in performing a most common task in almost any pharmacy—that of dispensing a patient's prescription. The changing health care environment requires pharmacists to critically examine risks in all aspects of their practice, especially as they look to take on more patient-oriented roles.

Historically, the primary risk exposure for pharmacists was related to traditional business risks (i.e., fire, theft, etc.), coupled with negligence related to prescription-filling errors. Modern pharmacy practice now must also consider new risks related to the use of technology and electronic data transmission, patient counseling and drug utilization review requirements, and protected private health information. As the practice of pharmacy continues to evolve, so do the risks associated with the changing environment and scope of pharmacy practice. Pharmacists must be aware of the inherent and evolving risks of delivering health care products and services and develop risk management strategies to deal with the risks. This chapter will review the concept of risk management and then focus on the new and developing risks associated with modern pharmacy practice in a technology-based environment.

DEFINITION OF RISKS

Risks are associated with negative outcomes. A *risk* is anything that threatens the ability of a person or organization to accomplish its mission. To fully understand risk in one's life or business venture, one must realize that there are several factors related to defining a risk as

a threat. A risk may best be described as some *degree of probability* that *exposure* to a *hazard* will lead to a *negative outcome or consequence* such as loss, damage, injury, or death (Ropeik and Gray, 2002). Exposures to some risks are a part of daily life. You could have an auto accident on any given day. For a risk to be a threat, there must be some statistical chance (probability) that a negative event will occur. One may or may not be exposed to a risk that may diminish or eliminate the risk as a real threat. You cannot drown if you are not near water. You cannot suffer an adverse reaction from a drug you have never consumed. To be a risk, it also must constitute a hazard (hence the sports phrase "No harm, no foul"). The severity or consequences also must be negative to be a risk. A drug may have a small probability of anaphylactic shock, but it may result in death. A new computer virus could destroy all the patient files and records stored in the pharmacy computer system.

From an insurance perspective, there are two basic types of risks: speculative risks and pure risks. A *speculative risk* involves a chance of gain or benefit as well as loss. Speculative risks are not insurable. Gambling is the prototypical speculative risk. When the $1 scratch-off lottery ticket you just bought didn't win the instant $1,000, you knew you had a very good chance of losing your dollar. The individual decides on the amount of risk he or she is willing to assume, including how much money to gamble and at what odds. Choosing to purchase shares of a mutual fund or common stock as an investment also involves speculative risk. Based on an investor's choices and a great number of other factors, his or her investment portfolio can experience substantial gains or suffer significant losses. Operating a pharmacy also involves speculative risk, in that there is no guarantee of success or failure. The number of independent community pharmacies in the United States declined from 31,879 in 1990, to 20,641 in 1998 (DHHS, 2000). In general, small-business ownership is inherently a risky venture. Data from the U.S. Bureau of Labor Statistics has found that only 45 percent of newly established businesses survive at least 4 years (Knaup 2005).

Pure risk involves a risk in which there is only the opportunity of sustaining a loss; there is no opportunity for gain. Pure risks are considered accidental, unanticipated, or unavoidable. Illness, death, fire, flood, and most accidents involve pure risk. Insurance is a product designed to assist people in managing their exposure to these unanticipated or accidental risks. Individuals and businesses can purchase insurance for risks involving health, death, and damage to home and business property. Damage to a place of business from fire or a tornado could cause catastrophic loss with little chance of gain for the owner and is therefore an insurable pure risk. The identification and management of pure risks are essential for a business to manage potential threats to its mission.

CRITERIA FOR INSURABLE RISKS

For a pure risk to be insurable, it must meet certain requirements (Schafermeyer, 2007):

- The loss must be measurable in dollar figures, easy to measure, and result in a substantial loss.
- The loss must have a defined time and place.
- The loss must be accidental for the insured. There should be no prospect of gain or profit for the individual.
- The probability of the event occurring in a population can be accurately calculated. There must be a sufficiently large number of homogeneous individuals with similar risks to make losses predictable.
- The insured must have an insurable interest. Compensation cannot be awarded to those not actually suffering the loss.
- The insurance premium must be available for a reasonable cost. One would not want to pay an insurance premium greater than the value of the item insured.

DEVELOPING A RISK MANAGEMENT STRATEGY

What strategies should pharmacists pursue to identify and minimize their risk exposure? A risk management process should be developed to analyze and identify strategies to manage risk threats. A risk management strategy should be designed to protect the vital assets of a pharmacy through coping with uncertainty. This process involves not only identifying risks but also assessing their threat potential and making decisions on managing those risks. Recall the definition of risk in this process—that some type of probability exists that exposure to some type of hazard will lead to a negative outcome or consequence.

THE RISK MANAGEMENT PROCESS

There are five steps that organizations should follow when developing a risk management process:

1. *Establish the context.* What are the goals of the risk management process? What are potential vulnerabilities of the business? Do employees or patients risk injuries? How might the reputation of the pharmacy suffer if a patient was injured owing to a prescription error or if his or her health condition was inadvertently made public by an employee? Could costly claims be avoided by not providing certain services or products?

2. *Identify and analyze risks.* Pharmacy managers should start by analyzing each dimension of their operation. Some examples of risks faced by pharmacies include the activities inherent in their business (i.e., filling prescriptions, counseling patients, and providing professional services). Other risks faced by pharmacies include making deliveries; maintaining the building, sidewalks, and parking lot; preparing sterile products; maintaining a computer system; and protecting patient health information. Problems in any of these could result in substantial losses for the pharmacy.

3. *Evaluate and prioritize the risks.* Pharmacy managers must prioritize their risks because every risk cannot be addressed at one time. Some risks are fairly common yet are not associated with a high degree of loss (e.g., prescription insurance claim rejections and shoplifting). Other risks are much less common yet are associated with substantial losses (e.g, catastrophic damage from a fire, flood, or storm or harm to a patient associated with a dispensing error). Pharmacies should prioritize managing risks

that have the greatest potential to result in substantial losses for their business.

4. *Select an appropriate risk management strategy and implement the technique.* Pharmacy managers must determine which risks could (and should) be avoided. Policies and procedures should be developed for appropriate risk prevention measures. Additional insurance policies or add-on riders should be secured as necessary. *Riders* are supplemental policies that provide additional coverage for something not covered in the original policy at some additional charge. There may be a ceiling or maximum amount the original policy will cover to replace personal property or equipment that may not provide adequate cost replacement for an asset(s). Thought should go into the level of deductibles to appropriately balance risk-sharing and risk-transfer issues (see "Techniques to Manage Risks" below). These strategies and the evaluation of which risks to avoid versus those that should be managed should be discussed with consultants or advisors (e.g., attorney, accountant, etc.) of the business operation.

5. *Monitor decisions and update the risk management program.* Pharmacy managers should monitor and update their risk management strategies to meet new challenges, threats, and opportunities. For example, when a pharmacy decides to offer immunizations to their patients, it not only creates new patient care and business opportunities, but it also exposes itself to additional risks (e.g., patients could experience an anaphylactic reaction to the immunization, patients could receive an inappropriate or incorrect immunization, and pharmacy employees could be exposed to pathogens). Once these new risks are identified, managers must create new strategies for their management.

■ TECHNIQUES TO MANAGE RISKS

Although risk is inherent to some degree in all our activities, there are different types of risks that require different techniques to manage. Each risk should be evaluated individually as to which technique(s) would be the most appropriate for that given risk.

1. *Risk avoidance.* While avoiding risks may sound like a logical approach, it is often impractical for most risks in a business environment. For example, most pharmacies cannot (and would not want to) avoid dispensing prescriptions despite the inherent risks involved in the process. However, there may be situations where not offering a specific good or service with an unreasonable risk may be the most prudent action. Many pharmacies choose simply not to perform sterile compounding services rather than incur the expense and risks associated with the preparation of these products.

2. *Risk prevention/mModification.* Pharmacy managers may not be able to eliminate a risk, but they can take steps to minimize the likelihood of its occurrence. All pharmacies take steps to avoid medication dispensing errors. This commonly involves the development of policies and procedures to prevent errors and improve patient safety (see Chapters 7 and 30).

3. *Risk absorption/retention.* Pharmacies often choose to retain or absorb some risks. Pharmacies commonly accept losses owing to shrinkage (i.e., shoplifting, employee theft, and unsalable products), usually by losing profits or passing on higher prices to consumers. A deductible on an insurance policy is absorption of risk. Some may choose to pay higher deductibles when losses occur in exchange for lower insurance premiums.

4. *Risk sharing or transfer.* Another technique to manage risk is to share or transfer the risk to another party. Insurance companies commonly share or transfer the risks inherent in paying for health care for their beneficiaries by entering capitated agreements with providers, paying them a set amount per member per month regardless of how much or how little their beneficiaries need health services. Another method to share or transfer risk is to purchase reinsurance (insurance for insurance companies). Health care providers can also purchase insurance to share or transfer the risks involved in providing care to patients whose costs may exceed the income provided in the capitated contract.

On an individual level, one can avoid some unnecessary risks (i.e., someone may never go swimming to avoid the risk of drowning), but from a business perspective, this strategy is impractical. One may choose to absorb certain risks if the cost of insurance is very high and the potential loss is small. Foregoing automobile collision insurance on a vehicle of minimal value would be an example (while retaining legally required liability insurance). Risk prevention is an important component of effective risk management strategies and is generally used in tandem with risk transfer. On the most basic level, risk prevention includes the use of smoke alarms, security systems, and theft detection. Additionally, for a business such as a pharmacy, employee training programs, education, and established policies and procedures are essential to deal with such risks as prevention of medication errors. With the possible exception of risk avoidance, most instances of conducting risk management will use some combination of each of the techniques of risk prevention, risk absorption, and risk sharing.

BASIC INSURANCE CONCEPTS

A pharmacy, like any other business entity, needs to protect itself, its employees, and its customers from physical and financial harm. No matter how careful a pharmacy is about preventing risks, it is practically impossible to eliminate accidents, such as when a customer or employee slips on the pharmacy's floor. At the same time, insuring for these risks does not eliminate the need for pharmacies to take effective risk prevention measures. Indeed, insurers commonly require that pharmacies have risk prevention measures in place to keep insurance policies in good standing for these risks or to reduce premiums. For instance, insurance for fire damage generally requires a sprinkler system or smoke detectors or alarms.

Common Insurance Terms

Insurance companies often use language that may be confusing to individuals not in the insurance industry. Pharmacy managers should have an understanding of the following terms commonly used in insurance policies (Insurance Information Institute, 2007):

Coverage   The scope (extent) of protection provided under an insurance contract.

Coinsurance   A provision that requires the insured party to share (absorb) some of the costs of covered services or losses on a fixed percentage basis. This may require the insured to pay 20 percent of the replacement costs, for example.

Deductible   The amount (a fixed amount specified in dollars) of an insured loss to be paid (or absorbed) by the policyholder. Deductibles may range from several hundred to several thousand dollars. $500 deductibles are common for automobile collision insurance.

Disability insurance   A type of health insurance that provides monthly income to the policyholder if he or she becomes unable to work because of an illness or accident.

Insured   The party covered by the insurance contract or persons entitled to benefits under the terms of the policy (e.g., family members may be covered under the employee's employer-sponsored health insurance plan).

Liability   Individual responsibility for causing injury to another person or damage to another's property through negligence.

Negligence   The failure to use reasonable care. The failure to do something a reasonably prudent person would do in like circumstances.

Peril   Insurance terminology for risk, possible cause of injury, or event causing damage or loss.

Policy   A written contract for insurance between an insurance company and the insured party.

Rider   Term used to describe a document that amends or changes the original policy.

Umbrella liability   A form of insurance protection in excess of the amount covered by other liability insurance policies. It also protects the insured in situations not covered by the usual liability policies.

Worker's compensation   A policy that pays benefits to an employee (or his or her family) for job-related injury or death.

Types of Insurance for a Pharmacy

Depending on the needs of the individual pharmacy, several different types of insurance policies may be required to provide adequate risk protection for the business. The geographic location, type of practice, and services offered will influence the types of insurance needed. The risk management process is a continuous process, and periodic evaluations are necessary to address new or emerging risk threats to the pharmacy. Emerging threats discussed later in this chapter exemplify how recent changes in health care practices (privacy issues) and technology create new and different risk threats to the pharmacy.

Property Insurance

This is one of the most common types of insurance for protecting the property and physical assets of any business entity. These policies generally cover losses owing to fire or lightning and theft and the costs of removing property to protect it from further harm. Property that should be insured include buildings (leased or owned), equipment, supplies, fixtures, inventory, money, accounts receivable records, computers and other data storage devices, vehicles, and intangible assets (e.g., goodwill and the value of a trade secret). Additional coverage can be purchased for specific "extended perils" such as windstorms, hail, floods, explosions, riots, or other specific events. A pharmacy manager should know exactly what is covered in his or her basic property insurance policy to determine if additional coverage is warranted owing to geographic location or local circumstances.

Liability Insurance (also Known as Casualty Insurance)

Liability insurance protects a business entity against claims when it is sued for damages or injuries caused by the negligence of the business or its employees. Liability insurance generally covers bodily injury, property damage, personal injury (including libel and interference with privacy), and advertising injury. Advertising injury may occur when advertising activities cause loss to another person through slander, defamation, libel, violation of privacy, or misuse of a copyright or trade-

mark (Rupp's, 2002). The legal expenses involved in a negligence suit (i.e., investigation, settlement, or trial) also should be covered by the policy. In today's litigious society, liability insurance is essential for any business entity, including pharmacies. Even fraudulent lawsuits brought by plaintiffs with little hope of success will result in expenses necessary for the pharmacy to defend itself. When a pharmacy is found to be negligent (such as in a dispensing error), a single judgment could result in a claim into the millions of dollars, resulting in financial ruin for an uninsured pharmacy. Liability insurance does not protect against nonperformance of a contract, wrongful termination of employees, sexual harassment, or race or gender lawsuits.

Business Owner's Policy

Insurance companies commonly bundle property and liability coverage together in the same policy for small-business owners. This policy allows for broader coverage, generally with less expensive premiums, than if property and liability insurance were purchased separately. Small businesses must meet certain criteria to qualify for these policies, such has having fewer than 100 employees and revenues not exceeding set amounts. These policies generally do not include professional liability coverage, worker's compensation, or employee health insurance. These must be purchased separately.

Individual Professional Liability Insurance

Pharmacists frequently purchase individual professional liability insurance policies in addition to what their business or employer may provide. This policy protects the individual against claims emanating from actual or alleged errors or omissions, including negligence, in the course of professional duties or activities. Individual policies are purchased because the business policy limits may not be high enough, and they will not cover the pharmacist outside that workplace. These policies commonly provide coverage of up to $1 milliom to $2 million per incident.

Key Person Insurance

This is insurance designed to protect a business entity from financial loss if key individuals (very likely the owner or partners) were to die or experience a disability. For instance, if the pharmacist-owner were to die suddenly or become disabled, this policy would pay to find and train a replacement or replace profits the company may have earned if the person had not died.

Umbrella or Excess Liability

It is possible that a lawsuit filed against a pharmacy could exceed the limits of the primary liability protection. For instance, a pharmacy's base liability policy may provide a maximum of $300,000 of coverage, but the pharmacy experiences a lawsuit in which the settlement or judgment reaches $1 million. The umbrella policy would cover the difference between the base liability limits and the judgment amount. An umbrella policy is activated only when the limits of the underlying base policy have been exceeded and exhausted. Umbrella liability policies can add substantial coverage for a relatively small additional cost.

Worker's Compensation

This statutory insurance covers medical expenses, disability income, and death benefits to dependents of an employee whose accident, illness, or death is job-related. Businesses are required to provide a safe working environment for their employees. Failure to provide a safe environment makes an employer liable for harm to their employees and may result in damage claim lawsuits from their employees. Worker's compensation can be a costly expense for some types of business in which the risk of injury to the worker is high, such as construction. Examples of injuries related to a pharmacy would be those owing to falls, overexertion, or repetitive motion, such as using a computer keyboard. Coverage rates depend highly on individual state laws and the type of work employees are engaged in.

There are a number of insurance companies that specialize in providing insurance coverage to pharmacies. It is a good idea for pharmacies managers to meet with representatives from these companies to discuss their specific insurance needs and compare policy offerings. Pharmacies may also purchase additional coverage for the specialty services they may offer. Examples include policies for home medical equipment, consultant pharmacist services, and professional liability insurance

for pharmacists. As previously mentioned, it is generally a good idea for pharmacists to purchase individual professional liability insurance for more comprehensive protection.

■ EMERGING RISKS ASSOCIATED WITH MODERN PHARMACY PRACTICE

The health care industry, including pharmacy, is one of today's most dynamic environments. Health care is a technology-rich environment, with pharmacy often leading the way in technological innovations and advancement. For example, pharmacies now commonly use robotics to assist in the prescription-filling process. They have long used computers in the transmission of third-party prescription claims and to share information between pharmacies. Today, prescriptions are increasingly transmitted electronically from the physician to the pharmacy, a process known as *electronic prescribing* (or *e-prescribing*). While advances in technology may offer many benefits in terms of patient safety and cost reductions, pharmacies need to incorporate these new technologies into their risk management processes. Employees need to be trained to become aware of new patient privacy regulations and requirements. Pharmacists may need to check and verify not only prescription dispensing activities by technicians but also computer input and data review. Ignoring or not understanding the impact of new professional requirements or technologies can place the pharmacy at risk. The Omnibus Budget Reconciliation Act of 1990 (OBRA 90) and the Health Insurabe Portability and Accountability Act (HIPAA) are examples of significant changes in pharmacy practice that present risk factors the pharmacy must consider in risk management.

Omnibus Budget Reconciliation Act of 1990 (OBRA 90)

The Omnibus Budget Reconciliation Act (OBRA) is enacted by Congress on an annual basis. It is used primarily to enact the budget for all the nation's governmental agencies and activities and generally has little to do specifically with pharmacy. However, the OBRA passed by Congress in 1990 (OBRA 90) had implications for pharmaceutical costs and state Medicaid pharmacy programs. In general, OBRA 90 specified what was expected of pharmacists in providing drug therapy to Medicaid patients. By 1993, pharmacists providing medications to state Medicaid recipients were required to provide prospective drug use review (Pro-DUR) and patient counseling and to maintain proper patient records. Most states quickly amended their state pharmacy practice acts to require that all patients receive this level of pharmacy services. Although patients had the option to refuse counseling, pharmacists now had the legal responsibility to provide information to their patients. While most pharmacists welcomed the legal acknowledgment of the professional responsibilities of modern pharmacy practice, OBRA 90 and the resulting changes in state pharmacy practice acts required that pharmacies reassess their risk exposure. Historically, pharmacists and pharmacy liability exposure had been limited to errors (negligence) when a prescription was filled incorrectly. A policy known as the *learned intermediary doctrine* traditionally held that pharmacist had no duty to warn patients against potential adverse reactions or other problems associated with a properly filled prescription. The duty to warn resided with the prescribing physician. However, with the advent of OBRA 90 and new professional standards of practice in pharmacy, courts have begun to abandon this doctrine (Dinardo, 2006; Holleran, 1995). While three-fourths of all claims against pharmacists are still related to dispensing the wrong drug or wrong strength, drug review claims against pharmacists (i.e., checking for interactions, allergies, and other problems), which virtually did not exist before 1991, now account for 9 percent of all claims (O'Donnell, 2005).

The Health Insurance Portability and Accountability Act (HIPAA) of 1996

The Health Insurance Portability and Accountability Act (HIPAA), which set standards for the privacy of individually identifiable health information, was signed into law in 1996 and went into effect in 2003. The Department of Health and Human Services (HHS) was required by Congress to promulgate the privacy standards and to set security standards for patient health information (DHHS, 2003). The standards for security and privacy are interconnected so that meeting the security standards would satisfy privacy concerns (Spies and Van Dusen, 2003). An individual's health information is referred to as *protected health information* (PHI) and is subject to the HIPAA privacy and security rules.

Pharmacies are affected by these rules in two ways. Pharmacies, by definition, deal with PHI (e.g., a prescription itself is PHI). If the pharmacy uses a computer, the information is then electronic and is known as *ePHI* (Barlas, 2004). HIPAA protects all "individually identifiable health information" held or transmitted by a covered entity or its business associate in any form or media, whether electronic, paper, or oral (DHHS, 2003). This covered information includes demographic data, including the individual's physical or mental health (past, present, or future); the health care provided to the individual; and payment information and common identifiers (e.g., name, address, birth date, and Social Security Number) that can be used to identify the individual. Pharmacies must have numerous policies and procedures in place to be in compliance with the HIPPA mandates. These include conducting risk assessments, appointing security and privacy officers to ensure compliance, and implementing policies and procedures to detect and prevent security violations.

There are a host of issues involving HIPAA that can place a pharmacy at risk. These include procedures for handling PHI in the event of fire, theft, system malfunctions, and disaster situations (Spies and Van Dusen, 2003). Even such seemingly benign events such as sticky-note reminders regarding customer requests in the pharmacy area or a technician verbally inquiring at the counter if the Zoloft for Mr. Jones prescription came in the morning wholesaler shipment are likely HIPAA violations. Risk exposure involving PHI goes beyond violations of federal law. Personal injury claims (nonbodily injury) are one of the fastest-growing areas of professional liability claims against pharmacists (O'Donnell, 2005). These claims involve libel, slander, or the unauthorized release of confidential records.

The release of a patient's protected health information constitutes the unauthorized release of confidential records.

Information Technology–Related Risks

The health care sector in general and community pharmacies specifically have become increasingly dependent on information technology. Almost all aspects of goods, services, and activities provided or conducted by community pharmacies have become interlinked with information technology. Many community pharmacies have invested heavily in information technology systems not only to dispense prescriptions and maintain patient records but also to digitize their financial and accounting systems, enterprise resource planning, human resources, and almost every other element of the business. Information technology has benefited community pharmacy in many ways. However, pharmacy's increased dependence on information technology has brought about a relatively new and increasingly important risk known as *information technology–related risk* (ITRR), often referred to as *digital risk*. Hardly a day passes without the report of some business losing confidential client information or having its computer network compromised by unauthorized intruders.

In addition to the usual ITRR that any business must confront, community pharmacies possess patient health, prescription, and financial data that can be an attractive target to unauthorized individuals wishing to gain access to those data. Therefore, risks owing to the implementation of and dependence on information technology potentially can offset the benefits derived if the implementation and management of information technology are not given sufficient attention. The ITRR incurred by community pharmacies can be grouped into several areas:

Strategic Risk

Strategic risk is the first and foremost risk confronted by pharmacies implementing information technology. To make any information technology project successful in the long run, pharmacies must assess the compatibility of the technology with their mission and goals

(see Chapter 3). Businesses must make choices between investing in information technology and other types of resources to achieve their overall goals and objectives. While the purpose of most information technology is to achieve efficiencies and competitive advantages, there are always risks that the organization would have been better off by pursuing other options. The costs of these risks are known as *opportunity costs*. Such risks even can result in failure to meet a pharmacy's goals and objectives and potentially can put the pharmacy at risk for significant financial loss.

Successful implementation of information technology projects can be difficult to achieve. According to the Standish Group's CHAOS Report (2003), an analysis of 13,522 information technology projects found that 15 percent "failed" and another 51 percent were considered "challenged." Further, a survey found that 30 percent of all application projects lasting more than a year "failed to meet business requirements" Lynch, 2007. In a survey of 82 Fortune 500 companies, 44 percent of respondents experienced "total abandonment" of an information technology project and another 16 percent experienced "substantial abandonment" (Ewusi-Mensah, 2003). Within community pharmacy, failures of this sort can be numerous and wide-ranging. For example, a new (or even existing) information technology system may fail to interface with pharmacy benefit manager (PBM) systems, resulting in an inability to process almost all third-party prescriptions. A pharmacy information technology system's failure to interface with a wholesaler's system may result in an inability to order and receive drugs and other goods in a timely manner. These are only two of many examples of system failures that a pharmacy can experience and that can seriously hinder its financial performance.

Organizational behavior problems can arise when integrating information technology into pharmacy practice. These often occur when stakeholders (i.e., employees and patients who interact with these systems) are not provided appropriate training before or after information technology implementation. The intended outcomes of information technology integration into pharmacy operations can occur only if there is good communication, commitment, cooperation, and coordination among all the stakeholders. Pharmacy managers incur risks associated with the acquisition and implementation of information technology resources when there is denial of the potential adverse events that can occur in the future. Pharmacy managers must "think outside the box" and consider each and every bad situation that can arise from the implementation and increased dependence on information technology.

Performance Risk

Performance risk is the degree of uncertainty inherent in the procurement and application of information technology solutions that may keep the system from meeting its technical specifications or from being suitable for its intended use and the consequences (Browning, 1999). The most important aspects of performance—those contributing most to performance risk—will vary with the needs and desires of the pharmacy (Barker et. al., 1998).

Performance risk arises from product complexity. Product complexity involves the number of components, functions, and interfaces in the pharmacy information system. There are several factors that contribute to product complexity:

SYSTEM REQUIREMENTS Specifications required by a pharmacy in its information technology are directly related to the degree of product complexity and performance risk. These challenges result from the various individual tasks pharmacies require of their information technology and the desire to integrate these tasks into a single piece of technology. Pharmacy information systems must handle a multitude of complex and interrelated elements, such as prescription entry, claim processing, prescription pricing, inventory, and financial management (see Chapter 6). These interrelationships make it difficult to balance optimal performance in all these areas and achieve the ultimate design goal of the system (i.e., enhanced operational efficiency and patient safety). For example, the information system must work to adjudicate third-party prescription claims and at same time check therapeutic substitution or drug–drug interaction for a particular patient. Another area of concern to pharmacies is data storage. Pharmacy information systems have become a huge repository of PHI for patients. The need to prevent unauthorized third-party access to sensitive patient data increases the chances of data becoming corrupted or lost owing to improper maintenance, decreased replication (backup), and complex encryption and decryption processes. Therefore, there is a tradeoff between data privacy and longevity data storage.

MODULARITY The ability of important components to function independent of the main application is preferable for information technology systems operated by pharmacies. The system should be decomposable into subsystems that make the product less complex. This provides room for individual component upgrades instead of redesigning the whole system when specifications change in certain areas, such as claim processing.

Operational Risk

Operational risk generally is defined as risk of loss resulting from inadequate or failed internal processes, people and systems, or external events (APRA, 2007; Erickson, 2001; McCuaig, 2005; Vaughn, 2005; Walker, 2001; Wikipedia, 2007). Information technology operational risks in today's digitized pharmacy are characterized by six event factors:

1. *Internal fraud* is an act committed by at least one internal party (typically an employee) that leads to data theft and/or loss. Information technology creates a tempting environment for employees to create fraud not only because the payoff from such activities can be high but also because the risk of detection is minimal.

   An *intranet* can help a pharmacy operate more efficiently by allowing information to be shared and communicated quickly and reliably. However, having a large number of users increases the intranet's vulnerability to internal threats. Intranet applications and their content may be exposed to a far greater audience than just those authorized users of the intranet. Recent research reports that more than 30 percent of all organizations report at least one security incident beginning within the organization, and an additional 24 percent reported a security incident but could not determine the origin (Allan, 2006). A pharmacy intranet can become more vulnerable as the user base becomes larger and more complex. Pharmacy intranet users commonly include employees, wholesalers, vendors, business partners, and other associated parties such as pharmacy students. Coincidentally, pathways from outside the intranet to the network can become less effective as the gateways needed to protect the organizational assets (mostly data) grow in scope and size. Finally, the degree of protection offered by firewalls can diminish as more and more exceptions to otherwise tight controls to the pharmacy's intranet are granted.

2. *External fraud* is an act committed by a third party that leads to data theft, data loss, and function disruption. People with technology skills can access (hack) the computer systems of pharmacies to steal or manipulate patient information for financial or nonfinancial reasons. For example, cell phone service provider T-Mobile experienced ongoing security problems that led to the publication of celebrity Paris Hilton's personal information and the telephone numbers of many Hollywood stars (Brian, 2005). One can only imagine the problems that could arise if patient data contained in a pharmacy's database were to be exposed, stolen, or manipulated.

In general, threats from external users can be classified into one of two groups: information attack and business-functions attack. *Information attack* can lead to Web site defacement, financial data theft, denial of service, and network performance degradation. *Business-function attack* may cause disruption of online refill requests, physician e-prescribing, and inventory management and interference with automated schedule actions. One of the most vulnerable areas of information technology for pharmacies are Web servers for Internet applications (e.g., pharmacy Web sites where patients can go to place refill orders or make other purchases). Web servers that have not been configured specifically to the pharmacy's needs (i.e., default configuration, insufficient input validation, poor encryption, improper cleaning of temporary files, and poor management of user sessions) are susceptible to serious attacks that may compromise these applications.

Another important tool of pharmacy automation is the barcode, which can be used to increase patient safety, facilitate inventory management, deliver checked prescriptions to patients, and refill automated stock cabinets (see Chapter 22). However, barcodes can be bypassed and are increasingly easy to exploit. To duplicate a barcode, one needs only the font of the barcode, a scanner, and the right software program. Pharmacy may be at great risk in maintaining the security of its supply system as the risk of counterfeit drugs becomes increasingly common. Radiofrequency identification (RFID) chips are now being developed to help maintain the security of the drug supply system (see Chapter 22).

3. *Computer homicide* is the use of information technology systems to perform a malicious act that results in the death of a patient (Brenner, 2001a, 2001b). A user could access the information technology system and alter a patient's health care or prescription data. Whenever a pharmacy's computer system is compromised, this kind of event could be very probable, and its impact on the pharmacy's business can be profound. While there are no documented incidences of this happening within the pharmacy setting, it is easy to see how it could be carried out. For instance, what if a patient is severely allergic to a drug such as penicillin? It could be possible that a malicious person could gain access via the pharmacy's information technology system to the patient record and alter the patient record such that the allergy is no longer documented? Further, if a prescription were written for penicillin or any penicillin-like product, the contraindication would not likely be caught by the computer software. While this is a very simplistic example, it is easy to see that without proper pharmacy information technology system safeguards, there is a great potential for patient harm or homicide because of the sensitive nature of patient data contained in the pharmacy's databases.

4. *Digital veil* is the term applied when the use of computer and automated machinery to execute business-related tasks creates a unique state of mind among the employees, resulting in complacency and blind trust in automation. This results in a mental disengagement with the work process, as if existing under a veil of digitization.

   In the summer of 1995, the Panamanian cruise ship *Royal Majesty* ran aground off the coast of Nantucket Island. The ship drifted off course because its satellite-based navigational system silently failed, and the crew did not monitor other sources of information that would have warned them they were in danger. Luckily, no one was hurt, but the mistake cost Majesty Cruise Lines $7 million in damages and lost revenue (Azar, 1998). Similar circumstances can occur in today's highly automated pharmacy. Employees can be become complacent, and the resulting mistakes in both patient and pharmacy safety and security can be catastrophic.

5. *The human–automation tradeoff* becomes more prominent as pharmacies become more dependent on automation. Years of experience and situational factors cannot be incorporated into software, which makes it less capable than humans to deal with emergency situations. Machines do not have the problem-solving capabilities that humans do for responding to new types of situations or threats.

6. *System failures* can occur in a multitude of ways once a pharmacy business is automated. System failures can have disastrous consequences. The use of sophisticated and intertwined Web services such as Internet refill request and processing, insurance processing, and inventory management create an overlay data-level network that ties multiple business functions together. If one function crashes, its failure potentially creates a cascading effect, causing other Web services to fail as well. Additionally, an attack against a single node supporting a purchase transaction in a supply chain could corrupt databases at several pharmacies, interfere with logistics and third-party shipping organizations, and create errors in financial reports and inventory management. The damage may not be localized to the node that was attacked initially. The damage could extend across a business network, spanning companies.

The examples of system failures just cited are general and can happen in any automated business. However, some system failures are unique to pharmacies because of time and regulation constraints. Automated dispensing devices have become increasingly common to enhance pharmacy efficiency and improve patient safety. Although the implementation of automated dispensing reduces personnel time for medication administration and improves billing efficiency, reductions in medication errors have not been uniformly realized (Murray, 2001). Further, a case study by Perry, Wears, and Cook (2005) provided vivid insight into the operational risk associated with automated dispensing unit failure. Automation failures can test the adaptive capability of practitioners. In this specific case, an automated dispensing unit in an emergency department failed to dispense medications in an emergency situation. The authors assert that the more reliable the technological system is, the less skilled workers become in responding to eventual system breakdowns. Finally, the desire to avert human error by practitioners can lead to fragile automation and unanticipated forms of failure that can be impossible to plan for.

Psychosocial Risk

Psychosocial risk involves the moral and legal issues related to the interaction of information technology and the safety and health hazards that technology poses to employees in the workplace (Burton, 2006). Pharmacies with an increased risk of these conditions also risk higher worker's compensation costs, absenteeism, short- and long-term disability, and decreased productivity. Highly automated businesses, such as pharmacies, may seem like a safe work environment but actually may have hazardous work conditions. Repetitive-motion injuries, known as *cumulative trauma disorders,* are common among employees who deal with automation on a regular basis. The most common cumulative trauma disorder is carpal tunnel syndrome, a painful injury that can debilitate the hands, wrists, and arms. Carpal tunnel syndrome stems primarily from the repetitive motions of typing and computer work (Sheehan, 1990). Other illnesses associated with pharmacy automation and computer usage include neck, shoulder, and lower back pain; headaches; irritability; difficulty sleeping; deteriorated vision; and eye strain (Daniels, 1995; English, 2001; Sodani, 2003).

RISK PARADIGM

Risk can be defined either as a negative outcome (e.g., lung cancer is a risk among smokers) or the cause for any negative outcome (e.g., smoking is a health risk). When there are several causes for a single outcome or several outcomes from a single cause, the qualitative assessment of risk becomes complicated. The *quantitative* approach in defining risk does not divide the events into causes and outcomes explicitly; rather, a probability is assigned to each possible relationship whose development is undesirable. The impact of the previously discussed four categories of risk associated with integration of information technology in pharmacies can be viewed as probability events (which are also risks) because they happen at a discrete time and have impact on financial and nonfinancial aspects of pharmacies, as described in Table 28-1.

The *qualitative* explanation for risk provides a better understanding of risk in terms of both cause and outcome. However, the identification of causes and predictions of outcomes is better rather than identifying the outcomes and predicting the causes to minimize the risk because the failure rate of information systems projects is high and is an ever-changing field bringing new and advanced solutions almost every year.

REVISITING THE SCENARIO

Bill Halsey clearly saw a huge task in front of him if he was to purchase Corner Drug. He started making a list of all the issues and risks he would have to address. Not only would he need to update most of the fixtures in the store, but he also foresaw problems with the current layout of the pharmacy department from a security standpoint. He would have to purchase a new computer system and install other information technology and then consider the security issues related to this new technology. Two local physicians were interested in having Bill monitor drug therapy for all their geriatric patients. Bill knew that he also would have to develop a training program for the store's employees to meet HIPAA requirements and for counseling and monitoring documentation. One of his first tasks would be to develop a risk management program to assess current and future risk threats and to ascertain which techniques would have to be employed to address the risks. Bill breathed a sigh of relief that his current employer had included him in meetings with his insurance agent and that he had become well versed in insurance terminology and planning. He would have a big job in front of him and a lot of additional learning

Table 28-1. Pharmacy Risk Paradigm

Cause/Effect	Financial Risk	Reputation Risk	Privacy Risk	Human Capital Risk
Strategic risk	Budget constraint; low or no return			Skill shortage; key personnel loss
Performance risk	Low or no return; patient injury	Loss of customers/ trading partners		
Operational risk	Data theft/loss; patient injury	Loss of customers/ trading partners	Data theft	
Psychosocial risk	Productivity loss; increased health benefits			

to do, but Bill thought he was prepared to know where to start and what needed to be done.

CONCLUSION

Just as with human beings in our daily lives, business entities such as pharmacies face risks that may threaten their financial health or ability to exist. Risk management is the process of identifying risks and developing strategies to manage or eliminate negative outcomes for the business. Risk management programs are an important component of business management. Risk management techniques include not only the use of insurance to transfer risk but also implementing strategies to minimize the likelihood of hazards occurring. Pharmacists need to be aware of these potential threats and seek assistance from their professional business consultants and experienced colleagues to develop and maintain appropriate risk management programs. Advice from experienced professionals may be crucial because most pharmacists have little training or experience in these areas.

The use of advanced information technology in community pharmacies continues to rise. Managers must be continually vigilant in safeguarding not only the pharmacy's own assets but also patient data from individuals both within and outside the pharmacy. As pharmacies grow more reliant on information technology and attacks on pharmacy systems grow more frequent and sophisticated, the successful pharmacy manager must manage the various risks brought about by this technology.

QUESTIONS FOR FURTHER DISCUSSION

1. Why is a risk management program an important component of a progressive patient-oriented pharmacy practice?
2. Many pharmacists have argued and fought for expanded roles in patient-oriented medication therapy management (MTM). These newer roles obviously increase the risk exposure of the pharmacists and the pharmacy. Should they therefore be avoided?
3. A local physician has approached you about the possibility of establishing a paperless e-prescribing system with your pharmacy. What are the risks involved, and how can you minimize those risks?
4. You have decided to establish a Web site that can be used by your patients to order both over-the-counter medications and prescription refills. You also would like to incorporate inventory management? What are the specific patient security risks? What are the pharmacy data security risks? Are other strategic, operational, performance, and psychosocial risks involved?

REFERENCES

Allan D. 2006. Web Risk Exposure: Don't Forget Your Intranet. A white paper from Watchfire. Waltham, MA: Watchfire.

APRA. 2007. Prudential Practice Guide: LPG 230—Operation risk. Available at www.apra.gov.au/Life/upload/Prudential-Practice-Guide-LPG-230-Operational-Risk.pdf.

Azar B. 1998. Danger of automation: It makes us complacent. *APA Monitor Online* 29(7). Available at www.apa.org/monitor/jul98/auto.html.

Barker K, Felkey B, Flynn E, Carper J. 1998. White paper on automation in pharmacy. Available at www.ascp.com/publications/tcp/1998/mar/feature2.shtml.

Barlas S. 2004. Securing electronic HIPAA data becomes hip. *P&T* 29:343.

Brian K. 2005. Paris Hilton Hack Started with Old Fashioned Con. *Washington Post,* May 5, 2005; www.washingtonpost.com/wp-dyn/content/article/2005/05/19/AR2005051900711.html.

Browning T. 1999. Sources of Performance Risk in Complex Systems. Available at http://sbufaculty.tcu.edu/tbrowning/Publications/Browning percent20(1999)–INCOSE percent20Perf percent20Risk percent20Drivers.pdf.

Brenner S. 2001a. State cybercrime legislation in the United States of America: A survey. *Richmond J Law Technol* 7(3).

Brenner S. 2001b. Cybercrime investigation and prosecution: The role of penal and procedural law. Available at http://npan1.un.org/intradoc/groups/public/documents/APCITY/UNPAN003073.pdf.

Burton J. 2006. Psychosocial risk management: What every business manager should know! Available at www.iapa.ca/pdf/2006_hwp_psychosocial_risk.pdf.

Daniels C. 1995. Computer ergonomics: Living with computers. Available at www.klis.com/computers+health/.

Dinardo JE. 2006. Your liability in filling Rxs correctly. *Drug Topics,* June 19.

Erickson J. 2001. IT trends: Operational risk. Available at www.forrester.com/Research/LegacyIT/Excerpt/0,7208,29917,00.html.

English T. 2001. One pharmacist's battle with work-related injuries. *Pharmacy Today* 7(5).

Ewusi-Mensah K. 2003. *Software Development Failures: Anatomy of Abandoned Projects.* Cambridge, MA: MIT Press.

Garvey PR, Cho C-C. 2003. An index to measure a system's performance risk. *Acquisit Rev Q* 10:188.

Lynch C. 2007. IT Value Methodologies: Do They Work? CIO WebBusiness Magazine, Apr. 10, 2007. Accessed at http://www.cio.com/article/103059/IT_Value_Methodologies_Do_They_Work_/1. (Accessed on 5/20/08).

Holleran MJ. 1995. Avoiding civil liability under OBRA 1990: Documentation is the key. *J Pharm Pract* 8:48.

Insurance Information Institute. 2007. Glossary of Insurance Terms. Available at www.iii.org/media/glossary/; accessed on December 3, 2007.

Knaup AE. 2005. Survival and longevity in the business employment dynamics data. *Monthly Labor Rev* May:50.

McCuaig B. 2005. The Case of Operational Risk Management. Available at www.cgservices.com/compliance/library/Case_for_Operational_Risk_Management.pdf.

Murray M. 2001. Automated Medication Dispensing Devices. Available at www.ahcpr.gov/clinic/ptsafety/pdf/chap11.pdf.

O'Donnell JT. 2005. Pharmacist practice and liability. *J Nurs Law* 10:201.

Perry SJ, Wears RL, Cook RI. 2005. The role of automation in complex system failures. *J Patient Saf* 1:56.

Ropeik D, Gray G. 2002. *Risk: A Practical Guide for Deciding What's Really Dangerous in the World Around You.* Boston: Houghton Mifflin.

Rupp's Insurance & Risk Management Glossary. 2002. Chatsworth, CA: NILS Publishing

Sammons M. 2003. Remarks at the NACDS Pharmacy & Technology Conference. Available at www.nacds.org/wmspage.cfm?parm1=3213.

Schafermeyer KW. 2007. Private health insurance. In McCarthy RL, Schafermeyer KW (eds), *Health Care Delivery: A Primer for Pharmacists,* 4th ed. Boston: Jones and Bartlett.

Sheehan M. 1990. Avoiding Carpal Tunnel Syndrome: A Guide for Computer Keyboard Users. Available at http://reporterbigskyoffice.com/content.php?id=36.

Sodani O. 2003. Computer-Related Injuries Guide. Available at www.help2go.com/Tutorials/Computer_Basics/Computer_Related_Injuries_Guide.html.

Spies AR, Van Dusen V. 2003. HIPAA: Understanding the security requirements. *U.S. Pharmacist* 28:42.

Standish Group. 2003. CHAOS. Available at www.projectsmart.co.uk/docs/chaos_report.pdf.

U.S. Department of Health and Human Services (DHHS). 2000. *The Pharmacist Workforce: A Study of the Supply and Demand for Pharmacists.* Rockville, MD: Health Resources and Services Administration.

U.S. Department of Health & Human Services (DHHS). 2003. OCR Privacy Brief: Summary of the HIPAA Privacy Rule. Available at www.hhs.gov/ocr/privacysummary.pdf.

Vaughn R. 2005. IT Hardware Disposal Risk Management. Available at www.blancco.com/binary/file/-/id/46/fid/500/.

Walker S. 2001. Operational Risk Management: Controlling Opportunities and Threats. Available at www.connleywalker.com.au/ORM.pdf.

Wikipedia. 2007. Operational risk. Available at http://en.wikipedia.org/wiki/Operational_risk.

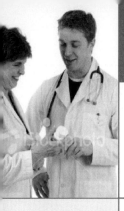

29

COMPLIANCE WITH REGULATIONS AND REGULATORY BODIES

Bartholomew E. Clark

About the Author: Dr. Clark is an Associate Professor in the Pharmacy Sciences Department at Creighton University School of Pharmacy and Health Professions. He earned a B.S. and an M.S. in pharmacy from the College of Pharmacy, University of Illinois at Chicago, and a Ph.D. in social and administrative sciences in pharmacy at the University of Wisconsin–Madison School of Pharmacy. Dr. Clark has practiced in a variety of community and institutional pharmacy settings and has served as professional affairs manager for the National Association of Boards of Pharmacy (NABP). His teaching and research interests include pharmacy practice management, pharmacy law, patient safety, pharmacists' work environments, and the pharmacy benefits management (PBM) industry.

■ LEARNING OBJECTIVES

After completing this chapter, students should be able to

1. Describe the reasons for the evolution of pharmacy and drug regulation that have created the current legal environment for pharmacy practice organizations.
2. Summarize and explain the basic provisions of the major pharmacy and drug laws discussed in this chapter.
3. Describe the manager's role in monitoring a pharmacy's compliance with applicable laws and professional standards.
4. Explain the role of the manager in developing and maintaining appropriate policies for the protection of patient privacy.
5. Analyze practice-based situations where laws and/or professional standards may have been violated. In these analyses, consider the implications (statutory, regulatory, and civil) of a manager's actions in resolving any problems presented by these situations and propose appropriate courses of action for the manager.

SCENARIO

Few examples of how much trust is put in the hands of a pharmacist and the extent to which that trust can be betrayed come close to the story of Robert Courtney, a former pharmacist from Kansas City. During the 9 years leading up to his arrest in August 2001, Courtney secretively diluted the chemotherapy drugs of over 4,200 cancer patients to increase the profits of his home infusion pharmacy business. Courtney broke the law while betraying the trust of his patients and damaging the reputation of his profession.

Patients place their trust in pharmacists to do and know things that they themselves do not understand. Patients trust pharmacists, whereas both state law and federal law provide additional layers of protection to shield the public from dangerous and/or contaminated drugs and from dangerous and/or dishonest professionals. As with any system, though, it can be breached. Consider how Courtney accomplished his deception.

Courtney began by diluting chemotherapy drugs for patients who were near death. He started out by diluting the drugs only a bit, thinking no one would notice. Later, he became more bold and diluted medications to the point that only a trace of the prescribed dose remained. He started out cheating "just a little" and then slid down a slippery slope until he was convicted of his crimes and sentenced to 30 years in prison. As stated in a newspaper feature about his case:

"The path to hell leads one step at a time," says Mike Ketchmark, the brash but persistent attorney who successfully litigated a $2.2 billion civil judgment against Courtney. "I think he started from the gray market and realized you could make a whole bunch of money. Then he'd get orders in from people who were on their deathbed, and he'd slice a little bit. Then he realizes he can just continue to cut it, and no one's going to notice. It's a felony once you engage in the gray market; you're then breaking down the barrier of a person's inhibition. You don't go from being John-Boy to Charles Manson overnight" (Draper, 2003).

While the Courtney case is an extreme example of just how far someone can go in betraying their professional duties and in breaking the law, it is important to understand that Courtney's transgressions started out small and were almost undetectable. Then his moral compass drifted further, and greed became his guide. His patients no longer mattered to him. Their trust in him was betrayed. Laws were broken. Courtney's crimes provide a hideous but poignant example of just how vulnerable patients are and exactly why there are pharmacy and drug laws in the United States to protect them.

CHAPTER QUESTIONS

1. How have standards and legal requirements for pharmacists evolved to the point where we see them today?
2. What is the significance of the current state of pharmacy and drug regulation for pharmacy managers?

INTRODUCTION

The purpose of this chapter is not to present a study guide for pharmacy law, an area to which entire texts have been devoted (e.g., Abood, 2007). Instead, its purpose is to provide an orientation to the professional and operational implications of food and drug law, pharmacy law, and professional regulation for pharmacy managers. This orientation should encourage pharmacy managers to think seriously about how the legal and regulatory environment external to a pharmacy practice organization can exert substantial influences on both the organization and its members. This encouragement includes a strong recommendation to know, understand, and follow applicable laws and professional standards in the operation of a pharmacy.

This chapter begins with a discussion of standards for pharmacists' professional performance and their importance to a manager. It continues with a brief overview of some key historical mileposts in the development of laws and regulations governing both the quality of drug products (at the federal level) and the conduct of pharmacy professionals (at the state level). Next, it concludes with an examination of how the existence of standards can affect what an organization should and/or needs to do. These concepts are then illustrated by case-study examples that apply the principles presented.

STANDARDS FOR PHARMACISTS' PROFESSIONAL PERFORMANCE AND THEIR IMPORTANCE TO A MANAGER

Webster's Dictionary defines a *standard* as "something established by authority, custom, or general consent as a model or example" and states that *standard* "applies to any definite rule, principle, or measure established by authority (standards of behavior)" (Webster's, 2003). From a contemporary managerial perspective, standards of conduct for a pharmacist and for the operation of a pharmacy are derived both from laws and from professional standards or values. Standards for professional conduct and the operation of a pharmacy, whether stated formally in statutes and regulations or present in professional codes of ethics, are important for managers to understand and apply. Violations of these standards can affect the licensure status of a pharmacy practice site and/or its pharmacists, may result in litigation if a patient is harmed subsequent to a violation, and in the most serious cases can result in criminal prosecution. Both criminal prosecution and civil liability resulted in the case of Robert Courtney, the pharmacist discussed in the scenario. Courtney was sentenced to 30 years in prison, fined $25,000, and ordered to pay $10.4 million in restitution to the patients and families affected. These penalties were in addition to the civil judgment of $2.2 billion (Stafford, 2002).

What Are Standards and Where Do They Come From?

Before there were laws in the United States for governing specifically the behavior of professionals, there were standards or codes of ethics established by professional guilds and associations. These codes of ethics stated in a formal way the type and level of professional performance that a professional association expected from its members. These expectations were derived from the kinds of expert services that society needed from members of that profession. The professional standards in codes of ethics helped to align the highest standards of a profession with society's expectations. Knowing that professionals worthy of their title and status should adhere to their profession's standards, society came to expect no less.

Bledstein (1976) discussed the evolution of the relationship between professionals and those whom they serve and noted that in mid-Victorian America there seemed to be a prevailing sense of insecurity among some members of the population. People who were seeking to expand their cultural horizons looked to professionals even for such things as recommendations concerning what should be considered appropriate reading material.

> A riot of words and a crisis of confidence alarmed a society which began placing its faith in professional persons. In mid-Victorian America, the citizen became a client whose obligation was to trust the professional. Legitimate authority now resided in special spaces, like the courtroom, the classroom and the hospital; and it resided in special words shared only by experts . . . . [T]he professions as we know them today were the original achievement of mid-Victorians who sought the highest form in which the middle class could pursue its primary goals of earning a good living, [and] elevating both the moral and intellectual tone of society . . . . Americans after 1870, but beginning after 1840, committed themselves to a culture of professionalism which over the years has established the thoughts, habits and responses most modern Americans have taken for granted [Bledstein, 1976, pp. 78–81].

The trust in the professional just mentioned came at a time in the history of American culture long before the existence of the commercial aspects of professional–client relationships sometimes seen today. This dichotomy was discussed by May:

> Contract and covenant, materially considered, seem like first cousins; they both include an

exchange and an agreement between parties. But, in spirit, contract and covenant are quite different. Contracts are external; covenants are internal to the parties involved. Contracts are signed to be expediently discharged. Covenants have a gratuitous, growing edge to them that springs from ontological change and are directed to the upbuilding of relationships.

There is a donative element in the upbuilding of covenant—whether it is the covenant of marriage, friendship, or professional relationship. Tit for tat characterizes a commercial transaction, but it does not exhaustively define the vitality of that relationship in which one must serve and draw upon the deeper reserves of another [May, 1988, p. 93].

Why Laws Governing Drugs and Professional Conduct Became Necessary

Despite such lofty expressions of the duties owed to society by those who served them, maximization of profits (rather than adherence to the highest standards) sometimes was the goal of those selling "medicinal" products. Stephen Hilts (2003) described in exhaustive detail the evolution of drug regulation in the United States beginning in the late nineteenth century through the present. During the late nineteenth century and well into the middle twentieth century, laws governing the content and quality of medicinal products provided, by today's standards, little or no protection to an unknowledgeable and unsuspecting public. Members of a relatively uninformed society were left to their own devices in making decisions for the purchase and use of medications. Subsequently, it took the occurrence of sentinel events such as the Elixir Sulfanilamide tragedy of 1937 and the thalidomide disaster of 1962 to raise consumer ire and prompt government action aimed at protecting the public from dangerous drug products.

The evolution of the pharmacy profession in the United States from colonial times to the present is rather astounding. During this time, pharmacy has made the transition from an unlicensed occupation that in many ways resembled a trade to its current status requiring a professional doctorate (Pharm.D.) degree to become eligible for licensure. At first, scant formal education and long periods of apprenticeship were required to attain full status as a pharmacist. During this period in the middle nineteenth century, the American Pharmaceutical Association (now the American Pharmacists Association) was established in 1852. Contemporaneously, the more classic definitions of professions and professionals applied. Professionals were expected to be ethical and honest in their dealings with the public, and the pharmacy profession was largely self-regulating, with sanctions from within its ranks as the only punishment for violation of the profession's standards. As schools and colleges of pharmacy emerged and became firmly established, the number of years required to earn a degree in pharmacy increased from as little as 2 to the present minimum requirement of 6 years of postsecondary education.

◼ HISTORICAL OVERVIEW OF LEGAL DEVELOPMENTS IN THE REGULATION OF DRUGS, PHARMACIES, AND PHARMACISTS

This section examines briefly some of the more pivotal pieces of legislation enacted during the last century and discusses how they have evolved to provide pharmacy with the current legal and regulatory environment for the regulation of drugs, pharmacists, and pharmacies.

Regulation of Food and Drug Safety: Standards for Foods and Drugs Sold at Retail

The authority to regulate foods and drugs sold in interstate commerce is given to the federal government by the commerce clause of the U.S. Constitution (U.S. Constitution, Article I, Sec. 8, Clause 3). Until the beginning of the twentieth century, the only federal law regulating drugs in the United States was the Drug Importation Act of 1848, which empowered the U.S. Customs Service to prevent the importation of adulterated (i.e., contaminated) drugs from other countries (FDA, 2002). Beginning in the early twentieth century, a series of highly publicized dramatic events provided the impetus for changes and improvements in the regulation of food, drug, and cosmetic safety.

Pure Food and Drug Act of 1906

The Pure Food and Drug Act of 1906 (59th Congress, Session I, Chap. 3915, pp. 768–772) was prompted by increased interest in the popular press concerning food safety that culminated in the publication of Upton Sinclair's exposé, *The Jungle,* a book that highlighted filthy and unsanitary conditions in meat packing plants. As stated in the 1906 act, the purpose of the new law was "for preventing the manufacture, sale, or transportation of adulterated or misbranded or poisonous or deleterious foods, drugs, medicines, and liquors, and for regulating traffic therein." In essence, this law required that foods and drugs be hygienic and accurately labeled. Before this law was enacted, there was a lack of standards and "traveling medicine shows," "patent medicines," and other unregulated products and activities were rampant. Products such as Lydia Pinkham's Vegetable Compound were nothing more than alcohol, whereas "soothing syrups" marketed as remedies for teething babies contained undisclosed and varying amounts of opium (Hilts, 2003).

The Food, Drug and Cosmetic Act of 1938 and Amendments

Passage of the Food, Drug and Cosmetic Act of 1938 was preceded by the Elixir Sulfanilamide tragedy of 1937. The 1906 act required drugs to be pure and labeled accurately but contained no requirement that drugs be safe. As one of the first effective oral antimicrobial drugs, sulfanilamide was very popular with physicians and was used widely to treat streptococcal infections. Bitter in taste, it was not easy to administer to children. Therefore, with some difficulty, the manufacturer developed a liquid dosage form called *Elixir Sulfanilamide.* Sulfanilamide powder is not soluble in either water or alcohol. Chemists at the manufacturer settled on ethylene glycol—the same chemical currently used as automobile antifreeze/coolant. This sweet-tasting chemical is highly toxic, causing painful kidney failure and death within a few days of ingestion.

In 1937, no safety testing was required prior to marketing a drug product, and no premarketing safety tests were performed on Elixir Sulfanilamide. Two hundred and forty gallons were shipped to physicians and pharmacies all over the country, and 107 children died after using the product. Despite the extreme danger that this product represented to the public, the only legal basis the Food and Drug Administration (FDA) had for removing it from the market was that the product label stated "elixir," whereas technically it was not an elixir because it contained no alcohol and therefore was misbranded. The danger of allowing drug products to enter the market without safety testing became obvious, and the public demanded that something be done. The result was the requirement for premarketing safety testing in the Food, Drug and Cosmetic Act of 1938.

The 1938 act was strengthened subsequently by amendments. The 1951 Durham–Humphrey Amendments created the separate categories of prescription-only and over-the-counter (OTC) drugs. Prior to passage of these amendments, there was no legal prohibition against selling drugs without a prescription. These 1951 amendments transformed pharmacy in ways likely unintended by their sponsors (Senator Hubert Humphrey was a pharmacist). There was a synergy between these amendments and the increased availability of finished-dosage forms in the post-World War II pharmaceutical industry boom that transformed the professional activities of neighborhood pharmacists. This transition from compounding and selling drugs at retail to "lick, stick, count, and pour" occurred simultaneously with the creation of the prescription-only market niche—a niche that only pharmacists were allowed to fill.

Next, the early 1960s saw another tragedy related to an unsafe drug product. Thalidomide was a drug marketed in Europe as a tranquilizer and used extensively to treat morning sickness in pregnant women. Although the manufacturer was eager to market this product in the United States, the efforts of FDA pharmacologist and reviewer Dr. Frances Kelsey prevented thalidomide from reaching the U.S. market. At the time, an FDA reviewer had 60 days either to approve or reject a new drug application (NDA) from a manufacturer. However, an FDA reviewer could request further information from the manufacturer and restart the 60-day clock—a tactic Dr. Kelsey employed several times because she was satisfied with neither the quantity nor quality of the data she had received about thalidomide's safety.

Tragedy in the United States was averted by Dr. Kelsey's efforts. Her refusal to approve the thalidomide NDA without further proof of safety occurred just as news from Europe revealed that thalidomide was responsible for a birth defect that caused infants to be born with flipper-like limbs. This near miss in the United States led to passage of the 1962 Kefauver–Harris Amendments to the 1938 act. These amendments established requirements that testing for *both* safety and proof of drug efficacy had to be conducted in well-controlled clinical trials before an NDA could be approved and a drug allowed to reach the market (Bren, 2001).

Establishment of State Pharmacy Practice Acts and State Boards of Pharmacy

Prior to 1870, when Rhode Island became the first in the nation to enact a state pharmacy practice act, regulation of the pharmacy profession was accomplished sporadically—generally at the local level or through the regulation of the medical profession (Green, 1979). States subsequently enacted their own pharmacy practice acts over the next several decades. The establishment of state pharmacy practice acts and the state boards of pharmacy created by these acts represents a legally binding codification of society's expectations of professional performance and a delineation of legal consequences for violation of these standards. The regulation of professional behavior by the states is pursuant to the police powers granted to the individual states by the U.S. Constitution. The establishment of state statutes and regulations governing the practice of pharmacy and operation of a pharmacy business not only provided a new layer of safety for the public but also created a real barrier to entry into the pharmacy profession. This was a significant step in increasing both the professionalism of pharmacy and the expectations that society had of pharmacists. Prior to establishment of such standards and legal requirements, practically anyone could operate a business and call it a pharmacy.

Currently, all states have some form of pharmacy practice act (a state statute) and state board of pharmacy regulations. These laws establish legally binding standards for the conduct of pharmacists and ancillary personnel, as well as standards for the physical facilities licensed as pharmacies. These statutes and regulations are not to be taken lightly. Violations can result in penalties ranging anywhere from reprimands and fines to the loss of licensure to practice the profession or maintain operation of a given pharmacy facility. Practicing pharmacy without a license is a violation of criminal law, so it is important for pharmacy managers to have a clear understanding of their responsibilities under these statutes and regulations and to communicate these responsibilities clearly to nonpharmacist management personnel involved in operation of the pharmacy. Consider, for example, the situation where a pharmacy is located within a larger store that is open when the pharmacy department is closed. If the nonpharmacist store manager decides to open the pharmacy to get someone's refill on a holiday when the store is open but the pharmacy department is closed (and, of course, there is no pharmacist on duty), this would violate the pharmacy practice act and board of pharmacy regulations in any state. A managing pharmacist has to make clear to nonpharmacist managers what they are not allowed to do under the law. Further, a pharmacist who allows such illegal practices also has committed a violation.

■ FEDERAL LAW AND THE CONDUCT OF PHARMACISTS

Omnibus Budget Reconciliation Act of 1990 (OBRA 90)

Until the passage of OBRA 1990 (Public Law 101-508), federal law in the pharmacy arena had been concerned primarily with drug product safety. OBRA 90, while not explicitly usurping the police powers of the states, required that to be eligible for federal matching dollars, states participating in the Medicaid program would have to establish standards for

- *Maintaining proper patient records.* Pharmacies must make reasonable efforts to obtain, record, and maintain at least the following patient information: patient name, address, telephone number; age and gender; individual history (where significant), including disease state or states, known allergies and/or drug reactions, and a comprehensive list of medications and relevant devices; and the pharmacist's comments about the patient's drug therapy.
- *Prospective drug use review (pro-DUR).* Prior to dispensing a prescription, a pharmacist must conduct an evaluation of a patient's medication record to detect potential therapy problems, such as therapeutic duplication, drug–disease contraindications, drug–drug reactions (including serious interactions with OTC medications), incorrect drug dosage or duration of drug treatment, drug–allergy interactions, and evidence of clinical abuse/misuse.
- *Patient counseling.* A dispensing pharmacist must offer to counsel regarding matters that are, in the pharmacist's professional judgment, significant, which include but are not limited to name and description of the mediation, route of administration, dose, dosage form, and duration of therapy. Additionally, such standards require pharmacists to discuss special precautions and directions, common severe side effects or interactions, therapeutic contraindications that may be encountered (including how to avoid them and what to do if they occur), proper storage, techniques for self-monitoring of drug therapy, what to do if a dose is missed, and refill information.

Not wanting to establish two separate legal standards of care—one for Medicaid patients and another for non-Medicaid patients—states generally adopted standards to meet the OBRA 90 criteria while extending the standards to benefit all pharmacy patients, not just Medicaid patients (Catizone, Teplitz, and Clark, 1993). Implications for pharmacy management include how the manager decides to structure employee duties and the organization of work in the pharmacy. It is the managing pharmacist's duty to maintain compli-

ance with applicable state and/or federal laws by ensuring that requirements for prospective drug use review and patient counseling are followed. From a management perspective, this means organizing work in the pharmacy and staffing the pharmacy to facilitate performance of these legal duties. Individual states may have their own requirements that may be stricter—but not more lenient—than federal law.

Health Insurance Portability and Accountability Act of 1996 (HIPAA)

This statute and its rules establish, for the first time, federal standards for protecting the privacy and security of patients' protected health information (PHI). These standards include, but are not limited to, how patient PHI must be stored, under what conditions it may be released, and to whom. This law has sweeping implications for pharmacies and pharmacists alike. The HIPAA privacy rules are designed to strike a balance between maintaining the flow of patients' health information among persons and entities providing health care to patients while simultaneously maintaining privacy for individuals. Essentially, this combination of statute and implementing regulations increases privacy and security for private information by establishing a "need to know" basis for who may have access to someone's PHI and to what extent they may have that access. Further, it establishes requirements for security of storage and for transmission of PHI by anyone who has access to the information. The purpose of this chapter does not include an exhaustive summary and explanation of this landmark legislation; entire volumes already have been devoted to the subject.[1] The rules implementing this federal statute became effective as of April 14, 2003. Suffice it to say that pharmacy managers are responsible for making sure that their staff and policies and procedures are in compliance with HIPAA.

---

[1] See (1) *HIPAA Privacy Standards: A Compliance Manual for Pharmacists.* National Association of Chain Drug Stores, Inc., and Mintz, Levin, Cohn, Ferris, Glovsky, and Popeo, P.C., 2003; and (2) Fitzgerald WJ. *The NCPA HIPAA Compliance Handbook for Community Pharmacy.* National Community Pharmacists Association, 2003.

From a pharmacy manager's perspective, it is essential to understand that HIPAA establishes transaction standards, security standards, and privacy standards for PHI. Transaction standards and security standards are concerned primarily with how data are handled and transmitted. In the day-to-day operation of pharmacy, a manager needs to understand and comply with the requirements for privacy standards. As stated in the summary of the HIPAA privacy rule:

> A major goal of the Privacy Rule is to assure that individuals' health information is properly protected while allowing the flow of health information needed to provide and promote high quality health care and to protect the public's health and well-being. The Rule strikes a balance that permits important uses of information, while protecting the privacy of people who seek care and healing. Given that the health care marketplace is diverse, the Rule is designed to be flexible and comprehensive to cover the variety of uses and disclosures that need to be addressed [DHHS, 2003b].

A pharmacy manager should know the answers to the following questions regarding these privacy standards:

1. *Who is covered by the privacy rule?* The privacy rule considers health plans, health care providers, and health care clearinghouses as covered entities. "Every health care provider, regardless of size, who electronically transmits health information in connection with certain transactions, is a covered entity" (DHHS, 2003b). This definition includes pharmacies.
2. *What information is protected?* According to the Department of Health and Human Services Office of Civil Rights,

> The Privacy Rule protects all *individually identifiable health information* held or transmitted by a covered entity or its business associate, in any form or media, whether electronic, paper, or oral. The Privacy Rule calls this information *protected health information* (PHI). Further, the Privacy Rule states that *individually identifiable health information* is information, including demographic data, which relates to

> - the individual's past, present, or future physical or mental health or condition,
> - the provision of health care to the individual, or
> - the past, present, or future payment for the provision of health care to the individual,

> and that identifies the individual or for which there is a reasonable basis to believe can be used to identify the individual. Individually identifiable health information includes many common identifiers (e.g., name, address, birth date, Social Security Number) [DHHS, 2003b].

3. *What must the covered entity do to protect information?* Every covered entity must have an individual designated as the facility's "privacy officer"—a person who is charged with the responsibility of keeping the site in compliance with HIPAA. Essentially, a covered entity may not release or disclose PHI except as allowed under the privacy rule. The following subsections summarize briefly what a pharmacy manager (a person who also may be the privacy officer) must be aware of.

Employee Training

Employees of a pharmacy should be trained in HIPAA rules and procedures as a condition of employment. Newly hired personnel should receive training before being allowed to work with PHI. This training should be documented as having been completed and repeated, if necessary, for employees who do not perform up to the standard. Although this may seem harsh, it is necessary to keep the pharmacy in compliance. At a minimum, the training should include making clear to employees (1) how, to whom, to what extent, and under what circumstances PHI may be released and (2) that PHI should not be included in casual conversations with others—even in conversations with other health care providers if they are not involved in the patient's care. Also, employee access to PHI should be restricted to what is necessary in the performance of their duties.

Notice of Privacy Practices

Under the HIPAA privacy rule, all covered entities are required to provide patients with a "notice of privacy practices." The covered entity must provide this notice to all patients, and it should be written in understandable language. The privacy officer, most likely the pharmacy manager, is responsible for documenting patient signatures acknowledging receipt of the notice and documenting the reasons for any patient refusals of the notice or any patient refusal to sign in acknowledgment of having received the notice. The covered entity must maintain records of these documents for 6 years. Again, the importance of maintaining well-organized and easily retrievable records cannot be overemphasized.

Business Associates

The HIPAA privacy rule definition of a *business associate* and requirements regarding business associates are as follows:

Business Associate Defined. In general, a business associate is a person or organization, other than a member of a covered entity's workforce, that performs certain functions or activities on behalf of, or provides certain services to, a covered entity that involve the use or disclosure of individually identifiable health information.

Business associate functions or activities on behalf of a covered entity include claims processing, data analysis, utilization review, and billing. Business associate services to a covered entity are limited to legal, actuarial, accounting, consulting, data aggregation, management, administrative, accreditation, or financial services. However, persons or organizations are not considered business associates if their functions or services do not involve the use or disclosure of protected health information, and where any access to protected health information by such persons would

be incidental, if at all. A covered entity can be the business associate of another covered entity.

Business Associate Contract. When a covered entity uses a contractor or other non workforce member to perform "business associate" services or activities, the Rule requires that the covered entity include certain protections for the information in a business associate agreement (in certain circumstances governmental entities may use alternative means to achieve the same protections). In the business associate contract, a covered entity must impose specified written safeguards on the individually identifiable health information used or disclosed by its business associates. Moreover, a covered entity may not contractually authorize its business associate to make any use or disclosure of protected health information that would violate the Rule [DHHS, 2003b].

In general, a pharmacy manager and/or privacy officer (in consultation with legal counsel) should tailor the pharmacy's relationships with business associates via the business associate contract. The overarching goals in an appropriately constructed business associate contract are to minimize the business associate's exposure to PHI while clearly establishing what uses of the PHI are permitted by the business associate. The privacy officer should have a clear idea of what business associates plan to do with any PHI they obtain and should make sure that any subcontractors have similar agreements. The privacy officer should monitor the business associate for any violations of the contract. In fact, the contract should stipulate that it is the responsibility of the business associate to report unauthorized disclosures of PHI. Finally, the privacy officer is responsible for the disposition of any PHI released to the business associate and should make sure that after it has been used by the business associate, PHI is either returned, held securely, or destroyed.

Patient Authorization Required for Release of PHI

A pharmacy, as a covered entity, needs to obtain a patient's written authorization for any disclosure or use of PHI that is not for treatment, payment, or health care operations. This authorization cannot be used as a precondition for benefits eligibility, payment, or treatment. The authorization document must be written in plain and specific language, and it may allow use and disclosure of protected health information by the covered entity. An example of a disclosure of PHI that would require a written authorization by a patient is disclosure of such information to a drug manufacturer for marketing purposes. All authorizations must specify what information may be disclosed and must identify the person(s) disclosing and receiving the information, must specify an expiration date for the authorization document, and must state that a patient has the right to revoke the authorization in writing. Patient authorization for the release of PHI is not required for circumstances where a pharmacist reports spousal abuse or child neglect, becomes involved in legitimate law enforcement situations (including compliance with workers' compensation laws), is avoiding a threat to health or safety, or is reporting an adverse drug reaction to the FDA Medwatch program.

Circumstances Where PHI May Be Released without Explicit Patient Authorization

PHI may be released without explicit patient authorization under certain circumstances defined in the law and rules. These circumstances (with examples) include treatment (e.g., when a pharmacist discusses a patient's condition with the patient's physician), payment (e.g., when a claim for payment is submitted to a third-party payer), regular health care operations (e.g., the transfer of PHI among departments within a hospital), and when the information has been "de-identified."

PHI is considered to be "de-identified" when the following data elements have been removed:

- Patient's name, Social Security Number, and telephone and/or fax numbers
- Patient's town, street address, and/or ZIP code (state of residence need not be removed)
- Any dates of service (except year)

- Medical record number, health plan number, account number, and/or prescription number
- Any vehicle identifiers (e.g., license plate number)
- Medical device identifiers and/or serial numbers
- Patient's Web site URL, computer IP address, and/or e-mail address
- Biometric identifiers
- Photographic images (identifiable)
- Any other unique characteristic or code

Remember, though, that "de-identification" of information is not necessary between covered entities involved in a patient's care. "De-identification" is also not necessary between a covered entity and a business associate with which the covered entity has a business associate contract.

The HIPAA statute and rules have created considerable confusion for pharmacy managers who have wondered about how these changes may affect normal operations in their pharmacies. Questions arise regarding situations such as when a neighbor is picking up a prescription for a patient. (*Note:* HIPAA rules allow the pharmacist to release a prescription to a patient's neighbor and counsel that neighbor as the patient's *agent.*) In response to these sorts of questions, the U.S. Department of Health and Human Services Web site has a search function that finds answers to many common questions about a wide variety of health care practice situations (DHHS, 2003c).

Prescription Drug Marketing Act

Pharmacy managers must also be aware of federal law regulating economic issues in pharmacy. The Prescription Drug Marketing Act of 1987 (PDMA) represents one area where some pharmacists have encountered considerable legal problems, resulting in large fines and/or prison sentences (Associated Press, 2000; Eiserer, 1999). In brief, the PDMA prohibits the diversion of drug samples into the retail market sector. Pharmacies may not have in their stock any prescription drug samples, and pharmacies may not possess or sell any drug samples. Further, the PDMA restricts the annual wholesale distribution of drugs by pharmacies to other pharmacies to no more than 5 percent of the annual dollar value of drug sales for the distributing pharmacy (e.g., one pharmacy providing drugs to another that has run out of stock of an item). Pharmacy managers must ensure compliance with the PDMA or be prepared to face stiff penalties. In a Nebraska case, a pharmacist violated the PDMA by colluding with a pharmaceutical manufacturer's sales representative to divert and profit from the sale of drug samples. In 1999, the pharmacist pled guilty to illegally selling prescription drug samples over a 15-year period (Eiserer, 1999). In 2000, the pharmacist was sentenced to 18 months in prison and ordered to pay nearly $147,000 in fines and restitution (Associated Press, 2000).

Civil Law and Liability Concerns

When a pharmacist or pharmacy organization is sued, the issue of negligence becomes the key to what the outcome of the lawsuit will be. Negligence theory revolves around either the failure to do something that a reasonable and prudent person *would* do or doing something that a reasonable and prudent person *would not* do. In this case, the person is the pharmacist. The pharmacist's role has changed over time because of the evolving nature of pharmacy practice (e.g., OBRA 90 ushered in the requirement to offer patient counseling). Case law also changes pharmacy practice standards. Case law is based on precedents established by the outcomes of civil cases. If, for example, the result of a lawsuit establishes that a pharmacist had a duty to warn a patient about certain dangers of a drug that was dispensed, then a new standard of behavior for pharmacists is established through case law, not by statute or regulation.

The thought of being sued for something one has done while practicing or the thought of a pharmacy manager being sued for the actions of his or her staff pharmacists is not at all pleasant. The first thing someone might think of is, "How can I prevent that from happening to me?" This question opens the door to a field of management called *risk management* that deals with how to reduce and manage exposure to risk (see Chapter 28). Sound practice site design, consistent adherence to applicable law, and a well-organized workflow system designed to detect errors before they can reach the patient are all essential to minimizing exposure to risk. As with all laws governing the activities of pharmacists, managers are encouraged to become familiar with these important provisions.

■ HOW DO LEGAL STANDARDS AFFECT WHAT AN ORGANIZATION SHOULD AND/OR NEEDS TO DO?

It is important for managers to understand that statutory and regulatory standards create an environmental context for an organization, a factor critical in determining whether or not the organization prospers and grows. The manager is a person embedded within an organization that is, in turn, embedded within the environment—an environment that is constantly changing. For pharmacists and pharmacies, statutes and regulations represent society's codification of standards beyond its normative expectations—beyond the sanctions implicit in not meeting the expectations of professional peers. Statutes and regulations also provide for enforcement by way of penalties if they are violated. Regulations are standards that are derived from statutes and have legal enforcement mechanisms (i.e., potential penalties) attached to them. For example, state pharmacy practice acts create a board of pharmacy and empower that board to establish rules and/or regulations to interpret and implement the practice act. Board of pharmacy regulations carry the full force of the law and establish penalties anywhere from warnings, to fines, and on to suspension and/or revocation of pharmacist or pharmacy licensure.

Performance Improvement versus Meeting Minimum Performance Standards

To avoid legal sanctions for practitioners and/or the pharmacy, the manager can take steps to prevent or avoid substandard practices that could lead to penalties. How should a manager approach such a task? One way some organizations approach making sure that they meet minimum legal standards is by setting up programs to foster performance improvement. Meeting minimum performance standards is compliance with the bare minimum legal requirement, whereas performance improvement goes beyond this and can provide additional protection in the risk prevention and risk management arenas. If a pharmacy and its pharmacists aim to establish standards for the performance of the organization that exceed the legal minimum, it is much less likely that performance quality will result in violations of the law or in performance so poor that it results in a civil lawsuit. For example, a pharmacist manager may decide to establish a policy that every patient visiting the pharmacy will receive a personal offer of counseling from a licensed pharmacist, even where state law may allow pharmacy interns or other pharmacy staff to perform this function. Further, if a lawsuit is filed against the pharmacy, it can work in a pharmacy's favor if the pharmacy has in place standards of care and policies and procedures that exceed the legal minimum and afford better protection for clients. Also, with such systems in place, it is much less likely that a pharmacy will encounter legal difficulties of either kind. Establishment of a practice environment and philosophy that are centered on doing what is best for the patient while knowing and obeying all applicable laws is essential to avoiding legal problems in either the civil or criminal realm.

CONCLUSION

This chapter began by reviewing the history of and motivation for the development of standards, statutes, and regulations governing the manufacture of drugs and the practice of pharmacy. Next, within this context, some of the milestones of pharmacy and drug regulation, such as HIPAA, OBRA 90, and the Prescription Drug Marketing Act, were summarized. Finally, civil law and its impact on pharmacy practice were considered. All these aspects of pharmacy and drug regulation were examined from the viewpoint of the pharmacy manager.

The chapter concludes with the following case examples for discussion of laws pertinent to the operation of a pharmacy. These cases are presented as starting points for discussion and analysis of practice-based situations a pharmacy manager is likely to encounter. Pharmacy and drug law, as well as civil law, all present managers with criteria on which to fashion their own management style in operating a pharmacy. Law, while quite explicit in its language, often can be silent on some issues and thus open to interpretation and the exercise of professional judgment. Pharmacy students reading this chapter are encouraged to work together in analyzing the situations presented here and to come up with their own plausible solutions to the problems presented.

QUESTIONS FOR FURTHER DISCUSSION

Case Examples for Discussion of Laws Pertinent to Operating a Pharmacy

Case 29.1: Why Won't the Pharmacist Just Refill My Prescription?

A FEDERAL DRUG LAW: THE CONTROLLED SUBSTANCES ACT OF 1970 Maureen Smith, R.Ph., the pharmacist manager of ABC Drugs Community Pharmacy, encounters the following situation within 10 minutes of arriving at the pharmacy on a Tuesday morning. She finds herself dealing with a complaint from a patient, Mr. Jones, about one of the staff pharmacists. Yesterday evening, Monday, at about 8:30 p.m., Mr. Jones came to the pharmacy and presented an empty prescription vial to the pharmacist on duty and asked for a refill of his acetaminophen with codeine no. 3 tablets. Acetaminophen no. 3 is a schedule III controlled substance, and the federal Controlled Substances Act limits prescriptions for such medications to a maximum of five refills within 6 months of the time they are issued. Mr. Jones had not seen the prescribing physician in about 7 months and was now experiencing pain unrelated to the reason for his visit 7 months ago. However, the label on his vial stated that he had three refills remaining, and he wanted one right away.

Sally Howard, Pharm.D., the pharmacist who was on duty Monday evening, explained to Mr. Jones that she would need further authorization from Mr. Jones' prescriber because the prescription had been written over 6 months ago and was now no longer valid for re-filling. Sally tried to reach Mr. Jones's doctor to obtain authorization but was unsuccessful in reaching the prescriber before the pharmacy closed at 9:00 p.m. Therefore, she informed Mr. Jones that the pharmacy would not be able to refill the prescription until it could reach the prescriber. Mr. Jones became angry when he heard this and remains very angry as he is telling Maureen about the situation.

DISCUSSION QUESTIONS

1. What are the essential legal issues involved?
2. How should the pharmacy manager handle this situation?
3. How might another manager deal with the problem presented by this difficult patient?

Case 29.2: The Grandmother Who Did Not Need an Easy-Open Prescription Vial

A FEDERAL CONSUMER PROTECTION LAW: THE POISON PREVENTION PACKAGING ACT The (federal) Poison Prevention Packaging Act requires that prescription medications (with very few exceptions, such as sublingual nitroglycerin tablets) be dispensed in child-resistant containers. Mrs. Mabel Brown, a 79-year-old great grandmother to 2-year-old Barbara Brown, is a long-standing patient at the community pharmacy where you are the manager. You have just been informed by Mrs. Brown's great granddaughter's pediatrician that little Barbara was treated at the local hospital emergency room yesterday evening. It seems that while Barbara and her parents were visiting Mabel at her house, Barbara climbed up on the kitchen counter and grabbed Mabel's prescription vial containing propranolol 80 mg long-acting capsules. Little Barbara had only been out of her mother's sight for about 2 minutes when her mother walked into the kitchen and found Barbara sitting on the kitchen counter munching away on Mabel's medicine. Although she became a bit lethargic, luckily she did not have enough time to consume a dangerous quantity and was treated and released.

After speaking with the pediatrician, you do some checking in Mabel's patient record, and you discover that all her medications have been dispensed in non-child-resistant containers (i.e., "easy open" flip-top containers). On further investigation, you discover that there is no request on file where Mabel or her physician actually asked for easy-open containers. While discussing this with your pharmacy staff, you learn that everyone just assumed that a 79-year-old patient would want the non-child-resistant containers but that no one had ever asked her if she wanted them.

DISCUSSION QUESTIONS

1. How would the pharmacy manager need to articulate and address the issues presented by this situation?
2. What are the key issues, and how should a pharmacy manager handle them with pharmacy staff?
3. What recommendations for change, if any, would be appropriate to assist the pharmacy in refining the pharmacy's policies and procedures?
4. What additional civil liability issues arise from situations like this one?

Case 29.3: The Supertechnician

A STATE PRACTICE ACT/BOARD OF PHARMACY PROVISION Trudy Hamilton, Pharm.D., is a licensed pharmacist and is currently the manager of a hospital pharmacy department. In the state where Dr. Hamilton is licensed, nonpharmacist personnel are prohibited by both statute (the state pharmacy practice act) and state board of pharmacy regulation from engaging in activities defined as the practice of pharmacy. The specific activities that fall within the definition of the practice of pharmacy are limited to being personally performed by licensed pharmacists only. Such activities include counseling patients about their medications and responding to drug information requests from other health care professionals (e.g., physicians and nurses).

Robert Allen recently earned his certification as a certified pharmacy technician (C.Ph.T.) and has been working as a technician in the pharmacy department for the past 3 years. Robert is rightly proud of his accomplishment and recently has expressed interest in applying for admission to pharmacy school. Today,

Dr. Hamilton received a phone call from Ann Brown, D.O., an attending physician at her institution. Dr. Brown was noticeably angry. Yesterday, Dr. Brown called the pharmacy with a drug-interaction question about a drug that is new to the hospital's formulary (i.e., the list of drugs that the hospital pharmacy regularly keeps in stock). She was told by the "pharmacist" who answered the phone that the pharmacy department's computer system showed no interactions. Today, Dr. Brown's patient experienced a severe interaction between the new drug and a medication that the patient was already taking.

At a recent continuing-education seminar, Dr. Hamilton and her staff pharmacists learned of the potential for a significant interaction between the two medications in question. She was puzzled as to why one of the pharmacists would have told a physician that there are no drug interaction problems with the new drug. Dr. Hamilton and the staff pharmacists are aware that the hospital information technology department has not yet updated the pharmacy department computer system to include this interaction. As she concludes her conversation with Dr. Brown, she promises to find out what happened and take corrective action.

In Dr. Hamilton's investigation, she discovers that technician Robert Allen in fact took the phone call and answered Dr. Brown's question. Dr. Hamilton calls a meeting of the pharmacists to discuss how to prevent such problems from occurring in the future. During the meeting, she discovers that a few of the staff pharmacists have, on occasion, observed Robert stepping outside his technician role because he was trying to be helpful. They tell her that they have attempted to correct his behavior but have had little success. This is the first time Dr. Hamilton has heard of the problem.

DISCUSSION QUESTIONS

1. How should Dr. Hamilton address this situation?
2. Are there problems with the way the department is functioning as a unit?
3. Is this situation simply a "personnel" issue confined to Robert's behavior?

4. Are there other issues or combinations of issues that should be addressed?

Case 29.4: The Poorly Written Prescription and the Hurried Pharmacist

CIVIL LIABILITY (TORT LAW) Stuart Johnson, R.Ph., is manager of Johnson's Apothecary, a community pharmacy. When he arrived at the pharmacy today, there was a frantic voice-mail message left for him in the middle of the night while the pharmacy was closed. It seems that a staff pharmacist, Dave, made a dispensing error yesterday, and Suzie Jones, a 3-year-old child, was taken unconscious by ambulance to the local community hospital emergency room at 2:00 a.m. Suzie and her family had just moved to town about 2 weeks ago, and yesterday was their first visit to Johnson's Apothecary.

In the process of both calling the hospital and interviewing Dave, the staff pharmacist, Stuart learns the following: Somehow Dave misinterpreted a poorly written prescription that was supposed to be for glycerin suppositories (Directions: "Use as directed") as a prescription for Glynase 5-mg tablets (a drug used to treat diabetes in adults). As a result of this error, Suzie's blood sugar dropped to dangerously low levels, and she is now in a coma. Dave was very busy when the error occurred and did not determine that the patient, Susan Jones, was in fact a 3-year-old child. He also did not speak to Suzie's mother, who brought in the prescription. Because he was very busy, he quickly checked a pharmacy technician's work and let her dispense the prescription to Mrs. Jones, an uninsured cash-paying customer. The sad truth is that the doctor had not even intended this written note to be a prescription (glycerin suppositories are available without a prescription); it just looked like one because it was on one of the doctor's prescription blanks.

DISCUSSION QUESTIONS

1. From this case, describe violations of both state and federal law and the tort law implications (i.e., potential for being sued).
2. What is the manager's role in determining what happened internally that was out of conformance

with standards, with external regulatory bodies, and with professional performance standards beyond the letter of the law?

3. How can all these be brought to bear on the pharmacy?

4. How should Stuart as the manager respond when the local TV station and newspaper want interviews?

REFERENCES

Abood RR. 2007. *Pharmacy Practice and the Law,* 5th ed. Boston: Jones and Bartlett.

Associated Press. 2000. Drug Representative, Pharmacist Sentenced. *Omaha World-Herald,* February 12, p 16.

Bledstein BJ. 1976. *The Culture of Professionalism,* p. 78. New York: Norton.

Bren L. 2001. Frances Oldham Kelsey: FDA medical reviewer leaves her mark on history. *FDA Consumer Magazine,* March–April.

Catizone CA, Teplitz J, Clark BE (eds). 1993. *NABP Survey of Pharmacy Law.* Park Ridge, IL: National Association of Boards of Pharmacy.

Draper R. 2003. The Toxic Pharmacist. *New York Times Magazine,* June 8.

Eiserer T. 1999. 2 Plead Guilty in Fraudulent Drug Sale Case. *Omaha World-Herald,* October 9, p. 34.

Green MW. 1979. Epilogue, Prologue. In *From the Past Comes the Future—The First 75 Years of the National Association of Boards of Pharmacy.* Chicago: National Association of Boards of Pharmacy.

Hilts PJ. 2003. *Protecting America's Health: The FDA, Business and One Hundred Years of Regulation.* New York: Knopf.

Longest BB, Rakich JS, Darr K. 2000. *Managing Health Services Organizations and Systems,* 4th ed. Baltimore: Health Professions Press.

May WF. 1988. Code and covenant or philanthropy and contract: Hastings Center report 1975. In Callahan JC (ed), *Ethical Issues in Professional Life,* p. 93. New York: Oxford University Press.

Stafford M. 2002. Ex-Pharmacist Gets 30 Years for Diluting Cancer Drugs. Associated Press, December 5.

U.S. Department of Health and Human Services (DHHS). 2003a. Covered Entity Decision Tools, Centers for Medicare and Medicaid Services, modified July 24, 2003; available at www.cms.hhs.gov/hipaa/hipaa2/support/tools/decisionsupport/default.asp.

U.S. Department of Health and Human Services (DHHS). 2003b. Office of Civil Rights (OCR) Privacy Brief: Summary of the HIPAA Privacy Rule, rev., May 2003; available at www.hhs.gov/ocr/privacysummary.pdf.

U.S. Department of Health and Human Services (DHHS). 2003c. HIPAA Questions and Answers. Available at http://answers.hhs.gov/cgi-bin/hhs.cfg/php/enduser/std_alp.php.

U.S. Food and Drug Administration (FDA). 2002. FDA Backgrounder: Milestones in U.S. Food and Drug Law History, updated August 5, 2002. Available at www.fda.gov/opacom/backgrounders/miles.html; accessed on March 21, 2003.

Webster's Online Dictionary. Available at www.m-w.com/cgi-bin/dictionary?book=Dictionary&va=standard+; accessed on March 20, 2003.

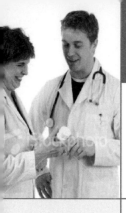

30

PREVENTING AND MANAGING MEDICATION ERRORS: THE PHARMACIST'S ROLE

Matthew Grissinger and Michael R. Cohen

About the Author: Mr. Grissinger is the Director of Medication Error Reporting Programs for the Institute for Safe Medication Practices (ISMP). Prior to joining ISMP, he served as a home care and long-term care pharmacy surveyor for The Joint Commission (TJC). Mr. Grissinger is a frequent speaker on pharmacy topics and current issues in medication safety. He has published numerous articles in the pharmacy literature, including regular columns in *P&T*, *Pharmacy Today*, and *U.S. Pharmacist*. He is also a clinical analyst for the Pennsylvania Patient Safety Reporting System (PA-PSRS). Mr. Grissinger serves on the U.S. Pharmacopeia's Safe Medication Use Expert Committee, the National Coordinating Council on Medication Error Reporting and Prevention (NCC MERP), the Editorial Board for *P&T*, and the Publications Advisory Board for *Davis' Drug Guide for Nurses*. He is also an Adjunct Assistant Professor at Temple University School of Pharmacy and Clinical Assistant Professor at the University of the Sciences in Philadelphia. Mr. Grissinger received a B.S. in pharmacy from the Philadelphia College of Pharmacy and Science and is a fellow of the American Society of Consultant Pharmacists.

Michael Cohen, R.Ph., M.S., Sc.D., is President of The Institute for Safe Medication Practices, a nonprofit health care organization that specializes in understanding the causes of medication errors and providing error-reduction strategies to the health care community, policymakers, and the public. He is editor of the textbook, *Medication Errors,* and serves as coeditor of the *ISMP Medication Safety Alert!* that reaches over 2 million health professionals and consumers in the United States, as well as regulatory authorities and others in over 30 foreign countries. Dr. Cohen is a member of the Sentinel Event Advisory Group for the Joint Commission and served recently as a member of the Committee on Identifying and Preventing Medication Errors for the Institute of Medicine. He is also a member of the National Quality Forum's Voluntary Consensus Standards Maintenance Committee (CSMC) on Safe Practices and served recently on the FDA Drug Safety and Risk Management Committee. Dr. Cohen has consistently been recognized by *Modern Healthcare* as one of the top 100 "Most Powerful People in Healthcare," and in 2005 he was recognized as a MacArthur Fellow by the John D. and Catherine T. MacArthur Foundation. Dr. Cohen received a B.S. in pharmacy and an M.S. in hospital pharmacy administration from Temple University. He has received Doctor of

Science degrees (*honoris causae*) from the University of the Sciences in Philadelphia and Long Island University in New York and a Doctor of Public Service from the University of Maryland.

■ LEARNING OBJECTIVES

After completing this chapter, students should be able to

1. Discuss the role of the pharmacist in preventing medication errors.
2. Define latent and active failures and the role each plays when a medication error occurs.
3. Determine the cause(s) of system breakdowns that result in medication errors.
4. Define the types of medication errors that can occur during the ordering and dispensing process.
5. State the 11 steps necessary for safe dispensing of medications.
6. List some commonly used drugs that can result in medication error–related deaths.
7. Define confirmation bias.
8. List steps that should be taken to minimize errors when receiving verbal orders.
9. Describe what changes are needed at the risk management level to better address medication safety issues, including the use of failure mode and effects analysis to reduce the potential for errors.
10. Identify specific problems in our approach to error prevention and what needs to be changed to ensure patient safety.

■ SCENARIO

This scenario is based on a true story that demonstrates the multiple breakdowns that can occur during the medication use process that led to the death of an infant. An infant was born to a mother with a prior history of syphilis. Despite having incomplete patient information about the mother's past treatment for syphilis and the current status of both the mother and the child, *a decision was made to treat the infant for congenital syphilis.* After phone consultation with infectious disease specialists and the health department, an order was written for one dose of "benzathine penicillin G 150,000 units IM."

The physicians, nurses, and pharmacists, unfamiliar with the treatment of congenital syphilis, also had limited knowledge about this medication. The pharmacist consulted *Drug Facts and Comparisons* to determine the usual dose of penicillin G benzathine for an infant. However, *she misread the dose* as

500,000 units/kg, a typical adult dose, instead of 50,000 units/kg. Consequently, the pharmacist also *incorrectly read and prepared the order as 1,500,000 units, a 10-fold overdose.* Owing to the lack of a consistent pharmacy procedure for independent double-checking, *the error was not detected.* The pharmacy *dispensed the 10-fold overdose in a plastic bag containing two full syringes of Permapen 1.2 million units/2 mL each,* with green stickers on the plungers to "note dosage strength." A pharmacy label on the bag indicated that 2.5 mL of medication was to be administered intramuscularly to equal a dose of 1,500,000 units. After glancing at the medication sent from the pharmacy, the infant's primary care nurse expressed concern to her colleagues about the number of injections required to give the infant the medication (since there a maximum of 0.5 mL per intramuscular injection allowed in infants, the dose would require five injections).

Anxious to prevent any unnecessary pain to the infant, the two colleagues *decided to investigate the possibility of administering the medication intravenously instead of intramuscularly.* The monograph on penicillin G did not specifically mention penicillin G benzathine; instead, it noted the treatment for congenital syphilis with aqueous crystalline penicillin G slow intravenous push or penicillin G procaine intramuscularly. Nowhere in the two-page monograph was penicillin G benzathine mentioned, and no specific warnings regarding "IM use only" for penicillin G procaine and penicillin G benzathine were present. Unfamiliar with the various forms of penicillin G, a nurse practitioner *believed that "benzathine" was a brand name for penicillin G* and concluded that the drug could be administered safely intravenously. While preparing for drug administration, *neither nurse noticed the 10-fold overdose, and neither noticed that the syringe was labeled by the manufacturer, "IM use only."* The nurses *began to administer the first syringe of Permapen as a slow intravenous push.* After about 1.8 mL was administered, the infant became unresponsive, and resuscitation efforts were unsuccessful (ISMP, 1998).

The three nurses involved in this case were indicted for criminally negligent homicide in the death of the baby. ISMP provided a systems analysis and expert testimony at trial and identified over 50 different failures in the system that allowed this error to occur, go undetected, and ultimately, reach a healthy newborn child, causing his death. Had even just one of these failures not occurred, either the accident would not have happened, or the error would have been detected and corrected before reaching the infant.

▪ CHAPTER QUESTIONS

1. At what stages of the medication use process do medication errors occur?
2. What types of contributing factors lead to medication errors during the ordering process?
3. What procedures should be followed when taking a verbal order?
4. What steps should be followed during the prescription-filling process to prevent medication errors?

5. What three important factors play a role in any patient interface?
6. Which types of patients are more at risk for noncompliance?

▪ INTRODUCTION

Patient safety has become a major concern since the November 1999 release of the Institute of Medicine's (IOM) report, "To Err Is Human." Health care practitioners may have been surprised to learn from this report that errors involving prescription medications kill up to 7,000 Americans a year. The IOM released a report in 2006 entitled, "Preventing Medication Errors" and indicated that medication errors are among the most common medical errors, harming at least 1.5 million people every year. The reports concluded that 400,000 preventable drug-related injuries occur each year in hospitals. Another 800,000 occur in long-term care settings, and roughly 530,000 occur just among Medicare recipients in outpatient clinics. Assuming conservatively an annual incidence of 400,000 in-hospital preventable adverse drug events (ADEs) yields an annual cost of $3.5 billion in 2006. The report noted that these are likely underestimates because the data excluded errors of omission such as the failure to prescribe medications for which there is an evidence base for the ability to reduce morbidity and morbidity (IOM, 2006).

With this increased attention to medication errors by the lay media, concern has intensified in both the public and health care sectors. Research demonstrates that injuries resulting from medication errors generally are not the fault of individual health care professionals but rather represent failures in a complex health care system. Medication error prevention starts with recognizing that errors are multifactorial and are faults of the system as a whole rather than results of the acts or omissions of the people in the system. Even when an error can be traced directly to a specific individual (e.g., the pharmacist dispensing the wrong medication or the nurse administering the wrong medication), further investigation often determines that a number of factors, such as poor order communication between the physician and pharmacist, dangerous storage practices in pharmacies, and look-alike labeling, may have played a role in the error. Protecting patients from inappropriate administration of medications has become an important focus for pharmacists and technicians, including those in ambulatory, acute care, long-term care, home care, and managed-care settings.

Pharmacists and technicians play a major role in medication safety in modern pharmacy practice. After summarizing several studies performed in hospitals and long-term care facilities, Allan and Barker (1990) estimated that medication errors occur at a rate of about 1 per patient per day. In a more recent study performed in ambulatory pharmacies, they found an overall dispensing accuracy rate for prescription medications of 98.3 percent (Allan, Barker, and Carnahan, 2003). While most of these errors probably have minimal clinical relevance and do not affect patients adversely, many experts believe that medication error rates may be higher in the ambulatory care setting because errors may not always be evident to the health professionals who work there. For example, medication errors can occur when a patient purchases nonprescription medications without speaking with the pharmacist about any potential interactions with his or her prescription medications or if patients fail to verify the appropriate dose of the over-the-counter (OTC) medication.

This chapter focuses on system enhancements and the checks and balances needed to proactively prevent medication errors as pharmacists and technicians prepare, dispense, and monitor the effects of medications in all practice settings. In addition, focus is placed on the importance of determining latent failures that contribute to mediation errors by developing effective medication error reporting programs to discover how latent failures occur and how they can be prevented.

▓ BACKGROUND

Currently, many organizations take an ineffective approach to preventing medication errors. Investigations tend to focus on the *front end* or *active end* of the error

(e.g., the front-line practitioner, such as the pharmacist dispensing the medication). When an error occurs, human nature needs to assign blame to someone or something. In addition, health care practitioners work in an environment where they strive for perfection. Individuals involved in the commission of an error may be considered inattentive, incompetent, lazy, and uncaring. They are often subject to punitive action such as disciplinary action, public or private reprimands, remedial education, suspensions, or termination. As a result, the practitioner develops feelings of inadequacy, denial, and embarrassment.

Effective approaches, on the other hand, consider factors that contribute to medication errors that occur at the organizational level, known as the *latent end* or *blunt end* of an error. Latent failures are weaknesses in organizational structure, such as faulty information management or ineffective personnel training, that may have resulted from decisions made by upper management (Reason, 1990). Latent failures can also stem from incomplete information, such as missing allergy or diagnosis information, unclear communication of a drug order, lack of an independent double check before dispensing, lack of computer warnings, ambiguous drug references, drug storage issues, and look-alike/sound-alike medications. These latent failures are properties of the medication use system. To prevent medications errors, we must change and improve the *system* and not rely on changing people. Latent failures are categorized by the key elements of the medication use system and include patient information; drug information; communication of drug information; drug packaging, labeling, and nomenclature; drug device acquisition and use; drug storage, stock, and distribution; environmental factors; staff competency and education; patient education; quality processes; and risk management (Cohen, 1999). By themselves, latent failures often are subtle and may not cause problems directly. The potential consequences are often hidden, becoming apparent only when they occur in a certain sequence and combine with the active failures of an individual.

Medication errors may also be the result of deficits in one of two areas: knowledge or performance.

Because no individual knows everything, and because everyone has occasional slips or lapses in performance, everyone makes errors. Medication use is a complex process that consists of subprocesses such as the ordering, preparing, dispensing, administration, and the provision of patient education.

ORDERING MEDICATIONS

Physicians or their designees—pharmacists, nurse practitioners, physician assistants, and nurses—initiate the drug dispensing and administration process through a medication order or prescription. Errors in ordering medications or writing prescriptions occur because of a lack of knowledge or poor performance by the prescriber. While computerized prescriber order-entry (CPOE) and electronic prescribing systems, each with clinical decision-support tools, are being implemented in more settings, as of 2007, most pharmacists still dispense from handwritten medication orders. Illegible, ambiguous, or incomplete handwritten prescriptions or medication orders contribute to many errors made by nurses, pharmacists, pharmacy technicians, and other health care workers.

Illegible Handwriting

To minimize the chance of misinterpretation, encourage physicians with poor handwriting to print prescriptions and medication orders in block letters. In the institutional setting, have physicians review orders with the nursing staff before leaving the patient care area. More important, ask physicians to include the purpose of the medication as part of the prescription or medication order to help readers distinguish drug names when handwriting legibility is less than ideal. Many medications have look-alike names, but very few name pairs that are spelled similarly are used for similar purposes. Preprinted orders, dictation, and direct order entry into the computer by physicians are other solutions for poor handwriting.

Because even skilled individuals can misread good handwriting, a system of independent double-checks for order/prescription transcription should be in place in which several individuals interpret and transcribe

an order. In many hospitals, each order is read by a unit secretary and reviewed by a nurse. At the same time, an exact copy of the order is sent to the pharmacy either directly or by facsimile. In the pharmacy, pharmacists and technicians have a number of opportunities to check the order, including a double-check against labels, printouts, and the drug containers. A technician often screens the order and sometimes enters it into the computer. After data entry, a label is printed, and a pharmacist interprets the original order/prescription and verifies the technician's computer entry by comparing it with the label. Later, the order and label will be read again by technicians and pharmacists as doses are prepared and dispensed. In the outpatient setting, this system should include a final check when providing counseling to the patient. In no case should pharmacy technicians interpret orders on their own because this process does not offer enough checks to prevent an error. In addition, orders must not be filled only from computer-generated labels. Rather, the original order should accompany the label to serve as another check.

Look-Alike Drug Names

Medications with names that are spelled similarly can be easily misread for one another. Pharmacists and technicians must be alert to this problem and should never guess about a prescriber's intent.

Study the handwriting in Figs. 30-1 and 30-2. Would you have had difficulty reading these medication orders correctly? These are actual examples of handwritten orders in both the inpatient and

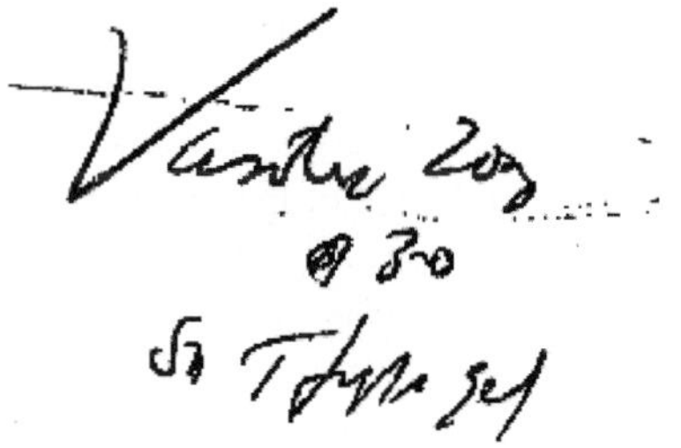

Figure 30-1. Order for Vantin 200 mg misread as Vasotec 20 mg.

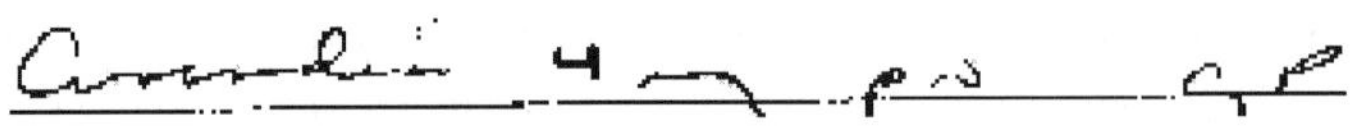

Figure 30-2. Order for Avandia 4 mg misread as Coumadin 4 mg.

outpatient settings, each of which led to medication errors. The problem was not uncertainty. On the contrary, each order was misread from the start. No consideration was ever given to the alternative drug because in each case the pharmacy staff members thought they were reading the order correctly.

When pharmacists and technicians interpret prescriptions and medication orders, newly marketed drugs are a particular problem. Staff members are not as familiar with names of the drugs, and they tend to misinterpret them as older drugs. It is important that up-to-date education on all new medications is provided to the pharmacy staff, including any potential for error that may exist with these new products. In the ambulatory care setting, physicians can write both the generic and trade names legibly on the prescription, and they can add the intended purpose of the medication to further alert pharmacy staff to the correct medication name.

Sound-Alike Names

Drug orders communicated orally are often misheard, misunderstood, misinterpreted, or transcribed incorrectly. Celebrex and Cerebyx sound alike, as do Celexa and Zyprexa, Sarafem and Serophene, Flomax and Volmax, and hundreds of other name pairs. Each of these drugs has been confused for the other, resulting in patients receiving incorrect medications. In many cases, serious injuries have occurred because of misinterpreted verbal orders. This is a good reason for health care facilities such as hospitals and long-term care facilities to establish policies that prohibit oral requests for medication without pharmacy review of a hard copy of the order. Sound-alike drug names present many of the same problems as look-alikes. Obviously, when uncertainties exist, the pharmacist must contact the prescriber for clarification.

To decrease the opportunity for misunderstanding, health care facilities and community pharmacies should discourage verbal orders. The Joint Commis-

sion (TJC), a national accrediting agency for health care organizations, required in its 2003 National Patient Safety Goals that accredited organizations improve the effectiveness of communication among caregivers by implementing a process for taking verbal or telephone orders that requires that a verbal order to be transcribed and then "read back" completely by the person receiving the order (TJC, 2003).

Greater use of facsimile machines among hospital areas, medical offices, pharmacies, and nursing units will help. When verbal communication is unavoidable, strict adherence to these procedures for verbal orders can minimize errors:

- Verbal orders should be taken only by authorized personnel.
- If possible, a second person should listen while the prescription is being given.
- The order should be transcribed and read back, repeating exactly what has been ordered, sometimes spelling the drug name for verification and the strength by using a digit-by-digit technique for the dose (1-5, not 15).
- In the acute care setting, record the verbal order directly onto an order sheet in the patient's chart whenever possible. Transcription from a scrap of paper to the chart introduces another opportunity for error. Obtain the prescriber's phone number in case it is necessary for follow-up questions.
- The prescribed agent must make sense for the patient's clinical situation.

To prevent sound-alike and look-alike errors, physicians must be encouraged to include complete directions, strengths, route of administration, and indication (purpose) for use. All these elements can serve as identifiers. It cannot be stressed enough that even if such information is lacking on orders, by knowing a drug's purpose, as well as the patient's problems, skilled health care professionals can judge whether the drug ordered makes sense for the patient in the context in which the order is written. For example, knowing that the patient has a diagnosis of diabetes would be an important clue in determining that Avandia is intended by the medication order in Fig. 30-2. Diagnostic procedures along with orders could also provide important information. This is why it is important for pharmacists to verify all orders processed by technicians. When in doubt, technicians should check with the pharmacist, who can contact the prescriber for clarification if the intent is not completely clear.

Ambiguous Orders

Errors can result when ambiguous orders are interpreted in a manner other than what the prescriber intended. Proper expression of doses is vital in a drug order. Pharmacists should be able to recognize improper expressions of doses, and the potential for error, when they see them. When the order is not clear, the pharmacist must contact the prescriber for clarification. Pharmacists and technicians should avoid using dangerous expressions of doses as they process orders, type labels, and communicate with others. The following examples include several improperly expressed orders that were reported to the Institute for Safe Medication Practices (ISMP):

- *Decreased doses.* A patient with diabetes had been receiving 80 mg prednisone daily for several months. After an office visit, the physician decided to decrease the daily dose by 5 mg, from 80 to 75 mg, and wrote the order, "Decrease prednisone—75 mg." The order was misinterpreted as meaning 80 mg minus 75 mg and was transcribed as, "Prednisone 5 mg PO daily." As a result, a 5-mg dose was given, and the unintentional sudden large decrease in dosage caused the patient to collapse. "Decrease prednisone by 5 mg daily" is clearer, but the safest way to write the order is, "Decrease prednisone by 5 mg daily. New dose is 75 mg daily."
- *Tablet strengths.* Orders specifying both strength and number of tablets are confusing when more than one tablet strength exists. For example, "Metoprolol

1/2 (one-half) tablet 25 mg once daily" appears clear enough. However, when you realize that this product is available in both 25- and 50-mg tablets, the ambiguity of this order becomes apparent. What is the intended dose, 25 or 12.5 mg? Orders are clearer if the dose is specified regardless of the strengths available (e.g., "Metoprolol 12.5 mg once daily"). For doses that require several tablets or capsules, the pharmacy label should note the exact number of dosage units needed. For example, the label on an 800-mg dose of Asacol (mesalamine), which is available only in 400-mg tablets, should read "2 × 400-mg tablets = 800 mg." For a 6.25-mg dose of captopril, which is available in 12.5-mg tablets, the label should read one-half ($^{1}/_{2}$) × 12.5-mg tablet = 6.25 mg." If your pharmacy prepares a computer-generated medication administration record (MARs) for nurses, this same type of notation should be used.

- *Liquid dosage forms.* Expressing the dose for liquid dosage forms in only milliliters or teaspoonfuls is dangerous. For example, acetaminophen elixir is available in many strengths, including 80, 120, and 160 mg per 5 mL. If the prescriber wrote "5 mL," the intended number of milligrams would be unclear. However, an order of "80 mg" states the appropriate dose. The amount of drug by metric weight, as well as the volume, always should be included on the pharmacy label (e.g., "Acetaminophen elixir 80 mg/5 mL"). Further, the patient dose should also be included. For a 320-mg dose, the label should read, "320 mg = 20 mL." The same holds true for unit-dose and bulk labels.
- *Injectable medications.* For injectable drugs, the same rule applies. List the metric weight or the metric weight and volume, never the volume alone, because solution concentrations can vary. An example of this error occurred at a hospital where hepatitis B vaccines were being administered. A preprinted physician's order form was used to prescribe the vaccine, listing only the volume to be given. When the clinic switched to another brand of vaccine, containing a different concentration of vaccine, the same preprinted forms continued to be used. This resulted in the underdosing of hundreds of children

until the error was discovered. This could have been avoided had the amount of vaccine been prescribed in micrograms rather than just the volume in milliliters.

- *Variable amounts.* A drug dose never should be ordered solely by number of tablets, capsules, ampules, or vials because the amounts contained in these dosage forms vary. Drug doses should be ordered with proper unit expression (e.g., "20 mEq potassium chloride"). A patient whose doctor orders "an amp" of potassium chloride might get 10, 20, 30, 40, 60, or 90 mEq. Under certain circumstances, the higher doses of this drug could be lethal.

- *Zeros and decimal points.* When listing drug doses on labels or in other communications, never follow a whole number with a decimal and a zero. For example, "Coumadin 1.0 mg" is a very dangerous way to express this dose. If the decimal point were not seen, the dose would be misinterpreted as "10 mg," and a 10-fold overdose would result. The same could happen when "Dilaudid 1.0 mg" is written. The proper way to express these orders would be "Coumadin 1 mg" and "Dilaudid 1 mg," respectively.

  On the other hand, always place a leading zero before a decimal point when the dose is smaller than 1. For example, the ISMP received a report where "Vincristine. 4 mg" was seen as "Vincristine 4 mg" when there was a poor impression of the decimal,

such as on faxes or carbons or no-carbon-required (NCR) copies of orders. Avoid using decimal expressions when recognizable alternatives exist because whole numbers are easier to work with. For example, "Digoxin 0.125 mg" would be good, but "Digoxin 125 mcg" would be better. Use "500 mg" instead of "0.5 g."

- *Spacing.* Two overdoses were reported because a lowercase *l* (ell) was the final letter in a drug name and was misread as the number 1. In one case, an order for 300 mg Tegretol (carbamazepine) twice daily appeared as "Tegretol 300 mg bid" and was misinterpreted as "1300 mg bid" (see Fig. 30-3). In another case, a nurse misread an order for 2 mg Amaryl (glimepiride) as 12 mg because there was insufficient space between the last letter in the drug name and the numerical dose. In addition, when labels are printed, make sure that there is a space after the drug name, the dose, and the unit of measurement. It is difficult to read labels when the drug name and dose run together.

- *Apothecary system.* Use the metric system exclusively. Although you may have learned about the apothecary system and its grains, drams, minims, and ounces, it is very inaccurate. For example, symbols for dram have been misread as "3," and minim has been misread as "55." Orders for phenobarbital 0.5 gr (30 mg) have been mistaken as "0.5 gram

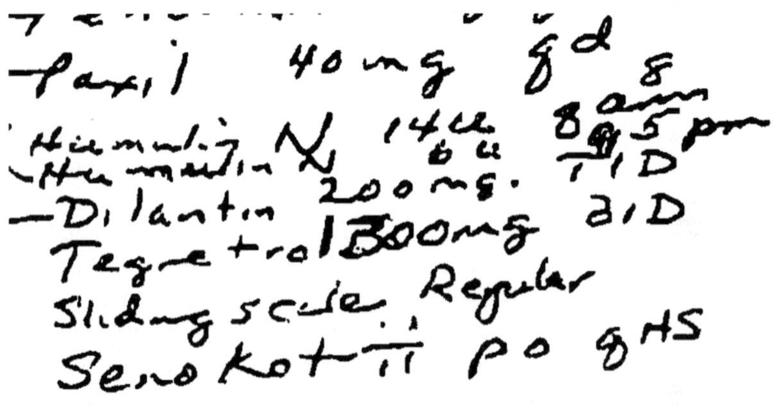

Figure 30-3. Order for Tegretol misread as 1300 mg instead of 300 mg.

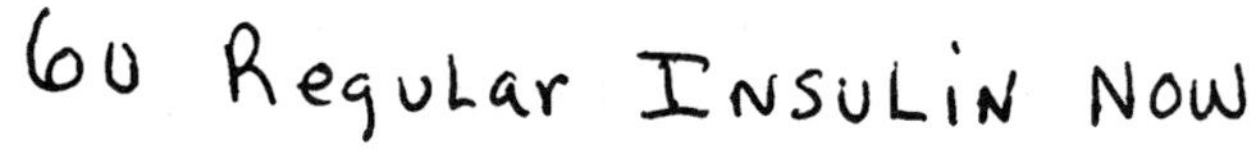

6U Regular Insulin Now

Figure 30-4. Misinterpretation of 6 units (U) regular insulin for 60.

(500 mg)." Use of the apothecary system is no longer officially recognized by the United States Pharmacopeia (USP).

Abbreviations to Avoid

Certain abbreviations are easily misinterpreted. Controlling dangerous abbreviations can reduce communication errors. Although many health care facilities have lists of abbreviations that are approved for use by professional staff, it would be far safer if each hospital also developed a list of abbreviations that never should be used. In fact, such a negative list is easier to maintain and enforce. In addition, The Joint Commission (TJC), has recommended that accredited organizations standardize abbreviations, acronyms, and symbols used throughout their facilities, including a list of abbreviations, acronyms, and symbols not to use.

The ISMP has developed a list that contains several easily misinterpreted abbreviations from actual medication errors reported to ISMP, some of which resulted in patient harm (ISMP, 2001a, 2001b). These abbreviations never should be used in medication orders, on pharmacy labels, in newsletters, or in other communications that originate in a pharmacy or pharmacy computer systems. The abbreviation *U* for units provides a good an example of what can go wrong. Errors have occurred when the letter *U* was mistaken for the numerals 0, 4, 6, and 7, and even cc, resulting in disastrous drug overdoses of insulin, heparin, penicillin, and other medications whose doses sometimes are expressed in units. For example, an order written as "6U regular insulin" has been misinterpreted as "60

regular insulin," with the patient receiving 60 units rather than the intended 6 units (see Fig. 30-4).

D/C is another example of an abbreviation that should not be used. It has been written to mean either "discontinue" or "discharge," sometimes resulting in premature stoppage of a patient's medications. In Fig. 30-5, the "d/c" order was incorrectly interpreted as "discontinuation" of an antibiotic that the patient had never even received. In reality, the "d/c" is really "OK," meaning that the drug was approved for use by the infectious disease physician.

Do not abbreviate drug names. For example, *MTX* means "methotrexate" to some health professionals, but others understand it as "mitoxantrone." *AZT* has been misunderstood as "azathioprine" (Imuran) when "zidovudine" (Retrovir) was intended. In one case, this misinterpretation led to a patient with AIDS receiving azathioprine, an immunosuppressant, instead of the intended antiretroviral agent. The patient's immune system worsened, and he developed an overwhelming infection. In another example, an order for "HCTZ50 mg" (hydrochlorothiazide) was mistaken for an order for "HCT 250 mg" (hydrocortisone).

■ PREPARING AND DISPENSING MEDICATIONS

An important safety enhancement for preventing dispensing errors is the development of a system of redundant checks from the time a prescription order first is written in the physician's office or on the nursing unit to receipt in the pharmacy and through dispensing and administration. Such a system is suggested in this

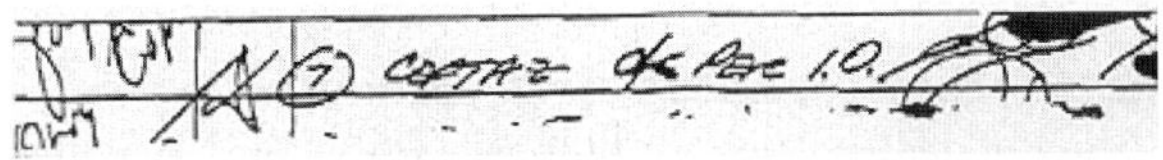

Figure 30-5. Ceftazidime "OK" per ID misread as ceftazidime "d/c" per ID.

section. Obviously, the more "looks" an order receives (while efficient workflow is maintained), the better. Health professionals can review orders at several checkpoints and thereby maximize the chances of errors being discovered. Pharmacies with computerized drug distribution systems have an advantage because labels and reports can be printed so that order interpretation and order entry can be verified at various steps.

Steps in Prescription Filling

It is important that all health care professionals, including prescribers, nurses, and the pharmacy, work together when filling prescriptions so that the lines of communication are kept open if questions should arise. The following describes a suggested workflow for reducing the risk of medication errors during the prescription filling process:

1. The prescriber sees the patient; performs an assessment; determines the appropriate medication, dose, route, and frequency; and writes the order or communicates the order verbally to nursing personnel or the pharmacy.

2. In the inpatient setting, a unit secretary reads and transcribes the order onto the medication administration record (MAR). This step is unnecessary in hospitals where computers generate the MAR or where prescribers can enter orders by computer, although the nurse and the pharmacist still must verify the order for appropriateness.

3. In the inpatient setting, a nurse checks the unit secretary's transcription for accuracy.

4. A direct copy of the order is transported or faxed to the pharmacy, or the prescriber's computer entry reaches the pharmacy. The pharmacist or pharmacy technician reads the order and enters it in the pharmacy computer system. If the technician finds a duplicate order, incorrect dose, allergy, or the like, it is documented and called to the attention of the pharmacist during the clinical screening in step 5.

5. A pharmacist reviews the technician's computer entry, compares it with the original prescription (handwritten or electronic), and performs a clinical screening of the prescription with respect to the need for the drug, allergies or other contraindications, proper dose, and proper route of administration.

6. A label and/or a medication profile is printed. A copy of the original prescription or medication order continues to accompany the label or medication profile while the order is filled. Orders never should be filled solely on the basis of what appears on the label or medication profile because the computer entry may have been in error.

7. To choose an item for dispensing, a technician reviews both the label and the medication order for possible discrepancies.

8. A pharmacist checks the technician's work, reviewing the label against the medication order and the dose that has been prepared. The drug is labeled and dispensed. In the institution, the nurse receives the drug and compares the medication and pharmacy label against the copy of the physician's order, as well as the handwritten transcription made earlier in the MAR.

9. In the community setting, the pharmacist uses the patient counseling session to further assess that the correct medication is being dispensed and that the patient has a condition treatable with the product being provided. Pharmacists should ask patients if they have any questions about their medication. For refills and medications patients have received in the past, patients should be encouraged to ask the pharmacist about any changes in the appearance of the product. If patients or caregivers are provided with devices, such as oral syringes for the administration of liquids or suspensions, in addition to providing patients with appropriate devices for measuring doses, practitioners must ensure that the patient or caregiver understands how to use them properly with the medication. Demonstrate for patients how to use the device, and follow with a return demonstration by the user.

10. Patients in the community setting should be educated about the common adverse effects of medications they are taking and understand what

clinical signs to watch for and report to health professionals. In institutional settings, the nurse administers the dose, giving the drug's name, explaining the drug's purpose and potential adverse effects, and answering questions and concerns raised by the patient.

11. The final step in the process is the assurance of adherence to medication therapy. If the patient is taking too much medication or is not taking the drug as frequently as prescribed, the pharmacist should speak with the patient to determine the reasons for and address the variation. In addition, patients should be asked about common adverse effects and about signs of serious drug toxicities. In an institution, pharmacy personnel check unit-dose bins and medication administration records (MARs) to make sure that nursing staff is administering the medication on the proper schedule.

Selecting Medications

The importance of reading the product label while selecting medications and filling prescriptions cannot be overemphasized. Too often the wrong drug or wrong strength is dispensed. Such errors often stem from failure to read the label thoroughly. During drug preparation and dispensing, the label should be read three times: when the product is selected, when the medication is prepared, and when either the partially used medication is disposed of (or restored to stock) or product preparation is complete. However, selecting the correct item from the shelf, drawer, or bin can be complicated by many factors. Similar labeling and packaging, as well as look-alike names, is a common trap that leads to medication errors (see Figs. 30-6 and 30-7). Restocking errors are quite common and can lead to repeated medication errors before being detected.

Automated dispensing machines have become common on nursing units in many hospitals. The nurse must enter a security code and a password into the dispensing device, along with the name of the patient and the name of the medication, before the machine will allow access to remove the medication. This system allows better control of items kept on the nursing unit and serves as a check for the nurse who retrieves the

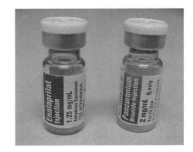

Figure 30-6. Similar packaging might lead to medication errors.

medication. One important feature that should be included in these dispensing units is online communication with the pharmacy system that allows a pharmacist to review medication orders before nursing accesses the medication.

Automated dispensing devices create several situations that can easily result in errors. While these machines are routinely restocked, the wrong drug still can be placed into the wrong bin during this process. Devices that have multiple medications in each drawer and/or that do not require pharmacist review of orders before access have drawbacks that are identical to the flaws in traditional floor-stock systems:

- The pharmacy can replenish the system with an incorrect medication.
- The nurse can retrieve either the wrong item or additional items to use for other patients.

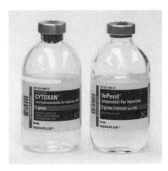

Figure 30-7. Another example of packaging that might lead to medication error.

- Lack of pharmacist double-checking and screening orders allows prescribing errors, wrong dosages, incorrect routes of administration, and other clinical errors to occur.

The term *confirmation bias* is used to describe the phenomenon that when choosing an item, people see what they are looking for, and once they think they have found it, they stop looking any further. Often health professionals choose a medication container based on a mental picture of the item. Staff members may be looking for some characteristic of the drug label, the shape and size or color of the container, or the location of the item on a shelf, in a drawer, or in a storage bin instead of reading the name of the drug itself. Consequently, they may fail to realize that they have the wrong item in hand.

A number of approaches can be used to minimize the possibility of such errors in the pharmacy and in automated dispensing machines. Physically separating drugs with look-alike labels and packaging reduces the potential for error. Some pharmacies also separate drugs with similar names and overlapping strengths, especially those labeled and packaged by the same manufacturer. For example, chlorpromazine 100-mg tablets and chlorpropamide 100-mg tablets, both from the same unit-dose packager (see Fig. 30-8), might pose a problem. So might morphine 10 mg and hydromorphone 10 mg. Another strategy would be to change the appearance of look-alike product names on computer screens, pharmacy shelf labels and bins, and pharmacy product labels by highlighting, through boldface, color, or the use of "tall man" letters, the parts of the names that are different (e.g., hydrOXYzine and hydrALAzine). In fact, the FDA Office of Generic Drugs requested that the manufacturers of 16 look-alike name-pair drug products voluntarily revise the appearance of their established names to minimize medication errors resulting from look-alike confusion. Manufacturers were encouraged to differentiate their established names visually with the use of "tall man" letters. Examples of established names involved include chlorproMAZINE and chlorproPAMIDE, vinBLASTINE

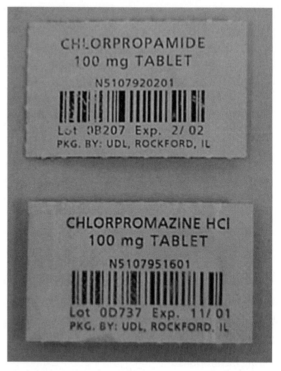

Figure 30-8. Similarity in labeling of two different medications.

and vinCRISTINE, and NICARdipine and NIFEdipine.

Pharmaceutical companies are aware of labeling and packaging problems, and many have responded to suggestions made by technicians and pharmacists. Health professionals can alert manufacturers about errors caused by commercial packaging and labeling problems by using the USP-ISMP Medication Error Reporting Program (MERP). Reports are forwarded to the individual pharmaceutical company and the FDA, and ISMP provides follow-up when appropriate. Call 1-800-FAILSAFE, visit ISMP's Web site at www.ismp.org, or complete a USP-ISMP MERP report (see Fig. 30-9). All reports are confidential.

In institutional and community pharmacies with several staff members, everyone should have input in deciding how and where drugs are available, how doses are prepared, who is responsible for preparing them, the appearance of the storage containers, and how they

MEDI-CATION ERRORS

REPORTING PROGRAM

USP MEDICATION ERRORS REPORTING PROGRAM
Presented in cooperation with the Institute for Safe Medication Practices

USP is an FDA MEDWATCH partner

Reporters should not provide any individually identifiable health information, including names of practitioners, names of patients, names of healthcare facilities, or dates of birth (age is acceptable).

Date and time of event:

Please describe the error. Include description/sequence of events, type of staff involved, and work environment (e.g., code situation, change of shift, short staffing, no 24-hr. pharmacy, floor stock). If more space is needed, please attach a separate page.

Did the error reach the patient? ☐ Yes ☐ No

Was the incorrect medication, dose, or dosage form administered to or taken by the patient? ☐ Yes ☐ No

Circle the appropriate Error Outcome Category (select one—see back for details): A B C D E F G H I

Describe the direct result of the error on the patient (e.g., death, type of harm, additional patient monitoring).

Indicate the possible error cause(s) and contributing factor(s) (e.g., abbreviation, similar names, distractions, etc.).

Indicate the location of the error (e.g., hospital, outpatient or community pharmacy, clinic, nursing home, patient's home, etc.).

What type of staff or healthcare practitioner made the initial error?

Indicate if other practitioner(s) were also involved in the error (type of staff perpetuating error).

What type of staff or healthcare practitioner discovered the error or recognized the potential for error?

How was the error (or potential for error) discovered/intercepted?

If available, provide patient age, gender, diagnosis. Do not provide any patient identifiers.

Please complete the following for the product(s) involved. (If more space is needed for additional products, please attach a separate page.)

	Product #1	Product #2
Brand/Product Name (If Applicable)		
Generic Name		
Manufacturer		
Labeler		
Dosage Form		
Strength/Concentration		
Type and Size of Container		

Reports are most useful when relevant materials such as product label, copy of prescription/order, etc., can be reviewed. Can these materials be provided? ☐ Yes ☐ No   Please specify:

Suggest any recommendations to prevent recurrence of this error, or describe policies or procedures you instituted or plan to institute to prevent future similar errors.

Name and Title/Profession	Telephone Number ( )	Fax Number ( )
Facility/Address and Zip		E-mail
Address/Zip (where correspondence should be sent)		

Your name, contact information, and a copy of this report are routinely shared with the Institute for Safe Medication Practices (ISMP). Copies of reports will be sent to third parties such as the manufacturer/labeler, and to the Food and Drug Administration (FDA). You have the option of including your name on these copies.

In addition to releasing my name and contact information to ISMP, USP may release my identity to these third parties as follows (check boxes that apply):

☐ The manufacturer and/or labeler as listed above   ☐ FDA   ☐ Other persons requesting a copy of this report   ☐ Anonymous to all third parties

Signature	Date

Return to:
USP CAPS
12601 Twinbrook Parkway
Rockville, MD 20852-1790

Submit via the Web at www.usp.org/mer
Call Toll Free: 800-23-ERROR (800-233-7767)
or FAX: 301-816-8532

Date Received by USP	File Access Number

PSF1190

©USPC 2003

Figure 30-9. Form used in reporting medication errors or problems to the ESP/ISMP Medication Reporting Program.

are labeled. In addition, staff members should be encouraged to use a technique known as *failure mode and effects analysis* (FMEA) to examine the use of new products to determine points of potential failures and their effects *before any error actually happens.* In this regard, FMEA differs from *root-cause analysis* (RCA). RCA is a reactive process, employed after an error occurs, to identify its underlying causes. In contrast, FMEA is a proactive process used to carefully and systematically evaluate vulnerable areas or processes. FMEA can be employed before the purchase and implementation of new products to identify potential failure modes so that steps can be taken to avoid errors before they occur (ISMP, 2001a, 2001b). Procedures to ensure safe medication use must be written, and the importance of adhering to the guidelines must be shared by all involved pharmacy, medical, and nursing personnel.

Selecting Auxiliary Labels

To help prevent errors and improve patient outcomes, pharmacists and technicians should apply auxiliary labels in certain circumstances, especially in the community setting. For example, amoxicillin oral suspension is available in dropper bottles for pediatric use. When the suspension is used for an ear infection, some parents have been known to place the suspension in the child's ear rather than to give it properly (orally). An auxiliary label, "For oral use only," would help to prevent this administration error. However, this practice can be unsafe if the patient is unable to understand the warning. A study that appeared in the *American Journal of Health-System Pharmacy* showed that there is a high level of misunderstanding of auxiliary labels among adults with low literacy, a reading level at or below the sixth-grade level (Wolf et al., 2006). The rate of correct interpretation of these labels ranged from 0 to 78.7 percent. With the exception of the label "Take with food," less than half of all patients were able to provide adequate interpretations of the warning labels' messages. In fact, none were able to correctly interpret the label, "Do not take dairy products, antacids, or iron preparations within 1 hour of this medication." Studies also have shown that a combination of a verbal description of a warning along with visual symbols

improves the overall comprehension of the warning (Lesch, 2003).

■ STERILE ADMIXTURE PREPARATION

In preparing fluids for injectable administration, the potential for grave error is increased for several reasons. First, patients often are sicker when they need intravenous drugs, so the medications used have more dramatic effects on the body's function and physiology. Further, most injectable solutions are clear, colorless, water-based fluids that look alike, regardless of what drug and how much of it are actually in the fluid. Therefore, in the sterile admixture preparation setting, the chance of dosage miscalculation or measurement error must be minimized by systems designed with procedures that require independent double-checks by two staff members. The independent double-check in some pharmacies might be required for all calculations or measurements, whereas others may require it only for calculations falling in special categories, such as dosage calculations for admixture compounding for any child under age 12, critical care drug infusions requiring a dose in micrograms per kilogram per minute, insulin infusions, chemotherapy, and patient-controlled analgesia. Calculators and computer programs may improve accuracy, but they do not eliminate the need for a second person to review the calculations and solution concentrations used.

Another important way to minimize calculation errors is to avoid the need for calculations. This can be accomplished by using the unit-dose system exclusively as follows:

- Using commercially available unit-dose systems such as premixed critical care parenteral products.
- Standardizing doses and concentrations, especially of critical care drugs such as heparin, insulin, dobutamine, dopamine, and morphine.

Similar steps can be taken in community pharmacies that provide sterile admixtures to physician offices, home care programs and patients, long-term care facilities, and other clients.

The use of standard dosage charts on nursing units in institutions and standard formulations in the pharmacy minimizes the possibility of error and makes calculations much easier. For example, in critical care units, physicians need to order only the amount of drug they want infused and list any titration parameters. No one has to perform any calculations because dosage charts can be readily available for choosing appropriate flow rates by patient weight (in kilograms) and dose ordered.

Standard concentrations for frequently prepared formulations should be recorded and be readily accessible for reference in the admixture preparation area of the pharmacy. Of course, all calculations must be double-checked and documented by the pharmacist. Diluents as well as active drugs must be checked. The stock container of each additive with its accompanying syringe should be lined up in the order it appears on the container label to facilitate the checking procedure. The final edge of the plunger piston should be aligned with the calibration marks on the syringe barrel, indicating the amount used.

In many hospitals and home infusion pharmacies, automated compounding equipment is being used for admixing both large- and small-volume parenterals. Automated equipment has been known to occasionally fail. Also, accidents can occur when solutions are placed in the wrong additive channel. These can result in serious medication errors. Therefore, it is important that the pharmacy have an ongoing quality assurance program for the use of automated compounding equipment. This program should include double-checks and documentation of solution placement within the compounder, final weighing or refractometer testing of the solution to ensure that proper concentrations have been compounded, and ongoing sampling of electrolyte concentrations. Pharmacists who prepare special parenteral solutions in batches (e.g., total parenteral nutrition base solutions or cardioplegic solutions) should have additional quality assurance procedures in place, including sterility testing and quarantine until confirmation.

PATIENT COUNSELING AND EDUCATION

The patient is the last individual in the medication use process. The pharmacist–patient interface can play a significant role in capturing medication errors before they occur. Unfortunately, many health care organizations do not take advantage of this key interaction. Three important factors play a role in any patient interface and often determine the outcome of error-prevention efforts. These include direct patient education, health care literacy, and patient compliance.

In 2001, the number of retail prescriptions was 3.3 billion, which is an increase from 2.7 billion in 2000. By 2005, this figure neared 3.4 billion prescriptions (NACDS, 2007). This increase in prescription volume, when combined with the shortage of pharmacists, often results in a decrease in the amount of time available for direct pharmacist involvement in patient education. A 1999 study involving community pharmacies in eight states revealed that 87 percent of all patients received written information with their prescriptions. However, only 35 percent of pharmacists made any reference to the written leaflet, and only 8 percent actually reviewed it with the patient (Svarstad, 2000). Contributing to this gap in patient education is the failure to provide patients with understandable written instructions.

The second factor is patient literacy, which includes general literacy levels and health care literacy. Many people have difficulty understanding their illness or disease, proper management of disease, and their role in maintaining their health. Whether limited by knowledge, socioeconomic factors, emotional or clinical state, or cultural background, patients' level of health literacy (i.e., the ability to read, understand, and act on health care information) often is much lower than many health care providers appreciate. Examples of patients who have had difficulty reading and understanding medication directions are plentiful according to medication error reports submitted to the USP/ISMP Medication Error Reporting Program, for example, an elderly patient who could not tell the difference between his bottle of Coumadin (warfarin) and Celebrex (celecoxib), a mother who, after reading the label on a bottle of acetaminophen, could not accurately state her child's dose, and a teenager who misunderstood directions for contraceptive jelly and ate it on toast every morning to prevent pregnancy.

According a report published by the American Medical Association Ad Hoc Committee on Health Literacy, more than 40 percent of patients with chronic illnesses are functionally illiterate, and almost a quarter of all adult Americans read at or below a fifth grade level. Unfortunately, medical information leaflets typically are written at or above a tenth grade reading level. It is estimated that low health literacy skills have increased our annual health care expenditures by $73 billion. Further contributing to the dilemma is the fact that an estimated three-quarters of patients throw out the medication leaflet stapled to the prescription bag without reading it, and only one-half of all patients take their medications as directed (AMA, 1999).

One reason for this lack of understanding may be that people who have difficulty reading or understanding health information are too embarrassed or ashamed to acknowledge their deficits. Instead, they refuse to ask questions and often pretend to understand instructions. In addition, low literacy is not obvious. Researchers have reported poor reading skills in some of the most poised and articulate patients (ISMP, 2001a).

Compliance is the third patient-related factor contributing to medication errors. One study found a 76 percent difference between medications patients actually are taking when compared with those recorded in their charts as prescribed. Two factors that contribute to this high rate of discrepancy include confusion that may accompany advancing age and the increase in the number of prescribed medications (Bedell et al., 2000). Another study demonstrated that patient noncompliance played a role in 33 percent of hospital admissions (McDonnell, Jacobs, and McDonnell, 2002).

Noncompliance may be exhibited by patients in many ways, such as not having a prescription filled initially or refilled, dose omission, taking the wrong dose, stopping a medication without the physician's advice, taking a medication incorrectly or at the wrong time, taking someone else's medication, and financial inability to purchase their medications. Patients at risk for being noncompliant include those taking more than one drug, those with a chronic condition who are on complex drug regimens that may result in bothersome side effects, those who take a drug more than once daily, and those who have a condition that produces no overt symptoms or physical impairment such as hypertension or diabetes (NCPIE, 2002). In addition, elderly patients are more at risk owing to factors such as decrease in mental acuity and increased confusion, lack of family or caregiver support, decreased coordination and dexterity, and impaired vision (Lombardi and Kennicutt, 2001). Pharmacy managers must consider these factors in the developing and providing patient education tools or methodologies.

■ EFFECTIVE MEDICATION ERROR PREVENTION THROUGH REPORTING AND MONITORING SYSTEMS

All drug-dispensing procedures should be examined regularly, and the cause of system breakdowns must be discovered so that prevention measures can be designed. Pharmacy staff needs to communicate clearly to managers what it takes to do the job correctly in terms of personnel, training programs, facilities design, equipment, drug procedures and supplies, computer systems, and quality assurance programs. In addition, reducing medication errors requires an effective, nonpunitive environment and a voluntary medication error reporting system.

Currently, many pharmacies have an ineffective approach to error reduction. Investigations that occur during the error reporting process tend to focus their attention on the front end or active end of the error such as the front-line practitioner (e.g., a technician preparing a prescription or a pharmacist dispensing the medication). Human nature tends to assign blame to these front-line practitioners involved in medication errors. It is easier and in our nature to blame individuals and resort to familiar solutions: disciplinary action, individual remedial education, placing error information into personnel files, or developing new rules. While these actions may not seem outwardly punitive, these forms of reprimand lead to underreporting of errors. In fact, punishing individuals for errors actually can be dangerous to an organization. It inhibits open discussion about errors, creates a defensive and reactive environment, and hinders careful and unbiased consideration of the system-based root causes of errors. Pharmacies are weakened further by punitive actions, especially if the sole responsibility for safe medication practices rests on individuals rather than on strong systems that make it difficult for practitioners to make errors. The goal of patient safety is best served with a nonpunitive environment that places more value on reporting problems so that they can be remedied rather than on pursuing the unprofitable path of disciplining employees for errors. A voluntary, confidential reporting program provides pharmacists and pharmacy technicians with the opportunity to tell the complete story without fear of retribution. The depth of information contained in these stories is critical to understanding the error. This information is critical to identification of system deficiencies that can be corrected to prevent future errors. However, successful and sustained improvement of error-prone processes cannot occur if there is little information available about factors that contribute to an error.

Many organizational factors inhibit the reporting of medication errors. Examples include inconsistent definitions of a medication error, a punitive approach to medication errors, mandatory reporting systems, failure to improve the medication system or address reported problems, lack of feedback to staff over concern with medication error rates, complex reporting processes, a perception that reporting is a low priority, concern for personal liability, and the need for pharmacy managers to look within when assessing errors. Practitioners who are forced to report errors in a mandatory reporting system are less likely to provide this depth of information because their motivation may be adherence to a requirement, not necessarily to help others avoid the same tragedy. Further, a voluntary program encourages practitioners to report hazardous situations and errors that have the potential

to cause serious patient harm. A confidential reporting system where everyone understands that errors will not be linked to performance appraisals is critical. Many pharmacy organizations have regular meetings where medication errors are addressed. The results of these meetings often are not shared with the front-line staff, therefore giving the impression that "nothing is being done" when errors are reported. In addition, busy practitioners tend to avoid reporting errors owing to the cumbersome nature of their organizations' reporting forms and processes. It is important to make error reporting easy, reward error reporting, and provide timely feedback to show what is being done to address problems. Consistently applying a nonpunitive approach to errors is important. If even one person is disciplined for an error, mistakes will be hidden. Employees should not be evaluated based on errors or lack of making mistakes but on positive measures that evaluate an employee's overall contribution to the organization. Armed with these tools, pharmacists can become aware of the deficiencies in their organizations and make performance-improvement changes. Without them, we are only addressing errors when they surface rather than at the root cause.

To be successful, medication error-reduction efforts must result in system improvements that are identified through a four-pronged analysis of errors. The first two prongs, both reactive in nature, include analysis of organization-specific errors that have caused some degree of patient harm and analysis of aggregate medication error data (e.g., trends by drugs or location of drugs involved in errors). Equally important, the other two prongs, both proactive in nature, include analysis of "near misses" (errors that have the potential to cause patient harm) and analysis of errors that have occurred in other organizations. Each prong contains valuable information about weaknesses in the system that, collectively, can lead to effective error-reduction strategies. Yet many organizations focus primarily on the first two prongs of error analysis and action. Most often proactive efforts are not given high priority. As a result, organizations may be busy "fighting fires" rather than preventing them. A near miss should be clear evidence that a tragic event could occur. Unfortunately, too often this wakeup call is not heard. Little attention is focused on thorough analysis of errors that, fortunately, do not cause actual patient harm, especially if organizations identify errors that require analysis by a severity rating that is based on actual patient outcome. For example, a serious overdose detected before administration may not be given the same priority and analysis as a similar error that actually reached and possibly harmed the patient. Worse, some organizations fail to use errors that have occurred elsewhere as a road map for improvement in their own organization. Staff will be more comfortable discussing a serious external error than one that has occurred within its own organization. Because blame is not an issue, defensive posturing and other obstacles to effective discussion will not be present. Staff can identify possible system-based causes of the error more easily and the likelihood of a similar error in their facility and make suggestions for improvement. As improvements are made, enthusiasm builds for identifying, reporting, and analyzing errors that are actually occurring within the organization. In the end, discussion about external errors leads to more effective analysis of internal errors.

Multidisciplinary educational programs should be developed for health care personnel about medication error prevention. Because many errors happen when procedures are not followed, this is one area on which to focus through newsletters and in-service training. It also is important for pharmacy staff not just to focus on their own internal errors but also to look at other pharmacies' errors and methods of prevention and to learn from them. Organizations such as the ISMP, USP, and many others provide ongoing features to facilitate these reviews in publications such as *Hospital Pharmacy, Pharmacy Today, U.S. Pharmacist,* and *Pharmacy and Therapeutics* or newsletters that report on current medication safety issues and offer recommendations for changes.

CONCLUSION

Pharmacists play a key role in the drug use process throughout any health care organization. Pharma-

cists and other members of the pharmacy department should lead a multidisciplinary effort to examine where errors arise in this process. Pharmacy managers should encourage their staff to collaborate in designing quality assurance programs to obtain information that helps to establish priorities and make changes. For example, joint reviews of the accuracy of unit-dose cart fills are of great help in detecting reasons for missing or inaccurate doses and changing the drug-dispensing system accordingly. Programs can be established to monitor the accuracy of order entry into computers in the pharmacy. Quality assurance efforts that include a review of medication error reports help to develop a better understanding of the kinds of systemic or behavioral defects being experienced so that necessary corrections can be identified. The medication error problem will never be eliminated completely, but pharmacy managers, working together with their staffs and other health care providers, can use their expertise to address issues of safety and thus ensure best outcomes in the safest environment possible.

QUESTIONS FOR FURTHER DISCUSSION

1. Have you witnessed or been involved in a medication error, and what actions did you take to prevent any future errors?
2. Have you counseled a patient whom you know did not understand his or her doctor's instructions? What steps did you take to ensure that the patient thoroughly knew his or her medication, directions, and indication for use?
3. Will you include medication error prevention strategies in the orientation process for new employees and ongoing education for pharmacy staff?
4. Do you think that you will be involved in reporting medication errors both internally within your organization and externally to reporting agencies such as the ISMP or the FDA? Do you think this will make a difference in your pharmacy practice setting?

REFERENCES

Allan EL, Barker KN. 1990. Fundamentals of medication error research. *Am J Hosp Pharm* 47:555.

Allan EL, Barker KN, Carnahan BJ. 2003. National observational study of prescription dispensing accuracy and safety in 50 pharmacies. *J Am Pharm Assoc* 43:191.

American Medical Association (AMA), Ad Hoc Committee on Health Literacy for the Council on Scientific Affairs. 1999. Health literacy: Report of the Council on Scientific Affairs. *JAMA* 281:552.

Bedell SE, Jabbour S, Goldberg R, et al. 2000. Discrepancies in the use of medications: Their extent and predictors in an outpatient practice. *Arch Intern Med* 160:2129.

Cohen MR (ed). 1999. *Medication Errors,* p. 20.4. Washington, DC: American Pharmaceutical Association.

Institute for Safe Medication Practices (ISMP). 1998. *ISMP Medication Safety Alert!* p. 3. Washington, DC: ISMP.

Institute for Safe Medication Practices (ISMP). 2001a. *ISMP Medication Safety Alert!* p. 6. Washington, DC: ISMP.

Institute for Safe Medication Practices (ISMP). 2001b. *ISMP Medication Safety Alert!* p. 6. Washington, DC: ISMP.

Institute for Safe Medication Practices (ISMP). 2003. www.ismp.org/MSAarticles/specialissuetable.html; accessed on April 30, 2003.

Institute of Medicine (IOM). 2007. www8.nationalacademies.org/onpinews/newsitem.aspx?RecordID=11623; accessed on June 10, 2007.

The Joint Commission (TJC). 2003. www.jcaho.org/accredited + organizations/patient + safety/npsg/npsg_03.htm; accessed on April 30, 2003.

Kohn LT, Corrigan JM, Donaldson MS (eds). 1999. To Err Is Human: Building a Safer Health System, Institute of Medicine Report, November 29; available at http://bob.nap.edu/html/to_err_is_human/; accessed on March 18, 2003.

Lesch, MF. 2003. Comprehension and memory for warning symbols: Age-related differences and impact of training. *J Saf Res* 34:495.

Lombardi TP, Kennicutt JD. 2001. Promotion of a Safe Medication Environment: Focus on the Elderly and Residents of Long-Term Care Facilities. Available at www.medscape.com/; accessed on May 14, 2001.

McDonnell PJ, Jacobs MR, McDonnell PJ. 2002. *Pharmacotherapy* 36:1331.

National Association of Chain Drug Stores. 2007. www.nacds.org/user-assets/pdfs/facts_resources/2005/Prescriptions 2005.pdf; accessed June 10, 2007.

National Council on Patient Information and Education. 2002. www.talkaboutrx.org/compliance.html; accessed on October 30, 2002.

Reason J. 1990. The contribution of latent human failures to the breakdown of complex systems. *Philos Trans R Soc Lond B Biol Sci* 327.

Svarstad B. 2000. FDA-Commissioned Research, University of Wisconsin–Madison. Presented February 2000, Rockville, MD, and June 2000, Kuopio, Finland.

Wolf MS, Davis TC, et al. 2006. Misunderstanding of prescription drug warning labels among patients with low literacy. *Am J Health-Syst Pharm* 63:1048.

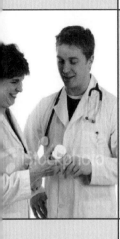

SECTION VIII

MANAGEMENT APPLICATIONS IN
SPECIFIC PHARMACY PRACTICE SETTINGS

SECTION VII

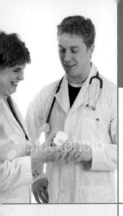

31

ENTREPRENEURSHIP

Bradley Tice

About the Author: Dr. Tice is Chief Clinical Officer of PharmMD Solutions, LLC. PharmMD is an early-stage medication therapy management delivery company based in Nashville, Tennessee. He earned a B.S. and a Pharm.D. from the University of Kansas. Prior to his current position, Dr. Tice was an Associate Professor at the Drake University College of Pharmacy & Health Sciences. His work has focused primarily on the development, implementation, and evaluation of innovative pharmacy services and has evolved into entrepreneurship. Dr. Tice attended the Experiential Classroom for Entrepreneurship Educators at Syracuse University and the Executive Management Program for Pharmacy Leaders at the Wharton School of Business and was a leader in the development of the DELTA Rx Institute at Drake University. Dr. Tice defined and introduced the concept of *entrepreneurial leadership* in pharmacy through his presentation and accompanying publication and was awarded the Alfred B. Prescott Leadership Award in 2005. He has been an advocate of the integration of entrepreneurship principles into pharmacy education. He has also developed a software product to enable pharmacists to deliver and document their services and subsequently started a company, RXInterventions, LLC. He has also served on numerous committees and in elected positions with the Iowa Pharmacy Association, the American Pharmacists Association, and the American Association of Colleges of Pharmacy.

▪ LEARNING OBJECTIVES

After completing this chapter, students should be able to

1. Define *entrepreneurship*.
2. Discuss characteristics and types of entrepreneurs.
3. Discuss the applicability of entrepreneurship principles in the profession of pharmacy.
4. Given an "opportunity concept," apply the process of entrepreneurship to evaluate, pursue, execute, and harvest the venture.

CHAPTER QUESTIONS

1. What are three common characteristics of entrepreneurs?
2. What are the four types of entrepreneur personalities, which one do you most identify with, and what leads you to identify yourself with this characterization?
3. Why is the understanding and use of the "process" of entrepreneurship an important component in the establishment of entrepreneurship as its own body of knowledge?
4. Why is it important for an entrepreneur to be able to clearly and succinctly communicate the business concept?

SCENARIO

Pharmacist John Adams works for a chain pharmacy in a large city with a population of over 1 million people. He has been out of school for several years and has worked through such positions as staff pharmacist and pharmacy manager. In the last year he has started focusing his work on patients with diabetes. He has incorporated a complete diabetes program into his practice that includes classes on blood glucose monitoring, sick-day management, insulin administration, meal planning and healthy eating for patients with diabetes, and a general overview of diabetes. He also has one-on-one counseling sessions that he offers in these areas. During the course of delivering these sessions, John has discovered that a recurring problem patients have is not getting enough blood for a measurement when they stick their fingers to check their blood sugar. Additionally, patients often find this painful and do not do this as often as they should. One day John develops a device that is very effective at getting the necessary blood sample from patients and is nearly pain-free. The device is very popular with his patients, and he starts to get referrals for the device.

While the high salary as a pharmacist was attractive to John at first, he now is starting to feel more confident in his abilities and would like a new challenge and opportunity. He wonders if this lancet device he has developed could be worth something. He did not take any business classes in pharmacy school, when he was growing up, his father ran the hardware store in their small town, so he has some exposure to running a business. He thought that his father might be interested in helping him out. John has developed a number of relationships with businesspeople through his involvement in the community and thinks that he might elicit their advice, too.

Some questions running through his mind are

- Should he pursue developing this idea into a product?
- If he does, should he do this through the company that he is currently with or on his own?
- If he chooses to do this on his own, would he need to completely quit what he is currently doing?
- How much money will he need, and is he really ready to commit his money to this?

BACKGROUND

Entrepreneurship has been a longstanding component of the profession of pharmacy, going back to the earliest days of the corner drugstore. Coca-Cola (Coca-Cola, 2007) and Dr. Pepper (Dr. Pepper, 2007) are two examples of products that arose from some of the earliest days of that practice setting. In an era when industrialized medicinal products did not exist, pharmacists were in the position of creating new recipes and formulations to meet physicians' orders and treat patients. As the industry evolved and more standardized and large-scale methods were developed, the profession of pharmacy evolved with it. Traditionally, independently owned pharmacies were started and run usually with one pharmacist opening up the store as an owner-operator. Some pharmacists saw opportunities beyond single-store ownership and pursued and developed multiple stores. This led to the development of what is now referred to as *chain store pharmacies*. These pharmacies are often thought of as not being entrepreneurial for pharmacists who enter as employees; however, chain pharmacy itself is an example of entrepreneurship, and as will be discussed later, there are opportunities for entrepreneurship within large companies. Within the hospital setting, clinical pharmacy was developed in the 1960s and eventually made its way into the community pharmacy practice setting. In the last 15 to 20 years, the concept of *pharmaceutical care* was established and transitioned into medication therapy management (MTM), which has led to many entrepreneurial activities and endeavors in disease-state management, immunization delivery, and other new businesses.

To date, the entrepreneurial endeavors within the profession have been undertaken largely without formal training in entrepreneurship within the pharmacy curriculum. It is likely that formal training in entrepreneurship can increase the success rate of these entrepreneurial endeavors. The ability to integrate this formal training is increasing because the field of entrepreneurship is a growing rapidly. In 1975, 104 colleges and universities offered courses in entrepreneurship (Kauffman Foundation, 2006). By 1990, this had increased to 370, and by 2005, the number of schools offering courses in entrepreneurship had exploded to 2,662 (1,194 two-year schools and 1,468 four-year schools). There are now over 895 programs in entrepreneurship for business students, 126 programs with undergraduate minors, and 463 programs for nonbusiness students.

WHAT IS ENTREPRENEURSHIP?

The word *entrepreneurship* has come to have many definitions. One commonly used definition is "the process by which individuals pursue opportunities without regard to resources they currently control." One of the key aspects of this definition is that entrepreneurship is a process. This has several implications. First of all, a process is something that can be taught and is something that is repeatable. It also implies characteristics of passion and perseverance. In pursuing opportunities without regard to resources currently controlled, the entrepreneur must believe in and have a passion to succeed that will carry him or her through difficult

times. The end goal is achieving the vision. As Michael Morris, Witting Chair of Entrepreneurship at Syracuse University, states and teaches, entrepreneurship is a "philosophy of life" (Morris, 1998). It is a way of approaching life to identify problems and proactively turning them into opportunities to improve the situation, whether that is society, individual life, or the profession.

Pharmacists work with patients every day to help solve their problems in managing their medications and health. Because of this, pharmacists are in an ideal position to identify opportunities that may be viable business opportunities.

WHO IS AN ENTREPRENEUR?

There are often misperceptions about *who* an entrepreneur is (Kuratko, 2003). Some common stereotypes are that an entrepreneur is someone who is lucky, highly charismatic, and greedy and often that they are just "born." The definition given earlier helps to debunk these misperceptions. The process orientation and ability to teach the process shows that entrepreneurship is not something a person is just born with or that just depends on luck.

Likely because of the misperceptions, the area of identifying who is an entrepreneur is one of the most heavily researched areas in the field. Some of the common characteristics of entrepreneurs include a high level of achievement motivation, an internal locus of control, and a tolerance for ambiguity. John Miner, is his book, *The Four Routes to Entrepreneurial Success* (Miner, 1996), identifies four types of entrepreneurs (Table 31-1). Each of these types has unique characteristics that can help to break through the stereotypes. For instance, the "super sales person" is the more charismatic individual typical of some stereotypes, but the other three types help to identify where less charismatic people fit as entrepreneurs. Additionally, "real managers" identifies the type of entrepreneur that can fit into corporate entrepreneurship. One characteristic that is not present in the descriptions of entrepreneurs is "high-risk gamblers." Entrepreneurs have been found to have a tolerance for ambiguity but not to be inclined

Table 31-1. Types of Entrepreneurs	
Personal Achievers	**Super Sales People**
Need for feedback	Capacity to understand others, empathize
Need for achievement	Belief that social processes are important
Strong commitment	Good at external relationship building
Internal locus of control	Belief in sales force
Expert Idea Generators	**Real Managers**
Build venture around new products	Desire to take charge, compete, be decisive, stand out
Involved with high-tech companies	Desire to be corporate leader, desire for power
Desire to innovate	Positive attitude towards authority
Intelligence as source of competitive advantage	

to take unnecessary risk and even have been found to be more risk-averse than people who are not entrepreneurs (Xu and Ruef, 2004).

An important aspect of entrepreneurs to recognize is that they are not necessarily experts in all areas of business (e.g., finance, accounting, marketing, operations, etc.). It is not possible for one person to be an expert in every area necessary to start, grow, and run a business. Entrepreneurs typically are very good at establishing networks of people who can help them in areas that are not their strengths. An example of this is Henry Ford (Hill, 1960). During World War I, a Chicago newspaper called Mr. Ford an "ignorant pacifist." Mr. Ford did not like this and took the paper to court. When Mr. Ford was on the witness stand, the attorney drilled him with questions to test his knowledge with the intent of showing that Mr. Ford was unable to answer the questions and was indeed "ignorant." After getting frustrated with the line of questioning, Mr. Ford stated that if he really wanted to know the answer to any question, he had a row of electronic buttons on his desk. By pushing the right buttons, he could summon to his aid someone who could answer any question he could think to ask, so why should he clutter up his mind with this knowledge. The attorney was stumped, and Mr. Ford showed that he was not an "ignorant" man. Knowing how to get access to the people and information needed and not being afraid to ask are important characteristics of entrepreneurs.

■ THE ENTREPRENEURIAL PROCESS

Understanding the process of entrepreneurship and its application is one of the most important aspects of "learning" entrepreneurship because it provides a structured approach that can repeated, analyzed, and improved on. For these reasons, integrating the process of entrepreneurship into pharmacy practice is likely to provide a methodology that can increase the success of entrepreneurial activities.

Identifying an Opportunity

Ideas can come in many different forms and from many different places. Table 31-2 lists categories where ideas can come from. While this table was not created specifically to address pharmacy, there are many opportunities in each category on the list that exist within pharmacy. Once trained to look at life through the lens of an entrepreneur, an individual likely will generate many ideas (e.g., the "expert idea generator" type) and see opportunity where others do not. McGrath and MacMillan (2000), in their book, *The Entrepreneurial Mindset,* indicate that entrepreneurs often generate and maintain an *opportunity register.* This is a list of ideas for opportunities that is ongoing. The entrepreneur then chooses which one to pursue and maintains the list to go back to when he or she is ready to move to the next opportunity. It is impossible to pursue every idea. The entrepreneur must be disciplined in the selection of

Table 31-2. The Entrepreneurial Process

Identify an opportunity	Changing demographics	Acquire the necessary	Debt
	Emergence of new	resources	Equity
	market segments		Leveraging
	Process needs		Outsourcing
	New technologies		Leasing
	Incongruities		Contract labor
	Regulatory change		Temporary staff
	Social change		Supplier financing
			Joint ventures
Develop the Concept	New products		Partnerships
	New services		Barter
	New processes		Gifts
	New markets		
	New organizational	**Implement and**	Implementation of concept
	structure/forms	**manage**	Monitoring of performance
	New technologies		Payback of resource providers
	New sales or		Reinvestment
	distribution channels		Expansion
			Achievement of performance
Determine the required	Skilled employees		goals
resources	General management		
	expertise	**Harvest the venture**	Absorption of new concept
	Marketing and sales		into mainstream operations
	expertise		Licensing of rights
	Technical expertise		Family succession
	Financing		Sell venture
	Distribution channels		Go public
	Sources of supply		Shut down the venture
	Production facilities		
	Licenses, patents, and		
	legal protection		

Source: Used with permission from Morris, 2001.

opportunities to pursue because resources likely will be limited and pursuit of an opportunity requires focus, perseverance, and dedication.

Developing the Concept

As the opportunities are identified, the next step is to develop the concept further and determine where the best market opportunity lies. Most ideas have multiple ways that they can be implemented. Table 31-2 lists some of the possible options. Determining which idea to pursue and how to execute the opportunity are key decisions for the entrepreneur to make. To guide these decisions, the entrepreneur often will perform a *feasibility analysis* (Barringer, 2006).

In the feasibility analysis, extensive research is performed on the product/service, industry, market, organizational feasibility, and financial feasibility of the opportunity. This is an extremely important component of the decision to pursue or not pursue opportunities and speaks to the risk-averse nature of entrepreneurs. Much of this research will go into the building of a business plan (see Chapter 4).

When pursuing opportunities within a corporation, the feasibility analysis can be used to weigh opportunities, or projects, against each other. This type of entrepreneurship is called *corporate entrepreneurship* or *intrapreneurship* (Morris, 2002).

Determining the Required Resources

As the definition at the beginning of the chapter describes, entrepreneurs typically will not have all the resources needed to pursue the identified opportunity. This step in the process, which can be a part of the feasibility analysis, will help to identify what resources are needed and help to determine if the entrepreneur can obtain those needed resources. The list in Table 31-2 identifies at least some of the areas to be included in the analysis. This is an especially important point for pharmacists to evaluate because pharmacists have a specialized body of knowledge and are often not diverse in their training in business, management, marketing, finance, and other areas important to pursuing an entrepreneurial venture. It is important to realize that this does not have to be a limiting factor but rather a factor that can and needs to be managed.

This step in the process will also help to identify the extent to which financial resources need to be acquired and at what stage in the business-development timeline they are needed. Generally, when outside financial resources are needed, they are not all acquired at the same time. To maintain an equity position for those starting the business, rounds of funding are established that enable the business to develop, having enough capital to operate but not an overabundant amount of money as to be wasteful. Acquiring capital from investors results in awarding those investors with shares of the business. The investors who are in at the earliest time are subject to the most risk and therefore get more shares for less money. Conversely, this early money is costing the business owner more equity for the dollars he or she is getting. Acquiring the money in stages lets the owner maintain a larger equity position in the business. It should be noted that one of the biggest mistakes entrepreneurs make is not being willing to give up equity to fund their venture. While it can be important to be smart about how and when to give up equity, one analogy in entrepreneurship compares equity to manure (yes, manure). The more manure is piled up, the more it smells, but the more it is spread around (on a field), the more it helps things to grow.

Acquiring the Necessary Resources

Once the entrepreneurial idea and venture have been well defined and researched through the feasibility analysis, resources are acquired to pursue the idea. Table 31-2 lists some of the ways to acquire resources. Usually, to help get others to invest, the entrepreneur will have to put some of his or her own money into the development. This is referred to as having "skin in the game." Entrepreneurs can get very creative in how to get their businesses started. Grants and small-business loans are used often, but grants can take longer to acquire than other methods. The benefit of not having to pay back the financing or to give up equity in the company can be very attractive. A lot of "sweat equity" (time put into developing the business without receiving payment for the time put in) is usually also required, and this typically does not translate into actual dollar equity. If the entrepreneur cannot identify enough resources himself or herself, identifying an *angel investor* may be the next best alternative. An angel investor is someone who can supply the money himself or herself. This person also often helps to mentor the entrepreneur to ensure success.

It can also be beneficial to go after *strategic money*. Once someone provides capital to the business, he or she is likely to have a vested interest in seeing the business succeed. Money from individuals who can help make connections to potential customers and other stakeholders can be an important part of getting the business established. Joint ventures and partnering also can help to speed up the adoption process and get buy-in to the business.

Financial resources are obviously not the only types of resources that will need to be acquired. One of the most important resources to be acquired is a management team. Finding key people who can drive the business idea forward is an essential component of

Table 31-3. The 5 + 5 + 5 Bernelli Entrepreneurial Learning (BEL) Method

Five Stages of Development	Five Skills to Teach at Each Stage	Five Steps How to Transmit the Information Effectively
Exposure	Self-starting skills	Continuity
Hands-on	People skills	Problem solution
Broadening experience	Marketing skills	Meet and greet
Formal entry	Money skills	Create networks
Leadership	Leadership skills	Recap

the success of the business. As implied earlier in the example of Henry Ford, having a strong network is an extremely powerful characteristic of an entrepreneur. Entrepreneurs who are able to identify key individuals and make connections through the people they know can get the right people to work for them, obtain funding, and get work done (e.g., marketing and business development/client recruitment) without having to spend as much money on regular outsourcing.

Implement and Manage

Implementation and management of the startup, growth, and ongoing operations are also critical components of the entrepreneurial process. The skills needed for this level of the process can be self-taught or learned in more formal training. Entire business degrees focus on the different areas where expertise is needed to run a business. Still, there are many successful business owners who do not have a formal degree in business. Decision-making abilities and experience are two of the most important attributes for success in this process. While some people may seem "born" with natural abilities in these areas, both decision-making ability and experience often are learned over time and can be learned within the profession of pharmacy after licensure. Pharmacists are put in many decision-making positions in professional practice. This experience, along with others that can be gained in managing a pharmacy, growing a practice, or working in a business unit of a large company, can serve as training and provide confidence to pharmacists to decide later in their career to pursue an opportunity. These same attributes can be acquired outside the profession and earlier as well.

Any exposure to running a business or decision-making positions can help to provide training that is beneficial to developing entrepreneurial abilities. The 5 + 5 + 5 BEL (Bernelli Entrepreneurial Learning) Method (Table 31-3) was developed by a pharmacist, Cynthia Ianerelli, now president of Bernelli University, who left the profession to help with the family business. In pursuing more formal training to run the business, she realized that many of the decisions in business school were easier for her than for others. She attributes this to her growing up around the family business and the subtle experiences she had in doing so. Her research has focused in this area and developed this method of teaching entrepreneurship that focuses on experiential learning, even starting as early as preschool, to train for entrepreneurship. As is seen in Table 31-3, the BEL Method identifies five stages of development and provides initially for exposure and hands-on experience. Once the individual has this, he or she can grow into broader experiences. It is not until after the person has these earlier experiences that he or she builds into formal entry and leadership stages. Research and reports (Hise, 2007) also support the value of experience in developing entrepreneurial thinking.

For any business, the key to implementing and managing the opportunity will center on cash flow. First, acquiring capital to get the business started, as discussed earlier, and then, once the business is started, balancing the expenditure of money with the need to obtain more to keep the business going. Businesses often fail because they do not have enough cash when they start. It is recommended that a business have enough cash to support it for 3 years when it is started. However, this is often difficult to obtain. Additionally, in opportunities where the business is obtaining funding through investors and venture capital and is giving up equity, it is typical for the business to pursue rounds of funding. The reason for this is that investors at the earlier stages get more equity for the money they put in because it is a riskier stage of the business. As the business develops and can demonstrate success, funding is not as risky and requires less equity to be given up.

Balancing the use of cash to operate the business with the need for funds to grow the business is delicate. Typically, the business is using funds to acquire supplies and resources to support the product. If the business is not paid expediently when sales are made, it can be difficult to replenish the supplies and resources for the next round of sales, and this can cause difficulty for the business in paying its bills on time.

Harvest the Venture

Harvesting the venture refers to how the entrepreneur will reap the rewards of the endeavor. There are many ways that an entrepreneur can "exit" the business. Some of these include selling the business to someone else, passing the business on to someone in the family, licensing the rights of the intellectual property developed in the business, going public with the business, or simply shutting the business down. To maximize the reward of the opportunity, it is important to develop the *exit strategy* or list of potential exit strategies early on in the concept-development process. Often the best time to cash in on a venture will be when the venture blossoming. This can be a difficult time to part with the venture unless a strategy is mapped out in advance. Having the exit strategy(ies) mapped out in advance can help in business planning and execution and in identifying opportunities to maximize reward.

▓ INTELLECTUAL PROPERTY

One of the most important aspects of entrepreneurship is protecting the idea, referred to as *intellectual property*. Intellectual property can take many forms, from logos, to products, to business processes, as some examples. Types of protection include copyrights, trademarks, and patents (Allen, 2003).

Copyright protection is the easiest and least costly to acquire. However, it also generally provides the least amount of protection. This protection does not protect the ideas, processes, or methods of the intellectual property. It only protects the form, or original work, which is the end result of the ideas, processes or methods. Copyrights can be obtained officially through the U.S. Copyright Office for as little as $30.

Trademarks are used to protect names, brands, logos, and other marketing devices that are distinctive. Trademarks are somewhat more expensive. They generally can be filed for $750. It is also possible to do a trademark search on your own on the Internet through the U.S. Patent and Trademark Office Web site (www.uspto.gov). It is also possible to pay attorneys to do the search for you.

Patents offer the highest level of protection. They take the most time and money to acquire, usually taking at least 2 years and $4,000 to file. It is generally necessary to hire intellectual property attorneys to assist with the filing and defense of the patent. Patents protect the idea, method, and design of products and businesses. (For a full description of patents and the filing process, go to www.uspto.gov.) It is important to research the timelines for filing—generally within 1 year of use—and to decide if you need only a patent in the United States or a patent filed in other countries as well (and there are specific timelines on when this needs to be done).

▓ INCUBATORS

A useful concept for entrepreneurs that may be especially applicable to pharmacist entrepreneurs is the *incubator*. This term describes an entity that exists to help get new businesses started. As stated earlier, entrepreneurs cannot be an expert in every area required of entrepreneurship. Incubators bring all or many of the necessary areas together (e.g., accounting, business plan development, legal, capital acquisition, etc.) to help entrepreneurs bring their ideas to market. As discussed previously, investment early in the idea-development process costs the most. Incubators usually take significant equity of the business to get started. The entrepreneur must assess how much is really needed and how much the incubator is really going to contribute before signing on. Incubators are often found connected to academic institutions, especially those with entrepreneurship programs. They can also exist within an area's business community and can serve as a method for local investors to formalize or outsource their investment process. For example, a person wishing to invest in new opportunities can use the incubator to screen opportunities and provide structure to the opportunities to lessen the risk of the investment. Locating an incubator can also be done by searching on the Internet.

TIMING AND COMPETITION

One of the most important aspects of bringing an idea to market is timing. No matter how good the idea is, if the market is not prepared for it, it will never reach its full potential. *First-movers,* the first person to bring a concept to market, can have what is called *first-mover advantage,* allowing them to gain the rewards of early entry into a market. At other times, the second person into the market can gain the advantage because the first-mover has had to go to all the effort to train and educate the market about the concept. Deciding exactly when an opportunity is ripe is one of the most important decisions an entrepreneur must make. Research, focus groups, forecasting, and competitive analysis can go a long way toward identifying when the timing is right. However, many companies spend enormous resources to identify when the timing is right and exactly what the product should be only to see their product fall flat or short of expectations. As is described by Zaltman (2002), people cannot tell in advance of a product offering what their true reaction to the product will be. Zaltman's research showed that 95 percent of people's thinking occurs in their subconscious mind, so while they may even desire to help, their true reaction can be seen only with exposure to the product and all the parallel decisions accompanying it. One often counterintuitive factor that can help to identify a product's success is whether or not a similar product offering exists. Competition, in general, can be a positive sign that the market is ready for the concept and can serve to

bring down the costs of bringing the product to market. The competition's presence and marketing can serve to validate the need for the product, increase awareness of the need for the product, and help tear down walls of resistance to the new product.

SELLING THE CONCEPT

To sell the opportunity effectively, the entrepreneur must be able to quickly communicate the value proposition associated with the product, service, or business. In entrepreneurship circles, this is referred to as the *elevator pitch.* The elevator pitch refers to the ability to pitch the concept to a potential investor in the amount of time it takes to get on an elevator and then get off. The idea behind this is for the entrepreneur to be ready to pitch the concept clearly and concisely at any time. This skill actually fits in well for pharmacists because it is similar to how pharmacists often must counsel patients and make drug therapy recommendations to prescribers. One method of getting additional training in doing this effectively is the book, *How to Get Your Point Across in 30 Seconds or Less* (Frank, 1986). Three key questions that may be helpful to address are

1. What is the benefit?
2. How is the opportunity new and different?
3. What is the reason to believe?

One common mistake that is made by inexperienced entrepreneurs and pharmacists in "selling" their product or service is to focus on its *features.* They describe these features or aspects of the product or service but do not relate to the customer or how the features provide benefit or value. Benefits relate directly to how the product or service will make buyers' lives better. Investors are looking for an obvious value proposition and preferably one that is recurring or leads to multiple selling opportunities.

ADDITIONAL RESOURCES

There are many resources for entrepreneurs. Searching the Internet can easily identify a number of resources.

Networking in the community with business owners also can identify mentors who can be a vital resource as well. Some recommended resources include

- *The DELTA Rx Institute* (www.deltarx.com). The DELTA Rx Institute is based at the Drake University College of Pharmacy & Health Sciences. DELTA stands for "Drake Entrepreneurial Leadership Tools for Advancement." The Web site provides resources on entrepreneurship, profiles pharmacy entrepreneurial leaders, and provides tools and courses that can help to get pharmacists started on the path to entrepreneurship.
- *The Stanford Technology Venture Program* (http://stvp.stanford.edu/). This is a Web site through the Stanford University School of Engineering that is "dedicated to accelerating high-technology entrepreneurship research and education to engineers and scientists." The Web site has many resources and podcasts from entrepreneurs, including many from successful entrepreneurs in Silicon Valley, that can provide great insights.
- *The Entrepreneurship and Emerging Enterprises Program at Syracuse University* (http://whitman.syr.edu/eee/). This Web site also has many resources that can assist in growing entrepreneurial capabilities and links to other sites targeted to entrepreneurship.

■ REVISITING THE SCENARIO

John Adams decides that the time is right to pursue this opportunity. He decides that to really give this opportunity the chance for success that it needs, he will focus his attention by fully researching the opportunity, identifying a mentor, and setting everything in place. Once that is accomplished (under a planned timeline), he will turn to this as a full-time opportunity, leaving his current employment. "Traditional pharmacist positions are easy to get back into, and I can probably get a sign-on bonus somewhere if I needed it, so why not?"

■ CONCLUSION

Entrepreneurship has strong roots in the pharmacy profession. The specialized knowledge, skills, and practice of pharmacy provide a solid foundation for identifying and pursuing entrepreneurial endeavors. While stereotypes often portray entrepreneurs as charismatic high-risk gamblers, evidence suggests that people can be successful entrepreneurs with a variety of personal characteristics. Importantly, identifying that entrepreneurship is a formal process that can be repeated and taught shows that it is not simply a trait individuals are "born with." Applying the described process of entrepreneurship can provide a framework for success and for quality improvement through refinement of the process. Financing the entrepreneurial endeavor requires a skillful balance of managing cash flow and equity to bring the opportunity to market successfully. Throughout pharmacy's history, entrepreneurship has been a strong component of the profession that has helped it to adapt and strengthen itself over the years. With the explosive growth of entrepreneurship education and the rapid change in today's world, there is no doubt that it will be just as vital in moving the profession forward.

■ QUESTIONS FOR FURTHER DISCUSSION

1. Describe the importance of networking for entrepreneurs, and identify methods of networking in the profession, community, and business world.
2. What, in your opinion, is the most difficult step in the process of entrepreneurship? Describe and explain why?
3. Describe an approach to financing an entrepreneurial venture. Include a discussion of the pros and cons of debt acquisition, using personal and "friends and family" funds, and venture capital.
4. After identifying an opportunity, develop a 30-second elevator pitch that clearly communicates the value of the concept.

5. Which category from Table 31-1 do you most readily identify with, and how would you see this leading toward your own individual entrepreneurship?

REFERENCES

Coca-Cola. 2007. The Chronicle of Coca-Cola. Available at www.thecoca-colacompany.com/heritage/chronicle_birth_refreshing_idea.html; accessed on October 7, 2007.

Dr. Pepper. 2007. A History of Dr. Pepper, the World's Oldest Major Soft Drink. Available at www.drpeppermuseum.com/dr-pepper-facts.html#history; accessed on October 7, 2007.

Allen KR. 2003. *Launching New Ventures: An Entrepreneurial Approach*, 3d ed. Boston: Houghton Mifflin.

Barringer BR, Ireland RD. 2006. *Entrepreneurship: Successfully Launching New Ventures*. Upper Saddle River, NJ: Pearson Prentice-Hall.

Frank MO. 1986. *How to Get Your Point Across in 30 Seconds or Less*. New York: Pocket Books.

Hise P. 2007. A chance to prove my worth. *Fortune Small Business* 17:1.

Hill N. 1960. *Think and Grow Rich*. New York: Ballantine Publishing Group.

Kauffman Foundation. 2006. Kauffman Panel on Entrepreneurship Curriculum in Higher Education, Report I on Research Projects. Kansas City, MO: Kauffman Foundation.

Kuratko DF, Hodgetts RM. 2004. *Entrepreneurship: Theory, Process, Practice,* 6th ed. Mason, OH: Thomson Learning.

McGrath RG, MacMillan I. 2000. *The Entrepreneurial Mindset*. Boston: Harvard Business School Press.

Miner JB. 1996. *The Four Routes to Entrepreneurial Success.* San Francisco: Berrett-Koehler.

Morris MH. 1998. *Entrepreneurial Intensity: Sustainable Advantages for Individuals, Organizations, and Societies.* Westport, CT: Quorum Books.

Morris MH, Kuratko DF. 2002. *Corporate Entrepreneurship.* Orlando, FL: Harcourt College.

Morris MH, Kuratko DF, Schindehutte M. 2001. Towards integration: Understanding entrepreneurship through frameworks. *Entrepreneurship and Innovation,* February:35.

Xu H, Ruef M. 2004. The myth of the risk-tolerant entrepreneur. *Strategic Organization* 2:331.

Zaltman G. 2002. *How Customers Think: Essential Insights into the Mind of the Market.* Boston: Harvard Business School Press.

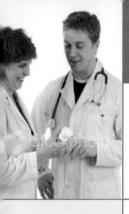

32

APPLICATIONS IN INDEPENDENT COMMUNITY PHARMACY

Joseph Bonnarens

A **bout the Author:** Dr. Bonnarens is currently Assistant Dean for Student Affairs and Associate Professor in Pharmacy Administration at Pacific University School of Pharmacy in Hillsboro, Oregon. He received a B.S. in general science and a B.S. in pharmacy from Oregon State University in 1990. He worked as a pharmacist in several practice settings, including independent, chain, and hospital pharmacies. In 1992 he completed the American Society of Health-System Pharmacists Executive Residency, followed by his employment with the National Community Pharmacists Association in Alexandria, Virginia, until 1996. Dr. Bonnarens pursued graduate education, earning an M.S. in 1999 and a Ph.D. in 2003 in pharmacy administration from the University of Mississippi. Dr. Bonnarens began his academic career as an Assistant Professor in the Social and Administrative Pharmacy Division at the University of Wisconsin School of Pharmacy, where we worked from 2003 to 2007. His research interests include entrepreneurship, patient care service development, workforce issues, and management issues facing pharmacy practitioners in various practice settings.

▉ LEARNING OBJECTIVES

After completing this chapter, students should be able to

1. Identify evolutionary changes leading to current independent community pharmacy practice.
2. Identify the characteristics of entrepreneurship and describe the opportunities that exist within independent community pharmacy practice.
3. Compare and contrast starting up a new independent community pharmacy versus purchasing an established pharmacy.
4. List and describe the steps necessary for starting an independent community pharmacy.
5. Identify methods of purchasing an established pharmacy.
6. List and discuss various issues facing independent community pharmacy practice.

■ SCENARIO 1

As Sue Franklin was completing her last rotation during her final year of pharmacy school, she began to think about where she wanted to work after graduation. As part of her required and elective rotations, Sue gained experience in a number of practice settings. She really enjoyed the critical care rotation at the University Medical Center. However, she knew that a residency probably would be required to land a position there. Sue had completed a rotation with the Indian Health Service and had thoroughly enjoyed her experience caring for a Native American population in New Mexico. She had also gained experience working at a chain pharmacy and then a supermarket pharmacy during holidays and vacations throughout pharmacy school. "What am I going to do?" thought Sue. She had so many great experiences and in some ways too many employment options. She had already received job offers from the chain and supermarket pharmacies, each paying a very good salary. She also had received an offer from Professional Pharmacy, a local independent community pharmacy in which she completed two rotations, community and administrative. Sue was surprised by the offer because she had spent only 10 weeks in the pharmacy. Prior to her rotations, Sue had never considered working in an independent community pharmacy. One of her favorite clerkship projects was the development of an immunization program for Professional Pharmacy. Sue loved the ability to create new programs and offer specialty services to patients in need. Darrel Burke, the owner of Professional Pharmacy, was very enthusiastic about the ideas Sue had shared with him regarding the development of other patient care specialty services. As Sue thought back about her experience, she was also impressed with Mr. Burke's management style. She remembered that the workflow was very organized and that the employees enjoyed taking care of patients and took pride in their jobs. Mr. Burke took great care of the entire staff. He was the only manager that Sue had worked with to hold brief staff meetings every couple of weeks to find out how things were going and to take action on issues raised during the meetings. Sue was also amazed at how much the customers cared for Mr. Burke and the staff, and vice versa. She could not remember receiving cookies from a patient whom she had helped on any other rotation. While the salary offered by Professional Pharmacy was slightly lower than those offered by other prospective employers, Sue realized how unique Professional Pharmacy is and began to see the value of working in a place that accepted and even encouraged its employees to seek creative strategies for enhancing customer service.

■ CHAPTER QUESTIONS

1. What is independent community pharmacy? From a practitioner's perspective? From a patient's perspective?
2. Historically, independent community pharmacies and the pharmacists owning them have been criticized as being "only in it for the money." How would you dispel this myth?
3. How can an independent community pharmacy owner of 15 years keep the entrepreneurial spirit alive in the pharmacy?
4. What are the advantages and disadvantages of starting a new pharmacy versus purchasing an existing one?

■ INTRODUCTION

As stated in Chapter 1, "The managerial sciences of accounting, finance, economics, human resources management, marketing, and operations management are indispensable tools for today's practitioner." Each of the tools referred to is critical to all pharmacy practitioners in varying degrees. This statement could not be more accurate when discussing independent community pharmacists. An independent community pharmacist works in an environment that demands a unique level of understanding of the proper use of each tool in providing patient care, in addition to running a respected business in a community. While a discussion of managing an independent community pharmacy practice could incorporate most of the concepts from this book, the goal here is to provide a cursory overview and discuss the application of management tools critical to this environment.

WHAT IS INDEPENDENT COMMUNITY PHARMACY?

What comes to mind when the word *pharmacy* is mentioned? Depending on your age, hometown size and location, personal health history, and experiences shared by family and friends, a number of examples might appear. While the descriptions would vary regarding the name and even the practice setting, many would envision a privately owned business that not only filled prescriptions but also took care of patients and their families. This type of pharmacy has been described in many ways: a "mom and pop" shop, a drug store, a chemist's shop, an apothecary, a prescription shop, or hundreds of brand names ranging from Abe's Drug to Zimmerman's Pharmacy. The business that is described by most is an independent community pharmacy.

A stereotypic description of an independent community pharmacy might include the existence of a small business with a prescription counter operated by the owner and located in the back of the store. The front of the store might contain a wide variety of offerings that could range from a small section of over-the-counter (OTC) medications, vitamins, and other health-related products to an expanded OTC area with additional offerings, such as greeting cards, candy, gifts, and health and beauty products. In general, one might find a relatively small but very helpful and friendly staff that know their customers by name and provide great service.

Historical Perspective

Pharmacy practice in the United States was founded on the shoulders of independent community pharmacy owners. Beginning with the earliest apothecary shops in colonial America, independent practices manufactured most medications that were provided to customers. In the early 1800s, apothecaries and drug stores became more prominent in cities and towns (Higby,

2003). Reasons surrounding this growth include the evolution of medicine and pharmacy into separate professions and the growing need for medications as the country and its population continued to expand. The drug store became recognized as the place to purchase medicine. These practices diversified and began to offer additional products and services to their respective communities.

In the late 1800s, the pharmacy began to stock and sell more products that were being created by pharmaceutical manufacturers. With this change, pharmacies needed less space for compounding products. The prescription department moved to the back of the store, with the front opening up for saleble goods and creation of the soda fountain. Since the pharmacist had a background in chemistry and experience with mixing and flavoring, the soda fountain was a perfect fit for the pharmacy. While the soda fountain attracted customers, events such as the prohibition movement greatly increased its popularity. A unique combination of prescription department, general store, and soda fountain established the drugstore as a cultural icon (Higby, 2003).

Independent community pharmacy practice evolved with the rest of the profession through the education reform of the early 1900s, increased competition from the development of chain and mass-merchandiser pharmacies, and the decreased need for practitioners compounding coinciding with the increased availability of mass-produced medications. The 1950s ushered in the "count and pour" era of pharmacy practice: a momentous surge in antibiotics and other medications coming to market, increases in the number of prescriptions dispensed, limited roles of pharmacists in patient care, and boom times for pharmacy businesses (Higby, 2003).

The 1960s witnessed a new era that dramatically changed the face of independent community pharmacy practice. Legislation created the Medicare and Medicaid programs and, with that, the birth of public pharmaceutical benefit programs (Williams, 1998). These events drastically changed the economics of independent pharmacy practice by introducing greater influence from government and private payers. Also during this time, the profession was beginning to embrace the concept of clinical pharmacy. Eugene White, an independent pharmacist, was advocating patient-oriented professional pharmacy practices by example with the development of a patient drug profile and an office-based practice (Ukens, 1994). The public, which had been viewed only as customers, now was recognized as patients (Higby, 2003).

Through the 1980s, community pharmacists began carving out their own niche in health care as drug information experts by expanding their scope of practice into patient care areas such as consulting, home health care, and long-term care. Independent community pharmacists began to accept this expanded role and fostered the pharmacist–patient relationship by continuing to provide high-quality, personalized service to all patients.

The dawn of clinical pharmacy provided the groundwork for the shift to the pharmaceutical care era. With significant changes in the areas of law (e.g., the Omnibus Budget Reconciliation Act of 1990 and the Health Insurance Portability and Accountability Act of 1996), health care reimbursement (e.g., the rise of managed care), and scope of practice (e.g., disease-state management programs, wellness programs, and collaborative practice agreements between pharmacists and physicians), independent practice has had to diversify and change to meet the needs of the various players in this environment. In addition, the independent community pharmacist has had to become a better manager in order to survive in such a competitive marketplace.

Today's Independent Community Pharmacy

According to various agencies, a strict definition of *independent community pharmacy* means that no more than three pharmacies are owned and operated by one person (Smith, 1986). Even with this established definition, other organizations have expanded the number of pharmacies that can be owned to as many as 11. A better sense of what independent community pharmacy is can be gained from the views of various stakeholders.

In a survey conducted by *Consumer Reports* (2003), over 85 percent of customers were very sat-

isfied or completely satisfied with their experience at independent community pharmacies. The article highlighted the fact that customers found independent pharmacists to be accessible, approachable, and easy to talk to while also being very knowledgeable about prescription and nonprescription medications (Consumer Reports, 2003). Independent community pharmacies also were recognized for offering additional patient care services, such as disease-state management education, health screenings, and specialty services such as compounding.

While the *Consumer Reports* survey provides a look at patient perceptions, it is important to get a sense of what independent community practitioners think. One of the principal advantages of this type of practice frequently pertains to personal control. Referred to in various ways, such as "being my own boss," "wanting to do things my way," and "besides my patients, I answer to know one but myself," the issue of personal control is a driving force for individuals to become owners. Other factors, such as involvement and recognition in the community and personal motivations, are also considered to be advantages of this practice setting (Smith, 1986). One of the predominant disadvantages of independent community pharmacy relates to the increased responsibilities assumed by the owner: financial, legal, and professional. Because the pharmacy is a business, in some sense everyone (e.g., customers, employees, payers, and regulators) is the "boss" of the independent (Smith, 1986). An additional disadvantage that also might be included are the long hours typically put in by the owner, especially during the business's formative years (Smith, 1986).

■ THE ENVIRONMENTS OF INDEPENDENT COMMUNITY PHARMACY

Overall Health Care Environment

Pharmacy continues to assume a larger portion of the health care dollar. According to projections for 2006, prescription drug expenditures were predicted to increase slightly to $213 billion (6.5 percent growth), following a steady decline into single-digit growth since 2000 (CMS, 2007). Spending for drugs is expected to reach nearly $500 billion by 2016 (Poisal et al., 2007).

Through 2003, Medicaid reimbursement had remained one of the best-paying third-party programs for independent community pharmacies. Additionally, Medicaid programs had been the active "laboratories" for pilot projects paying community pharmacists fees for managing the therapy of select groups of patients based on their disease state, such as diabetes and asthma (English, 1998). As the costs of each state's Medicaid program continued to grow, additional changes were looming on the horizon that would affect the rev-

enue stream of independent community pharmacies dramatically.

The Medicare Modernization Act (MMA) of 2003 (CMS, 2005) introduced a major change to the entire health care environment, with millions of beneficiaries eligible for this new program. This influx of individuals with an opportunity for prescription drug coverage can be shown by examining the changes in prescription drug spending by payer from 2005 through 2006 (Fig. 32-1) (CMS, 2005; Poisal et al., 2007). Medicare, as a payer, jumped from 2 to 22 percent in spending for prescription drugs, whereas Medicaid and out-of-pocket expenditures decreased. Although

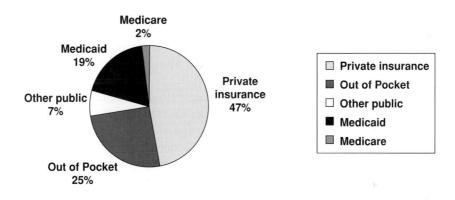

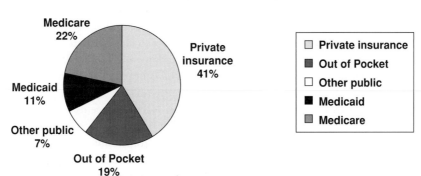

Figure 32-1. Changes in payers with implementation of Medicare Part D.

it has been suggested that Medicare Part D will not have much impact on the future prescription drug growth rate, the immediate impact in a variety areas has been significant and will be long lasting (Poisal et al., 2007).

Independent community pharmacies/pharmacists were the front-line professionals dealing with the issues leading up to and far after January 2, 2006—the first day of Part D. Such major change in the payment structure for prescription drugs has significant repercussions. Leading up to "Part D Day," there was great concern regarding the profitability of pharmacies with the shift in payers and subsequent reimbursement rates (Ukens, 2006). A July 2006 survey of over 500 independent community pharmacists revealed that 89 percent of respondents reported a worsening of cash flow, 55 percent reported that they had to obtain outside financing to supplement their cash flow, and 33 percent admitted to considering closing their pharmacy (Edmondson, 2007). A major factor relating to the cash-flow issues was the slow reimbursement rates related to the Part D program. A 2007 study confirmed the slow reimbursement rates to pharmacies (Medical News Today, 2007). The researchers found that 50 percent of community pharmacy claims were being paid more than 30 days after adjudication and that over 17 percent experienced delays over 60 days (Sheppard, Richards, and Winegar, 2007). These delays are critical considering that pharmacies must pay their wholesalers/supplies every 2 weeks to receive added benefits and within 30 days to avoid penalties.

Internal Pharmacy Environment

A unique publication provides financial benchmarks for independent community pharmacies. The *NCPA-Pfizer Digest* is an annual survey that compiles and summarizes financial data from independent pharmacies nationwide (NCPA, 2007). Data from the past 2 years of the *NCPA-Pfizer Digest* are used as a benchmark to describe the typical independent community pharmacy, as shown in Table 32-1. In general, the typical independent community pharmacy has a total sales volume of over $3.6 million, of which 92 percent is derived directly from prescription sales. Over

61,000 prescriptions are filled annually, with 91 percent of those prescriptions being paid for by a third party: 15 percent by Medicaid, 24 percent by Medicare Part D, and 52 percent by other third-party payers.

Independent community pharmacies have incorporated various elements of technology into the practice setting, including specialized software that checks for medication errors, fills and labels each prescription, and even the processes the sales transaction. Additional uses have grown to include automated dispensing machines, specialized compounding and intravenous mixing equipment, and customized software that can be used in the management of patients with particular disease states such as diabetes. One of the major technological growth areas is electronic prescribing. These capabilities refer to the connectivity between a prescribing physician and a community pharmacy, allowing for the electronic transmission of a patient's prescription from the physician to the patient's pharmacy of choice. This trend is relatively new, occurring within the past 3 to 5 years. The 2007 *NCPA-Pfizer Digest* reported that 51 percent of participating pharmacies were connected and capable of receiving electronic prescriptions, with 1.9 percent of prescriptions received electronically (NCPA, 2007).

A typical *NCPA-Pfizer Digest* pharmacy offers patients a number of specialized services, including but not limited to nutrition, delivery, patient charge accounts, compounding, herbal medicine, hospice, and durable medical goods, as well as scheduling of patient appointments and speaking to local organizations (NCPA, 2007). The trend to offer disease-state specialty services in independent community pharmacies continues to increase. Based on a survey conducted by the National Institute for Pharmacist Care Outcomes (NIPCO), nearly 15,000 community pharmacists have completed disease-state management programs accredited by NIPCO since its formation in 1995 (NCPA, 2003b). The most frequently offered programs are blood pressure monitoring, diabetes training, and immunizations (NCPA, 2007).

In addition to patient care services, another area that has been expanded by Medicare Part D has been

Table 32-1. Characteristics of a Typical Independent Community Pharmacy

	2006*	2005†
Total pharmacy size	4,623 sq ft	3,779 sq ft
Prescription area	1,275 sq ft	1,003 sq ft
Prescription volume (annually)	61,087 Rxs	61,071 Rxs
New	28,089 (46%)	29,284 (48%)
Refills	32,998 (54%)	31,787 (52%)
Third-party prescription coverage	91%	87%
Medicaid	15%	28%
Medicare Part D	24%	NA
Other third-party programs	52%	59%
Hours and days/week open	54 hours	60 hours
	6 days	6 days
Total sales (100.0%)	$3,612,000	$3,745,000
Prescription sales	92.4%	92.1%
Gross margin	22.8%	23.6%
Total expenses	20.0%	19.9%
Net profit (before taxes)	2.8%	3.7%
Cost of dispensing	$10.63	$10.53

*Based on 2007 *NCPA-Pfizer Digest.*
†Based on 2006 *NCPA-Pfizer Digest.*

medication therapy management (MTM) services and programs. MTM programs are designed to improve medication use, enhance patient safety, and increase patient adherence to their medication regimens (NCPA, 2007). Many of these initial MTM programs offered in independent community pharmacies do not include the service of a pharmacist; however, this trend is changing. The 2007 *NCPA-Pfizer Digest* reported that over 52 percent of independent community pharmacies offer MTM services, with an average charge of $40, and that 48 percent of the pharmacies are receiving reimbursement under Medicare Part D.

CHARACTERISTICS OF THE INDEPENDENT COMMUNITY PHARMACIST

Independent community pharmacy provides a unique venue for an individual pharmacist. Opportunities exist to be an owner and run the pharmacy, a part-time employee interested in staying in touch with community pharmacy practice, an entrepreneur with ideas for creating new service offerings for patients, or an employee working for the owner/manager. In this venue, the individual is limited only by his or her imagination. Thus, with this in mind, who chooses a career path in independent community pharmacy?

Whether one is interested in ownership or not, one of the key characteristics for a pharmacist in this practice setting is the importance of interacting with people. The independent community pharmacy provides pharmacists with a great opportunity to help patients. Problem-solving skills are critical as a pharmacist, and this setting provides constant challenges that require those skills. Other characteristics that are fostered by the independent setting are the ability to embrace change, deal with risk, and adapt to an ever-changing environment.

It is important that stereotypes sharing a negative connotation of independent community pharmacists be addressed. In some cases, pharmacists who are business-oriented have been viewed in a negative light. Additionally, many individuals interested in independent community pharmacy practice have been falsely accused of generalities such as "They are only going into business for the money," "They are not very clinical," and "They have a lack of professionalism."

Based on the descriptions of independent community pharmacy practice and the characteristics of the individuals who pursue this career path, several points must be made. First, independent pharmacists are placed in a difficult situation because of their need to possess expertise in pharmacy practice and business. All pharmacy organizations must stay in business so that they may provide goods, services, and care to patients. Second, independent community pharmacy practice represents one of the most accessible health care venues for patients. Because of this, there exist numerous clinical opportunities for pharmacists in the provision of quality patient care and positive patient outcomes. Third, independent community pharmacists contribute to the overall health of any community not only in the care provided but also in contributions to the economic and civic health of the community. As a health care provider, the pharmacy adds a stable business to any town's economic structure. Additionally, through involvement of the owner and other staff members in civic organizations, these individuals serve as volunteer leaders in activities ranging from school and hospital boards to elected offices.

Today's Independent

In visiting one of over 23,000 independent community pharmacies across the country, one might find the following two individuals. The first individual is the younger of the two. This pharmacist received a doctor of pharmacy (Pharm.D.) degree from an accredited program. There is a chance that this individual completed an MBA in conjunction with the pharmacy degree or at least had the chance to take some business courses. During his or her professional education, this individual took the required courses that introduced issues such as management, marketing, and economics into pharmacy practice. If available at the alma mater, any electives focusing on subjects ranging from pharmacy management and economics to entrepreneurship and ownership also would have been taken. While not a requirement, this individual probably was active in pharmacy school organizations. After graduation, this individual may have gained work experience at various practice settings or may have completed a community pharmacy residency. The individual has gained a variety of experiences from the practice settings worked, which ranged from one independent pharmacy to a variety of jobs that included experiences in hospital, chain, and other specialty practice areas, such as long-term care, home infusion therapy, or compounding pharmacy. This individual is in the process or has already established a specialty patient care service, such as an immunization program or disease-specific monitoring program in diabetes or asthma. The individual, along with other staff members, has received certification in these various specialty areas.

The second individual has been an owner for over 15 years. This individual received a bachelor of science degree. More than likely, this individual also completed course work pertaining to management and ownership. This individual may even have taken a class or two from the business school. This individual has a vast background of practice experience, often focused in community practice. This individual may have spent time working in a chain, a hospital clinic, or even another independent before pursuing ownership of his or her own practice. This individual manages a staff of pharmacists, technicians, clerks, delivery personnel, and other individuals, such as bookkeepers, accountants, part-time help, and contract employees. The owner has been a preceptor and has provided a recognized rotation site for the state's college or school of pharmacy since opening the store. This individual has always felt that the students provide the pharmacy with as much as the pharmacy gives to them. This individual also may have additional training experiences available, such as an administrative clerkship or a community residency program. In addition, this individual is an active member of several civic groups in the community, such as Rotary and the Chamber of Commerce. The owner is politically active, knowing the state and federal senators and representatives and voicing concerns to them regarding issues related to independent pharmacy practice. The owner supports various activities of the local schools, such as speaking at career days and sponsoring various programs. The pharmacy may sponsor a little league team in the summer and a basketball team in the winter. The owner knows his or her patients and is now taking care of several generations of families. He or she continues to participate in various certificate training programs and has implemented a variety of specialty services.

It is clear that both individuals enjoy their jobs from a professional, clinical, and personal perspective. They value the freedom to care for their patients through the variety of services they provide. Their career choice provides them with a salary that can support them individually and their families if appropriate. They are constantly learning and growing as practitioners, managers, and businesspeople. For both individuals, management plays an important role in their lives. The application of management tools is critical to the success of these individuals, as well as to the success of the independent community pharmacy.

SCENARIO 2

Sue has been on staff at Professional Pharmacy for 6 months. She is beginning to feel comfortable with the employees, customers, and flow of the business. The immunization program that she helped institute while a student has continued to grow, now offering vaccinations year round for influenza, diphtheria, and tetanus, in addition to miscellaneous travel and childhood vaccinations.

Sue began to realize that a large portion of Professional Pharmacy's patient population was diabetic. As she learned more by participating in diabetes-related continuing-education programs, Sue started to see opportunities for enhanced patient services that could

be provided to this specific population of patients. In one of the continuing-education programs that she attended, Sue learned how to create a business plan for the development of a diabetes care center. Sue created a business plan for a service that would help patients to identify whether they were diabetic, as well as to help educate and train those with diabetes to care for themselves and enhance their quality of life.

ENTREPRENEURSHIP/ INTRAPRENEURSHIP

In Scenario 2, Sue has formulated an idea, developed the idea through education and analysis, and created a business plan to test the strength of the idea. The process that Sue progressed through and the steps she took to develop her idea implicate her as a potential entrepreneur (see Chapter 31).

It is easy to see why most small-business owners, including independent community pharmacy owners, are categorized as entrepreneurs. There is more to being an entrepreneur, however, than just setting up a business. Entrepreneurs typically demonstrate the effective application of a number of enterprising attributes such as creativity, initiative, risk-taking, problem-solving ability, and autonomy and often will risk their own capital to set up a business (Bloomsbury Publishing, 2002).

Prior to a more descriptive discussion regarding the characteristics of an entrepreneur, Scenario 2 must be reexamined. Although it was suggested that Sue may be a potential entrepreneur, she is not really starting a business. She is an employee of Professional Pharmacy, and Sue's idea will provide a new business opportunity for the pharmacy and Mr. Burke, the owner. A more accurate definition of Sue in this scenario is as an intrapreneur. An *intrapreneur* is an employee who uses the approach of an entrepreneur within an organization (Bloomsbury Publishing, 2002). As a business ages and grows, the original entrepreneurial spirit can diminish. Intrapreneurs are critical to any established business in that they question the establishment and provide the internal spark to pursue innovation and new opportunities.

Characteristics of Entrepreneurs

Entrepreneurship is a growing area of research. A major area of interest is in identifying that magic combination of characteristics that makes a successful entrepreneur. Over 40 traits believed to be associated with entrepreneurship have been identified. Five of the more frequently identified characteristics include the following (Daft, 1994; Gartner, 1985):

- *Internal locus of control.* A belief by individuals that they are in control of their future and that other external forces will have little or no influence.
- *Need to achieve.* A human quality in which people are motivated to excel, so they pick situations in which they will be challenged but where success is likely.
- *Tolerance for ambiguity.* The psychological characteristic that allows a person to be untroubled by disorder and uncertainty.
- *Risk-taking propensity.* The likelihood of being a risk-taker no matter the circumstance.
- *Demographics factors.* These factors focus on a number of characteristics, including past work experience (experience in independent settings supports entrepreneurial tendencies), entrepreneurial parents (more likely to be entrepreneurial when parents have been as well), and age (most businesses are launched between the ages of 25 and 40).

▓ ENTREPRENEURIAL OPPORTUNITIES IN INDEPENDENT COMMUNITY PHARMACY

The history of independent community pharmacy provides a wealth of examples of entrepreneurship. Independent practitioners were some of the first to provide and use (Gumbhir, 1996)

- Complete patient medication profiles
- Total parenteral nutrition

- Delivery of products and care to prisons and long-term care facilities
- Home infusion services
- Veterinary pharmacy
- Specialty compounding services

In today's marketplace, entrepreneurial opportunities are everywhere. Individuals are limited only by their imagination in developing new services or other innovations. The biggest concern for any business is the ability to keep the entrepreneurial spirit alive. To continue that spirit, the owner/manager must create a climate that will support and foster the entrepreneurs and intrapreneurs in the pharmacy. Some rules that can be used in creating that climate in the pharmacy include (1) encourage action, (2) tolerate failure and use as a learning example, (3) be persistent in getting an idea to market, (4) use informal meetings to provide opportunities to share ideas, (5) provide challenges with the staff to help problem-solve given situations, and (6) reward and/or promote innovative personnel (Daft, 1994).

▓ SCENARIO 3

Sue loves her job. In the 3 years that she has been at Professional Pharmacy, she has developed patient care services in such areas as immunizations and osteoporosis, created a disease-state management program in diabetes, and successfully marketed the pharmacy's services to other health care providers in town. She has a great relationship with Mr. Burke, the owner, and thoroughly enjoys the people she works with and the patients she cares for in the community. While she is pleased with her accomplishments, she is also beginning to detect the emergence of several obstacles. Mr. Burke has been very supportive of her ideas, and even when he has disagreed, he has carefully explained his position against an idea. Over the past year, Sue has become more involved in the area of specialty compounding. A new dermatologist recently moved to the area, and during one of Sue's "detailing" visits to the Midtown Physicians Group, she struck up a conversation that has evolved into a steady stream of prescriptions for his "special" ointments and creams. Mr. Burke, although appreciative of the new business, is not interested in any expansion of the pharmacy to incorporate additional technology for use in compounding specialty items. Sue has been thinking so much about the potential for such a service that she sketched out a rough business plan one night when she could not sleep. Sue believes that this is a major local market that is going untapped; however, she knows that Mr. Burke wants no part in this venture. If she were her own boss, she could direct the business in the direction she saw fit. "Hmmm," she thought, "should the idea be shelved for a while, or is it time to look at the potential for owning her own business?"

■ INDEPENDENT COMMUNITY PHARMACY OWNERSHIP

While working for an independent owner can be a very fulfilling experience for many, one of the most attractive aspects of the independent setting is the opportunity to own a pharmacy. Interest in ownership has peaked and waned over the past 30 years. A significant decline in the number of independent community pharmacies occurred between 1990 and 1997 (NACDS, 2003). From the late 1990s to 2005, the number of independent practices has hovered around 24,000 sites. However, 2006 marked the first decline of independent community pharmacies in over 5 years, and even with that, this group represents 40 percent of all retail pharmacies in the United States (NCPA, 2007).

Some of the top reasons for wanting to go into business include self-management, creative freedom, and financial independence (SBA, 2003a). Other reasons include (1) not having to answer to others regarding the focus of the pharmacy, (2) being recognized and playing an important role in the business and health care needs of the community, (3) achieving a level of self-fulfillment and pride, and (4) continuing the legacy of pharmacy ownership established by family and/or mentors (Smith, 1986, 1996). Each individual who pursues ownership is driven by his or her own reasons. Once the decision of pharmacy ownership is made, the prospective owner must do the following: identify available pharmacies for sale or suitable locations for a new pharmacy, determine a satisfactory purchase price, evaluate and determine capital needs, and investigate and select the best source of capital (Gagnon, 1996). He or she must determine whether to start a new independent practice or purchase an established pharmacy.

Option 1: Starting from Scratch

Sue is determined to pursue her idea of creating a compounding specialty service. After her discussions with Mr. Burke confirmed his lack of interest, she realized that she has two options: Find another pharmacy that would be interested in pursuing this specialty service or start her own business. Sue decides that despite how well things have been for her at Professional Pharmacy, the time is right to start her own business.

The act of starting a new independent community pharmacy practice in a given community follows a long and rich history. As mentioned previously, a new pharmacy appears for various reasons, ranging from support of unmet health care needs for a particular patient population to taking advantage of a potentially lucrative business opportunity. Starting a new pharmacy, as with any business, requires considerable planning.

A number of distinct advantages are available to an owner opening a new independent community pharmacy. The opportunity to select and purchase each item of this new venture, such as fixtures, equipment, and inventory, is a great advantage. Also, hiring your own personnel, finding a great location, creating sound policies and procedures, and avoiding paying for intangible assets are additional advantages.

One of the intangible assets that requires further attention is goodwill. By definition, goodwill is an intangible asset of a company that includes factors such as reputation, continued patronage, and expertise, for which a buyer of the company may have to pay a premium (Bloomsbury Publishing, 2002). For an independent community pharmacy, specific factors that contribute to goodwill include the prescription files and accounts receivable (Smith, 1996). Since goodwill is related to the profitability of the pharmacy, the most frequently used method to estimate goodwill is some multiple of the annual net profit. The most recent year's net profit generally is considered the minimum price for goodwill, whereas a common value for goodwill is estimated at 1 to 2 years of net profit (Smith, 1996; Jackson, 2002).

If the venture is not planned carefully, the advantages of opening a new pharmacy can turn into disadvantages. There is a greater amount of risk that must be assumed by the owner and an increased chance of experiencing unforeseen events. For one, the lag time between startup and profit tends to be longer. Moreover, the challenge to secure capital is a formidable one.

How to Get Started

An individual interested in starting a new business can find a great number of books on the topic. While there are few books that specifically relate to the opening of a pharmacy, the general topics covered in the new business development literature are pertinent to any business type. This section offers a list of steps that can be followed on the path toward independent community pharmacy ownership:

1. Decide on the type of pharmacy.
2. Assess the potential market.
3. Develop a detailed business plan.
4. Determine the organization's structure.
5. Identify financing options.
6. Select a location.
7. Obtain licenses, permits, and insurance.
8. Develop a marketing and promotion plan.
9. Establish the management philosophy of the business.

Decide on the Type of Pharmacy

This question can only be answered by the potential owner. While it seems a very simple question, the answer requires considerable contemplation. As in Sue's

case, most individuals have a general idea of what type of business they want to start. For Sue, a compounding specialty pharmacy is her wish. Now Sue must begin to evaluate her idea thoroughly by resolving such questions as

- What products and services will I sell?
- From what base will I derive my customers?
- What skills do I bring to this business?
- Where should I be located?
- Will I have any competition?

Assess the Potential Market

Based on her evaluation of the type of pharmacy she would like to open, Sue has decided that she will start a compounding prescription business in the community where she currently lives. She has had a great deal of specialized training in this area and believes that there is a need for this type of pharmacy in the community. Now she must assess the potential market.

As described in the Chapter 24, Sue must undertake a complete market assessment of the area in which she plans to locate. Some of the questions to resolve include

- What is the potential customer base?
- How many physicians are in the community? Specialists?
- What is the competition? Other pharmacies? Other businesses?

Develop a Detailed Business Plan

It is important that the plan is well thought out and that due diligence is paid to eliminate as much uncertainty as possible when starting a new pharmacy (see Chapter 4).

Determine the Business Structure of the Pharmacy

A decision regarding the legal structure of the pharmacy must be made fairly early in the business development phase. Deciding on the legal structure of the pharmacy is critical to the overall success of the business. Each business venture is unique, and there is no one single ownership structure that suits every situation. The prospective owner should consult with an accountant

Table 32-2. Comparisons Between Business Structures

	Sole Proprietor	Partnership	S Corp	C Corp	LLC
Number of owners	One	Two or more	No more than 75 shareholders	Unlimited	No maximum, 1 person LLC permitted in most states
Level of liability	Unlimited, no personal liability	Unlimited, all partners jointly liable for actions of other partners	Limits personal liability to the amount invested to the limit of assets of the company	Limits personal liability to the amount invested to the limit of assets of the company	Limits personal liability to the amount invested
Tax issues	Owner pays tax on personal returns	Profits divided among partners; individuals must pay taxes	Profits flow to shareholders; individual pays taxes	Corporation pays tax on profit; shareholders pay on dividends	Profits flow to members; individual pays taxes
Can deduct losses on personal tax returns?	Yes	Yes	Yes	No	Yes
Ability to tranfer ownership	Totally transferable	May need consent of other parties	May be limited in order to preserve S status.	Totally transferable	Generally need concent of all owners

Sources: Tootelian and Gaedeke, 1993; Anthony, 2003a; SBA, 2003a, 2003b.

and an attorney to help select the ownership structure that will best meet her needs.

In general, three legal structures are available to pharmacy owners: sole proprietorship, partnership, and corporation. Table 32-2 identifies some of the unique characteristics of each legal structure (Anthony, 2003a; SBA, 2003a, 2003b; Tootelian and Gaedeke, 1993).

SOLE PROPRIETORSHIP This is the simplest ownership form because the business is owned by one individual. The sole proprietor owns all the assets, receives all profits, and is responsible for all aspects of the busi-

ness. While the owner receives all the profits generated from the business, there is also no legal distinction between the business and the owner, making the owner completely responsible for any liabilities and debts. This form of ownership is ideal for starting a business (Anthony, 2003b). However, as a business grows, there are other ownership forms that provide more security to the owner and the business.

PARTNERSHIP By definition under the Uniform Partnership Act, a partnership is an association of two or more persons to carry on as co-owners of a business for profit (Tootelian and Gaedeke, 1993). While seemingly straightforward, partnerships have the potential to be complex. Because of this, it is strongly recommended that a written legal agreement between the partners be executed. The agreement, also referred to as *articles of partnership,* should outline issues including, but not limited to, profit sharing, business decisions, resolving disputes, adding additional partners, and dissolving the partnership.

There are two types of partnership for consideration: general and limited. A *general partnership* entails all partners to divide the responsibility for management and liability, as well as profit or loss (Tootelian and Gaedeke, 1993). In addition, partners are jointly and individually liable for the actions of one another. While this is usually considered the least favorable form of ownership, a partnership can be less complicated than a corporation. For example, a payroll is not required for the partners in this relationship, and this provides for less paperwork and similar tax benefits to a sole proprietor (Anthony, 2003c). A *limited partnership* consists of at least one general partner and one or more "limited" partners (Tootelian and Gaedeke, 1993). *Limited partners* are individuals who provide capital to the business but are held liable only for the amount of their investment. These same individuals are not involved in any of the management decisions or operational issues of the business.

CORPORATION A *corporation* is a business that is chartered by the state and legally operates as a separate entity from its owners. The Supreme Court defined the corporation in 1819 as "an artificial being, invisible, intangible, and existing only in contemplation of the laws" (Tootelian and Gaedeke, 1993). This means that a corporation can be sued, taxed, own property, and enter into contractual agreements, whereas the owners of the corporation, the stockholders, are protected from liability. The stockholders elect a board of directors to oversee the entity and adopt bylaws to govern the corporation during its existence.

While incorporating a business seems like good move with regard to the limited personal liability experienced by the owners, there are detractors. The complexity of corporations requires a great deal of time and money for the setup and running of such an organization. Based on this structure, operating in accordance with local, state, and federal governments may result in higher taxation and require additional resources.

There are three forms of corporations that most businesses use: the S corporation, the C corporation, and the limited-liability corporation (LLC) (Table 32-3). Over 82 percent of average *NCPA-Pfizer Digest* pharmacies identified their structure as a corporation, with approximately 25 percent of those pharmacies further identifying themselves as S corporations (NCPA, 2002). Overall, the trend toward LLCs is recent because this corporate form is relatively new.

Identify Financing Options

Once the business plan has been outlined and the organizational structure has been selected, the next step for the soon-to-be owner is financing the pharmacy. Some questions that must be resolved include

- What are the financial needs for this venture?
- What type of financing will be best for the given situation?
- Where does one go to obtain capital for such a venture?

FINANCIAL NEEDS Every business has financial needs. These needs vary with the type and individualistic nature of each business. A pharmacy located in an urban area will have different financial needs than one located in a rural area. The buyer must understand the needs of the business venture. These financial needs refer to capital. *Capital* is wealth, in the form of cash, equipment, property, or a combination of these factors, that can be used in the production or creation of income (Kelly, 1996).

There are three areas of capital need: setup capital, startup capital, and operating capital (Tootelian and Gaedeke, 1993). Each area represents a period of time in the life of a business during which particular activities that require capital are conducted.

Establishing a pharmacy, whether starting new or making changes to an existing business, often requires

Table 32-3. Summary of Corporation Types

Type of Corporation	Advantages	Disadvantages
S corporation	• Limited personal liability • Corporate losses can pass through to shareholders • No corporate taxes • Shareholders and employees do not pay Medicare or FICA on profits/dividends	• Shareholder restrictions • Employee benefit expenses are included in gross income • All shareholders must agree to the election of S corporation status
C corporation	• Deduct 100 percent of health insurance paid for employees • Deduct fringe benefits such as qualified education costs, portion of life insurance, and employer-provided transportation for work • Profits up to $50,000 annually are taxed at lower rate if left in corporation rather than pay higher personal income tax rate	• If corporation loses money, owners cannot deduct on personal income tax • Corporate taxes on profit • If profits distributed to shareholders, they must pay personal income tax on dividends • More complicated and requires close monitoring
LLC	• Owners (members) receive limited liability as with corporation • As with partnership, income or losses are reported on member's individual tax return • One-person LLCs are treated as sole proprietor • In general, fewer restrictions and more flexibility	• Owners experience same self-employment tax treatment as partners and sole proprietors • States may differ in tax treatment • Newer corporation formless precedents

Source: Anthony, 2003d, 2003e, 2003f.

a considerable amount of capital. The activities that represent the largest initial capital expenditure focus on the physical aspects of the business. The remodeling and renovation of the pharmacy, purchasing of fixtures and equipment, finalizing the building's lease deposit if it is not owned directly, and purchasing the beginning inventory, prescription and nonprescription merchandise, are the major sources of capital expenditure. Most of the other activities in the area of startup relate more to paperwork and attention to detail. Such activities include prepaying insurance and utilities, obtaining the appropriate licenses and permits, and covering the professional fees of hired advisors (e.g., attorneys and accountants).

Types of financing Having identified a number of financial needs that come with the purchase of a pharmacy, the next step is to identify the type of funding available. Three main types of financing will be discussed: personal, debt, and equity.

Personal financing is just what it sounds like, the use of personal funds to finance the purchase of the pharmacy. It is no different from saving money for that first bicycle, car, or even one's retirement; personal savings is an important type of funding. This type of funding provides the buyer with the best possible funding source because there is no cost or payback terms, the amount can be unlimited, and it is relatively easy to use, whereas the only detractor is that there is a risk of loss (SBA, 2003a). However, in most cases, the buyer will need additional funds for the purchase, setup, startup, or operation of the pharmacy.

A common type of funding for a pharmacy is debt financing. *Debt financing* can be defined as something of value such as money that is borrowed at interest for a specified period of time (Kelly, 1996). Debt financing provides a buyer with an advantage by allowing him or her to borrow the needed capital without having to share any of the profits with the lender and to keep control of the management of the pharmacy. The disadvantages of debt financing highlight the fact that if something is borrowed, it must be returned. Loans must be repaid, with some measure of interest, over a defined period of time. Additionally, the amount of debt incurred is limited by the value of assets and earning record of the borrower (Tootelian and Gaedeke, 1993). Debt financing can consist of either or a combination of short- and long-term strategies (see Chapter 18).

Used less frequently, *equity financing* results in the buyer sharing ownership with investors who contribute funds. This level of investor ownership brings with it varying degrees of involvement in management of the business. Depending on the structure of the pharmacy, investors could be recognized as anything from a partner to a stockholder in the business. An advantage to equity financing is the chance to reduce the debt that must be repaid on a particular scale. Depending on the fiscal health of the business, partners or stockholders may or may not receive paid dividends. A significant disadvantage is that ownership of the pharmacy is spread among a larger group of individuals, thus reducing the owner's decision-making abilities (Tootelian and Gaedeke, 1993). Most small businesses, such as a pharmacy, are unable to attract much funding in this manner owing to the risk of small business survivals.

SOURCES OF FINANCING Banks are not the only source for obtaining capital. In fact, establishing an entirely new independent community pharmacy may not be appealing to a bank. Banks view the purchase of an established pharmacy as less risky, but there is no guarantee of obtaining a loan.

The choice of a funding source is critical to the future of a business venture and should be made carefully. The buyer must thoroughly weigh the options regarding the types of financing and the specific requirements provided for by each funding source. Table 32-4 provides a brief list of potential lenders (Kelly, 1996; SBA, 2003a; Tootelian and Gaedeke, 1993).

Select a Location

The familiar mantra Sue hears consists of three words: Location! Location! Location! The selection of the trade area, as well as the actual physical site of the pharmacy, is a primary factor in determining the success of the business. Sue has already incorporated the idea of location into her planning process by deciding on the type of pharmacy she wants to start and in conducting a market analysis.

Sue must evaluate the location of her pharmacy thoroughly with regard to population, potential customers, competition, physician availability, and community trends ranging from general health to economic issues (Kelly, 1996). To help Sue in accomplishing this task, a number of information resources are available to help analyze her pharmacy's location, including, but not limited to, public libraries; realty companies; utility companies; local, state, and federal documents and Web sites; state and national Small Business Administration (SBA) offices; and individually conducted or contracted surveys, interviews, or traffic counts. Sue is also reminded time and time again that this is a process that will be time-consuming and hard work. She should not depend solely on what the computer provides in the way of information. By putting in the work on the front end, the next steps will be smoother.

Obtain Licenses, Permits, and Insurance

As the owner of this new pharmacy, Sue will need to obtain specific licenses and permits to operate. While local zoning laws, building permits, and standards set by health, fire, and police are requirements that must be met by all businesses in a given community, Sue must also ensure compliance with a variety of state and

Table 32-4. Potential Capital Sources for Financing a New or Established Pharmacy Business

Source	Type	Positive	Negative
Personal savings	Personal	Easy, cheap	Risk of loss
Family	Personal, debt, or equity	Flexible	Can cause problems
Friends	Personal, debt, or equity	Flexible, usually good rate	Problems
Granting agencies	Personal	Cash awarded	Few, competitive, restricted regarding use
Credit cards	Debt	Easy to qualify, no collateral	Small amounts, high interest
Banks/savings & loans	Debt	Most common debt source	Hardest to qualify for
Commercial finance companies	Debt	More flexible alternative to banks	More expensive, collateral more important
Consumer finance companies	Debt	Personal loan, not loan to business; no restrictions on use of funds	High interest, personal collateral, not business
Wholesalers/suppliers	Debt	Line of credit, sometimes loans	Terms and conditions, requirements for use as wholesaler/supplier
Small business association	Debt	Longest payback time	Complex and competitive process
Venture capitalists	Equity	Can be large amounts	Hard to find, share ownership

Sources: Tootelian and Gaedeke, 1993; Kelly, 1996; SBA, 2003a.

federal regulations that pertain specifically to pharmacy (NABP, 2007; Tootelian and Gaedeke, 1993). Insurance is of critical importance to a pharmacy. Sue will need to find an insurance agent to help with creating a comprehensive insurance plan that covers events ranging from natural disasters and physical accidents to employee health and workers' compensation. In addition, professional liability insurance for Sue, professional staff members, and the business must be examined and obtained.

Develop a Marketing and Promotion Plan
How will Sue inform the community of her new pharmacy and the innovative services that she will be offering? Using the techniques and tools provided in Chapter 21, Sue will be able to develop a specific marketing plan to educate the community. Through the use of the local media outlets, such as newspapers, radio, television, and local Web site sponsorship, Sue will be able to execute a specific promotion plan for the new pharmacy. Sue should not focus all her marketing and promotional efforts on potential customers. A critical area for her specialty pharmacy will be the community of health care professionals, ranging from physicians and nurse practitioners to specialty practices such as dermatologists and veterinarians.

Establish the Management Philosophy of the Business
The owner of an independent community pharmacy sets the tone for the business. The owner has been involved in virtually every aspect of the business, from conceptualization and planning to development and completion. As the new owner, Sue will be involved in all aspects of the business. In addition to the potential

tools available in print, the experience that she has gained from working in an independent community pharmacy will be even more valuable to the dissemination of her management philosophy.

Option 2: "Why Reinvent the Wheel?"—Purchasing an Established Pharmacy

Sue has worked for Professional Pharmacy for 3 years. As she was closing up the pharmacy one night, Mr. Burke, the owner, brings up the idea that he is starting to think about retirement. He and his wife Helen eventually would like to move into a beachfront property. There they could take out their boat and have a place for their kids and grandchildren to visit. Sue is shocked by this sudden revelation. Mr. Burke reassures her that retirement is in the near future, but he wants to chat about her future career goals and whether those goals might include pharmacy ownership.

For a potential buyer, looking for the right pharmacy may seem like a daunting task. There are a number of places to begin a search. In many cases, the potential buyer already may have identified several businesses either through research or as a result of his or her current job. Local and state pharmacy associations are excellent resources for initial listings and referrals. A common section in the flagship publications of these organizations is a "pharmacy for sale" listing. The journals of most national pharmacy organizations have similar pharmacy listings. In addition, professional brokers who deal on the business side of the real estate market can be contacted and hired. There also exist specialty services provided by organizations. One example of this is the Independent Pharmacy Matching Service (IPMS) that is coordinated by the National Community Pharmacists Association (NCPA). The IPMS helps to match prospective buyers and sellers on various criteria, including geographic location.

Once a potential pharmacy is identified, an important question to ask is, "Why is this pharmacy for sale?" (Cotton, 1984). Is the owner retiring? Has the neighborhood changed owing to increased competition or economic changes to "sour" the location? Is the pharmacy on the verge of bankruptcy? These are just a few of the many questions that should be asked re-

garding the pharmacy. These questions reinforce the importance of researching the business and obtaining advice from various sources.

Purchasing an established pharmacy can provide an excellent opportunity to a potential buyer. Identifying the advantages and disadvantages of this ownership alternative will provide valuable insight into an individual's decision-making process regarding ownership (SBA, 2003c; Smith, 1986, 1996; Tootelian and Gaedeke, 1993).

Advantages and Disadvantages

According to many in the pharmacy and business literature, there are a number of advantages to purchasing an established pharmacy (Table 32-5). An established pharmacy already has eliminated a number of the unknowns that face the startup of a new pharmacy. There is a lower level of risk on the buyer's part because the pharmacy has an established history. Pending thorough

---

Table 32-5. Advantages and Disadvantages of Purchasing an Established Pharmacy

Advantages

Lower level of risk for the buyer

No additional competition added to the current marketplace

Reduced startup costs/less risk

Less time required to show a profit

Buyer receives established goodwill

Business has an established clientele

Business provides buyer with trained employees, inventory, physical facilities, and established relationships area healthcare providers

Disadvantages

Inadequate facilities

Old/outdated fixtures and equipment

Inventory that is too large and/or unsalable

Established policies and procedures do not match with new ownership's philosophy

Inflated sale price

Problems with the location

Undesirable established leases

research and assessment, the buyer should have fewer uncertainties regarding the pharmacy, ranging from the physical facility, inventory, and equipment to the personnel and patient base of the pharmacy. Based on this transfer of ownership, the pharmacy obtains new management while not adding another business to a competitive marketplace. Another advantage is that an established pharmacy provides the buyer with great potential for reducing startup costs and decreasing the length of time between startup and profitability. Additionally, the buyer receives the goodwill and reputation of the pharmacy.

The advantages related to this method of ownership can just as easily become disadvantages. The established assets, such as facilities and equipment, may be outdated or inadequate to meet the needs of the interested parties. The inventory of the business in question could consist of a large amount of out-of-date and unsalable items or even be too large for the pharmacy to support. The previously established policies and procedures could be in direct conflict with what the potential owner has in mind, thus creating potential human resources management problems. Additionally, the pharmacy's location may not be optimal, and the purchase price may be overinflated by goodwill.

During the negotiation of such a transfer of ownership, the careful review of all leases is a critical factor that is often overlooked. A *lease* refers to a long-term agreement to use or rent a fixture, a piece of equipment, the physical structure in which the pharmacy is located, or the land the business occupies (Gagnon, 1996).

Value Assessment and Price Determination

Once the decision has been made to purchase an established pharmacy and a specific property has been identified, the next step is to determine the value of the business. Prior to a value assessment, the future owner should conduct a thorough review of the external environment of the business, that is, the community in which the business is located.

The predominant method of determining the value of a business is through financial analysis. Chapter 15 discussed the basic principles of financial anal-

ysis. In determining the fiscal health of the business, its financial records (income statements and balance sheets) from at least the past 3 to 5 years should be reviewed. From these data, the various facets of financial analysis—solvency, liquidity, efficiency, and profitability—can be determined for the business, and trends can be projected based on the time frame analyzed. A number of financial formulas are used to provide a range of values that serve as a guide for either the buyer or seller to begin the negotiation process (Jackson, 2002). It is important to note that while there is no single formula that must be used, each formula determines the value of the business from various perspectives, providing a range of values that can be used to determine an initial buying or selling price.

Based on the preceding discussion, it should be obvious that determining the value of a business is not an exact science. While a number of established techniques may be used, each business is unique. In fact, the value of a business ultimately is determined through negotiation between the buyer and the seller (Jackson, 2002). The agreed-on price usually will lie somewhere between the initial price of the seller and the initial offer of the buyer. The valuation of a business is based on the assessment of facts about the business, informed judgment, and some common sense (Jackson, 2002).

Purchasing Methods

The next step for the prospective owner is to finance the cost of purchasing the pharmacy.

Financing

As was done during the preceding discussion regarding the financing of a new pharmacy, similar questions regarding the needs of the business, the type of financing, and the sources of capital must be addressed for the purchase of an established pharmacy. Whether purchasing an established pharmacy or starting one from scratch, a significant amount of capital will be needed to cover the cost of the venture. In this case, the buyer has a significant advantage over someone starting a new business because the established pharmacy will have lower startup costs and should take less time to begin making a profit.

From a buyer's perspective, various types of financing are available for purchase of a pharmacy. While personal, debt, and equity financing are examples available to the buyer, the main question that must be determined is will the pharmacy be bought outright, or will there need to be some financial arrangement made for purchasing over a period of time. In most cases, an individual buyer would have great difficulty in securing financing to buy a pharmacy outright. With this in mind, the following discussion illustrates a transfer of ownership that provides a win-win scenario for both the buyer and the seller.

Junior Partnership

A junior partnership provides an opportunity for a buyer to purchase a pharmacy with little or no initial capital and a seller to ease out of ownership and keep the legacy of the independent pharmacy alive in the community (Jackson, 2002). Instead of trying to figure out a way to sell the pharmacy when the owner is ready for retirement, this option allows the current owner to transfer ownership to a buyer, continue to have an income, and prepare for retirement.

The advantages of a junior partnership range from less risk and less initial capital needed by the potential buyer to the continued presence of an independent pharmacy to the economic and health care needs of the community. A junior partnership has disadvantages that are similar to those of any partnership arrangement. However, in this situation, because of the established relationship, the chance for both parties to determine compatibility, and the detailed nature of the agreement, a junior partnership proves beneficial.

▦ SCENARIO 4

It has been 4 years since Sue entered into a junior partnership with Mr. Burke, and at the end of next year, she will be majority owner of Professional Pharmacy. While the time has just flown by, Sue marvels at all she has learned about pharmacy practice from both the business and professional sides. Sue came to this realization shortly after her first scheduled meeting with this year's community pharmacy resident, Cindy Ryan.

Cindy had asked Sue to describe a typical workday. After laughingly explaining to Cindy that there is no such thing as a typical day when you are in the business of caring for patients, Sue offered the following description:

As the owner, I am responsible for the 40-member staff that makes up Professional Pharmacy Incorporated. This includes the main pharmacy, Professional Pharmacy West, and the compounding/home infusion pharmacy, Professional Pharmacy East. My day usually begins at East, where I check in with Jerry, the manager, to review the workload for the day and take care of any problems, usually human resources issues. I am usually at East for most of the morning, taking care of e-mail, mail, etc. I usually spend the afternoons at West. There I meet with Lois, the store manager, to go over things for the day and take care of problems. In each facility, on a weekly basis, a morning all-staff meeting is conducted to update staff regarding procedure changes and new third-party coverages, address employee concerns, and check in with everyone. The meeting can last up to 20 minutes. As the owner, I have had to spend more time managing the business and less working with the compounding center and the diabetes care program that we established several years ago. While I miss the time with patients, I have come to realize that becoming the best manager I can be helps to ensure that the patients we serve receive the best possible care.

▦ CURRENT ISSUES/ OPPORTUNITIES FACING INDEPENDENT PHARMACY PRACTICE

The life of an independent community pharmacy owner provides numerous challenges and can be highly rewarding. As Sue pointed out, most of her responsibilities have evolved into a management role. As a manager, the success or failure of the business is that individual's responsibility, and that success is dictated by the decisions made and actions taken.

The owner must balance a number of issues and ideas related to the pharmacy. Today's owner must be able to evaluate the issues, determine the feasibility of ideas, and take action. The following is a list of four issues that require a great deal of attention by an owner of an independent community pharmacy: competition, third parties, patient care service development, and niche development.

Competition

Independent community pharmacy practices operate in one of the most dynamic and competitive marketplaces. Most competition is readily apparent, such as traditional chain drug stores, supermarket pharmacies, and mass merchandisers. Independent community pharmacies also have experienced competition from other less obvious entities. This additional group of competitors consists of mail-order pharmacies, managed-care pharmacies, hospital ambulatory clinics and pharmacies, and even Internet pharmacies. Figure 32-2 illustrates the competitive retail market and provides an interesting look at a 10-year period of time. While the total number of retail pharmacies has remained relatively steady, the marketplace portrait has changed. Independents have experienced a decline in total numbers, whereas chains, defined as outlets including traditional chain drug stores, supermarket pharmacies, and mass merchandisers, have become more prolific. One contributing factor to this

role reversal has been competition in the prescription market. A number of independents that closed were unable to compete in certain markets for reasons ranging from third-party reimbursement rates that were too low to individuals being unable to embrace the changes that were taking place in the market. Those remaining continue to compete successfully.

Third-Party Issues

For an independent community pharmacy, addressing third-party issues is critical not only to the success of the business but also to its very survival. Addressed previously in this chapter, the average *NCPA-Pfizer Digest* pharmacy reported that 91 percent of prescriptions filled were paid for by a third party (NCPA, 2003a). This relationship identifies the importance of understanding third-party issues for owners and managers.

Third-party issues are wide-ranging. One of the most prominent issues from this arena focuses on the reimbursement rates for prescription medications that are received by independent community pharmacies from third parties. It is a constant struggle between third parties, who want to lower costs by lowering reimbursement rates to pharmacies, and independent practitioners, who must monitor the rates constantly to ensure that the pharmacy will be able to cover costs and have some profit margin.

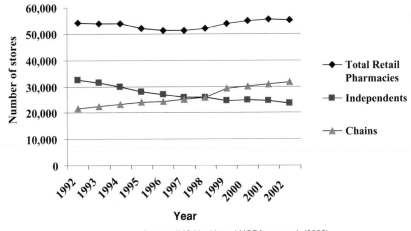

Source: IMS Health and NCPA research (2003)

Figure 32-2. Population of retail pharmacies, 1992–2002.

Again, Medicare Part D has added an additional issue to an already complex topic. While some of the problems have been improved, the difficulties for independent community pharmacy still remain (Chi and Paul, 2006). The issues of prompt payment and reimbursement rates will continue to contribute to an already complex and stressful environment, keeping everyone's focus on the continued evolution of the Medicare Part D program.

Patient Care Service Development

Independent community pharmacies have a rich tradition of service to patients. This tradition has evolved into a number of identifiable patient care services that are offered in many pharmacies. Patient care services can range from home delivery and patient charge accounts to specialized patient care such as disease-state management programs focusing on diabetes or asthma. The development of such services usually is based on the fact that patients needed to be cared for and the pharmacist began stocking the product and creating the service to help their patients. In areas such as herbal medicine, homeopathy, and nutrition, patients not only obtain specific products but also receive valuable information and learn that the pharmacist is a valuable information resource. As a complement to this continued development of patient care services comes the MTM programs and services (NCPA, 2007). All of pharmacy is striving to develop quality and cost-effective services that will continue to provide their patients with exceptional customer service while also helping to further secure the means to receive compensation directly for such services. Only through continued political and professional pressure will pharmacy earn the right to bill for the patient care services provided, as well as the ever-shrinking compensation for the medication itself.

Niche Development

The nature of independent community pharmacies and pharmacists is to develop and offer patient care services. In specific cases, certain services may be developed to fill a niche in the community. In Scenario 4, Sue identified and developed a niche with the creation of her compounding specialty business. The specialty service was created and succeeded because there was an unmet need for compounding services in the community. As was discussed in the entrepreneurship section of this chapter, independent community pharmacies provide a wealth of opportunities to develop specialty services based on an idea, such as patient monitoring programs focusing on anticoagulation therapy, AIDS services, or anticoagulation therapy. The development of niches provides the pharmacy and its staff with new challenges and opportunities for additional business success through the introduction of potential revenue streams.

CONCLUSION

Independent community pharmacy practice provides a vast array of opportunities for professional development and personal satisfaction. This venue accommodates all types of practitioners, ranging from allowing entrepreneurs and intrapreneurs the freedom to develop their ideas into actual goods or services to offering individuals interested in "being their own boss" the chance to start their own pharmacy and pursue unique practice niches. The independent community pharmacy continues to evolve from its earliest appearance in the United States to the technologically advanced patient care service entities of the twenty-first century. Independent pharmacists will continue to deal with unique issues facing their practices, and yet they will continue to innovate and provide quality patient care.

QUESTIONS FOR FURTHER DISCUSSION

1. Do you consider yourself to be entrepreneurial? Intrapreneurial? Why or why not? Can you identify another individual as being entrepreneurial and/or intrapreneurial? Explain why you selected that person.

2. After reading this chapter, what interests (or what does not interest) you about a career in independent community pharmacy practice?

3. Imagine that you are the owner of a new independent community pharmacy. If money were no

object, where would you be located? What patient care services would you offer? Would you have a general or specialized practice?

4. What is the most difficult management responsibility for the owner of an independent community pharmacy?

5. In your opinion, what is the future of independent community pharmacy? What are the largest challenges facing independent practice this year? In 5 years? In 10 years?

REFERENCES

Anthony J. 2003a. Money Matters: Pick the Business That's Right for You. Available at www.bcentral.com/articles/anthony/133.asp.

Anthony J. 2003b. Money Matters: Sole Proprietorships: Simple but Not Very Flexible. Available at www.bcentral.com/articles/anthony/107.asp.

Anthony J. 2003c. Money Matters: Start Your Business Partnership Off Right. Available at www.bcentral.com/articles/anthony/130.asp.

Anthony J. 2003d. Money Matters: More Pros than Cons to Becoming an S Corporation. Available at www.bcentral.com/articles/anthony/114.asp.

Anthony J. 2003e. Money Matters: C Corporations: Benefits Are a Big (Deductible) Benefit. Available at www.bcentral.com/articles/anthony/117.asp.

Anthony J. 2003f. Money Matters: Is LLC the Best Entity for Your Business? Available at www.bcentral.com/articles/anthony/132.asp.

Bloomsbury Publishing (ed). 2002. *Business: The Ultimate Resource.* Cambridge, MA: Perseus Publishing.

Centers for Medicare and Medicaid Services (CMS). 2002. Medicare Program: Medicare Prescription Drug Benefit. *Federal Register* 70(18). Available at www.cms.hhs.gov/statistics/nhe/projections2002/highlights.asp.

Centers for Medicare and Medicaid Services (CMS). 2003. National Health Expenditures Projections: 2002–2012. Available at www.cms.hhs.gov/statistics/nhe/projections2002/highlights.asp.

Centers for Medicare and Medicaid Services (CMS). 2007. National Health Expenditures Projections: 2006–2016. Available at www.cms.hhs.gov/NationalHealthExpendData/downloads/proj2006.pdf.

Chi J, Paul R. 2006. NCPA: Independents are down, but don't count them out. *Drug Topics,* November 6.

Consumer Reports. 2003. Time to switch drugstores? *Consumer Reports* 68:30.

Cotton HA. 1984. Pharmacy for sale: How to arrive at a fair price. *Curr Concepts Retail Pharm Manag* 2:2.

Daft RL. 1994. *Management.* Fort Worth, TX: Dryden Press.

Edmondson M. 2007. Viewpoint: Three ways to fight reduced reimbursement. *Drug Topics,* February 5.

English T. 1998. Mississippi Medicaid will pay for pharmacy services. *Pharmacy Today* 4:17.

Gagnon JP. 1996. Establishing and financing a community pharmacy. In Huffman DC Jr (ed), *Effective Pharmacy Management,* p. 87. Alexandria, VA: National Association of Retail Druggists.

Gartner WB. 1985. A conceptual framework for describing the phenomenon of new venture creation. *Acad Manag Rev* 10:696.

Gumbhir AK. 1996. Entrepreneurship. In Huffman DC Jr (ed), *Effective Pharmacy Management,* p. 1. Alexandria, VA: National Association of Retail Druggists.

Heffler S, Smith S, et al. 2003. Health spending projections for 2002–2012. *Health Affairs* 22:W54.

Higby GJ. 2003. From compounding to caring: An abridged history of American pharmacy. In Knowlton CH, Penna RP (eds), *Pharmaceutical Care,* p. 19. Bethesda, MD: American Society of Health-System Pharmacists.

Jackson RA. 2002. Maintaining our independents. *America's Pharmacist* 124:54.

Kelly ET III. 1996. Location analysis and lease evaluation. In Huffman DC Jr (ed), *Effective Pharmacy Management,* p. 29. Alexandria, VA: National Association of Retail Druggists.

Medical News Today. 2007. University of Texas Study Details Lengthy Payment Delays for Medicare Part D Prescription Drug Claims, Confirming Need For Legislative Fix. *Medical News Today,* September 8; www.medicalnewstoday.com/articles/81802.php.

National Association of Chain Drug Stores (NACDS). 2003. Industry Statistics. Available at www.nacds.org/wmspage.cfm?parm1=507.

National Community Pharmacists Association (NCPA). 2002. *NCPA-Pharmacia Digest.* Alexandria, VA: National Community Pharmacists Association.

National Community Pharmacists Association (NCPA). 2003a. *NCPA-Pfizer Digest.* Alexandria, VA: National Community Pharmacists Association.

National Community Pharmacists Association (NCPA). 2007. *NCPA-Pfizer Digest.* Alexandria, VA: National Community Pharmacists Association.

National Community Pharmacists Association (NCPA). 2003b. Independent Pharmacy Today: Prospering in the New Millennium. Available at www.ncpanet.org/about/pharmacytoday.shtml.

National Association of Boards of Pharmacy (NABP). 2007. *Survey of Pharmacy Law*. Mount Prospect. IL: National Association of Boards of Pharmacy.

Poisal JA, Truffer C, et al. 2007. Health spending projections through 2016: Modest changes obscure Part D's impact. *Health Affairs* 26:W242 (published online February 21, 2007).

Sheppard M, Richards K, Winegar A. 2007. Prescription Drug Payment Times by Medicare Part D Plans: Executive Summary. Available at www.ncpanet.org/pdf/leg/ut_study_exec_sum_090607.pdf; accessed on November 1, 2007.

Small Business Association (SBA). 2003a. Small Business Startup Guide. Available at www.sba.gov/starting_business/startup/guide.html.

Small Business Association (SBA). 2003b. Forms of Business Ownership. Available at www.sba.gov/starting_business/legal/forms.html.

Small Business Association (SBA). 2003b. Essential Elements of a Good Business Plan for Growing Companies. Available at www.sba.gov/managing/strategicplan/guide.html.

Smith HA. 1986. *Principles and Methods of Pharmacy Management*. Philadelphia: Lea & Febiger.

Smith HA. 1996. Purchasing an established pharmacy. In Huffman DC Jr (ed), *Effective Pharmacy Management*, p. 57. Alexandria, VA: National Association of Retail Druggists.

Tootelian DH, Gaedeke RM. 1993. *Essentials of Pharmacy Management*. St Louis: Mosby–Year Book.

Ukens C. 1994. Whatever happened to pharmaceutical care? *Drug Topics* 138:38.

Ukens C. 2006. Medicare part D off to rocky start. *Drug Topics* 150(2):12.

Williams CF. 1998. *A Century of Service and Beyond*. Alexandria, VA: National Community Pharmacists Association.

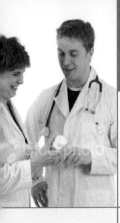

33

APPLICATIONS IN CHAIN COMMUNITY PHARMACY

Michele Belsey

About the Author: Ms Belsey is Vice President of College Relations and Professional Recruitment for Rite Aid Corporation. Michele received a B.S. in pharmacy from Duquesne University in 1992. She has been with Rite Aid Corporation since that time and has been involved with the company's development training and recruitment since 1998. Her department specializes in domestic and international pharmacy relations. Ms Belsey has served on 11 schools of pharmacy advisory boards.

▪ LEARNING OBJECTIVES

1. Describe the ways a chain community pharmacy can create and build corporate culture.
2. Evaluate contemporary management culture and how it can apply or applies to chain community practice.
3. List the steps in identifying and creating management positions for pharmacists in chain community practice.
4. Identify unique opportunities for pharmacists in chain community practice.

▪ SCENARIO—COMPANY CULTURE

Emily Bancroft and Tony Dinardo are staff pharmacists in a chain community drugstore, Remedies, located on Central Avenue. They graduated from pharmacy school 3 years ago and have worked at the same location since graduation. Perry Coleman is the pharmacy manager of Remedies on Central Avenue, and he has been the pharmacy manager for 6 years. Elizabeth Bailey is the pharmacy district manager at Remedies, and she oversees the pharmacy operations for 25 pharmacies including the pharmacy on Central Avenue. Elizabeth has worked for Remedies for 10 years and was promoted to pharmacy supervisor 2 years ago. Elizabeth reports to the vice president for pharmacy operations, Vicki Corbo, who was brought into the company 2 years ago from an outside pharmacy corporation. On Monday, April 2, Emily enters the pharmacy to begin her week. Today, Emily is aware that this will be a busy day not only because it is a

Monday but also because it is first of the month. In community pharmacy practice, Monday and the first of the month are typically busy days because physicians usually schedule patient appointments on Mondays, and because prescriptions are written for a 30-day supply, many patients are ready for refills on the first of the month.

"Good morning, Emily," says Perry.

"Good morning, Perry," says Emily.

As Emily prepares herself for the day by putting on her freshly pressed white pharmacist's jacket, she notices that Tony has not yet reported to work. "Where is Tony this morning? I thought he was supposed to start at 8 a.m. with us." said Emily.

"You are right Emily, Tony was supposed to be here this morning, but he called to say he had a flat tire and he would be a few minutes late. It is so nice to work with such a great team, especially when they respect each other to call when there is a problem," said Perry.

Emily began to think to herself, "I really enjoy working here, to have a pharmacy manager who is understanding and who respects us as well. It is great to work within such a professional atmosphere."

Tony made his way into the pharmacy about 20 minutes later, short of breath and apologizing for not being on time. "My car had a flat tire this morning, and I fixed it as fast as I could."

Perry responded, "Don't worry. These things happen. You have always been on time, and you are an excellent pharmacist. I really appreciate the fact that you called to let me know what was happening. That type of behavior demonstrates a sign of respect for who you work with and where you work."

Tony thought to himself, "I really enjoy working here because our company has a culture of respecting each other and appreciating the contributions each of us brings to the pharmacy and to the organization."

CHAPTER QUESTIONS

The culture in which a community pharmacy operates defines the workday. Based on the scenario, answer the following questions.

1. What steps did the pharmacist take to demonstrate the behavior of respecting coworkers?
2. With what you have learned in previous chapters on personnel management, how would you characterize the culture in which this Remedies pharmacy operates?
3. Would you be able to work effectively within this type of culture?
4. What type of company culture would you create within your own company? How would you go about doing so?
5. Would you have treated the tardiness of the pharmacist differently? If yes, how so?

INTRODUCTION

This chapter explores applications in company culture and career path opportunities. These two topics coexist when a company is defined by its most important asset—its people. Chain practice can be demanding, but the daily rewards can be quite fulfilling. Just one to two decades ago, it could be argued that the opportunities for pharmacists were not very diverse; however, there now exist an extraordinary number of opportunities that are only expected to grow as the profession evolves. When a company has pharmacist positions available at multiple levels, this speaks volumes about the company's culture and how the company recognizes the value a pharmacist brings to the organization. But how does an organization arrive at the level of recognizing the benefits a pharmacist brings to it? It is through the company's culture that the tone is established for such recognition.

UNDERSTANDING, DEFINING, AND DEVELOPING COMPANY CULTURE

How does a company define its culture, and what does company culture really mean? By applying information from previous chapters, there are ways to develop company culture. For example, the first step is for the company to decide exactly what it represents. It can define what it represents through a mission statement and a set of core values that focus on the daily objectives of each associate's function. An *associate* is company terminology for an employee, but by using the word *associate,* it creates the impression that the employees are business partners in the company. The use of this term is designed to foster a sense of ownership by each member of the organization and to instill a value in them that the company is their responsibility and that their business actions are relative to the health of the company.

The mission statement and the core values are the two major factors in molding the culture of the company. There are many ways to organize the development of the mission statement and core values, but the company that cares about its associates should define a method for receiving feedback from its associates. For example, forming internal advisory committees where pharmacists, interns, and clerks are voted for by their peers to represent their respective area brings the various cultures that are important to the associates of the company to the table. Holding quarterly and yearly internal advisory committee meetings brings the company into touch with what is important to its associates. Developing an open-door communication policy and a method by which associates can communicate through company e-mail or through memos to their peers and to executives can help to drive the company into an associate-orientated culture.

As mentioned earlier, a successful company recognizes that its culture should be developed by the people who will live the culture daily, and these people are voted into representative positions by their peers. With regard to the management team, though, how can it be validated that the right people have been selected at the top of the company? A corporation guided by stockholders and its board of directors has a decision-making process to elect who leads the daily functions of the company. Individuals who are not only excellent business candidates but who also reflect the culture the board wants the company to have are interviewed and voted on by the board to determine if they would be the appropriate executive. An excellent resource for learning more about selecting the right person for an execu-

tive management position is the book *Execution—The Discipline of Getting Things Done,* by Larry Bossidy and Ram Charan (2002). This book focuses on the concept of the building blocks of business execution. Two of these very important building blocks are creating the framework for cultural change and having the right person in the right position (Bossidy and Charan, 2002). The company associates who are selected to develop the company culture should be evaluated just as the board of directors evaluates the executives and how each executive continuously evaluates his or her team. Developing company culture sets the foundation for the future of the company; thus the people who are creating it should be representative of the company itself. This concept should be applied from the highest levels in the organization. Examples of business effectiveness in a community pharmacy are maintaining appropriate inventory levels, meeting prescription sales objectives, increasing the percentage of generic prescriptions filled, meeting payroll objectives, understanding the third-party payments from the most frequently filled prescriptions, quality assurance, and providing excellent customer and patient service. The team's composition is critical because its members are responsible for meeting the pharmacy's business objectives in addition to providing care and service for patients.

At every level in the company, each person is being evaluated by his or her capabilities and the requirements for his or her position. This is the sign of a strong company because it does not rest on its good fortune—it continues to strive for excellence.

Exploring the trendiest management culture concepts and recognizing the ones that are most applicable to defining the organization is a management process that many corporations are moving toward. Working in a corporation, managers are always challenged to stay on top of the latest trend in company culture, to develop new ways to define what type of culture would work best in the company, and to decide how to engender that culture. But the best culture goes beyond the company and should be a code of everyday values each person lives by regardless of whether they are at work or away from work. A successful company culture helps associates transcend taking pride in a job well done and imbues in them a continuous desire for personal and team development. Company culture is an evolving process, and like the people who create it, the culture itself always should be evaluated to make sure that it is in step with what the associates expect from their company.

There are excellent resources that define relationships and culture and explain ways of recognizing associates through approaches that are meaningful to those associates. For example, one large national retail organization maintains a "Suggested Reading List." These easy-to-read books define the basic concepts of how to respect and recognize associates. They emphasize personal development methods that can be applied at work. These concepts are delivered in short parables and help employees to understand how to fulfill peoples' expectations in the business world and can be applied in personal and social contexts as well. Our lives are more demanding than ever, and because we are focused on projects and deadlines, we can forget about people. In poorly conceived company cultures, people are not recognized or rewarded for the wonderful and productive work they have done.

For example, from the "Suggested Reading List," the books by Ken Blanchard provide a reminder about how we can not forget the important steps in building positive relationships. In the book *Whale Done!* Blanchard discusses how we live in a "GOTcha" society and that this type of society is catching people doing things wrong. "If you grew up being GOTcha'd a lot, maybe you tend to perpetuate it with others. But if your goal as a manager is performance improvement, it is vitally important you start using the WHALE DONE Response" (Blanchard, 2002). "We need to create and ultimately live in a "WHALE DONE!" society where we catch people doing things right"(Blanchard, 2002). When we see behavior that is pleasing to us or is in the direction of achieving the objective of the corporation, we need to reward this behavior so that the correct behavior is reinforced and recognized.

The "WHALE DONE Response" is

- Praise people immediately.
- Be specific about what they did right or almost right.

- Share your positive feelings about what they did.
- Encourage them to keep up the good work (Blanchard, 2002).

Another example from the "Suggested Reading List" is the book, *Winning Ways,* by Dick Lyles. Lyles provides pointers on how to work well with people and to get great results. In the book, there are four secrets of "Winnings Ways":

- Make people feel stronger rather than weaker.
- Camels are okay—today's camel builders will be tomorrow's leaders (camels cross the finish line every time).
- Avoid two-valued thinking traps because very few decisions are choices between right and wrong or good and bad.
- Influence for the future rather the present or the past (Lyles, 2000).

In summary, the concepts in this book can be used to develop company culture and to continue this development into personal development that one can strive for everyday.

Another company culture that many corporations are adopting or have adopted is the concept behind Six Sigma (Chowdury, 2001). Six Sigma represents a statistical measure and a management philosophy that gives people well-defined roles and a clear structure to their tasks.

It works best when everyone in the company is involved. . . . Six Sigma is a management philosophy focused on eliminating mistakes, waste, and rework. It establishes a measurable status to achieve and embodies a strategic problem-solving method to increase customer satisfaction and dramatically enhance the bottom line. It teaches employees how to improve the way they do business, scientifically and fundamentally, and how to maintain their new performance level. It gives you discipline, structure, and a foundation for solid decision making based on simple statistics. It also maximizes your return on investment and your Return on Talent—your people. . . . Good companies focus on not making mistakes, not wasting time or materials, not making errors in production or service delivery, and not getting sloppy in doing what they do best [Chowdhury, 2001]

By creating this type of culture, it focuses the associates on the quality of work performed.

What do all these examples mean? They provide successful foundations for companies who have decided through their mission statement and core values that define company culture that their company is going to recognize the associates who build and operate the company on a daily basis.

How can these cultures be applied in chain community practice? It is the responsibility of management to learn about the various types of operating cultures and to decide if they want to apply a particular culture to their company. However, when applying culture to an organization, such as a corporation, management personnel who have a proven work record in a certain type of operating culture typically are selected by the board to instill this operating culture and to have it reflected in their associates. Applying the culture to the company can be done through a corporate training department, which consists of training specialists, human resources representatives, and potentially pharmacists. Each executive level, from senior management to field operators, would be provided an opportunity to attend management training and development classes. Reinforcement of the company culture can also happen through e-learning modules and either monthly or quarterly training classes. By infusing management into the culture training, the management team would then work with the associates to ensure that they are learning the culture of the company through everyday correspondence or learning through example when management visits the pharmacy for a team meeting.

■ SCENARIO—CAREER PATH

Emily Bancroft is working in the pharmacy, and she sees a woman dressed in a very nice suit. Emily begins to wonder what her life would be like if she was more involved in the business or "corporate" aspect of the pharmacy. Just then Elizabeth Bailey and Vicki Corbo enter the pharmacy for a surprise visit. During the visit, the pharmacy supervisor's (Elizabeth) objective is to talk with the pharmacy team, observe the overall workflow of the pharmacy, and review the corporation's operational objectives with the pharmacy team, including compliance with the training on company culture.

Emily thinks to herself, "This is my opportunity to talk with the supervisor to see what types of career opportunities are available for me."

The pharmacy supervisors continue their observation of the pharmacy team and noticed that Tony seems very happy. Elizabeth inquires, "Tony, you seem to be catching on here at the company, and every time I meet you, your attitude is very positive." Tony and Perry began talking about the flat tire early in the morning and how Tony is very lucky to be working with such a wonderful team and at a great company.

Elizabeth then asks Perry, "May I have a word with you privately?"

"Sure," Perry replies.

Perry and Elizabeth go into the pharmacy office, and Perry begins to tell Elizabeth about how learning the company's culture of respecting and treating associates has made it easier for him to operate the pharmacy since he understands the cultural operating expectations of the company.

Elizabeth says to Perry, "You have always been a wonderful pharmacist and an even better manager. It is the people who make this company, and we value, appreciate, and respect you and all the work you have done as a pharmacy manager. If you are interested in learning about promotions and other opportunities within the company, please do not hesitate to ask me."

Elizabeth thought to herself that the company culture training that each manager and pharmacist attends has really paid off. As she was exiting the office, Emily approached her and said, "I have always been fascinated about your job, but I'm not sure if it is just through personal admiration of you, simple curiosity, or if what you do is something I could really see myself doing. I think I may be interested in the corporate aspect of the organization. I know all our operational goals for the year, I have some great ideas on how we can expand our business through taking care of our patients, and I am at a point in my career, although it is a very young career, where I feel like I should get moving if I would like to be promoted."

"Well Emily, we have many opportunities for pharmacists both in the field and at the corporate office. Typically, a pharmacist works on staff for about 2 or 3 years until they master the transition into a pharmacist practitioner, feel comfortable in their role of pharmaceutical knowledge, and learn to provide effective patient care and efficient business operations."

"How does a pharmacist move up in the company? What should I be doing to make myself ready for a promotion?" asks Emily.

Elizabeth responds, "Well, Emily that is a great question. You have made the first step already."

"How so?" asks Emily.

Elizabeth responds, "Just by letting me know that you are interested in learning more about a career with the company. You see, as your pharmacy supervisor, if you do not mention to me that you are interested in moving up with the company, I am pretty much going to think you are happy right where you are, but by letting me know you are interested in other projects, I can begin to plan how we can help you to achieve your goal."

"That sounds great," replies Emily.

Elizabeth reaches into her briefcase for some documents.

"What is this?" Emily askes.

"This is our company organization chart for pharmacists," replies Elizabeth. "Each of the boxes represents an area where we have a pharmacist or multiple pharmacists employed. Emily, what is important is that we are a drug store, and when working with a drug store, pharmacy is a greater percentage of the overall business. For the most part, it *is* the business. We promote many pharmacists internally, and very rarely do we go outside the company to search for candidates to place in management positions."

"I did not know that we had this type of career path for a pharmacist in our company," says Emily. "It makes me feel like I have a chance at becoming very successful here."

■ CHAPTER QUESTIONS

1. What steps are taken to identify and develop positions for pharmacists within a corporation?
2. In what departments/capacities may a community chain pharmacist work?
3. What are some self-development goals for someone who is interested in working at the corporate office of a chain community pharmacy?
4. Identify various levels of executive management from pharmacy intern to senior vice president.

■ CAREER PATHS IN CHAIN COMMUNITY PHARMACY

Organizational Structure

Positions in a corporation are determined by their importance and responsibility in fulfilling the business objectives of the corporation. For instance, if the executives in the company determine that the company's focus is going to be within the marketing department, the company will determine how to dedicate resources to fulfilling that focus. Resources can be defined as anything from providing greater budgetary priority for supplies and new materials to creating an entirely new department with multiple positions in order to complete the company's business goals.

Once the goals of the company have been determined and the corporation has made a decision as to where to dedicate its resources, actual position descriptions should be developed. It is important to note that the company's size and cultural objectives can determine the importance a pharmacist has within the company. For example, if the pharmacy department in an organization represents 70 percent of the company's total gross profit, this company would be more sensitive to recognizing and developing its pharmacists compared with an organization in which pharmacy represents only 10 percent of the company's total gross profit. The actual description of a position is called a

Table 33-1. Components of a Job Description
Title of Position
Reporting lines
Location
Job number
Work status
Level of supervision received
Work pace
Internal customer contact
External customer contact
Creation/revision date
Job description summary
Essential duties and responsibilities
Supervisory responsibilities
Qualification requirements
Education and/or experience
Language skills
Mathematical skills
Reasoning ability
Other skills, abilities, and/or training
Certificates, licenses, and/or registrations
Physical demands
Work environment

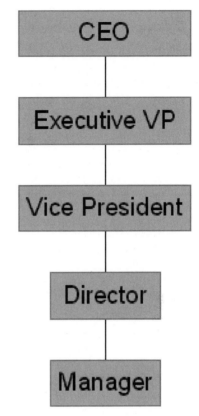

Figure 33-1. An abbreviated organizational chart.

job description. Table 33-1 illustrates components of a job description.

Additional items may be added to a job description based on the characteristics of the corporation and the specific needs that determine a position. For instance, a corporation that has multiple jobs in areas of distribution, marketing, and operations will have job descriptions that vary considerably based on the work performed.

The hierarchy in a corporation is also defined by position titles. Figure 33-1 is a "typical" abbreviated organizational chart within a corporation.

Positions may have prefixes added to them that can alter their significance within the organization. For example, the word *assistant* may be added to the beginning of the title *manager* to make it *assistant manager,* which would rank below the actual manager. In contrast, placing the word *senior* before the manager title

results in *senior manager,* which would rank above the actual manager. This technique can be used for any position within the organization. Once a title is changed, the job description for that position likewise should comply with the hierarchy. If the position created has a higher rank within the organization, the job description should reflect the additional responsibilities over the previous position, and vice versa.

Organizational charts become more complex as the organization grows (Fig. 33-2). Departments may be created based on the organization's needs and goals for the fiscal year. Many organizations typically operate on the calendar year January 1 to December 31 as their fiscal year. Some organizations, however, owing to the nature of their business or possibly when they went public (issued public stock), may operate on an alternative schedule.

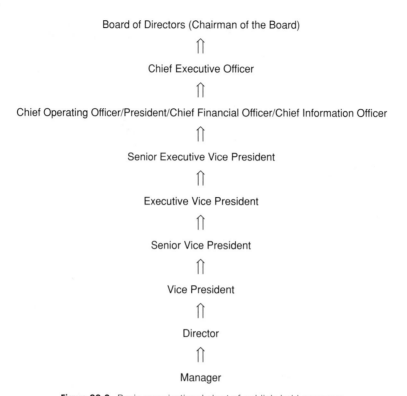

Figure 33-2. Basic organizational chart of publicly held company.

Some departments, such as marketing, accounting, distribution, human resources, information systems, legal, and operations, are common to most any organization. Each of these departments should have a department head who oversees its direction. The department head then reports to the chief executive officer (CEO) or another person at the top of the organization, such as a chief operating officer (COO) or president.

The board of directors defines the overall operating guidelines of the corporation. The board of directors is the governing body, consisting of various representatives who are either internal or external to the company. The board of directors is responsible for taking a strict look at the operating functions of the business without being immersed in its day-to-day operations. Boards typically meet quarterly but may meet more frequently. There may be emergency meetings called to vote on more urgent issues. Boards have a se-

nior representative, the chairman of the board, who is elected by the board members. When working with a public company, it is very important to recognize that the board of directors is responsible to government organizations such as the Securities and Exchange Commission (SEC).

The Case of Retail Chain Pharmacy

What about the career path for a pharmacist? Which positions can a pharmacist aspire to within a chain pharmacy? A lot of this depends on the company and its operating culture. Is the company focused on pharmacy, and does it promote internally? If both these answers are "Yes," then there is a very good chance that a pharmacist can rise to almost any position within the company. Figure 33-3 shows an organizational chart for the Rite Aid Corporation, illustrating various areas wherein pharmacists may work.

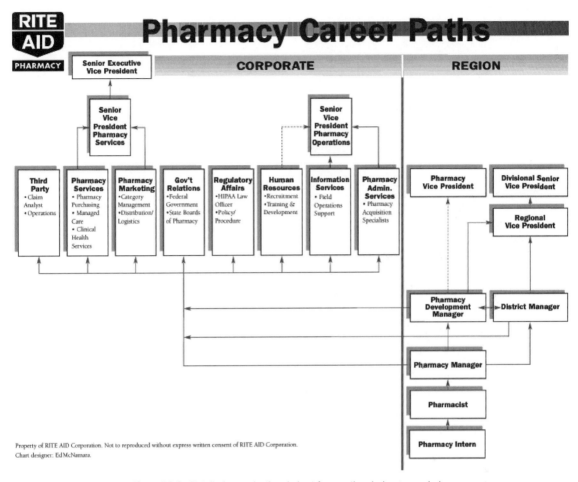

Figure 33-3. Detailed organizational chart for a national pharmacy chain.

Pharmacists have significant upward mobility prospects in many chain pharmacy organizations. For example, pharmacists occupy 100 percent of the pharmacy development manager (PDM) positions shown in Fig. 33-3. A PDM oversees the operation of about 25 pharmacies in an area. A district manager (DM) is a field management position; however, unlike a PDM, a DM oversees the operation of merchandising of the products in the front of the store. It is not a requirement to be a pharmacist to secure a DM position, but some district managers are pharmacists. The DM works closely with the merchandising department and vendors who have products represented in

the DM's specific operating area. The PDM and the DM positions have specific job descriptions, but job descriptions and position requirements change as titles change. For example, the title *vice president* does not have a department focus until the department is added to the title, such as *vice president, pharmacy operations.*

Based on the preceding example, there are a number of positions within retail chain pharmacy to which pharmacists may aspire. Figure 33-4 shows how a degree in pharmacy can grow into multiple career opportunities within an organization. The key to all these positions is to begin a career as an intern or as a graduate intern for the organization. These positions lend

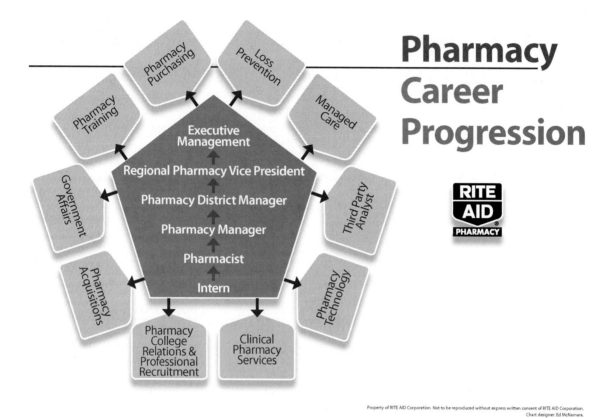

Figure 33-4. Pharmacy career progression chart.

themselves to the candidate learning more about the organization and the characteristics, responsibilities, and behaviors required to make the organization successful.

Once an intern has graduated from pharmacy school and becomes a graduate pharmacy intern, the next hurdle is to take and pass the national licensure examination plus any additional examinations required to practice in a particular state. Once verification of licensure has been made, the former intern now can practice as a pharmacist. For a pharmacist to move to the next level within the corporation, such as to pharmacy manager, or for the pharmacy manager to move to a pharmacy development manager level, a series of evaluations takes place. Many organizations in pharmacy are emphasizing annual performance appraisals of associates. An appraisal may be scheduled more fre-

quently than once per year as well. Reviews may be scheduled at 3, 6, or 9 months if the employee requires guidance or if he or she desires promotion within the organization. One of the best contemporary appraisal systems is one that contains three parts, such as

1. The performance appraisal from the supervisor
2. A self-appraisal from the associate who is being evaluated
3. A performance appraisal addendum that contains action plans for training and education for the candidate

Appraisals are not always performed by an associate's supervisor alone. Appraisals can be performed by a second superior with whom the candidate works with but does not report to, by peers of the associate (especially if they work in an environment that involves constant team projects), or a vendor or outside customer if the work entails frequent communication and relationship building with outside company partners.

The acquisition of significant knowledge about drugs and drug therapy is the expectation of a newly licensed pharmacist, but it is the demonstration of excellent management and human resources skills that is often necessary for a pharmacist to become recognized and evaluated for promotion. Important aspects in the operation of a chain community pharmacy that are reviewed during an associate evaluation are

- Customer satisfaction
- Containment of costs—profit and loss statements, more commonly referred to as P&Ls
- Personnel management

Customer satisfaction is different from customer service. Customer service is an aspect of customer satisfaction. Satisfying a customer involves anticipation of the items a customer is looking to buy, inventory of the product, location of the product in the store, availability of personnel to service the customer in a timely and friendly manner, convenience, and price of the product.

Chain pharmacy practice is challenging because of the diverse needs of various customers. One of the best ways to rate customer satisfaction is to continuously survey customers through electronic surveys, comment cards, or a Web site where customers can voice their opinions about pharmacy personnel. Once the comment cards have been received at a destination for evaluation, entering the results into a computer database for quick analysis can provide a platform for the pharmacy to determine how it can improve its customer satisfaction skills and how it will schedule the training for associates.

For example, at least one national pharmacy chain has a customer satisfaction training program for associates. Pharmacy managers are responsible for all new associates and for the experienced associates to participate in the training. There is a rewards program wherein associates are given company gift cards when they provide excellent customer satisfaction. This is an example of "catching" people doing the right behavior and rewarding them for that behavior.

The profit and loss statement is a management tool used to gauge how the company is performing financially. Each store has its own profit and loss statement. When a pharmacist and pharmacy manager are visited by the pharmacy development manager, the profit and loss statement is reviewed to make sure that the company is on or within plan. If the pharmacy is not operating to plan, the area of concern is evaluated, an action plan is developed, and then it is put into play to achieve the desired results.

Personal management is the third factor when evaluating a pharmacy for performance. When an associate is going through the appraisal process, it is not uncommon for his or her peers to evaluate his or her progress as well. Part of this evaluation is designed to encourage team leadership and interaction skills. Companies have become more inclined to offer management development courses to associates who aspire to become promoted. For example, live training may be provided for associates to understand about how important communication skills are to working in pharmacy. Courses delivered through CD-ROM, the Internet, or self-directed study offer a number of options for associates to design their development. If a supervisor or peer feels that an associate who is being evaluated could benefit from one of the courses, a recommendation can be made on the associate's evaluation, or a supervisor could suggest the course options to the associates so as to focus him or her on such development.

The beginning of a new career can be very exciting but can also be confusing if the pharmacist is not aware of the potential career path. A typical human resources benchmark for determining if someone has become a professional is if he or she remains in a position for about 3 years. The first 3 years in a career can set the tone of success or struggle. In human resources, it is recognized that a person's best performance is typically within the first year he or she is in a position. Performance can be accomplished in a short amount of time (known as the "quick win"). If the candidate continues to exceed the operating goals in years 2 and 3, he or she is ready to take on more business responsibility, such as the financial and other aspects of managing a store.

Once the pharmacist has become a pharmacy manager, he or she has the responsibility to maintain the manager's position based on pharmacy state law and the organization's expectations. Once the pharmacy manager has proven that he or she can comply with and then exceed expectations, then he or she can become a candidate for promotion. In the organizational chart shown in Figs. 33-3 and 33-4, the pharmacy manager has the opportunity to move into the corporate office or to move up into a field operations position. The more typical career path for a pharmacy manager is into the field operator position, but once in a while a corporate position will open up for a pharmacy manager. The field operator position may have multiple bosses, and the lines describe the reporting responsibility one has to those higher up. A straight reporting line means that the position reports directly to the position above it, and a dotted reporting line means that the position has some reporting responsibility to the position above it, but that the position is not a direct boss. When the corporate position is available, there are many points to take into consideration, such as possible relocation, variable work hours, a salaried position (work until you accomplish your project goals regardless of how many hours it takes to complete), politics, and overall increased responsibility.

A career path is a combination of self-management, fiscal management, and operations management. When all three of these are accomplished, the candidate has the potential for a great career. Quite frequently executives are asked, "How do I move up in your organization?" The following are some helpful suggestions:

- Read a newspaper every day.
- Read a current business management book.
- Read a current-events magazine each week.
- Become involved in pharmacy organizations.

- Become involved in charitable organizations.
- Learn multiple languages.
- Become a mentor to a pharmacy intern, technician, or high school student.
- Enroll in a management class or take a certificate course in a pharmacy specialty.
- Prepare/update a current résumé—be very careful of any spelling errors
- Enroll in a business etiquette course.

In addition to self-development, there are some common pitfalls to avoid:

- *Never be late for work.* Always report to work at least 10 minutes before you are scheduled and stay until the work is cleaned up from your shift. This will create the impression that you are a responsible partner in the work environment, and your partner will not walk into a mess the following morning.
- *Always leave a place in better condition* (cleaner, more organized) than how it was when you arrived.
- *Never bite the hands that feed you.* This includes not only your boss's hand but also your department head's hand and, most important, the company that signs your paycheck.
- When you are required to turn in a project for your supervisor, *turn it in before the deadline.*
- Always remember to *ask your coworkers how you can help them* instead of not extending help.
- *Be courteous when working with printers, staplers, and other office equipment.* For example, do not leave printers without paper, a copier without paper, or if you used the last staple, refill the stapler.
- *Always follow company dress code policy and represent yourself as the professional you are or going to be in the future.* This includes appropriate name badge or identification.
- *Always make sure that you are properly groomed as a professional.* Hygiene is recognized not only by coworkers and supervisors but also by customers/patients.
- *Always greet your coworkers every morning and say "Good night" when leaving work* regardless of the position they hold within the company. You never know

who tomorrow's next boss is going to be, so be nice to everyone.

- *Do not gossip about other people.* It is unprofessional and can damage their reputation. Remember that the old axiom "What comes around goes around" could not be more truthful in the corporate world.
- *Keep personal information personal.* Do not discuss your issues at work or with coworkers. This includes the amount of pay you receive and additional benefits.

▓ REVISITING THE SCENARIO

Emily said to Elizabeth, "Thank you so much for taking the time to show me where a pharmacist can aspire to within our company. This really helps me understand our company better, and I would love to work more in the field operator's position."

"Great," said Elizabeth. "The next time I am in town, let's plan to go on an audit for a third-party company, tour some pharmacies, and work on preparation for an inventory."

"Thanks," said Emily. "I am looking forward to it."

▓ QUESTIONS FOR FURTHER DISCUSSION

1. What would you find the most challenging aspect of creating a culture that reflects each associate's point of view?
2. Which opportunities in community chain practice would you be most interested in?
3. Could you see yourself moving up the corporate ladder in a chain pharmacy organization? Why or why not? If not, what could you do to make yourself a more suitable candidate to do so?

REFERENCES

Blanchard K. 2002. *Whale Done!—The Power of Positive Relationships,* pp. 40 and 42. New York: Free Press.

Bossidy L, Charan R. 2002. *Execution—The Discipline of Getting Things Done,* pp. 85–86, 109–113. New York: Crown Business.

Chowdhury S. 2001. *The Power of Six Sigma,* pp. 19, 22, 24–25. Chicago: Dearborn Trade.

Lyles D. 2000. *Winning Ways–4 Secrets for Getting Great Results by Working Well with People,* pp. 48, 62, 75, 86. New York: Putnam.

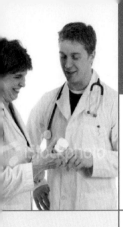

34

APPLICATIONS IN HOSPITAL PHARMACY PRACTICE

Frank Massaro and William A. Gouveia

About the Author: Frank Massaro is Pharmacy Practice Manager at Tufts-New England Medical Center. Dr. Massaro manages clinical programs for the Department of Pharmacy and is responsible for the professional development of the pharmacist staff. He is a member of the General Internal Medicine patient care team and an active member of several interdepartmental performance improvement committees. Dr. Massaro received both a B.S. in pharmacy and a D.Pharm. from the Philadelphia College of Pharmacy and Science. He completed a residency in hospital pharmacy at New England Medical Center. Dr. Massaro's current faculty appointments include Tufts University School of Medicine, Northeastern University's Bouvé College of Health Scinces, and the Massachusetts College of Pharmacy and Health Sciences.

Mr. Gouveia has served as Director of Pharmacy at Tufts New England Medical Center for the past 35 years. Mr. Gouveia has served in a number of editorial positions with the *American Journal of Health-System Pharmacy,* most recently as senior contributing editor, pharmacy practice management. Mr. Gouveia received a B.S. in pharmacy and an M.S. in hospital pharmacy administration from the Northeastern University College of Pharmacy. He has been Chairman of the American Society of Health-System Pharmacists (ASHP) Commission on Goals and was named Fellow of the ASHP in 1993. He received the ASHP Research and Education Foundation Award for Achievement for Sustained Contributions to the Literature and the Outstanding Alumni Award in Health Sciences from Northeastern University. In 1999, he received the Harvey A. K. Whitney Lecture Award, health system pharmacy's highest honor, from the ASHP. Mr. Gouveia's current faculty appointments include Tufts University School of Medicine, Northeastern University's Bouvé College of Health Sciences, and the Massachusetts College of Pharmacy and Health Sciences.

■ LEARNING OBJECTIVES

After completing this chapter, students should be able to

1. Describe a typical organizational chart, management structure, and flow of information for a hospital and a hospital's pharmacy department.

2. Describe the integration of clinical and managerial roles assumed by pharmacists in the hospital setting.
3. Identify and describe models for managing clinical pharmacist services in a hospital.
4. Describe budgetary issues confronting a hospital's pharmacy department. Identify strategies undertaken by the department's director and staff pharmacists to reduce operating costs without compromising patient care.
5. Identify strategies for managing personnel, including clinical pharmacists, in a hospital pharmacy.

■ INTRODUCTION

Every hospital pharmacist is a manager. Every pharmacist must acquire, maintain, and constantly update a unique and specialized body of knowledge. Every pharmacist must learn to direct, support, persuade, discipline, and collaborate with others. Every pharmacist is expected to understand and use the principles of accounting, finance, economics, marketing, and informatics. Indeed, optimal patient care depends on a pharmacist's ability to thoughtfully apply the science of therapeutics and on his or her ability to manage people and information.

In many situations, a pharmacist with excellent management skills and average clinical knowledge is more effective than a pharmacist with poor management skills and an excellent knowledge base. Consider the clinical pharmacist who appears to approach and solve problems with ease compared with the pharmacist who has difficulty gathering even basic information to make an informed decision. This paradox has led some to ascribe this skill in managing to "experience" or "judgment." To be sure, the ability to manage improves with study and experience. However, managing a budget or a group of individuals is not a mysterious process. It is a method that parallels the clinical problem-solving process. It is a method that can be both taught and learned. It requires both knowledge and skill. And these skills can be refined only through practice.

■ SCENARIO 1

As a critical care clinical pharmacist for 10 years, Ken had performed all the functions of a hospital pharmacist. He had provided pharmacy care to individual patients, worked in a satellite pharmacy, served as a preceptor for pharmacy students and residents, taught the critical care section of a course at a school of pharmacy, and published journal articles. He was a successful clinician and was highly regarded by his peers, by the medical community, and by nursing staff. At some point Ken decided that it was time for a change. While he still enjoyed caring for individuals, he yearned for the chance to influence a larger number of patients. He wanted to make a contribution to the broader context of the health system. Thus, when the opportunity arose to develop a hospital-wide antimicrobial management program, Ken gladly accepted the challenge. After only a year in his new position, Ken was able to show improvements in the appropriate use of anti-infective drugs while reducing drug costs and to describe a comprehensive plan for the future. He was able to engender the support of the hospital's senior managers, physicians, and pharmacists. He was able to document a positive impact on patient outcomes. The quality of pharmacy services provided and the hospital's financial position improved. How was all this possible in such a short time?

■ THE HOSPITAL ENVIRONMENT

The pharmacist in Scenario 1 is, like many practitioners, a skilled clinician. His successes as a critical care pharmacist were supported by his formal education and his close working relationship with the medical and surgical staffs. His successes as the leader of a hospital-wide program are no more surprising. Ken simply applied the same skills he used in caring for patients to the

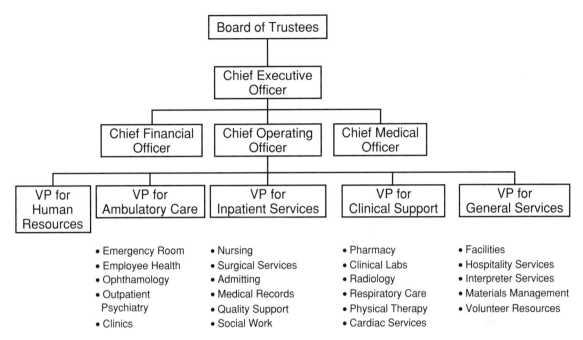

Figure 34-1. Hospital organizational chart.

development of a new clinical service. He worked to identify the types of information he needed to make informed decisions. He generated a list of clearly articulated goals and gathered the necessary resources to reach the stated goals. His first step, however, was to understand how the hospital is organized.

Figure 34-1 shows a typical hospital organizational chart. The chart shows the reporting structure and formal lines of communication within the institution. It is important to realize that the position of the pharmacy department and the administrator to whom the director of pharmacy reports can significantly affect how senior managers and others view the pharmacy. If, for example, the director of pharmacy reports to an ancillary services administrator along with housekeeping, maintenance, and security, pharmacy is more likely to be viewed as a service department not directly involved in patient care. On the other hand, if the pharmacy falls under the patient care division along with radiology, the clinical laboratory, and the emergency department, then the pharmacy is more likely to be viewed as a participant in direct patient care. Figure 34-2 shows an organizational chart for a typical department of phar-

macy. The chart hints at the information-, product-, and outcome-oriented nature of the profession. It also gives some indication of a key goal of the pharmacy, that is, to control the acquisition and use of drugs so that a patient's drug therapy is appropriate, safe, and cost-effective and achieves the proper outcome.

When a pharmacist accepts his or her first job in a hospital pharmacy, it is important that he or she fully understand the structure of the drug control system. Control implies accountability, not for its own sake, but to promote safety, effectiveness, and economy as drugs are used in patient care. This accountability for drug therapy can be achieved through a variety of pharmacy functions. Pharmacists decide how drugs are selected and obtained, how drugs are ordered for individual patients, and how drugs are prepared for administration. Pharmacists monitor the therapeutic benefit or possible harm that may result from the use of drugs and the costs associated with these services.

While the scope of pharmacy services varies from hospital to hospital depending on the needs of the patients served, there are certain minimum standards to which a hospital must conform. These published

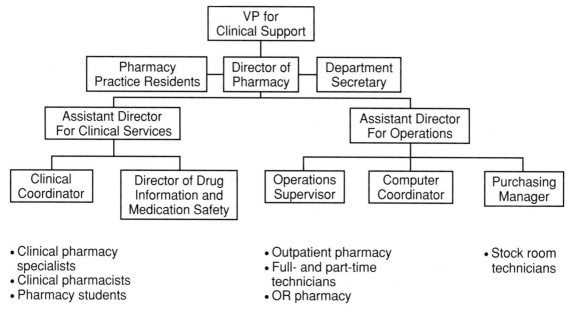

Figure 34-2. Organizational chart of the department of pharmacy.

standards provide a basis for evaluation, review, and goal setting for the hospital pharmacy director. The American Society for Health-System Pharmacists (ASHP) has developed a list of practice standards that define acceptable professional practices (American Society of Health-System Pharmacists, 2006a, p 297). The six basic standards are

1. The pharmacy shall be managed by a professionally competent, legally qualified pharmacist. The director of pharmacy service must be thoroughly knowledgeable about hospital pharmacy practice and management.
2. The pharmacist shall provide patient-specific drug information and accurate and comprehensive information about drugs to other pharmacists, health professionals, and patients as appropriate.
3. The pharmacist, in concert with the medical and nursing staffs, must develop policies and procedures for ensuring the quality of medication therapy. This must include processes designed to ensure the safe and effective use of medications and to increase the probability of desired patient outcomes.

4. The pharmacy shall be responsible for the procurement, distribution, and control of *all* drug products used in the hospital.
5. To ensure optimal operational performance and quality patient care, adequate space, equipment, and supplies shall be available for all professional and administrative functions relating to medication use.
6. The pharmacist should initiate, participate in, and support medical and pharmaceutical research appropriate to the goals, objectives, and resources of the specific hospital.

State boards of pharmacy and departments of public health also influence hospital pharmacy practice. The state boards serve as licensing bodies for both the location of pharmacies and those individuals able to practice. The primary duty of the department of public health (DPH) is to uphold the public interest in quality pharmacy service within the laws and regulations of the state. In fulfilling these obligations through an evaluation of the pharmacy, the board of pharmacy and the DPH assure the public that minimum standards of practice are met. These regulatory bodies also review citizens' complaints and investigate reports of drug loss and diversion.

The major nongovernmental regulatory body to which many hospitals must conform is the Joint Commission. The Joint Commission is an independent, not-for-profit organization governed by a board that includes physicians, nurses, and consumers. The Joint Commission sets the standards by which health care quality is measured. A team of Joint Commission surveyors can visit acute care hospitals without warning. The surveyors compare a department's performance to a set of published standards in the context of the larger hospital organization (Joint Commission, 2006). The purpose of the review is to evaluate a hospital's performance and to improve the safety and quality of care provided to the public through health care accreditation.

The hospital organization, external regulatory bodies, and standards of pharmacy practice define the formal structure within which a pharmacy manager must operate. However, the real hospital environment is much more complicated. The skilled manager also recognizes the informal relationships within the hospital and works to develop a good rapport with influential clinicians, key hospital administrators, and physician leadership. Pharmacy managers who display a genuine concern for patients and can work effectively with the hospital's professional staffs will achieve the pharmacy's mission more easily. The development of such relationships should be a priority for every pharmacist. One way to demonstrate knowledge and to cultivate strong bonds with other professionals is to participate in a variety of patient care committees (Table 34-1).

Table 34-1. Patient Care Committees

Antibiotic Control
Cancer Care
Human Investigation Review Board
Infection Control
Patient Safety and Quality
Pharmacy and Therapeutics

In Scenario 1, the pharmacist's success was due in part to his ability to develop relationships with members of the hospital's pharmacy and therapeutics committee, the medication safety committee, and the antibiotic control committee.

Committees dealing with patient care always include members of the medical staff. To conduct its business, the medical staff, with approval of the board of trustees, elects officers and organizes itself into various committees, as outlined in its bylaws. The hospital usually has two kinds of committees, standing and special or ad hoc committees. Standing committees are permanent and cannot be dissolved without changing the bylaws. Such committees usually have ongoing business to conduct throughout the year and therefore must meet regularly. Examples include the hospital's committee on credentialing and the pharmacy and therapeutics committee. Ad hoc committees are chartered as needed to solve special problems and then are dissolved when the task is completed. All committees of the medical staff report their activity and make recommendations to the medical board or executive committee.

Most medical staff bylaws call for a pharmacy and therapeutics (P&T) committee consisting of physicians, nurses, pharmacists, and administrators. The primary purposes of the P&T committee are (American Society of Health-System Pharmacists, 2006b, p 92)

1. *Policy development.* The committee formulates policies regarding evaluation, selection, and therapeutic use of drugs and related devices.
2. *Education.* The committee recommends or assists in the formulation of programs designed to meet the needs of the professional staff (i.e., physicians, nurses, pharmacists, and other health care practitioners) for complete current knowledge on matters related to drugs and drug use.

One of the P&T committee functions is to develop a *formulary* of drugs accepted for use in the hospital. The formulary is a continually revised compilation of drug products that reflects the current clinical judgment of the medical and pharmacy staffs. The selection of items in the formulary is based on an extensive literature review and evaluation. The written monographs presented to the committee for analysis include the relative therapeutic merits of a drug, its safety, and its cost. The committee tries to minimize duplication of basic drug types, drug entities, or drug products. Limiting the number of drug products available from the pharmacy can produce substantial patient care and financial benefits. These benefits are increased greatly through use of *generic equivalents* (drug products considered to be identical with respect to their active components, e.g., two brands of amoxicillin capsules) and *therapeutic equivalents* (drug products differing in composition that are considered to have very similar pharmacologic and therapeutic activities, e.g., two different first-generation oral cephalosporins). The P&T committee must make clear the policies and procedures governing the dispensing of generic and therapeutic equivalents. The pharmacy department, working through the P&T committee, must make certain that the medical and nursing staffs are informed about the existence of the formulary system and the policies and procedures governing its operation.

The safety of the medication system is the primary concern of every hospital pharmacist. Recently published reports of the incidence, causes, and cost of injury resulting from medication errors have led many hospitals to critically evaluate their quality assurance systems (Bates et al., 1996, 1997; Classen et al., 1997; Kohn, Corrigan, and Donaldson, 1999; Leape et al., 1991, 1995; Poon et al., 2006; Stelfox, et al., 2006). Written incident reports were once the standard for gathering information about medication misadventures. This method is now believed to lack sufficient completeness and reliability for identifying weaknesses in a medication system (Classen et al., 1991; Cullen et al., 1995; Leape, 1994, 2002; Leape et al., 1995).

Deficiencies in reporting have spawned the formation of new standing committees in many hospitals. Medication safety committees are charged with developing processes to identify and quantify medication errors and adverse drug reactions. Pharmacists, physicians, nurses, risk management personnel, legal counsel, administrators, and patients work together to implement specific changes to improve the medication system. Most programs are designed to gather information about *potential errors* (i.e., mistakes in prescribing, transcribing, dispensing, or planned administration that are detected and corrected *before* actual administration to the patient) and *actual errors* (i.e., mistakes identified *after* the drugs are administered or failure to administer a scheduled drug).

Well-designed systems can (1) describe the stage in the medication process where the error occurred (i.e., prescribing, transcription, pharmacy computer entry error, dispensing, and administration), (2) the nature of the error within each stage of the process, and (3) the therapeutic category of the drug involved. Such systems provide meaningful data about medication errors and adverse drug reactions and allow for the development of strategies to prevent recurrences. For example, early in the development of the infection control program described in Scenario 1, the pharmacist noticed a trend in prescribing errors reported through the medication safety committee. Physicians consistently chose the correct antibiotic to treat a suspected or known infection, but the prescribed dose frequently was inappropriate. Physicians often failed to consider the site of the infection, the likely virulence of the pathogen, possible antibiotic resistance, and the patient's organ function. The pharmacist used the information to focus his educational efforts to improve patient care and to demonstrate his clinical expertise. The pharmacist's active involvement in the medication safety committee served to (1) promote safe and effective drug therapy, (2) improve the performance of the medication system, and (3) promote a positive image of the pharmacist, the pharmacy department, and the profession.

■ SCENARIO 2

Suburban General is a 350-bed community hospital located just outside a major metropolitan area. The department of pharmacy at Suburban General is well respected within the institution for its financially efficient operation and its use of cutting-edge technology. It was the first community hospital in the state to install automated dispensing machines in all patient care areas.

Decentralized pharmacists use radiofrequency laptop computers to enter medication orders into the pharmacy computer system, and nurses rely on the pharmacists to accurately manage an electronic medication administration record for every patient.

The department of pharmacy is directed by a visionary with the ability to get others to look into the future with her. Interestingly, her vision of the future includes helping to raise her many grandchildren. Thus, after 27 years of service, the director of pharmacy decided to arrange an early retirement. Before leaving Suburban General, the outgoing director convinced senior management that the new director should be someone who could bring a level of clinical sophistication to the department that could match its operational efficiency. The incoming director of pharmacy was charged with maintaining the current level of operational efficiency while developing and implementing clinical pharmacy services.

▓ MANAGING CLINICAL PRACTICE

Two models, the *generalist model* and the *specialist model,* can describe traditional approaches to the management of clinical pharmacy services in a hospital. The generalist model evolved as a result of the decentralization of hospital pharmacy practice that began in the 1960s. Decentralization relocated many pharmacists from the basement to patient care areas, sometimes without additional training. This model maintains that for the pharmacist to affect the care of patients, it is necessary to be present where and when drug therapy decisions are made. The defining feature of the generalist model is that pharmacists are responsible for both clinical and drug distribution services. For this model to work, some of the pharmacist's activities must be supported by the use of qualified pharmacy technicians.

The definition of clinical pharmacy services may vary considerably under the generalist model. Services may consist of departmentally defined drug monitoring, collection of data for drug-use reviews, and target drug class screening. Pharmacists provide clinical ser-

vices that are predefined, assuming that product preparation and drug distribution needs have been satisfied first. Providing clinical oversight might depend on whether a particular drug is prescribed because many services are in reaction to a physician's order for a target drug. All too often the service is drug-specific rather than patient-specific. The decision to provide a higher level of clinical oversight should be based on what a patient needs rather than on what is prescribed.

Some pharmacy departments use the *specialist model,* in which a distinction is made between clinical pharmacists and staff pharmacists. The specialists are responsible for providing clinical pharmacy services throughout the hospital. However, unless there are sufficient resources, it is not always possible to provide comprehensive clinical care to all patients. Therefore, the only patients who receive clinical pharmacy services are those who conform to specialty categories (e.g., critical care, oncology, or pediatrics) defined by the clinical manager. Under the specialist model, clinical pharmacy services may not be coordinated with drug distribution services. Without coordination between clinical activities and drug distribution, the entire system is less than optimally efficient, and this can lead to confusion about the role of the pharmacist. The greatest problem for patient care under this model is that the patient may not even receive clinical pharmacy services. Whether a patient receives a particular service may depend on the patient care area to which the patient was admitted, the practice in which the pharmacist is most interested, and whether a specific pharmacist is scheduled on a particular day. Sometimes a full-time college of pharmacy faculty member serves as the specialized clinician.

Many departments have moved pharmacists from the central pharmacy to patient care areas with the expectation that they will provide pharmacy care automatically. These relocated pharmacists are expected to define their roles without a sense of a departmental mission. Without a clear definition of clinical services and without the use of a mission statement that reflects this definition in actual practice, pharmacists are placed in an ambiguous situation. They have the desire to care for patients but do not clearly understand the priorities. The immediacy of drug distribution may give these tasks priority. Also, the pharmacists may not have the vocabulary to define their expanded role to patients, nurses, and physicians.

The generalist and the specialist models have been successful in many hospitals, provided that there has been a systematic approach to the development, implementation, and evaluation of the clinical services provided. There must be a clearly articulated philosophy of practice that describes why a pharmacist provides clinical services and a clear definition of the work to be done. We must remember that the patient is central to any endeavor. If the clinical service is defined in terms of patient need, it becomes easier to define priorities, resource requirements, and optimal outcomes. The primary focus of a clinical service should be the patient and not a medical service or a drug category. Full integration of clinical practice into drug distribution services optimizes the chances for success.

The first priority in any clinical service must be to achieve desired patient outcomes—that is, to promote health and prevent disease by ensuring rational drug therapy. The second priority is efficient procurement, preparation, and distribution of drug products for the purpose of supporting the clinical service. The successful integration of patient- specific clinical pharmacy services with an efficient drug distribution operation will result in the best care possible. Pharmacists can identify, resolve, and prevent both clinical and distributive drug-related problems. An integrated practice allows pharmacists to collect data, access patient needs, decide what tools are needed to resolve problems, and then proceed to do so.

The change in focus of a department of pharmacy from production- and distribution-centered services to patient-centered clinical services requires major adjustments in administrative thinking. Strand and colleagues (1990) described five departmental requirements:

- *Mission statement.* The pharmacy department needs a concise mission statement that reflects how the staff will provide patient-specific services designed to achieve (1) optimal therapeutic outcomes by ensuring safe and effective drug therapy and (2) quality procurement, preparation, and distribution of drug products. The department's mission statement must be consistent with the hospital's mission.

- *Organizational structure.* It is necessary to develop an internal organization structure that allows pharmacists to focus on the individual patient, exercise clinical judgment, and be supported in a manner consistent with their work. Training and education of pharmacy technicians must be provided to make possible the development of clinical services. Financial resources must be directed toward clinical functions with as much enthusiasm as that shown for distributive functions.

- *Practice standards.* Practice standards are needed to ensure consistent, comprehensive pharmacy services for each patient. According to the mission statement, the goal is for each patient to be free of drug-related problems. And drug products must be procured, prepared, and distributed cost-effectively, efficiently, and safely. The standards must be designed so that the pharmacist is reasonably able to maintain them. Career advancement opportunities should be made available within clinical practice and not be confined to a managerial track. Career ladders should be constructed to institutionalize and formalize department expectations for the development of clinical practice skills.

- *Staff development.* There should be a staff development and skills advancement program for making the individual pharmacist competent to identify, resolve, and prevent drug-related problems. Educational experiences (i.e., continuing-education requirements) for the sole purpose of maintaining a pharmacy license are inadequate. The patient must benefit directly from the pharmacists' training. Successful staff development means that the pharmacist will be able to achieve (1) the necessary knowledge and skills in clinical pharmacology and therapeutics, (2) the capacity to mobilize the drug distribution system to meet a patient's needs, and (3) the relationships with patients and health care professionals that are necessary for executing clinical work.

- *Documentation.* The work of the pharmacist must be documented in writing so that the unique knowledge and contributions of the pharmacist are available to physicians, nurses, and other providers. If the pharmacist does not perceive the identification, resolution, and prevention of drug-related problems to be important enough to be documented, then society cannot be expected to support such functions with human and financial resources.

◼ SCENARIO 3

Hospitals are big business. And like many privately owned companies, final responsibility for the fiscal integrity of a private not-for-profit hospital rests with the board of trustees. Bayside Medical Center (BMC) is no different.

BMC has been in business for more than 100 years. Its financial success is due in part to strong leadership by the chief executive and a very active board of trustees. Until recently, BMC has generated enough revenue to meet operating expenses and to expand services to outlying communities. Unfortunately, in the past 3 years, dramatic decreases in investment income and reductions in reimbursement from third-party payers have almost eliminated the cash available for expansion. If the trend continues, there will be a shortage of operating capital within the next 2 years.

Ever vigilant, the board of trustees identified the problem early. To better understand the cost of providing service, the board hired the services of a health care consulting firm. The consultants are charged with meeting with key hospital department heads to identify opportunities for reducing the cost of doing business. Of course, the director of pharmacy and his staff are on the list.

◼ BUDGETING AND FINANCE

Financial control of a hospital is of utmost importance in maintaining the institution's solvency. The hospital will not survive unless there is adequate income to cover operating expenses and capital improvements. This survival requires that every senior administrator and every department director be highly skilled finan-

cial managers. What is unique about the department of pharmacy is the disproportionate cost of supplies (e.g., drugs) versus wages compared with other hospital departments. Typically, 90 percent of a pharmacy's budget is for drugs, whereas less than 10 percent is for employee wages. The reverse is true for most other departments. The overall cost of medications and the proportion of the drug expenditures that are under the influence of each clinical pharmacist require that every hospital pharmacist understands the principles of financial management. A review of the usual financial administrative structure within a hospital, the budget process, and the difference between cost and charge may be helpful.

As described in Scenario 3, the board of trustees is ultimately responsible for the fiscal health of a private not-for-profit hospital. It has a financial responsibility to the public. The board typically delegates all routine responsibilities to the chief executive officer (CEO) of the institution. The board also appoints a finance committee of the board to advise the CEO on overall financial management. The finance committee is responsible for overseeing the financial position of the hospital to ensure that there is adequate operating and long-term capital available. The committee advises the board of trustees on all fiscal and investment matters.

Although the board delegates day-to-day financial matters to the CEO, it is impossible for one person to supervise all aspects of the hospital's operations. The number of internal and external demands that require the CEO's personal attention and the highly technical nature of operations require the CEO to delegate many tasks to the hospital's senior managers and department directors. Indeed, financial management is a principal function of all administrators and managers.

An important and fundamental part of financial control is budgeting. Each hospital department will have an annual budget, and a good department manager will be able to anticipate revenue and predict expenses for the coming year. To estimate next year's budget, it is useful to review the current budget and the budget for the past 2 or 3 years carefully. By observing the trends in cost for major items (e.g., intravenous solutions and specific therapeutic categories of drugs), it is easier to forecast future expenses. Experienced directors of pharmacy also gather information from two additional sources to predict the future: published reports and clinical pharmacy specialists.

Published reports in the lay press and in health care journals continue to predict increasing drug expenditures. Financial analysts speculate in the *Wall Street Journal* on sales of soon-to-be marketed drug products. Group purchasing organizations (GPOs) publish annual drug price forecasts for use by their members to plan for the coming year. And national professional organizations such as the American Society of Health-System Pharmacists support the development and publication of estimates of future drug prices (Hoffman et al., 2007). The astute pharmacy manager gathers predictive data from a variety of sources and applies the information to the development of the department's drug budget. An understanding of market forces gathered through scanning the literature helps the manager to be prepared for the future and to educate hospital senior management about drug costs.

Clinical pharmacists working in the hospital are an often-underutilized source of information about future trends in drug expense. They care for patients and participate in drug therapy discussions with staff physicians every day. They see first hand the effects of investigational drug products and of marketed drugs used in novel ways. They keep up with the scientific literature. The pharmacy director and the clinical pharmacy staff should share information from a variety of sources frequently to get a better look into the future. For example, in many hospitals, pharmacy managers and clinicians were able to predict the economic impact of a new drug to help manage sepsis before the drug was on the market. They also were able to develop widely accepted guidelines for use to ensure appropriate prescribing and reasonable expenditures. As a result, costs were managed, and only those patients who would benefit from the drug received it.

The budget process begins with a directive from the board of trustees regarding the general policies and goals for the next year. These policies may include changes to the physical plant or capital equipment or approval to provide new services. Next, the budget department outlines departmental guidelines consistent with the directives from the board of trustees. Basic operating statistics and assumptions, such as patient days, anticipated admissions, and the impact of inflation, are prepared. Target expenses and revenues are identified for each department and are rolled up into the hospital's consolidated budget. The third step is for each department to prepare its budget based on the budget guidelines. Next, a final review is conducted. The department budget is compared with the established targets, and senior management conducts negotiations of the final figures. A final roll-up of actual budgets is then prepared and submitted to the board of trustees for approval or modification.

Most hospital pharmacy budgets contain three major components: (1) salary and wage expense, (2) drugs, supplies, and equipment expense, and (3) revenue. Every hospital will have its own format of financial reporting and budgetary summary. Table 34-2 is a hypothetical income and expense report compared with a budget for a 6-month period.

- *Salary and wage expense.* This includes payroll expense for regularly scheduled hours and for salaried employees. The salary subsection also includes a budgeted amount for overtime, sick, vacation, and holiday pay. Remember that sick, vacation, and holiday pay represents nonproductive expenses. While most department budgets do not represent benefits (e.g., health insurance, disability insurance, etc.), the hospital's overall budget will. Benefits generally are 20 to 30 percent of total salary and wage costs.
- *Supplies and equipment expense.* This nonsalary section of the budget usually is sufficiently detailed so that the manager can monitor it by category. The supplies and equipment budget may include expense categories such as drugs, office supplies, and maintenance contracts (see Table 34-2). Many pharmacy directors subdivide the drug expense category into therapeutic classes to better monitor new services or trends in therapy. For example, the economic impact of a newly marketed drug to treat pancreatic cancer is easier to track if the expense is shown in the

Table 34-2.   Six-Month Financial Analysis

	YTD Actual	YTD Budget	Variance
Expenses			
Regular salary & wages	1,089,584	1,072,966	(16,618)
Overtime	13,738	35,669	21,931
Holiday pay	15,791	18,667	2,876
Weekend premium	8,501	10,397	1,896
Evening differential	9,387	11,979	2,592
Night differential	4,693	4,291	402
Contract labor	77,854	33,857	(43,997)
Total salary & wages	**1,219,548**	**1,187,826**	**(31,722)**
Drugs	8,985,727	9,462,991	477,264
Service contracts	0	24,000	24,000
Dues/subcriptions/books	5,711	4,100	(1,611)
Software contracts	16,119	64,016	47,897
Med/surg supplies	37,016	46,767	9,751
Drug packaging supplies	22,729	45,745	23,025
Office supplies	17,156	4,380	(12,776)
Repairs	0	1,500	1,500
Telephone	11,863	8,295	(3,568)
Equipment rental	58,878	61,275	2,397
Printing	4,783	4,684	(99)
Total nonlabor expenses	**9,159,982**	**9,706,153**	**546,171**
Revenue			
Inpatient revenue	16,053,087	18,021,933	(1,968,846)
Outpatient revenue	10,691,251	12,054,596	(1,363,345)
Miscellaneous revenue	5,995	0	5,995
Total revenue	**26,750,333**	**30,076,529**	**(3,326,196)**
Net operating income (loss)	**16,370,803**	**19,182,550**	**(2,811,747)**

antineoplastic category of the drug section of the expense budget.

- *Revenue.* Revenue is sometimes used interchangeably with charges. Generally, a department's charges must cover its expenses. However, in some hospitals, pharmacy department charges are used to subsidize non-revenue-producing departments. This component of the budget differs widely among hospitals. Generally speaking, depending on the particular payers that a hospital has, the pharmacy may be a cost center or a revenue center or a mixture of both. The department manager must clearly understand the mechanism for establishing pharmacy charges, whether by a fee structure or a percent markup, so that revenue can be reported and compared with the various expense categories in the expense budget.

The system for establishing pharmacy charges must be fair, economically sound, and explainable to patients and third-party payers. Some hospitals use a simple *percent markup* on drug cost strategy. The charge for a drug is the product of the acquisition cost and the markup. Higher-cost drugs theoretically yield a higher return. The *professional fee* concept is based on the fact that a prescription medication is not an article of trade capable of being bought and sold by anyone and that the cost of dispensing, including the skill and knowledge involved, is not related to the cost of the ingredients used. A professional fee may be applied to doses dispensed or on a per-diem or per-patient basis. This approach has particular merit for nondistributive clinical services. Hospitals may choose a combination of approaches, using a percent markup for drugs dispensed and a professional fee for services, such as drug information or patient education, which are not necessarily related to a specific drug product.

Most important to this discussion on hospital revenue is the fact that the true economic cost of a medical service seldom is reflected by its charge. Because hospital accounting in the United States has been designed for the purposes of maximizing third-party payment and thus hospital reimbursement, the charge for a service may be very different from the true costs of the resources that are actually consumed in providing it. Hospital overhead and other shared expenses usually are allocated systematically and are not necessarily allocated according to the way the overhead is actually used.

In Scenario 3, it is likely that the external consultants will be asked to evaluate the potential cost savings and the reduction in revenue that would result from eliminating a patient care service. Since charges do not accurately reflect the average cost of providing a service, the expenses would not necessarily be saved if the service were not provided. The only costs that would be saved if the service were not given to a particular patient are the costs that are incurred by providing that one additional unit of service. For example, a clinical laboratory in a hospital that reduces the number of laboratory tests it performs will save only the portion of its expenses that would have been added by each additional test (e.g., the cost of the reagents). The laboratory will not save expenses that are incurred independent of the number of tests performed (e.g., purchasing expensive pieces of equipment) if only a few tests are eliminated. It is only the *marginal costs,* those incurred because of the provision of the additional units of service, that can be saved. These costs are also described as variable costs because they vary with the volume of services provided. In contrast to variable costs, another set of costs is incurred regardless of the volume of services. These are described as *fixed costs.* The expensive equipment that a clinical laboratory might purchase, such as a multichannel autoanalyzer, are examples of fixed costs. The elimination of a few laboratory tests will not reduce the expense that was incurred in buying the equipment.

In calculating the savings that a hospital might enjoy if it were able to reduce the frequency with which a drug is given, fixed and variable costs should be distinguished. Only the variable costs will be avoided. For example, a laminar flow ventilation hood is required in the pharmacy for sterile product preparation whether a few or many units of a particular drug are dispensed. The cost of the hood is independent of volume and, therefore, can be described as a fixed cost. Other costs may be incurred as a result of the initiation of a new program (e.g., hiring new pharmacy technicians to prepare and deliver sterile products) but remain independent of the volume of activity once the program has been set up (within limits, of course). A very large increase in the number of patients requiring parenteral drugs might require hiring another technician. Other costs of drug administration may be obviously variable, such as the number of intravenous piggyback bags that contain a dose of an antibiotic. The more doses that are administered, the larger will be the number of bags used. Other costs are not so simply variable. If the number of doses that need to be prepared is decreased, will the pharmacy be able to employ fewer personnel? Because reductions in costs such as personnel require relatively large decreases in volume, they are often described as *stepped-variable costs.* In reviewing the economic impact of any service, it is important to be sure that the assumptions of certain costs as variable and others as fixed costs are acceptable.

▪ SCENARIO 4

Joan has been serving as the clinical coordinator for the department of pharmacy in a 500-bed hospital for more than 9 years. She provides clinical services to patients admitted to the general medicine service, manages clinical programs for the department, and is responsible for the continued professional development of 12 clinical pharmacists. Joan is a member of the pharmacy and therapeutics committee, the nutrition support committee, and an ad hoc committee to improve the patient discharge process. She also chairs the hospital's smoking-cessation campaign.

This morning Joan began her day like every other. She got to the office early to review her scheduled appointments:

7:00–8:30 a.m.	Patient care rounds
9:00–9:30 a.m.	Meet with architect to review pharmacy office renovation
11:00–12:00 noon	Pharmacy steering (management) committee
12:15–1:00 p.m.	Third-year medical student talk
2:00–2:30 p.m.	Meet with vendor to discuss TPN deliveries
3:00–4:00 p.m.	Mark's performance review

▪ MANAGING HUMAN CAPITAL

The role of any hospital pharmacy manager is complicated by his or her broad span of responsibility. Managers are expected to allocate hospital resources, supervise professionals and nonprofessionals, control drug distribution, and influence prescribing. These middle managers accomplish their goals by cultivating relationships in multiple dimensions. They relate to superiors as a subordinate: They take orders. They relate to their team as a superior: They direct. And they relate to peers in the organization as their equal: They cooperate. Pierpaoli (1987) contends that hospital pharmacy

managers must be "bilingual." He believes that managers must effectively relate to two major (and at times competing) organizational constituencies within the hospital: the hospital's corporate administration (for day-to-day management) and the medical staff and patients (for issues related to drug use and control). The "bilingual" manager must be able to span the boundaries of professional ideology and bureaucratic necessity. The successful pharmacy manager must participate in multiple pairs of "bilingual" communication every day to ensure that the department meets its goals while maintaining its flexibility.

Effective hospital pharmacy managers are, above all, good leaders. Shortell (1985) described a new management paradigm for high-performing health care organizations that puts the focus on leadership through the development of one's subordinates. He maintains that hospitals should be organized to maximize learning, that is, to push information down to the lowest possible level. He suggests that organizations should exhibit a loose coherence, where members are allowed considerable autonomy while coordinating individual contributions. He believes that employees must be held to the overall goals and mission of the organization while they are allowed to experiment and to try novel approaches to solving problems.

Pharmacy clinicians and managers must develop sound leadership qualities if they are to succeed in today's hospital environment. Good leaders are intelligent, flexible, creative, enthusiastic, socially and psychologically mature, willing to take risks, and good communicators (Bennis, 2003). While most hospitals do not have formal educational programs for those interested in becoming department heads, well-managed departments do include leadership training in their staff development plans. A department's success depends ultimately on the motivation and competence of its employees. And it is the responsibility of the department managers to ensure their competence.

Today's workforce is the best educated and best informed in history. The number of pharmacists entering the workforce with an entry-level doctor of pharmacy degree increases every year. Many of these graduates are investing another year or two in residency or fellowship programs or both. Young people who have devoted so much time and effort to preparing for a career will not be satisfied with assigned jobs with narrow responsibilities that are performed under close supervision. What they want is to have a positive influence on the outcomes of patient care in an environment that values quality and continued learning. Successful departments of pharmacy are able to attract and retain competent personnel and to use those staff members to respond creatively to the needs of patient care.

The primary duties and responsibilities of clinical pharmacists vary among hospitals. A representative job description and performance appraisal is included in Figure 34-3. Most hospital pharmacists are responsible for supervising drug distribution, providing patient-specific clinical services, educating students and residents, conducting research, and administering the programs of the department. While pharmacists will continue to have ultimate responsibility for drug distribution and drug control activities, certified pharmacy technicians should carry out as many of these functions as is permitted by law. This will free the major portion of pharmacists' time for clinical services. Further, drug distribution should be automated and mechanized to as great an extent as possible.

Pharmacy managers should consider the mission of the department to determine the composition of the workforce needed. This human resources plan usually allows for (1) identification of the right number of people with the proper skills that will be needed, (2) acquiring or training and developing the people who will be needed, and (3) motivating them to achieve their highest level of performance and become long-term employees. Pharmacy managers should consider that clinical services become more specialized as they expand. A mature clinical program requires pharmacists with more advanced and specialized training or experience or both.

One of the most important duties of a manager is to work with employees to develop them in such a way that they better meet the needs of the department while fulfilling their own desires and ambitions. Periodic written evaluations of an employee's skills and accomplishments should be performed. Employees should be encouraged to make self-assessments of their assets and to develop a career plan. Through discussions between the employee and manager, a development plan can be devised to help the department accomplish its business goals and the employee to grow professionally. For example, in Scenario 4, the pharmacy manager is scheduled to meet with a clinical pharmacy specialist to finalize his yearly performance evaluation. The manager and the employee recognize the need for the clinician to gain more experience speaking in public. Since the hospital is planning to institute new sedation guidelines for use in the adult intensive care unit, and since the clinical pharmacist practices in the adult ICU, the perfect opportunity exits for several goals to be meet. The pharmacist agrees to present a lecture to the pharmacy and nursing staffs about conscious sedation and the new sedation guidelines.

■ CONCLUSION

The fundamental purpose of pharmaceutical services in a hospital is to ensure the safe and appropriate use of drugs. Fulfillment of this responsibility is enhanced through the pharmacist's involvement in all aspects of the use of drugs. These goals will be met only if the pharmacy is well organized and is staffed by professionals, all of whom work to manage the department. This chapter describes how the environment, professional relationships, regulatory agencies, practice standards, finances, and human resources influence the effectiveness of hospital pharmacy managers.

■ QUESTIONS FOR FURTHER DISCUSSION

1. How might some of the roles and responsibilities of hospital pharmacists identified in the chapter differ from what you envisioned or experienced thus far?
2. Do you think that you have or will acquire the skills necessary to effectively manage clinical pharmacist services in a hospital? What sort of contributions

JOB TITLE: Clinical Pharmacist   **GRADE:**

DEPARTMENT: Pharmacy   **JOB CODE:**

FLSA: Exempt   **DATE:**

REPORTS TO: Pharmacy Clinical Coordinator   **APPROVED BY:**

TYPE OF EVALUATION: **New Employee** ☐   **Annual Evaluation** ☐

Employee Name: _____   **Date:** _____

JOB SUMMARY: Clinical pharmacists work closely with other health practitioners to meet the various needs of our patients. Pharmacists review and approve medication orders, monitor drug therapies, and provide drug information. Pharmacists supervise and direct support personnel. In the absence of the pharmacy manager, a clinical pharmacist may be required to assume the essential responsibilities and perform the duties of the pharmacy manager.

JOB REQUIREMENTS: Ability to work independently with minimal direct supervision. Ability to work with hospital and pharmacy staff. Ability to handle frequent interruptions and adapt to changes in workload and work schedule. Ability to set priorities, make critical decisions, and respond quickly to emergency requests. Ability to exercise sound professional judgement. Ability to meet the pharmaceutical care needs of neonatal, pediatric, adolescent, adult, and geriatric patients.

To perform this job successfully, an individual must be able to execute each duty satisfactorily and be able to use various computer systems proficiently. The candidate must be able to communicate effectively in English (orally and in writing).

CREDENTIALS: Graduate of an accredited college or university with a BSc in Pharmacy or a PharmD degree. Hospital experience preferred but not required.

LICENSURE: Licensed to practice pharmacy in the state or eligibility.

WORK SCHEDULE: Full-time employment is 40 hours per week; hours may be long and irregular. Includes evenings, nights, weekends, and holidays as necessary.

WORKING CONDITIONS/PHYSICAL DEMANDS: Repetitive use of hands and fingers (e.g., use of computer keyboard). May require lifting and carrying light loads, including boxes, equipment, and stooping or kneeling. Sitting, walking, or standing for long periods of time is often necessary. Must be able to physically operate equipment used for the job.

The above statements are intended to describe the general nature and level of work being performed. They are not intended to be construed as an exhaustive list of all responsibilities, duties and skills required of personnel so classified.

Figure 34-3. Clinical pharmacist job description and performance evaluation.

Scoring Guide:

(E)   Excels: This category identifies areas where an employee is consistently recognized as a role model relative to the effectiveness of his/her performance.

(M)   Fully Meets Expectations: This category conveys a high standard of performance, especially in response to continued efforts to maintain and improve the highest levels of quality.

(N)   Needs Improvement: This category reflects our commitment to respond to staff with a constructive means for professional growth and continued performance improvement.

I.   PRINCIPAL DUTIES/RESPONSIBILITIES

Performance Criteria/Standards   Rating   Comments

A. Supervises the preparation and distribution of medications from the pharmacy according to established policies, procedures, and protocols.

1. Interprets medication orders (verbal and written) and transcribes to computerized patient medication profiles accurately. Maintains accurate, complete patient medication profiles.

2. Compounds and dispenses pharmaceuticals including, sterile, chemotherapy, and parenteral nutrition products accurately.

3. Issues controlled substances to patient care areas and maintains records as required by law.

4. Supports drug therapy research programs by preparing and dispensing drugs under investigational protocols.

5. Serves as preceptor to pharmacy interns.

B. Ensures safe, appropriate, cost effective medication therapies for patients according to established policies, procedures, and protocols.

1. Monitors drug therapy regimens for contraindications, drug–drug interactions, drug–food interactions, allergies, and appropriateness of drug and dose.

2. Reads, extracts, and interprets information in patient charts and electronic databases accurately.

3. Detects and reports suspected adverse drug reactions accurately and in a timely manner.

4. Detects and reports medication errors accurately and in a timely manner.

5. Sustains the formulary by minimizing nonformulary procurements, utilizing therapeutic substitution protocols, and promoting rational drug therapy selection.

6. Supports the rational use of drugs by adhering to departmental anti-infective control and monitoring programs.

Figure 34-3. *(Continued)*

Performance Criteria/Standards	Rating	Comments

7. Provides clinical consultation and clarification to practitioners. Suggests appropriate, cost effective alternatives to medical staff as needed.

8. Provides accurate, adequate, and timely drug information to the professional staff.

9. Provides drug information to patients and their families.

10. Documents all clinical activities and interventions accurately and completely.

11. Participates in the quality improvement and medication use review activities of the department. Collects data; conducts quality monitoring and inspections; maintains logs, records, and other documentation assigned.

12. Completes and documents all Pyxis medications prior to loading and restocking.

13. Participates in the development and presentation of orientation, education, and training programs to the pharmacy, medical, nursing, and other staffs.

C. **Contributes to the quality and effective operation of the department.**

1. Supervises and directs pharmacy support personnel. Verifies the daily activities of pharmacy technicians. Participates in the performance appraisal of pharmacy support personnel.

2. Works independently with minimal supervision. Organizes and prioritizes work assignments. Ensures pharmacy services are provided in a timely manner.

3. Answers the telephone, identifying self and department. Directs calls to appropriate personnel.

4. Keeps pharmacy areas and equipment clean, neat, and well organized.

5. Performs essential duties of the pharmacy managers in their absence.

D. **Maintains competence required for current job title/position.**

1. Maintains current pharmacist licensure.

2. Participates in pharmacy staff meetings and pharmacist patient care rounds.

3. Attends orientation, education, and training programs. Reviews literature and other materials pertinent to the practice of pharmacy.

4. Completes all competence/skills assessment requirements (see attached competence assessment/skills list).

E. **Performs other duties as assigned by supervisor.**

Figure 34-3. *(Continued)*

II. DEPARTMENTAL STANDARDS

Performance Criteria/Standards   Rating Comments

1. Is punctual and dependable; reports to work as scheduled. Fulfills on-call obligations per pre-arranged schedule. Absenteeism and tardiness are within policy guidelines.

2. Maintains a neat, professional, well-groomed appearance. Observes pharmacy dress code. Wears identification badge at all times.

3. Performs work within specified time frames. Adapts to frequent interruptions and changes in workload and/or work schedule.

4. Provides courteous, cooperative, and timely service to patients, visitors, and staff. Demonstrates good oral and written communication.

5. Works cooperatively with all staff. Voices concerns and suggestions to appropriate persons in a positive manner.

6. Demonstrates sound professional judgement consistent with clinical/academic background.

7. Maintains strict confidentiality of patient, visitor, and employee information.

8. Fosters a team environment by providing orientation and training to new team members. Assists coworkers in tasks, as time permits.

9. Adheres to health system and departmental policies and procedures. Complies with all requirements related to risk management, safety, security, fire, and infection control. Complies with all applicable federal, state, and local laws, rules, and regulations.

III. ORGANIZATIONAL STANDARDS

Performance Criteria/Standards   Rating Comments

1. Performance demonstrates efforts to improve patient satisfaction, lower cost, and improve quality.

2. Understands and meets customers' needs and expectations. The patient and family members always come first.

3. Demonstrates the ability to address problems in a group setting using tools and techniques for identification and resolution of problems.

4. Demonstrates the values and behaviors of the organization.

Figure 34-3. *(Continued)*

IV. GOALS AND ACCOMPLISHMENTS

A. Describe status of goals set at previous evaluation.

_____

_____

_____

B. Describe special accomplishments achieved since previous evaluation.

_____

_____

_____

_____

PERFORMANCE GOALS AND OBJECTIVES

Provide an assessment of your own needs for growth and development. Develop a plan to meet educational and professional growth within the next 12 months.

_____

_____

_____

_____

V. COMMENTS

A. Supervisor's comments:

_____

_____

_____

B. Employee's Comments:

_____

_____

_____

Figure 34-3. _(Continued)_

1. can you make toward effective patient care while holding operating budgets in check?

3. The chapter mentions issues such as the acquisition of capital and loss of various opportunities resulting from poor investment income. From what sources might a hospital acquire capital, and why is capital so important to a hospital's solvency? How can declines in investment income affect a hospital's operations and indirectly affect patient care?

4. What sorts of skills, knowledge sets, and experiences are necessary to become the manager of a hospital pharmacy department? Is this something you can see yourself doing, someday?

REFERENCES

American Society of Health-System Pharmacists (ASHP). 2006a. ASHP guidelines: Minimum standard for pharmacies in hospitals. In *Best Practices for Hospital and Health-System Pharmacy*, p. 297. Bethesda, MD: American Society of Health-System Pharmacists.

American Society of Health-System Pharmacists (ASHP). 2006b. ASHP statement on the pharmacy and therapeutics committee. In *Best Practices for Hospital and Health-System Pharmacy*, p, 92. Bethesda, MD: American Society of Health-System Pharmacists.

Bates DW, Cullen DJ, Laird N, et al., for the ADE Prevention Study Group. 1996. Incidence of adverse drug events and potential adverse drug events. *JAMA* 274:29.

Bates DW, Spell N, Cullen DJ, et al., for the Adverse Drug Events Prevention Study Group. 1997. The costs of adverse drug events in hospitalized patients. *JAMA* 222:307.

Bennis W. 2003. *On Becoming a Leader.* Cambridge: Perseus Publishing.

Classen DC, Pestonik SL, Evans RS, et al. 1991. Computerized surveillance of adverse drug events in hospitalized patients. *JAMA* 266:2847.

Classen DC, Pestotnik SL, Evans RS, et al. 1997. Adverse drug events in hospitalized patients: Excess length of stay, extra costs, and attributable mortality. *JAMA* 277:301.

Cullen DJ, Bates DW, Small SD, et al. 1995. The incident reporting system does not detect adverse events. *Joint Comm J Qual Improv* 21:541.

Hoffman JM, Shah ND, Vermeulen LC, et al. 2007. Projecting future drug expenditures—2007. *Am J Health-Syst Pharm* 64:298.

Joint Commission. 2006. *2007 Accreditation Process Guide for Hospitals.* Oakbrook Terrace, IL: Joint Commission Resources.

Kohn LT, Corrigan JM, Donaldson MS. 1999. *To Err Is Human: Building a Safer Helath System.* Washington, DC: Institute of Medicine.

Leape LL. 1994. Error in medicine. *JAMA* 272:1851.

Leape LL. 2002. Reporting of adverse events. *N Engl J Med* 347:1633.

Leape LL, Brenan TA, Laird N, et al. 1991. The nature of adverse events in hospitalized patients: Results of the Harvard medial practice study II. *N Engl J Med* 324:377.

Leape LL, Bates DW, Cullen DJ, et al., for the ADE Prevention Study Group. 1995. Systems analysis of adverse drug events. *JAMA* 274:35.

Pierpaoli PG. 1987. Management diplomacy: Myths and methods. *Am J Health-Syst Pharm* 44:297.

Poon EG, Cina JL, Churchill W, et al. 2006. Medication dispensing errors and potential adverse drug events before and after implementing bar code technology in the pharmacy. *Ann Intern Med* 145:426.

Shortell SM. 1985. High-performing health care organizations: Guidelines for the pursuit of excellence. *Hosp Health Serv Admin* 30:8.

Stelfox HT, Palmisani S, Scurlock C, et al. 2006. The "To Err is Human" report and the patient safety literature. *Qual Saf Health Care* 15:174.

Strand LM, Guerrero RM, Nickman NA, Morley PC. 1990. Integrated patient-specific model of pharmacy practice. *Am J Health-Syst Pharm* 47:550.

INDEX

Page numbers with *t* and *f* indicates table and figure